Synopsis of Neuropsychiatry

Synopsis of Neuropsychiatry

Edited by

Stuart C. Yudofsky, M.D.
D. C. and Irene Ellwood
Professor and Chairman,
Department of Psychiatry and Behavioral Sciences,
Baylor College of Medicine;
Psychiatrist-in-Chief,
The Methodist Hospital,
Houston, Texas

Robert E. Hales, M.D.
Clinical Professor of Psychiatry,
University of California, San Francisco;
Chairman, Department of Psychiatry,
California Pacific Medical Center,
San Francisco, California

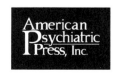

Washington, DC
London, England

Copyright © 1994 American Psychiatric Press, Inc.
ALL RIGHTS RESERVED
Manufactured in the United States of America on acid-free paper.

American Psychiatric Press, Inc.
1400 K Street, N.W., Washington, DC 20005

Library of Congress Cataloging-in-Publication Data
Synopsis of neuropsychiatry / edited by Stuart C. Yudofsky, Robert E.
　Hales.—- 1st ed.
　　　p. cm.
　　Includes bibliographical references and index.
　　ISBN 0-88048-691-0 (alk. paper)
　　1. Neuropsychiatry.　　I. Yudofsky, Stuart C.　II. Hales, Robert E.
　　[DNLM:　1. Nervous System Diseases.　2. Neuropsychology.
　3. Organic Mental Disorders.　　WM 220 S993 1994]
　RC341.S96　　1994
　616.8—dc20
　DNLM / DLC
　for Library of Congress　　　　　　　　　　　　　　　　　93-44844
　　　　　　　　　　　　　　　　　　　　　　　　　　　　　CIP

British Library Cataloguing in Publication Data
A CIP record is available from the British Library.

Contents

Section I: Basic Principles of Neuroscience

Section II: Neuropsychiatric Assessment

Section III: Neuropsychiatric Symptomatologies

Section IV: Neuropsychiatric Disorders

Section V: Neuropsychiatric Treatments

Contributors

D. Frank Benson, M.D. The Augustus S. Rose Professor of Neurology, Department of Neurology, University of California, Los Angeles, School of Medicine, Los Angeles, California

William Borden, Ph.D. Assistant Professor, Department of Psychiatry and School of Social Service Administration, The University of Chicago; Research Associate, Illinois State Psychiatric Institute, Chicago, Illinois

George T. Brandt, M.D. Instructor, Department of Psychiatry, Uniformed Services University of Health Sciences, Bethesda, Maryland; Assistant Chief, Psychiatry Consultation Liaison Service, Walter Reed Army Medical Center, Washington, DC

William G. Brose, M.D. Assistant Professor, Department of Anesthesia, Director, Pain Management Service, Stanford University School of Medicine, Stanford, California

Jeffrey L. Cummings, M.D. Associate Professor of Neurology, Psychiatry, and Biobehavioral Sciences, University of California, Los Angeles, School of Medicine; Chief, Behavioral Neuroscience Section, Psychiatry Service, West Los Angeles Veterans Affairs Medical Center, Los Angeles, California

David G. Daniel, M.D. Associate Clinical Professor of Psychiatry, George Washington University; Guest Researcher, Clinical Brain Disorders Branch, Division of Intramural Research Programs, National Institute of Mental Health, Washington, DC; Director, Clinical Neuroscience Service, HCA-Dominion Hospital, Falls Church, Virginia

Steven L. Dubovsky, M.D. Professor of Psychiatry and Medicine, Vice-Chairman, Department of Psychiatry, University of Colorado School of Medicine, Denver, Colorado

David V. Forrest, M.D. Associate Professor of Clinical Psychiatry, Consultation-Liaison Psychiatrist in Neurology, Faculty, Columbia Psychoanalytic Center, Columbia University College of Physicians and Surgeons, New York, New York

Richard J. Frances, M.D. Professor of Clinical Psychiatry, Vice-Chairman, Department of Psychiatry, New Jersey Medical School, Newark, New Jersey

John E. Franklin, Jr., M.D. Assistant Professor of Clinical Psychiatry, Department of Psychiatry, New Jersey Medical School, Newark, New Jersey

Robert P. Friedland, M.D.   Associate Professor of Neurology, Psychiatry, and
Radiology, Case Western Reserve University School of Medicine;
Clinical Director, Alzheimer Center, University Hospitals of Cleveland,
Cleveland, Ohio

Felicia B. Gershberg, Sc.B.   Graduate student, University of California,
Berkeley, Berkeley, California

Kenneth L. Goetz, M.D.   Assistant Professor of Psychiatry, Medical College of
Pennsylvania, Allegheny Campus; Associate Director, Inpatient Psychiatry,
Allegheny General Hospital, Pittsburgh, Pennsylvania

Morris B. Goldman, M.D.   Assistant Professor of Psychiatry, Pritzker School of
Medicine; Associate Director for Research, The University of Chicago
Research Program at Illinois State Psychiatric Institute, Chicago, Illinois

Lawrence S. Gross, M.D.   Associate Professor of Clinical Psychiatry and the
Behavioral Sciences, University of Southern California School of Medicine;
Director, Adult Psychiatric Outpatient Clinic, Los Angeles County and
University of Southern California Medical Center, Los Angeles, California

Robert E. Hales, M.D.   Clinical Professor of Psychiatry, University of California,
San Francisco; Chairman, Department of Psychiatry, California Pacific
Medical Center, San Francisco, California

Diane B. Howieson, Ph.D.   Assistant Professor of Neurology and Medical
Psychology, Oregon Health Sciences University; Head, Neuropsychology
Section, Portland Department of Veterans Affairs Medical Center, Portland,
Oregon

Charles A. Kaufmann, M.D.   Associate Professor of Clinical Psychiatry,
Columbia University, College of Physicians and Surgeons; Head, Laboratory
of Molecular Neurobiology, Scientific Director, Schizophrenia Research Unit,
New York State Psychiatric Institute, New York, New York

David J. Kupfer, M.D.   Professor and Chairman, Department of Psychiatry,
University of Pittsburgh School of Medicine, Western Psychiatric Institute and
Clinic, Pittsburgh, Pennsylvania

Muriel D. Lezak, Ph.D.   Associate Professor of Neurology, Psychiatry, and
Neurosurgery, Head, Neuropsychology Section, Department of Neurology,
Oregon Health Sciences University, Portland, Oregon

Mark R. Lovell, Ph.D.   Assistant Professor of Psychiatry (Psychology), Medical
College of Pennsylvania, Allegheny Campus; Chief of Neuropsychological
Services, Allegheny General Hospital, Allegheny Neuropsychiatric Institute,
Pittsburgh, Pennsylvania

Robert W. McCarley, M.D.   Professor of Psychiatry, Director, Neuroscience Laboratory, Department of Psychiatry, Harvard Medical School, Brockton Veterans Affairs Medical Center, Brockton, Massachusetts

Dolores Malaspina, M.D.   Assistant Professor of Clinical Psychiatry, Columbia University, College of Physicians and Surgeons; Unit Chief, Schizophrenia Research Unit, New York State Psychiatric Institute, New York, New York

John C. Markowitz, M.D.   Assistant Professor of Psychiatry, Cornell University Medical College, New York, New York

Frederick E. Miller, M.D., Ph.D.   Assistant Professor, Department of Psychiatry and Behavioral Sciences, Northwestern University, Chicago, Illinois

Robert M. Nagy, M.D.   Assistant Professor of Clinical Psychiatry and the Behavioral Sciences, University of Southern California School of Medicine; Ward Chief, Psychiatric Hospital, Los Angeles County and University of Southern California Medical Center, Los Angeles, California

Henry A. Nasrallah, M.D.   Professor of Psychiatry and Neurology, Chairman, Department of Psychiatry, The Ohio State University College of Medicine, Columbus, Ohio

Vernon M. Neppe, M.D., Ph.D.   Associate Professor of Psychiatry and Behavioral Sciences, Director, Division of Neuropsychiatry, University of Washington School of Medicine, Seattle, Washington

Thomas C. Neylan, M.D.   Medical Director, Inpatient Psychiatry, California Pacific Medical Center, San Francisco California

Fred Ovsiew, M.D.   Assistant Professor of Clinical Psychiatry, Chief, Clinical Neuropsychiatry, Department of Psychiatry, The University of Chicago, Chicago, Illinois

Samuel W. Perry, M.D. *(deceased)*   Professor of Psychiatry, Cornell University Medical College, Associate Chair for Research, The New York Hospital, New York, New York

Trevor R. P. Price, M.D.   Professor of Psychiatry and Medicine, Chairman, Department of Psychiatry, Medical College of Pennsylvania, Allegheny Campus, Pittsburgh, Pennsylvania

H. Matthew Quitkin, A.B.   Stanley Scholar, Columbia University, College of Physicians and Surgeons; Research Associate, New York State Psychiatric Institute, New York, New York

Stephen G. Rayport, M.D., Ph.D.   Assistant Professor of Psychiatry, Neurobiology and Behavior, Anatomy and Cell Biology, Columbia University; Director, Laboratory of Neurophysiology, New York State Psychiatric Institute, New York, New York

Charles F. Reynolds III, M.D.   Professor of Psychiatry and Neurology, Director, Sleep and Chronobiology Center, Western Psychiatric Institute and Clinic, University of Pittsburgh School of Medicine, Pittsburgh, Pennsylvania

Robert G. Robinson, M.D.   Professor and Head, Department of Psychiatry, University of Iowa College of Medicine, Iowa City, Iowa

Arthur P. Shimamura, Ph.D.   Associate Professor, Department of Psychology, University of California, Berkeley, Berkeley, California

Jonathan M. Silver, M.D.   Assistant Professor of Clinical Psychiatry, College of Physicians and Surgeons, Columbia University; Director of Neuropsychiatry, Columbia-Presbyterian Medical Center, New York, New York

Robert I. Simon, M.D.   Clinical Professor of Psychiatry, Director, Program in Psychiatry and Law, Georgetown University School of Medicine, Washington, DC

David Spiegel, M.D.   Professor, Department of Psychiatry and Behavioral Sciences, Director, Psychosocial Treatment Laboratory, Stanford University School of Medicine, Stanford, California

Sergio E. Starkstein, M.D., Ph.D.   Chief, Department of Behavioral Neurology, Director, Institute of Neurological Research Raúl Carrea, Buenos Aires, Argentina

Christopher Starratt, Ph.D.   Assistant Professor of Psychiatry (Psychology), Medical College of Pennsylvania, Allegheny Campus; Director of Neuropsychology, Allegheny Neuropsychiatric Institute, Pittsburgh, Pennsylvania

Milton E. Strauss, Ph.D.   Professor, Departments of Psychology, Neurology, and Psychiatry, Director, Clinical Psychology Program, Case Western Reserve University, Cleveland, Ohio

Richard L. Strub, M.D.   Clinical Professor of Neurology, Tulane University; Chairman, Department of Neurology, Ochsner Clinic, New Orleans, Louisiana

Daniel Tranel, Ph.D.   Associate Professor of Neurology, Chief, Benton Neuropsychology Laboratory, Division of Behavioral Neurology and Cognitive Neuroscience, Department of Neurology, University of Iowa, Iowa City, Iowa

Gary J. Tucker, M.D.   Professor and Chairman, Department of Psychiatry and Behavioral Sciences, University of Washington School of Medicine, Seattle, Washington

Daniel R. Weinberger, M.D.   Chief, Clinical Brain Disorders Branch, Division of Intramural Research Programs, National Institute of Mental Health, Neurosciences Center at Saint Elizabeths, Washington, DC

Peter J. Whitehouse, M.D., Ph.D.   Associate Professor of Neurology, Director, Alzheimer's Center, University Hospitals of Cleveland; Chief, Division of Geriatric and Behavioral Neurology, Case Western Reserve University, Cleveland, Ohio

Michael G. Wise, M.D.   Clinical Professor of Psychiatry, Tulane School of Medicine; Chairman, Department of Psychiatry, Ochsner Clinic, New Orleans, Louisiana

Stuart C. Yudofsky, M.D.   D. C. and Irene Ellwood Professor and Chairman, Department of Psychiatry and Behavioral Sciences, Baylor College of Medicine; Psychiatrist-in-Chief, The Methodist Hospital, Houston, Texas

Jeffrey R. Zigun, M.D.   Senior Staff Fellow, Clinical Brain Disorders Branch, Division of Intramural Research Programs, National Institute of Mental Health, Neurosciences Center at Saint Elizabeths, Washington, DC

Preface

Ten years ago we began to conceptualize and to craft the first edition of *The American Psychiatric Press Textbook of Neuropsychiatry*. At that time, we believed that the field of neuropsychiatry, which had both its origin and principal span of influence in the 19th century, was reemerging. The growing acceptance of the importance of biological interventions in the assessment and treatment of many neuropsychiatric illnesses combined with new electrodiagnostic and neurobiological assessments to implicate the prominent role of the brain in severe psychiatric illnesses such as major depression, bipolar disorder, and schizophrenia. Additionally, as the American population aged, there emerged an increased prevalence of disorders such as Alzheimer's disease, Parkinson's disease, and stroke, whose symptomatologies and treatments required the bridging of the specialties of psychiatry and neurology.

The overall result of these advances was an explosion in the scientific information required for a clinician to diagnose and treat patients with neuropsychiatric disorders. In teaching medical students and residents in the general hospital and outpatient clinical settings, we referred frequently to key articles about neuropsychiatric disorders that were to be found in a broad range of medical and other scientific journals, as well as to excellent "single-author" textbooks, including Lishman's classic book, *Organic Psychiatry: The Psychological Consequence of Cerebral Disorder;* Pincus and Tucker's excellent *Behavioral Neurology,* and Cummings' *Clinical Neuropsychiatry.*

Notwithstanding these valuable contributions and those of several other volumes by both psychiatrists and neurologists that emphasized the interface between neurology and psychiatry, we became convinced that the database, complexity, and relevance of the field of neuropsychiatry had expanded to the point that a new format was required. We ultimately decided on a textbook that used as chapter authors many individual investigators and clinicians with specialized knowledge of critical areas of neuropsychiatry. As a result, the first edition of *The American Psychiatric Press Textbook of Neuropsychiatry* was published in 1987. Comprising approximately 500 pages, the first edition was divided into 25 chapters, in which individual authors focused on practical issues related to the understanding, diagnosis, and treatment of patients with neuropsychiatric disorders. Our guiding principle was that if Lishman's classic textbook of neuropsychiatry could be conceptualized as an elegant English Rolls Royce, we desired to develop a practical and utilitarian American Jeep. The acceptance of the first edition of the *Textbook of Neuropsychiatry* exceeded our fondest expectations, as it was purchased by the equivalent of one in five American psychiatrists.

Over the years subsequent to the publication of *The American Psychiatric Press Textbook of Neuropsychiatry,* professional interest in and the influence of the neuropsychiatric perspective increased at a rapidly accelerating rate. Advances in brain imaging enabled, for the first time, brain function to be evaluated in living people with neuropsychiatric disorders, and major strides were made toward elucidating neuronal function on molecular terms, which also had broad implications and importance for neuropsychiatry. At both the basic and clinical levels, new journals focusing on neuropsychiatry—including the *Journal of Neuropsychiatry and Clinical Neurosciences*—and new organizations such as the American Neuropsychiatric Association were initiated and began to flourish. Additionally, curricula in medical schools and in neurological and psychiatric residency training programs increasingly emphasized the neuropsychiatric perspective, and fellowships in neuropsychiatry and behavioral neurology were developed across the country.

The second edition of *The American Psychiatric Press Textbook of Neuropsychiatry* was formulated not only to reflect, but to help advance, the growth of the field of neuropsychiatry. The number of pages of the text was expanded by over 40%, and the number of contributors increased from 42 to 56. Whereas the first edition had four sections—Evaluation and Basic Principles; Organic Mental Disorders; Neuropsychiatric Disorders; and Treatment Issues in Neuropsychiatry—the new edition was reconceptualized to encompass the rapid growth and knowledge in the basic neurosciences with the addition of a section entitled Basic Principles of Neuroscience.

Along with the many advantages afforded by the expanded and more comprehensive edition of the *Textbook,* certain disadvantages emerged. Directors of medical student education communicated to us that the second edition contained more information than was required at the medical student level, and they added that the cost of the *Textbook* was, for many students, prohibitive. Additionally, residency training directors believed that a condensed version of the second edition would be valuable for residents in both neurology and psychiatry to use in introductory courses to the field of neuropsychiatry. Clinicians in both neurology and psychiatry whose clinical practices did not focus primarily on patients with neuropsychiatric disorders also told us that they believed a condensed version of the *Textbook* would have value for purposes of updating their knowledge, as well as for use as a clinical reference.

For these reasons we have now gone "full circle" through the conceptualization and development of the *Synopsis of Neuropsychiatry.* We have endeavored to condense and distill the most relevant data from almost every chapter of the second edition of the *Textbook of Neuropsychiatry* and to present the information in a cohesive, interesting, and clinically applicable format.

We express appreciation to the authors of each chapter who have assisted us in the determination of the difficult, and sometimes, nearly impossible decision about what information should be included and what would be excluded. We thank Jude Berman, our text editor, who did the lion's share of rewriting and integrating this text. Consistent with previous projects and experiences, Ron McMillen and his excellent staff at the American Psychiatric Press were extraordinarily helpful and responsive to us. We particularly thank Claire Reinburg, Editorial Director for the books division, who worked closely with us on both the second edition of *The American Psychiatric Press Textbook of Neuropsychiatry,* as well as on the *Synopsis of Neuropsychiatry.* Finally, and most importantly, we wish to thank the many psychiatrists, neurologists, neuropsychologists, other mental health professionals, and students at all levels who have given us suggestions and encouragement to continue our work in this area through their communication to us that they have found these texts on neuropsychiatry useful in their clinical practices, for their teaching responsibilities, and for learning. It is our hope that our efforts and those of our chapter authors will be translated into another practical and enjoyable book for students and professionals who wish to learn more about how to understand, diagnose, and care for patients who have neuropsychiatric disorders.

Stuart C. Yudofsky, M.D.
Houston, Texas

Robert E. Hales, M.D.
San Francisco, California

Introduction

WHAT IS NEUROPSYCHIATRY?

Although there is considerable disagreement about just what neuropsychiatry comprises, fundamental to any definition is the indelible inseparability of brain and thought, of mind and body, and of mental and physical. Neuropsychiatry spans these interrelationships to enlarge our understanding of cognitive, emotional, and behavioral function and dysfunction. It is a fascinating paradox that modern neuropsychiatry, which derives from 19th century social dissension, anatomical dissection, and nosological differentiation, should, as manifested by its very name, be essentially a collaborative and integrative enterprise. Neuropsychiatry bridges the conventional boundaries imposed between mind and matter, between intention and function, and between the guildlike clinical considerations of the professional disciplines of neurology and psychiatry. Most importantly, however, neuropsychiatry vaults the limiting and misleading demarcations of traditional conceptual models of illness.

For example, although Parkinson's disease is classified as a movement disorder under the professional aegis of neurology, selected scientific studies show that more than one-third of patients with this disorder have depression (Mayeux 1981) and that dementia and other prominent behavioral and cognitive impairments occur, depending on the study, in from 10% to more than 50% of afflicted patients (Brown and Marsden 1984; Mayeux 1981). Similarly, schizophrenia, conventionally considered a psychiatric illness, is associated with elevated dopamine, subtype 2 (D_2), receptors in caudate nuclei (Wong et al. 1986) and with pathology in frontal, midbrain, diencephalic, and other regions of the brain (Andreasen et al. 1986). Scientific efforts using animal models have succeeded in determining the nucleotide sequence of the genes that code for D_2 receptors that have been implicated in both Parkinson's disease and schizophrenia (Bunzow et al. 1988). The future consequences of such scientific advances may be to compel a clinical reconceptualization of both Parkinson's disease and schizophrenia as neuropsychiatric disorders. This would help cast light and focus on disabling symptomatologies that often remain dimly recognized and untreated in the shadowy margins of psychiatry and neurology when the disorders or the specialties are too narrowly defined.

Conditions and Symptomatologies Subsumed

Although there is no universally accepted definition of neuropsychiatry, it is our hope that the *Synopsis of Neuropsychiatry*, through its considerations and emphases, will define and strengthen this concept. A prominent focus of neuropsychiatry is the assessment and treatment of patients with psychiatric illnesses or symptoms associated with brain lesions or dysfunction. These include neuropsychiatric aspects of the following: traumatic brain injury; cerebral vascular disease; seizure disorders; central nervous system (CNS) degenerative diseases, including Alzheimer's disease and other dementias; brain tumors; infectious and inflammatory diseases of the CNS; alcohol and other substance-induced organic mental disorders; and developmental disorders involving the brain. Neuropsychiatry also encompasses those symptoms that lie in the "gray zone" between the specialties of neurology and psychiatry: impairment of attention, alertness, perception, memory, language, and intelligence. Fundamental to neuropsychiatry is the effort to link psychopathology with measurable brain deficits. Where psychiatric symptoms are likely to stem from brain disorders, but where the state of technology has not developed sufficiently to establish brain-syndrome linkages, neuropsychiatry must assume the leadership in pursuing such associations.

There are several syndromes that currently are conceptualized as neuropsychiatric disorders, and for many of these conditions recent discoveries in even the basic neurosciences are also effecting far-reaching reconceptualizations.

For example, new molecular biological techniques have characterized the amino acid sequence associated with the synthesis of the amyloid protein that is found in neurofibrillary tangles in the brains of certain (although not all) patients with Alzheimer's disease (Kang et al. 1987). The gene responsible for the synthesis of this amyloid protein has been localized on chromosome 21 (St. George-Hyslop et al. 1987). In that the presence of amyloid and other brain pathology similar to that found in Alzheimer's patients are nearly always present in brains of older individuals with trisomy 21 disorder (Down's syndrome), this genetic localization could have implications for the diagnosis, treatment, and perhaps even the prevention of both illnesses. Thus modern molecular genetics may redefine two neuropsychiatric disorders—one conceptualized as a developmental disorder of young people (i.e., Down's syndrome) and the second conceptualized as a dementing illness of old age (i.e., Alzheimer's disease)—that heretofore were loosely linked by symptomatologies (dysfunction of memory, cognition, social judgment, and so on) and neuropathology (amyloid protein and neurofibrillary tangles).

Many human conditions that currently are not considered to be in the province of medicine, will, by virtue of neuroscience discovery, eventually become regarded as neuropsychiatric disorders. This reconceptualization will be of historic and monumental significance to the individuals who have these conditions and to society. Examples range from impulsive murderers and other types of criminal offenders to people with chemical dependencies. Presently, people with alcoholism are cared for by professionals and programs largely outside traditional medical specialties and hospital structures. Nonetheless, recent evidence is associating alcoholism with the D_2 receptor gene (Blum et al. 1990; Cloninger 1991; Comings et al. 1991). If such a link is ultimately established, the door will open wider to more fundamental involvement by psychiatrists and other medical specialists in the diagnosis and treatment of people who are alcohol dependent.

The Clinical and Philosophical Approach

Neuropsychiatry is a historic clinical discipline—arising in the mid-19th century and falling from prominence early in the 20th century—that is currently reemerging as a subspecialty of psychiatry and neurology. Not dissimilar to the clinical approaches of most other medical specialties or subspecialties, the following is considered by us to be the essence of neuropsychiatric intervention: 1) prevention (e.g., prenatal counseling and treatment of alcoholic expectant mothers to obviate alcohol-induced encephalopathy in infants); 2) early detection of neuropsychiatric symptoms (e.g., recognizing major depression in a poststroke patient with aphasia); 3) focused assessment and operationalization of neuropsychiatric dysfunction (e.g., use of the Overt Aggression Scale [Yudofsky et al. 1986] to describe, quantify, and monitor the dyscontrol of rage and violent behavior secondary to traumatic brain injury); 4) specific localization, where possible, in brain tissue, chemistry, physiology, and so on, of "causative" deficits (e.g., detecting an epileptogenic focus in the temporal lobe of a patient who experiences depersonalization and fugue states) and early and specific treatment, where possible, of such deficits; and 5) the use of multiple therapeutic modalities to enable the patients to adapt to those neuropsychiatric deficits that are not reversible.

One philosophical perspective of neuropsychiatry advanced in the *Synopsis of Neuropsychiatry* is that neuropsychiatric treatment is inherently complex and must, therefore, be comprehensive and collaborative. Thus clinical neuropsychiatry should be an organized, integrated, and multidisciplinary approach that includes not only many professional disciplines, the patient, and the patient's family, but also the enlightened organizations that act as advocates for individuals who are ravaged by neuropsychiatric disorders.

WHY THE RENAISSANCE OF NEUROPSYCHIATRY?

Neuropsychiatric Disorders Are Common and Disabling

Among the many reasons for the revival of neuropsychiatry is that the disorders subsumed under this rubric are so common and disabling. Although documentation of the prevalence of neuropsychiatric disorders and the comparison of their prevalence to those of other medical illnesses are beyond the scope of this introduction, compelling statistics and confirmatory data are included in the introductions to many of the chapters in the *Synopsis of Neuropsychiatry*.

In addition, the neuropsychiatric aspects of most of these disorders, including traumatic brain injury, alcohol-induced organic mental disorders, cerebral vascular disease, and seizure disorders, have been shown by many investigators to be among their most prominent, disabling dimensions (Oddy et al. 1985; Robinson and Starkstein 1990; West et al. 1984). With the aging of the population, many of these conditions will become even more prevalent.

A Neuropsychiatric Paradigm Reduces Stigma

A second reason for revitalizing the neuropsychiatric paradigm is to reduce the stigma associated with psychiatric symptoms like delusions, hallucinations, manic and depressive mood changes, confusion, impaired memory, disinhibited behavior, and so on. Appropriate focus on the underlying brain lesions and the biochemical or pathophysiological processes that produce psychiatric symptoms bolsters reconceptualization of symptom complexes as neuropsychiatric disorders. A neuropsychiatric conceptualization not only enlarges and refines the understanding and treatment of such disorders, but also avoids limiting and damaging misconceptions that stem from too-narrow, discipline-based perspectives.

A notorious example is schizophrenia—an illness with a predominantly psychiatric conceptualization—wherein the concept of the schizophrenogenic mother erroneously emerged and became widely accepted as a prominent cause of the disorder. This conceptualization incorrectly ascribes causality and, therefore, painful culpability to families who were already under great stress from a tragic and relentless disease. Fortunately, scientific evidence indicating genetic transmission of schizophrenia and the effectiveness of psychopharmacological treatment eventually resulted in the abandonment of the "schizophrenogenic causality" by our field—but not before psychiatry had alienated many patients and family members. A neuropsychiatric reconceptualization of schizophrenia would place greater emphasis on the underlying genetics and disorders of brain tissue, chemistry, and physiology, thereby rendering iatrogenic stigmatization far less likely.

Let us recall that before 1914, when Lewy (see Roth and Kroll 1986) traced the neuropathology of paralysis agitans (Parkinson's disease) to the basal ganglia of the brain, this illness was generally considered to be a mental disease, often associated with disparaging religious overtones. For example, even the great neurologist Charcot considered the disease to develop from "violent moral emotions" caused by political unrest prevalent in France in 1877. Even though today's better understanding of Parkinson's disease has documented prominent "mental" symptoms—dementia, depression, and psychosis—our acceptance of the neuropathological basis of the disorder discourages stigma and renders such damaging conceptualizations as a "parkinsonogenic parent" untenable. Although many psychiatrists (including us) have profound concerns that an increased focus on biology could cause the conceptual pendulum to swing to a reductionist extreme wherein psychosocial aspects of neuropsychiatric disorders are dangerously deemphasized, we nonetheless believe that neurobiological emphasis has, on balance, more advantages than disadvantages for our profession and the patients we serve. As Sir Martin Roth and Jerome Kroll so persuasively argued in their brilliant treatise *The Reality of Mental Illness* (Roth and Kroll 1986), critics of psychiatry (i.e., those who contend the profession "invents" mental illness to advance our own interests and material status) separate the mind from the body to bolster their contention that mental illness does not exist. Not only does the neuropsychiatric paradigm parry such attacks (i.e., stigmatization of the patient and the psychiatrist) from "outside" the profession, but, more importantly, it reduces "the attacks from within" (i.e., shame and embarrassment of the patient and family).

Although the psychobiological conceptualization of mental illness was clearly formulated and promulgated by Adolf Meyer over 65 years ago (see Winters 1951) and although a biopsychosocial model was brilliantly advanced for all of medicine almost two decades ago by George Engel (1977), the stigmatization of mentally ill people today remains pervasive. Those who work in the general hospital setting experience daily the reluctance of many individuals with highly disabling psychiatric disorders (e.g., major depression secondary to stroke or dependence on narcotic analgesics) to be transferred from general medical units to excellent, dedicated psychiatric services because "I'm not crazy." It is not uncommon for a patient with symptoms originally thought to be derivative of chronic, disabling disorders such as multiple sclerosis or even a brain tumor to express disappointment when told the underlying disorder is a treatable psychiatric condition such as depression. Political candidates in the United States vehemently deny ever having received psychiatric treatment and refrain from publicly stating, "So what if I, as have millions of other Americans, received treatment for a psychiatric disorder? Does this make me any less qualified to serve?" The unqualified protestations of politicians are obvious indications of their own and their advisers' perceptions of the voting public's negative views of mental illness and its treatment. Could it be that we have been far more successful in communicating and convincing ourselves of the integrity and applicability of our models of mental illness than we have our patients, their families, and society—all of whom still feel that shame is associated with our labels and paradigms? Is it not possible that, where appropriate and accurate, new models and paradigms, based on neuropsychiatric perspectives, would be not only more precise but also more palatable to those who have such illnesses?

The Revolution in Neuroscience Research

Lewis Judd, while Director of the National Institute of Mental Health in 1988, stated at the American Psychiatric Association Annual Meeting that 95% of what we know about the brain as it relates to behavior has been discovered in the past 5 years. This statement highlights the recent, unprecedented advances in the brain sciences. In many important respects, progress in medicine is linked to technological advancement. Before the refinement of the lens and the development of the microscope, a cohesive and broadly accepted conceptualization of infectious illness was not likely to occur. Likewise, without the technological capacity to measure brain waves through the electroencephalogram, a modern conceptualization of seizure disorders—with the many ensuing social and therapeutic benefits— would not be possible. An explosive proliferation of technological advances is under way, the rate and implications of which are heretofore unparalleled. Applied to neuropsychiatric assessment, these advances have resulted in useful innovations such as computed tomography (CT), magnetic resonance imaging (MRI), positron-emission tomography (PET), single photon emission computed tomography (SPECT), regional cerebral blood flow (rCBF), and a large array of neuroimmunological techniques. The net result of future applications of technological advances will be the inexorable transformation and redefinition of illnesses that had previously been conceptualized as *mental* or *functional* into the neuropsychiatric paradigm.

Coincident with this transformation and redefinition, it is critical that the sensitivity, humanity, and ethical bases so inherent to psychosocial models continue to remain prominent. The challenges presented by acquired immunodeficiency syndrome (AIDS) clearly demonstrate how technological, psychological, and interpersonal perspectives are inseparable in understanding and intervening in this devastating disorder. For the *Synopsis of Neuropsychiatry*, we have chosen topics and chapter authors who incorporate both recent discoveries and technological advances related to neuroscience research and psychosocial and ethical considerations into their chapters.

The renaissance in neuropsychiatry, for the reasons expressed above, will not only enhance the efficacy and integrity of the fields of psychiatry and neurology, but also will have even broader implications. For the silver lining of the scourge of neuropsychiatric illness is that these devastating diseases provide both the impetus and substrate whereby we can explore ourselves. Through understanding Alzheimer's disease, we will eventually gain vital insights into the minute particles of matter and complex spatial and electrical arrangements that regulate unimpaired memory and learning. Through our neurobiological investigation of bipolar illness, we will gain vital insights into the chemistry and physics of healthy feelings, temperament, and mood. It is thus one of life's bitter paradoxes that, through the painful and disabling lesions treated by psychiatrists and neurologists, we are discovering ourselves. In the course of such discovery, we will ultimately not only approach relief from illness, but we may also free ourselves from the limitations—ranging from anxiety to aging—that have been accepted for millennia as the human condition.

Stuart C. Yudofsky, M.D.
Houston, Texas

Robert E. Hales, M.D.
San Francisco, California

REFERENCES

Andreasen N, Nasrallah HA, Dunn V, et al: Structural abnormalities in the frontal system in schizophrenia. Arch Gen Psychiatry 43:136–144, 1986

Blum K, Noble EP, Sheridan PJ, et al: Allelic associations of human dopamine D_2 receptor gene in alcoholism. JAMA 263:2055–2059, 1990

Brown ER, Marsden CD: How common is dementia in Parkinson's disease? Lancet 2:1261–1265, 1984

Bunzow JR, Van Tol HHM, Grandy DK, et al: Cloning and expression of a rat D_2 dopamine receptor cDNA. Nature 336:783–787, 1988

Cloninger CR: D_2 dopamine receptor gene is associated but not linked with alcoholism. JAMA 266:1833–1834, 1991

Comings DE, Comings BG, Muhleman D, et al: The dopamine D_2 receptor locus as a modifying gene in neuropsychiatric disorders. JAMA 226:1793–1800, 1991

Engel GL: The need for a new medical model: a challenge for biomedicine. Science 196:129–136, 1977

Kang J, Lemaire H-G, Unterbeck A, et al: The precursor of Alzheimer's disease amyloid A4 protein resembles a cell-surface receptor. Nature 325:733–736, 1987

Mayeux R: Depression and dementia in Parkinson's disease, in Neurology 2: Movement Disorders. Edited by Marsden CD, Fahn S. London, Butterworth, 1981, pp 75–91

Oddy M, Coughlan T, Tyerman A, et al: Social adjustment after closed head injury: a further follow-up seven years after injury. J Neurol Neurosurg Psychiatry 48: 564–568, 1985

Robinson RG, Starkstein SE: Current research in affective disorders following stroke. J Neuropsychiatry Clin Neurosci 2:1–14, 1990

Roth M, Kroll J: The Reality of Mental Illness. Cambridge, England, Cambridge University Press, 1986

St. George-Hyslop PH, Tanzi RE, Polinksy RJ, et al: The genetic defect causing familial Alzheimer's disease maps on chromosome 21. Science 235:885–889, 1987

West LJ, Maxwell DS, Nobel EP, et al: Alcoholism. Ann Intern Med 100:405–416, 1984

Winters EE (ed): The Collected Papers of Adolf Meyer, Vol 3: Medical Teaching. Baltimore, MD, Johns Hopkins Press, 1951

Wong DF, Wagner HN Jr, Tune LE, et al: Positron emission tomography reveals elevated D_2 dopamine receptors in drug-naive schizophrenics. Science 234:1558–1563, 1986

Yudofsky SC, Silver JM, Jackson M, et al: The Overt Aggression Scale: an operationalized rating scale for verbal and physical aggression. Am J Psychiatry 143:35–39, 1986

Section I

Basic Principles of Neuroscience

Chapter 1

Cellular and Molecular Biology of the Neuron

Stephen G. Rayport, M.D., Ph.D.

We now have an increasingly comprehensive understanding of neurons as cells. Major strides are being made toward elucidating neuronal functioning in molecular terms. These advances in neural science have tremendous importance for neuropsychiatry (Barondes 1990; Pardes 1986). They provide a language to describe how neuropsychiatric diseases arise and evolve. Already, knowledge of neurons and their synapses provides the basis for understanding psychopharmacology (Cooper et al. 1986). In time, knowledge of how neurons function is certain to provide insights into higher mental functioning. It also will be essential to identifying the genes that likely underlie the major neuropsychiatric disorders (see Chapter 8).

To understand how abnormal genes affect higher mental functioning, we need to know how they affect the development and function of neurons. Nonfatal genetic mutations of the sort underlying neuropsychiatric disease probably act by coding for subtly altered molecules made in brain cells. Neuropsychiatric disorders also may arise from aberrant experience that permanently alters neuronal connectivity. This is most likely to occur during development when normal environmental input is essential for the fine-tuning of neuronal connections.

It will be crucial to understand how groups of neurons interconnect to form systems for the control of behavior and how these may be affected by pathological experience. Developments in information theory, semiotics, and neural network research have clarified the relationship between the brain and mind and shown how computer-based assemblies of digital elements might produce brainlike behavior (Sejnowksi et al. 1988). Already, neural network approaches have offered a way of understanding complexities in higher mental functioning that have eluded previous conceptualizations, such as the distinction between the thought disorders of schizophrenia and mania (Hoffman 1987) and insight into thought-processing abnormalities in schizophrenia (Servan-Schreiber et al. 1990). As we extend our insights into the cellular workings of the human brain, we will better know what therapeutic interventions best counter aberrant neuronal connections produced by pathological experiences during development or offset genetic defects. This chapter focuses on the properties of neurons: how they develop, connect, and communicate with one another. From the rapid pace of developments, we can be confident that molecular genetic interventions or therapies based on knowledge of how to normalize patterns of neuronal connectivity will lead to better treatments and eventually prevention of neuropsychiatric disease.

CELLULAR FUNCTION OF NEURONS

Individual neurons in the brain receive signals from thousands of neurons and in turn convey information to thousands of other neurons. Central nervous system (CNS) neurons may be seen as part of ephemeral, ever changing networks, shifting their participation from network to network as information is drawn from one task and used in another, often simultaneously following a parallel-distributed processing model. The sophistication of these networks depends in part on the neurons that make them up.

Neurons are the most differentiated and among the largest cells in the body, with processes stretching as long as a meter. There are also a great number of them in our brains, and the number of interconnections is astronomical. The human brain has 10^{12}–10^{13} neurons; this means that, if each neuron forms an average of 10^3 connections, the human CNS has as many as 10^{15}–10^{16} synapses. Our mental capacities arise primarily from the large number of neurons in our brains and the complexity of their interconnections.

Neurons share a common organization dictated by their function, which is to process and convey information. They come in various sizes and shapes, but all have four well-defined regions: dendrites, cell body, axon, and axon terminals (Figure 1–1). Dendrites receive signals from other neurons. From the dendrites, the signals spread passively, or with an active boost, to the cell body. The cell body serves as an integrating site for signals coming from all the dendrites. In addition, as in other cells, the cell body in a neuron contains the genetic information (in the nucleus) that codes for the fabrication of all the necessary elements of cellular functioning, as well as sites for their manufacture, processing, and transport. The axon conveys information from the cell body to other neurons, often over long distances. At the axon terminals, the neuron makes contact with other neurons or effector cells, in turn eliciting signals in their dendrites. For central neurons, the flow of information is initiated by synaptic input onto dendrites.

Signaling Mechanisms Within the Neuron

The neuron carries information electrically. Information enters the cell through synapses on its dendrites. In the cell body, signals from several dendrites combine. This grand postsynaptic potential (PSP) depolarizes the initial segment of the axon (the part of the axon closest to the cell body), which has the lowest threshold for activation. When threshold is reached, the striking all-or-none electrical explosion of the action potential is initiated. The action potential, or spike, propagates as an

Figure 1–1. *(at right)* Basic shape of the neuron. Neurons have four well-defined cellular regions: dendrites, cell body, axon, and axon terminals. Electrical signals from other neurons impinge on the dendrites. An integration of signals from all dendrites occurs in the cell body and initial segment of the axon. When signals exceed the threshold of the initial segment, an action potential is initiated that travels down the axon to reach the terminal zone. Axon terminals synapse with postsynaptic cells, starting the cycle of information flow anew.
Source. Reprinted from Kandel ER, Schwartz JH: *Principles of Neural Science,* 2nd Edition. New York, Elsevier, 1985, p. 15. Used with permission.

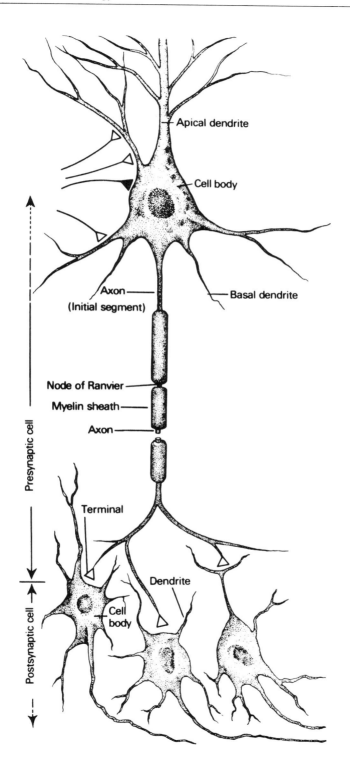

electrical wave down the axon at high speed, ultimately spreading into the axon terminals. At specialized sites in the terminals called active zones, electrical activity triggers the release of chemical neurotransmitters, which activate closely apposed postsynaptic receptors on the dendrites of other neurons.

The ability of neurons to generate an action potential derives from the presence of ionic gradients across the membrane, in particular of sodium (Na^+) and chloride (Cl^-), which are high outside, and potassium (K^+), which is high inside. These gradients are generated by the continuous action of membrane pumps. Also in the membrane are specialized proteins called membrane channels which regulate the flow of ions, such as Na^+, K^+, Cl^-, and calcium (Ca^{2+}) across the membrane. At rest, the membrane is selectively permeable to K^+ and Cl^-, which causes the cell to be negative inside by about -50 to -75 mV. When the cell is active, this permeability is reversed in favor of Na^+, causing the cell membrane to be depolarized to about $+50$ mV.

The permeability of Na^+ channel proteins depends on membrane voltage and time. Because inflow of Na^+ depolarizes the membrane, this confers a regenerative property; once a threshold potential is reached, increased Na^+ influx leads to depolarization, which further opens Na^+ channels, further enhancing Na^+ influx, and so on. The result is that at threshold, the membrane potential rapidly switches to $+50$ mV. The membrane potential only stays so depolarized for about a millisecond because the Na^+ channels then show a time-dependent inactivation. Additionally, voltage-dependent K^+ channels, which are also activated by depolarization (but more slowly), increase the K^+ permeability and repolarize the membrane. Therefore, the membrane potential peaks at a depolarized level determined by the Na^+ gradient and then rapidly returns to the resting potential, determined once again by the K^+ gradient. Once the neuron is repolarized, the Na^+ inactivation wears off (the time this takes accounts for the refractory period of the neuron, a brief period when the threshold for firing an action potential is elevated), and the cell can fire again.

The regenerative property of the action potential confers long-distance signaling capabilities (Figure 1–2). When the membrane potential peaks under the control of the increase in Na^+ permeability, adjacent regions of the axon become sufficiently depolarized so that they are in turn brought to threshold and generate an action potential. As successive axonal segments are depolarized, the action potential conducts at great speed down the axon, like a wave. This is further enhanced by myelination, which increases the rate of conduction severalfold by limiting the amount of current flow required for action potential conduction. Because of its all-or-none characteristics and ability to conduct over long distances, the action potential provides a high-quality digital signaling mechanism in the neuron.

Although the information that a neuron integrates depends on its synaptic input, how the neuron processes that information depends on its intrinsic properties (Llinás 1988). Many CNS neurons have the ability to generate their own patterns of activity even in the absence of synaptic input, firing either at a regular rate (pacemaker firing) or in clusters of spikes (burst firing). This endogenous activity is driven by specialized ion channels, with their own voltage and time dependence, which periodically bring the initial segment of the axon to threshold (Tank et al. 1988). These channels giving rise to autorhythmicity may be modulated by the membrane potential of the cell or second messenger systems. Further, CNS neurons may profoundly change how they respond to a given synaptic input as a function of slight changes in resting potential

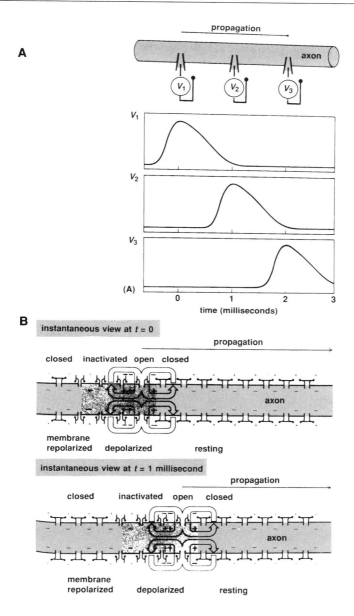

Figure 1–2. Action potential conduction. The regenerative property of ion channels in neuronal membranes mediates the rapid spread of the action potential down the axon. *Panel A:* Electrodes (V_1, V_2, and V_3) placed along the axon show the action potential traveling unchanged down the axon at high speed. *Panel B:* The action potential conducts as a wave. As each segment of the axon is depolarized, the spike it fires in turn depolarizes the subsequent segment. Therefore, as the action potential travels to the right, channels go from closed to open to inactivated to closed. In this way activation of the initial segment of the axon initiates an action potential that conducts all the way to the axon terminals.

Source. Reprinted from Alberts B, Bray D, Lewis J, et al: *Molecular Biology of the Cell,* 2nd Edition. New York, Garland, 1989, p. 1071. Used with permission.

(Llinás and Jahnsen 1982). For instance, a thalamic neuron fires as a pacemaker when stimulated from slightly depolarized levels, whereas it fires in bursts of action potentials when stimulated from somewhat hyperpolarized levels. Changes in second messenger levels may also profoundly affect the activity or response properties of neurons. This confers a much greater repertoire to the functioning of individual neurons. So, in addition to evoking a response in a postsynaptic neuron, synaptic activity can shape intrinsic firing patterns, causing a cell to shift from one mode of activity to another, or alter the cell's response to other synaptic inputs.

Signaling Between Neurons

Neurons communicate with one another by releasing chemical neurotransmitters at specialized sites of close membrane apposition called synapses. Most CNS synaptic connections are chemically mediated. Chemical synapses allow for a significant amplification of signals; they may be inhibitory as well as excitatory, are susceptible to a wide range of modulation, and can through the release of transmitters activating second messenger cascades in turn modulate the activity of other cells. One can think of chemical synapses as highly specialized microglands—ones that release their contents just in the synaptic zone (Figure 1–3). Like glands, they hold neurotransmitter molecules (their secretory substance) in numerous, small membrane-bound granules or synaptic vesicles, each containing several thousand molecules. When the action potential invades the axon terminal, it causes a near synchronous fusion of synaptic vesicles with the plasma membrane and release of transmitter into the synaptic cleft. Transmitter then has to diffuse only a short distance before it binds to postsynaptic receptors.

Transmitter action is typically limited in duration by one of several mechanisms that rapidly remove the released transmitter from the postsynaptic region (Cooper et al. 1986). Transmitter may be broken down as is the case for acetylcholine, which is hydrolyzed by the enzyme acetylcholinesterase. The monoamine and amino acid neurotransmitters are also metabolized, but, in addition, they are removed from the synaptic cleft by rapid reuptake mechanisms. Specific membrane pumps carry the transmitter back into the presynaptic terminal, the postsynaptic cell, or adjacent glial cells where it is repackaged in synaptic vesicles or metabolized or both.

Rapid Postsynaptic Response Mechanisms

Postsynaptic receptors activated by the binding of neurotransmitter fall into two classes. In the case of ligand-gated channel receptors, the channel is an intrinsic part of the receptor protein complex. Receptor activation directly increases the ionic permeability of the postsynaptic membrane through a change in the shape (allosteric) of the receptor complex. This results in either depolarization giving rise to an excitatory postsynaptic potential (EPSP) or hyperpolarization generating an inhibitory postsynaptic potential (IPSP). The neuromuscular junction is the prototypic excitatory synapse; simultaneous binding of two acetylcholine molecules opens a receptor channel permeable to both Na^+ and K^+. This results in a strong depolarization of the postsynaptic membrane mediated by Na^+ influx and moderated by K^+ efflux. Ligand-gated channels are found at synapses such as the neuromuscular junction where rapid and reliable activation of the postsynaptic cell is

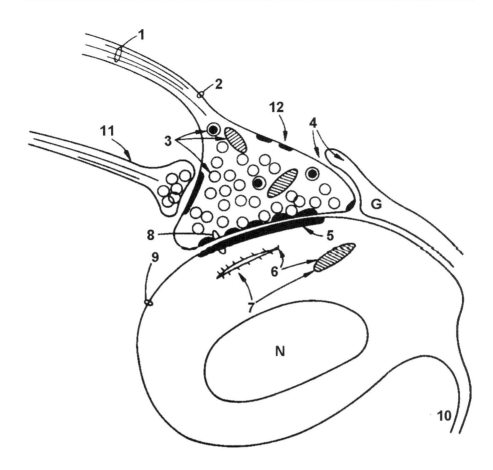

Figure 1–3. Chemical synaptic transmission. The essentials of the chemical synapse are revealed in 12 steps: 1) molecular components of the synapse get to the terminal by axonal transport; 2) an action potential invades the terminal, leading to a local influx of calcium (Ca^{2+}, which
triggers release of synaptic vesicles into the cleft; 3) synaptic organelles and enzymes synthe-
size and package neurotransmitter; 4) extracellular enzymes and glia (G) and neurons limit
transmitter action by degradation and reuptake of transmitter; 5) released transmitter impinges
on postsynaptic receptors to initiate postsynaptic signals; 6) organelles in the postsynaptic neuron respond to transmitter binding by release of Ca^{2+}, for example; 7) second messengers initiated by receptor binding may influence DNA transcription (in the nucleus [N]) leading to
longer-term responses and structural changes; 8) patterns of activity may lead to transient or
enduring changes in the efficacy of the synapse; 9) electrical activity in the postsynaptic membrane continues the cycle of information flow; 10) this may lead to generation of action potentials in the postsynaptic cell and signaling to other cells; 11) the functioning of the presynaptic
terminal may be influenced by presynaptic modulatory inputs; and 12) the presynaptic terminal
may be regulated by its own transmitter through autoreceptors (receptors to the cell's own
transmitter).

Source.   Reprinted from Cooper JR, Bloom FE, Roth RH: *The Biochemical Basis of Neuropharmacology,* 5th Edition. New York, Oxford University Press, 1986, p. 44. Used with permission.

required. For motor neurons, the coupling between pre- and postsynaptic cells is strong enough that one motor neuron spike reliably causes muscle contraction.

In the CNS, glutamate receptors mediate most fast excitatory transmission; γ-aminobutyric acid (GABA) and glycine are the most common inhibitory transmitters. GABA and glycine receptors are members of a superfamily of receptors modeled on the nicotinic acetylcholine receptor (Schofield et al. 1990); glutamate receptors form a separate family (Keinänen et al. 1990). Unlike motor neurons, central neurons function in groups so that generally no individual cell has so strong a synaptic connection with another cell that it alone brings it to threshold; rather, groups of neurons—active in concert—converge on a postsynaptic neuron to generate several PSPs. These may summate within regions of the postsynaptic neuron (spatial summation) if they occur close enough together in time (temporal summation) to cause the postsynaptic neuron to fire. As a rule, fast ligand-gated channels mediate the flow of detailed information, such as patterns of sensory input, associations between sensory modalities, or motor output.

Longer-Term Postsynaptic Response Mechanisms

Longer-term modulatory effects are generally mediated by non-channel-linked receptors. This class of receptors is akin to cell-surface hormone receptors where agonist binding regulates cell function via second messenger cascades. G proteins are the first link in signaling cascades that achieve their effects either through activation of protein kinases, enzymes that phosphorylate cellular proteins (Huganir and Greengard 1987), or via changes in the level of intracellular Ca^{2+}, which in turn can trigger protein phosphorylation (Kennedy 1989a). Phosphorylation of cellular proteins may either activate or inactivate them or change their shape profoundly. Proteins affected may include membrane channels, structural elements, and transcriptional regulators for the expression of genes. In this way modulatory actions mediated by second messengers may affect most cellular processes. The potential for amplification, combined with divergence and convergence of signals, provides the requisite mechanisms for enduring changes in neuronal function, in particular the changes essential in learning and memory and during development.

G proteins are links in four major second messenger cascades (Figure 1–4) (Neer and Clapham 1988); although in some cases a cascade may function in isolation, most often they interact, conferring a complexity of action (Role and Schwartz 1989), our knowledge of which is still incomplete.

1. G proteins may link directly to nearby membrane channels to regulate their permeability.
2. They may either up- or down-regulate adenylate or guanylate cyclase to change cyclic adenosine monophosphate (cAMP).
3. G proteins may activate the inositol phospholipid system (Berridge and Irvine 1989). In this case, two second messengers are generated. Binding of transmitter by the receptor activates phospholipase C (PLC) via a G protein that hydrolyzes the membrane phospholipid phosphatidylinositol-bis-phosphate (PIP_2) to produce inositol triphosphate (IP_3) and diacylglycerol (DAG). IP_3 stimulates the release of Ca^{2+} from intracellular stores.

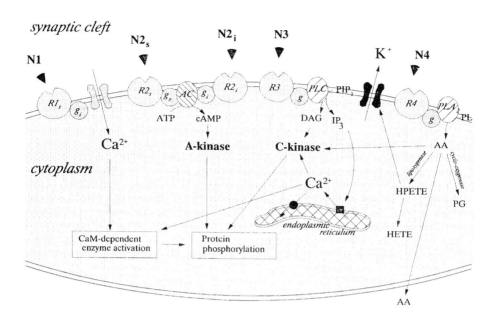

Figure 1–4. Second messenger cascades in neuronal signaling. Neurotransmitters (N1, N2, N3, and N4) activate specific receptors (R1, R2, R3, and R4). These receptors are coupled by G proteins to four postsynaptic signaling systems:

1. N1 inhibits membrane channels through its G protein (g_i) link; among those that may be inhibited are those regulating calcium (Ca^{2+}) entry, which serves as a second messenger with many effects mediated by calmodulin (CaM)-dependent enzyme activation.

2. Adenylate cyclase (AC) can be either stimulated ($N2_s$) or inhibited ($N2_i$) through separate G protein links (g_s and g_i); these actions can lead to an increase in synthesis of cyclic adenosine monophosphate (cAMP), which in turn controls the activity of A-kinase. A-kinase, like other kinases, controls cellular functions through protein phosphorylation.

3. N3 activates phospholipase C (PLC), which hydrolyzes phosphatidylinositol-bis-phosphate (PIP$_2$) producing two second messengers, diacylglycerol (DAG) and inositol trisphosphate (IP$_3$). IP$_3$ triggers the release of Ca^{2+} from the endoplasmic reticulum. Ca^{2+} in turn triggers the translocation of C-kinase to the cell membrane where it is activated by DAG. Because it becomes membrane bound with activation, C-kinase may be especially important in the modulation of membrane channels. Ca^{2+} released from intracellular stores may act similarly to Ca^{2+} that enters from outside the cell; however, because cells maintain Ca^{2+} at low levels, increases in Ca^{2+} levels are generally restricted.

4. N4 works through phospholipase A$_2$ (PLA$_2$) to trigger the production of arachidonic acid (AA) by hydrolysis of membrane phospholipids (PL). Unlike other second messengers, AA and its metabolites (hydroxyeicosatetraenoic [HETE] acids) and (hydroperoxyeicosatetraenoic [HPETE] acids) are membrane permeable so they can leave the postsynaptic cell to influence nearby cells; this may be important in long-term potentiation. K^+ = potassium ion; ATP = adenosine phosphate; PG = prostaglandins.

Source. Adapted from Piomelli et al. 1987; Ross and Gilman 1985.

4. G proteins may couple to phospholipase A_2 forming arachidonic acid (AA) by hydrolysis of membrane phospholipids (Axelrod et al. 1988; Piomelli and Greengard 1990; Piomelli et al. 1987).

Synaptic Modulation in Learning and Memory

Second messengers profoundly increase the range of responses a neuron may show to synaptic input. They activate kinases, which by phosphorylating other proteins act to both amplify and prolong signals. Receptor activation may induce kinase activity that lasts beyond agonist binding, enduring until the kinase is inactivated and phosphatases reverse phosphorylation. Because second messengers trigger numerous cellular functions, activation of a single receptor may trigger a coordinated cellular response involving several systems. This may include activity-dependent modulation of genomic transcription leading to enduring changes in cellular function. Learning and memory require both short- and long-term changes in neurons, which occurs at synapses.

Simple learning in *Aplysia*. Animals such as the marine mollusk *Aplysia californica* have proved fundamental to studies of cellular mechanisms of learning and memory because changes in such animals' behavior can be traced to specific alterations in signaling between neurons (Kandel 1989). Behavioral studies have shown that *Aplysia* exhibits a simple defensive behavior called the gill withdrawal reflex, which can be modified by experience. Stimulation of the siphon leads to habituation of the reflex. If on the other hand the animal is aroused by a shock, the reflex shows sensitization, and subsequently the gill is withdrawn more briskly. If the same shock is administered to *Aplysia* when the reflex is habituated, the responsiveness also increases, showing dishabituation. Habituation and sensitization show both short and long memory. A single training trial may alter the reflex for at most a period of hours, but if training is repeated several times, habituation and sensitization may last for weeks. The animal is also capable of associative learning. If siphon stimulation is immediately followed by tail shock, it will show an increased gill withdrawal to siphon stimulation. In effect, it learns that siphon stimulation signals tail shock.

The essential features of the neural circuit for gill withdrawal reflex are encompassed in a 3-cell circuit (Figure 1–5). Gill withdrawal is triggered when siphon stimulation elicits action potentials in the peripheral branches of sensory neurons. These spikes conduct to the abdominal ganglion where sensory cells make synaptic connections with motor neurons. At the sensory axonal terminals, Ca^{2+} influx triggers the release of neurotransmitter, producing an EPSP in the motor neuron. If the sensory-motor connection is strong enough, the motor neuron fires and its action potential conducts to gill muscle producing contraction and withdrawal. More often, however, several nearly synchronous spikes in one or more sensory neurons are required to bring the postsynaptic motor neuron to threshold. The increases in Ca^{2+} resulting from repeated activation of sensory neurons cause inactivation of presynaptic Ca^{2+} channels, resulting in a reduction of Ca^{2+} influx and a decrease in transmitter release. This process, whereby repeated activation of a synapse leads to a reduction in efficacy, is called homosynaptic depression—it is the cellular basis of habituation.

Sensitizing stimuli activate facilitatory interneurons. These cells release serotonin and peptide cotransmitters at synapses on the sensory neuron terminals. Firing of the facilitator cells does not in itself cause gill withdrawal. However, when the siphon is subsequently stimulated, the efficacy of the sensory transmission is increased. This process in which activity in a third neuron increases the strength of the connection between another pair of neurons is termed *heterosynaptic facilitation*—it underlies sensitization and results from increased transmitter release by the sensory neuron. The facilitatory transmitters mediate facilitation via activation of adenylate cyclase

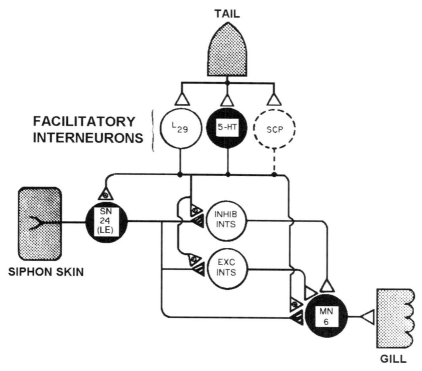

Figure 1–5. *Aplysia* gill withdrawal neural circuit. The marine snail *Aplysia* exhibits a simple defensive behavior, the gill withdrawal reflex, which shows habituation, sensitization, and associative learning. The reflex is mediated by a small number of neurons falling into three classes; the essential cells are shown by *dark circles*. These are sensory, motor, and modulatory interneurons. Sensory neurons (SN; of which there are a total of 24 in the LE cluster) pick up stimuli from the siphon skin. They activate gill motor neurons (MN; of which there are 6), to cause gill contraction. Facilitatory interneurons control the strength of the contraction; sensitizing stimuli to the tail activate neuron L_{29}, and other neurons that use 5-hydroxytryptamine (5-HT; serotonin) or small cardioactive peptide (SCP) as transmitters, to presynaptically increase transmitter release from the sensory neuron terminals (*shaded*), producing heterosynaptic facilitation. Other inhibitory (INHIB INTS) and excitatory interneurons (EXC INTS) may shape the response or mediate a heterosynaptic component of habituation or sensitization. The site of plasticity underlying learning in the reflex is in the presynaptic terminals of the sensory cells (*shaded*).

Source. Reprinted from Kandel ER: "Genes, Nerve Cells, and the Remembrance of Things Past." *Journal of Neuropsychiatry and Clinical Neurosciences* 1:103–125, 1989. Used with permission.

through a G protein link. cAMP binds to the regulatory subunit of A-kinase, releasing the catalytic subunit, which phosphorylates a class of voltage-dependent K^+ channels, sensitive to serotonin, known as S-K^+ channels. Because the falling phase of the action potential is mediated by an influx of K^+, closing S-K^+ potassium channels results in an action potential of increased duration, one that evokes a greater influx of Ca^{2+} and thus more transmitter release. This mechanism only works when Ca^{2+} channels are active (as in sensitization).

When the sensory-motor synapse is depressed, and Ca^{2+} channels are largely inactivated, another mechanism becomes primary. Serotonin activates C-kinase, which is thought to increase the pool of readily releasable sensory neurotransmitter, enhancing the action of a reduced Ca^{2+} influx and thus boosting transmitter release. Associative learning appears to result from a synergistic action of spike-triggered Ca^{2+} influx and serotonin-activated second messenger systems, leading to enhanced C-kinase activity (Braha et al. 1990). In sensitization, dishabituation, and activity-dependent enhancement of presynaptic facilitation (the cellular mechanism of associative learning), the penultimate effect is mediated by a phosphorylation of existing proteins. A covalent modification of existing proteins thus appears to be the molecular basis for short-term memory in *Aplysia*.

In contrast, long-term memory appears to require changes in transcription. Intriguingly, the mechanisms for short-term sensitization (which has been best studied) also contribute to long-term memory, in a continuum. In long-term, as in short-term, sensitization, the memory is encoded by a strengthening of sensory-motor synapses, there is increased transmitter release, S-K^+ channels are closed leading to increased Ca^{2+} influx, serotonin and cAMP are the first and second messengers, and a characteristic set of proteins are phosphorylated (Sweatt and Kandel 1989). For long-term memory there is an absolute requirement for gene transcription and the synthesis of new proteins, which leads to structural changes at sensory-motor synapses. Blocking transcription triggered by cAMP-responsive elements blocks mechanisms underlying long- but not short-term sensitization (Dash et al. 1990). Ultimately the changes triggered by repeated stimulation, activation of facilitatory interneurons, serotonin application, or cAMP injection lead to structural changes involving the growth of new processes and increased numbers and size of active zones. These structural changes are likely to be orchestrated by interactions among several second messenger systems, through regulation of transcription.

Hippocampal long-term potentiation.   In examining learning and memory in the mammalian nervous system, the hippocampus has been a particular focus because of its essential role in memory—bilateral hippocampectomy almost completely blocks the establishment of long-term memories. Brief high-frequency activation of hippocampal synapses permanently increases their strength through a phenomenon called *long-term potentiation* (LTP) (Kennedy 1989b; Malenka et al. 1989). LTP has thus proved particularly intriguing as a model of cellular plasticity that is likely to mediate memory function in the mammalian CNS.

The crucial initiating step in the induction of LTP is Ca^{2+} entry localized to the postsynaptic zone. Glutamate released from presynaptic CA3 cells acts on two classes of postsynaptic receptors on CA1 cells, the *N*-methyl-D-aspartate (NMDA) and α-amino-3-hydroxy-5-methyl-4-isoxazole propionic acid (AMPA) receptors (also known as kainate or quisqualate receptors). AMPA receptor activation causes depolarization via Na^+ influx, whereas NMDA receptors do so via both Na^+ and Ca^{2+} entry. NMDA receptors differ crucially from AMPA receptors in requiring an initial depolarization before they will respond to neurotransmitter. Both NMDA and AMPA receptors are localized to postsynaptic dendritic spines, but because of the NMDA receptor's depolarization requirement, only AMPA receptors are activated by low-frequency firing of the presynaptic cell, so that little Ca^{2+} enters. In contrast, stronger or higher-frequency activation activates more AMPA receptors, causes a larger postsynaptic depolarization, and is then able to also activate NMDA receptors. NMDA receptors then mediate a localized increase in intracellular Ca^{2+} in the postsynaptic dendritic spine. Ca^{2+} acting as a second messenger initiates a selective enhancement in synaptic efficacy. Because they operate only during strong stimulation, NMDA receptors are crucial for the triggering, but not the expression, of LTP. Their requirement for the conjunction of transmitter and postsynaptic depolarization appears to confer both the specificity and associativity of LTP.

Increased postsynaptic Ca^{2+} activates a cascade of intracellular messengers, which could mediate LTP (Figure 1–6). These include Ca^{2+}/calmodulin-dependent protein kinase II (CaM-KII), C-kinase and Ca^{2+}-dependent proteases. The relative importance of each remains open to question. For example, CaM-KII is localized to the postsynaptic membrane where it could phosphorylate postsynaptic AMPA receptors, increasing their response to transmitter. Because CaM-KII can be autoactivating once activated by Ca^{2+}, it might serve to maintain an increased receptor response over a course of minutes to hours. LTP also requires C-kinase activation; C-kinase may mediate transcriptional changes necessary for more permanent synaptic strengthening. Ca^{2+}-dependent proteases may also be important; they may induce structural changes in the postsynaptic spine to increase the effectiveness of synapses on just that spine.

Whereas LTP is triggered postsynaptically, the expression of LTP appears to be mediated presynaptically through an increased release of glutamate (Bekkers and Stevens 1990; Malinow and Tsien 1990). Indeed, tetanization sufficient to elicit LTP is associated with an increased glutamate release that can be measured for several hours (Bliss et al. 1986); this would most likely occur if each presynaptic action potential elicited more transmitter release. Another line of evidence reveals that although both induction and expression of LTP can be blocked by protein kinase inhibitors, injection of a kinase inhibitor into just the postsynaptic cell blocks the induction of LTP, but not its continued expression (Malinow et al. 1989). These results suggest that immediately after the tetanus, postsynaptic mechanisms triggered by a rise in intracellular Ca^{2+} and involving protein kinase activity boost synaptic strength. Later on, presynaptic kinase activity appears to be crucial, acting to increase transmitter release.

A membrane-permeable second messenger that could diffuse across the synapse and act on the presynaptic terminal seems to be required if postsynaptic signals are to trigger presynaptic changes (Lynch et al. 1989). Among the several second messengers considered in this chapter, only arachidonic acid (AA) is membrane permeable. Furthermore, AA levels rise after stimulation that induces LTP (Lynch et al. 1989). Specificity of action would be explained, if simultaneous presynaptic activity (this would be a second associative site) was required for its action. Indeed, AA application alone is ineffectual. However, delivery of a weak tetanus (one not sufficient to generate LTP itself) in combination with AA results in a slowly developing potentiation occurring over a course of 15–30 minutes (Williams et al. 1989). Potentiation occurs despite blockade of AA metabolism, indicating that the effect is mediated by AA itself and not its metabolites. Furthermore, potentiation cannot be blocked by NMDA antagonists (which block LTP), showing that AA production is a subsequent step in the pathway after NMDA receptor activation. As in LTP, AA application leads to an activity-dependent increase in glutamate release. Either maximal stimulation or AA-induced potentiation precludes further potentiation by the other intervention, supporting further the key role of AA as a membrane-permeable second messenger. How AA mediates increased release is not known, but its activity dependence seems to assure that only simultaneously tetanized presynaptic terminals will show increased glutamate release and thus LTP.

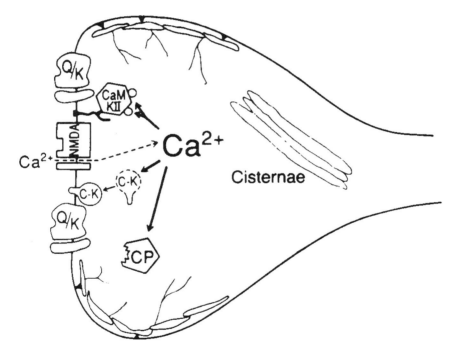

Figure 1–6.   Initiation of long-term potentiation (LTP). CA1 cells have two classes of glutamate receptors, those responding to quisqualate or kainate (Q/K)—also known as α-amino-3-hydroxy-5-methyl-4-isoxazole propionic acid (AMPA) receptors—and those selectively activated by *N*-methyl-D-aspartate (NMDA) when the membrane is depolarized. AMPA receptors mediate a sodium (Na+) dependent excitatory postsynaptic potential; with lower frequency synaptic activity no calcium (Ca^{2+}) enters. However, the conjunction of depolarization and glutamate activates NMDA receptors, which mediate Ca^{2+} entry. Postsynaptic Ca^{2+} may trigger LTP through several mechanisms. It may activate calmodulin-dependent protein kinase II (CaM-KII), C-kinase (C-K), or calpain (CP). C-kinase may also trigger arachidonic acid production (not shown), which may increase presynaptic transmitter release and appears to be essential for the maintenance of LTP.
Source.   Reprinted from Kennedy MB: "Regulation of Neuronal Function by Calcium." *Trends in Neuroscience* 11:417–420, 1989a. Used with permission.

NEURONAL DEVELOPMENT

How neurons are able to modify their connections with experience probably reflects a small fraction of the mechanisms harnessed during CNS development. If synapse modification in the adult resembles or uses developmental mechanisms, other forms of plasticity may exist in the adult that are vestiges of development. Neuropsychiatric disorders might result from aberrant activation of such mechanisms. Numerous developmental disorders result from aberrant growth of neurons forming deficient or aberrant connections. Schizophrenia has been suggested to be rooted in a failure of mesocortical dopaminergic neurons to connect with frontal cortex (Weinberger 1987). Thus, an insight into developmental mechanisms is likely to be fundamental to elucidating the causes of neuropsychiatric diseases.

Birth and Migration of Neurons

Neurons are largely defined by the place and timing of their birth. Cells destined to become CNS neurons arise from stem cells in the neural tube on a very exact schedule. Within a region, those neurons sharing the same birthday generally follow the same pattern of differentiation, remaining members of a distinct class of cells. Stem cells disappear once they have generated their sets of cells, so there is no further neuronal proliferation in the mature CNS. The adjustment of cell numbers to the requirements of different functions occurs through selective cell death.

Having completed their final cell divisions, neurons migrate to their definitive locations, guided by physical and chemical signals (Figure 1–7). Migration requires cell-adhesion molecules (Jessell 1988; Takeichi 1991). For example, astrotactin, produced by migrating neurons, mediates their attachment to radial glial guides (Hatten 1990). After arriving at their definitive locations, neurons elaborate processes and complete their maturation.

Process Outgrowth

Having migrated to their definitive locations, neurons start to elaborate processes. A specialized structure called the growth cone forms at the end of extending processes. The growth cone controls the insertion of new membrane elements into the cell membrane, it releases proteolytic enzymes to open a pathway through the extracellular matrix, and it extends very fine processes (filopodia) to guide the growing process to its proper target (Purves and Lichtman 1985).

Growing processes depend on several cues acting in concert to reach their targets. At different stages, different cues become important. Initially, growth cones depend on intrinsic adhesiveness of neighboring cells. Later on, they are guided by their targets or intermediate stepping-stone cells. Targets may release signaling factors, thereby establishing chemoaffinity gradients, or direct cell-to-cell contact may provide the signal. The definitive target ultimately validates correctly connecting cells by provision of trophic substances that support the survival of the innervating neurons. Cells that fail to make the appropriate connections die for lack of such substances.

The formation of specific connections has been extensively studied in grasshopper limb sensory neurons. These cells are born in the periphery and subsequently send

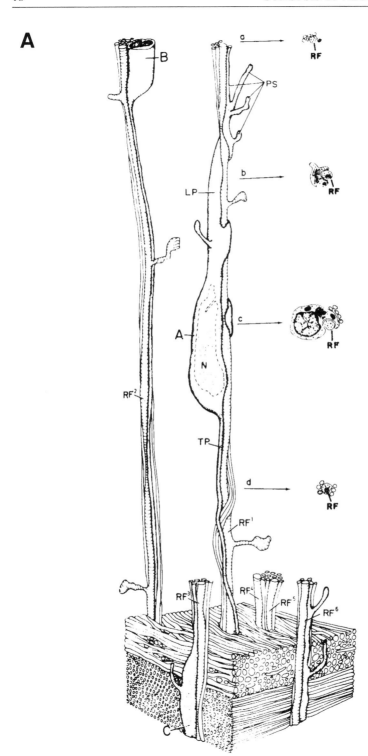

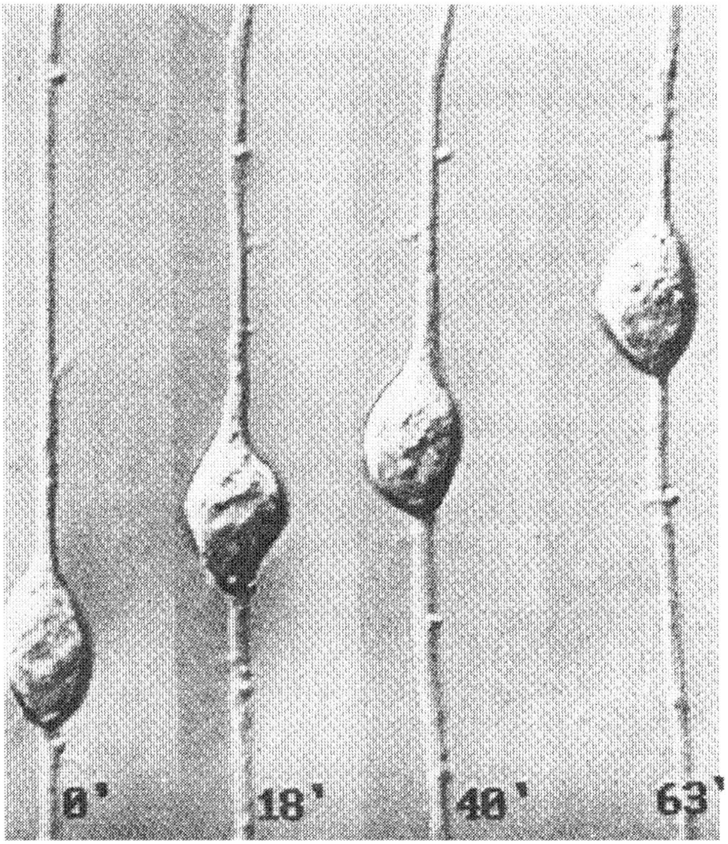

Figure 1–7. Neuronal migration during development. *Panel A: (at left)* Three-dimensional reconstruction of migrating neurons in the developing cerebral cortex. Neurons (A, B, and C) arise deep to the cortex (*bottom of schematic*) in the subventricular zone and migrate superficially along radial glial fibers (RF^{1-6}). The migratory neuron (A) is characterized by a leading process (LP) with filopodia (PS), a trailing process (TP), and a nucleus (N) pushed back toward the trailing end of the cell body. Cross-sections of the migratory profile (a, b, c, and d) shown at different levels reveal the close association between neuron and glial cell characteristic of migration.
Source.   (Reprinted from Rakic P: "Mode of Cell Migration to the Superficial Layers of Fetal Monkey Neocortex. *Journal of Comparative Neurology* 145:61–84, 1972. Used with permission.)
Panel B: (above) Developing neurons and glia recombined in culture show migration profiles. Successive frames (at about 20 minute intervals) of a migrating hippocampal neuron are shown. The neuron moves in a stop-and-go fashion along the radial glial fiber. A leading process (extending above the cell) has numerous highly active filopodial extensions. As in the reconstruction (*Panel A*), both a TP and posteriorly displaced N are also evident. Neurons will migrate on glia from different brain regions (glia in this figure are from the developing cerebellum), suggesting that there is a general molecular recognition system used throughout the brain in guiding neuronal migration.
Source.   Reprinted from Hatten ME: "Riding the Glial Monorail: A Common Mechanism for Glial-Guided Neuronal Migration in Different Regions of the Developing Mammalian Brain." *Trends in Neuroscience* 13:179–184, 1990. Used with permission.

axons into the developing CNS (Goodman et al. 1984). The first neurons to send out processes form the pioneer fibers. Later-developing neurons are guided by adhesive interactions with pioneer fibers. Recent work has shown that similar developmental mechanisms operate in the formation of the mammalian CNS. In developing spinal cord, commissural neurons in the dorsolateral spinal cord orient chemotactically to the floor plate in the ventral cord; on reaching the floor plate, they change direction and grow into the contralateral spinothalamic tract (Tessier-Lavigne et al. 1988). Similarly, in the developing brain stem, after corticospinal pioneer fibers have extended into the spinal cord, secondary processes arise that innervate the pons; during just this developmental stage, the pons releases a trophic factor that stimulates the outgrowth of pontine collaterals (Heffner et al. 1990).

Neurotrophic Factors

Several neurotrophic factors have now been characterized. These proteins stimulate the outgrowth of neuronal processes, attract growth cones, and support the survival of cells that take them up. Nerve growth factor (NGF) was the first discovered. Brain-derived neurotrophic factor (BDNF) followed; its amino acid sequence shows a significant homology with that of NGF. Together they begin to define a superfamily of neurotrophic factors (Barde 1989).

NGF is the best studied of the neurotrophic factors (Barde 1989). It is released peripherally by the targets of sensory and sympathetic neurons and is necessary for their survival. Indeed, the injection of anti-NGF antibodies into neonatal mice results in a chemical sympathectomy. Among sympathetic targets, NGF is found in extremely high concentration in mouse and snake salivary glands; these have provided quantities sufficient for extensive study. Processes of developing neurons will grow into areas where NGF concentration is high. NGF receptors bind NGF, leading to its endocytic uptake. It is then transported back to the cell body (by retrograde fast axonal transport), where it supports neuronal survival.

Neurotrophic and Neurotoxic Actions of Neurotransmitters

Neurotransmitters themselves may have trophic or toxic roles in the shaping of neurons and their interconnections (Lipton and Kater 1989). The progress of growth cones is regulated by local intracellular levels of Ca^{2+}. Ca^{2+} acts within a narrow window. When levels are low, growth cones are quiescent; they move when levels rise. Past a certain level, Ca^{2+} arrests growth and leads to retraction or destruction of neuronal processes (Kater et al. 1989; Silver et al. 1989). Glutamate can regulate the growth of neuronal processes through the control of Ca^{2+} influx. This can be countered by inhibitory neurotransmitters, as well as by provision of increased amounts of trophic factors (Mattson and Kater 1989; Mattson et al. 1989).

Higher levels of glutamate produce excitotoxicity, perhaps reflecting the pathological functioning of these developmental signaling systems (Kater et al. 1989). Alternatively, excitotoxicity might have a normal function in regulating cell numbers and connectivity. Excitotoxicity appears to be mediated acutely by the entry of Na^+ (through AMPA channels), which leads to neuronal swelling (resulting in brain edema) and, in a delayed mode (through NMDA receptor channels), by sustained Ca^{2+} entry, which kills neurons probably by activation of intracellular proteases. In addition to mediating Na^+ influx and swelling, AMPA receptors may be coupled to the IP_3-DAG pathway, leading also to increases in intracellular Ca^{2+} and C-kinase activation. The NMDA receptor, which is most strongly implicated in excitotoxicity (Choi 1988; Choi and Rothman 1990), is coupled to a high conductance channel for Na^+ and Ca^{2+}, which is blocked by magnesium ions (Mg^{2+}) at resting membrane potentials. Activation of the NMDA receptor requires membrane depolarization (which dislodges the Mg^{2+}) in conjunction with glutamate binding. Competitive antagonists that block NMDA receptors include 2-amino-5-phosphonovalerate (APV). Noncompetitive antagonists block the open channel; these include phencyclidine (PCP), dextrorphan, and MK-801.

Excitotoxicity is likely to underlie neuronal loss in strokes, status epilepticus, hypoglycemia, and head trauma (Choi and Rothman 1990). These brain insults are linked in that all lead to neuronal depolarization, which results in excessive electrical activity, evoking excessive increases in glutamate release. In each case, elevated extracellular glutamate levels can be detected in experimental models. The cytopathology can be mimicked by intracerebral injections of excitatory amino acids. The same neurons spared in the disease states are also less affected in the experimental models, probably because they have fewer excitatory amino acid receptors or have better intracellular Ca^{2+} buffering abilities. Injured neurons show increased intracellular Ca^{2+} levels, and excitatory amino acid antagonists, especially those blocking NMDA receptors or channels, prevent or dramatically reduce neuronal loss in these conditions.

Suggestive evidence supporting a role for excitatory amino acid toxicity in neurodegenerative disorders is less complete (Choi 1988). For example, a rare neurological disease, uniformly fatal in childhood, appears to be due to a deficiency in sulfite oxidase, resulting in elevations of the excitatory amino acid l-sulfo-cysteine (Olney et al. 1975). Two geographically localized neurodegenerative disorders have been tied to the ingestion of excitotoxins. Guam amyotrophic lateral sclerosis-parkinsonism-dementia results from ingestion of the excitatory amino acid β-n-methyl-amino-l-alanine (BMAA) found in the cycad plant (Spencer et al. 1987). Lathyrism, found in regions of Africa fraught with famine, is causally related to ingestion of the chick pea excitotoxin, β-n-oxalylamino-l-alanine (BOAA) (Spencer et al. 1986).

Similarities between other neuropsychiatric disorders and idiopathic neurodegenerative disorders suggest a role for excitotoxic mechanisms. A growing body of findings implicate excitotoxic mechanisms in Huntington's disease. The neuropathology of Huntington's disease is mimicked by excitatory amino acid injections; in particular, certain classes of striatal neurons are spared in both cases (Choi 1988; Wexler et al. 1991). Furthermore, measures of striatal NMDA receptors in patients dying of Huntington's disease revealed a selective loss of cells bearing these receptors, supporting the role of NMDA-mediated excitotoxicity in the pathogenesis of the disorder (Young et al. 1988).

Synapse Formation

When the growth cone approaches the target cell, a complex series of interactions commences. The growth cone functions like a protosynapse in that it releases neurotransmitter when its parent cell is electrically active. Uninnervated postsynaptic cells have transmitter receptors distributed over much of their surface (that later concentrate with innervation). Within minutes of initial contact, a rudimentary form of synaptic transmission starts. Over subsequent days, connections become stronger and stabilize as the growth cone matures into a presynaptic terminal, gathering the cellular elements that are necessary for focused release of neurotransmitter at active zones. In parallel, the postsynaptic cell concentrates receptors opposite the innervating process, removing them from other regions, and over the course of days, postsynaptic specializations develop. Maturation of the postsynaptic cell requires de novo protein synthesis, much as do learning dependent long-term changes. Immediate early response genes (Morgan and Curran 1989) are among the first genes activated with postsynaptic depolarization by elevations in Ca^{2+}, cAMP, cGMP, IP_3, or DAG. The prototype of this family of proto-oncogenes is c-fos. The transcription of these proto-oncogenes leads to the synthesis of proteins (e.g., fos) that modulate or induce transcription of other genes that directly or indirectly induce structural changes in the cell.

The provision of NGF or other neurotrophic factors by postsynaptic cells ensures the survival of successfully innervating presynaptic neurons. More subtle regulation of presynaptic cells occurs as well. In the developing sympathetic nervous system, young neurons are exclusively noradrenergic before synapse formation. Depending on the target tissue, they may become cholinergic, retaining only traces of the noradrenergic phenotype (Landis 1990). This target-dependent effect is mediated by the release of a soluble cholinergic differentiation factor (CDF) by the postsynaptic cells. Once synaptic contact is established, cholinergic activation of the postsynaptic cell by presynaptic spikes suppresses CDF release. Thus synapse formation may trigger far-reaching changes both pre- and postsynaptically, extending as far as the choice of neurotransmitter by a presynaptic neuron.

As in associative learning, simultaneous electrical activity of pre- and postsynaptic elements leads to the strengthening of connections, whereas discordant activity results in the elimination of synapses. As a general pattern, both an excessive number of neurons and synaptic connections arise in the developing nervous system; then, through a combination of activity-dependent competition, trophic factor requirements, and possibly excitotoxic mechanisms, cells and synapses are pruned until the highly defined pattern of innervation of the adult is formed (Purves 1988).

Sensory Input and Synaptic Plasticity

Sensory experience is essential to the normal maturation of specific neural connections. In the visual system, where this has been most extensively studied, overlapping visual input from the eyes must be combined in an orderly way to maximize acuity and stereopsis. In animals with binocular vision (e.g., humans, monkeys, and cats), visual stimuli striking the retina activate neurons in the ipsilateral visual cortex. This means that neurons in the left hemiretinas of right and left eyes both convey signals to the left cortex, and similarly neurons in the right hemiretinas do so to the right cortex (Figure 1–8; *panel A*). Thus visual information emanating from the same external source ends up in the contralateral hemisphere despite the fact that it is temporarily separated into right and left eye specific pathways.

How is this converging visual information recombined? In visual cortex, inputs from the two eyes project alternately to stripes dominated by one eye or the other forming ocular dominance columns (Hubel and Wiesel 1977). The pattern of stripes resembles those of a zebra (Figure 1–8; *panel B*). Output neurons in the ocular dominance columns project to prestriate visual areas where the visual information derived from inputs to both eyes is recombined and stereopsis clues extracted. How separate signals from each eye are handled in parallel, recombined, and separated again is representative of a more general pattern in the processing of visual information (Livingstone and Hubel 1988).

During development, the ocular dominance columns arise in a crude way independent of visual input (Hubel et al. 1977). Initially, axons carrying information from both eyes extend over all of visual cortex, after which during a critical period they begin to segregate out. During this period, the pattern of sharp stripes, evenly divided between the two eyes, depends on normal visual experience. If vision in one eye is impaired or there is strabismus, input from the normal or dominant eye comes to control most of visual cortex and the other eye becomes functionally blind (Figure 1–8; *panel C*). In the cortex, the ocular dominance columns of the normal or dominant eye expand at the expense of those of the impaired eye. The segregation of the optic fibers into columns is activity dependent (Constantine-Paton et al. 1990; Miller et al. 1989). It depends on discordant inputs from the two eyes; segregation fails if either visual input to cortex is blocked (with the Na^+ channel blocker tetrodotoxin) or it is artificially synchronized in both eyes (by simultaneous electrical stimulation).

Different patterns of electrical activity in each optic radiation, as occurs normally, mediate segregation. Segregation also requires activity of postsynaptic cortical cells; infusion of the inhibitory drug muscimol (a GABA-A agonist) causes a reversal of dominance so that, paradoxically, the weak rather than the strong eye gains the larger columns (Reiter and Stryker 1988). Apparently, appropriate segregation of cortical inputs requires both normal presynaptic activity and postsynaptic responses.

Pairing of presynaptic activity with postsynaptic depolarization appears to be required for activity-dependent segregation of sensory inputs, perhaps just as it is necessary for the induction of LTP (Constantine-Paton et al. 1990). As in LTP, this pairing dependence is mediated by the NMDA receptor, which requires both agonist and depolarization (to remove the Mg^{2+} block of the channel) for activation. Infusion of the specific NMDA antagonist APV into developing visual cortex prevents both normal segregation of visual inputs and the effects of unbalanced activity from the two eyes during the critical period (Kleinschmidt et al. 1987).

PERSPECTIVES

A shared molecular language is emerging for activity-dependent segregation of visual inputs, LTP, excitotoxicity, and the shaping of growing neurites (Brown et al. 1990; Choi and Rothman 1990; Constantine-Paton et al. 1990; Hawkins and Kandel 1984; Lipton and Kater 1989). The key player is the NMDA receptor, which requires both agonist and depolarization for activation. This appears to be the essential requirement for pairing specificity, a mode of synaptic plasticity initially postulated by Hebb (1949), whereby simultaneous activation of pre- and postsynaptic elements strengthens connections. Correlation of presynaptic activity with postsynaptic inhibition may selectively weaken connections (Reiter and Stry-ker 1988). The Ca^{2+} influx mediated by the NMDA receptor may trigger changes in the effectiveness of synapses, in time leading to structural changes. At higher levels, Ca^{2+} may arrest the growth of neurites, cause their retraction, or selectively lesion the susceptible cell.

The cellular and molecular language of neurons has powerful explanatory power with respect to the action of psychotropic drugs (Barondes 1990; Cooper et al. 1986). The early antipsychotic reserpine acts in the presynaptic terminal to reduce stores of catecholamine neurotransmitters (which in excess may underlie psychotic symp-toms). Current antipsychotics block synaptic transmission in the mesolimbic dopa-mine system (reducing the effects of catecholamines), possibly specifically at the newly discovered D_3 receptor (Sokoloff et al. 1990). Tricyclic antidepressants block catecholamine reuptake, whereas monoamine oxidase inhibitors block their break-down, both leading to increased synaptic levels. Anxiolytics modulate the GABA receptor. Lithium modulates the inositol phospholipid system, thereby reducing its activity when it is overactive (Baraban et al. 1989; Berridge et al. 1989). Agents se-lectively acting in second messenger pathways may prove to be the next generation of psychotropics.

Neuropsychiatric disorders will increasingly come to be understood in the lan-guage of neurons. Among the examples mentioned above, striatal degeneration in Huntington's chorea may be a result of NMDA receptor mediated excitotoxicity (Wexler et al. 1991). In Parkinson's disease, a selective loss of dopaminergic neurons in the substantia nigra may be the delayed result of a viral process, lesioning by dopaminergic neurotoxins exemplified by 1-methyl-4-phenyl-1,2,3,4-tetrahydro-pyridine (MPTP), or a deficiency in the neurotrophic factor BDNF, which may be

Figure 1–8. *(at right)* Ocular dominance columns in visual cortex. *Panel A:* Human visual pathway. Optic fibers from each eye split at the chiasm with half going to each side of the brain. Fibers conveying visual information from the right or left sides of each retina project to the lateral geniculate nucleus on the same side of the brain and subsequently to ipsilateral cortex. In this way, left visual field information goes to the right cortex and vice versa. This arrange-ment raises the question of how the optic radiations from each eye combine in cortex to produce a single image and stereopsis.
Source panel A.   Reprinted from Alberts B, Bray D, Lewis J, et al: *Molecular Biology of the Cell,* 2nd Edition. New York, Garland, 1989, p. 1129. Used with permission.
Panel B: Visual inputs form ocular dominance columns. In a normal monkey, one eye was injected with a radioactive tracer which is transported transsynaptically along the visual path-ways. Cortical areas receiving input from the injected eye show up as white. An alternating pattern of stripes is revealed, equally divided between the two eyes. *Panel C:* Monocular depri-vation alters ocular dominance column development. Although alternating stripes of ocular dominance arise in the absence of visual input, the sharpening of the pattern depends on expe-rience and activity-dependent competition. Blocking vision in one eye places it at a disadvan-tage in such a process so that it ends up controlling a minority of cortex. In this plate, the nondeprived eye was injected with the transsynaptic tracer showing that it has come to control most of cortex. Normal visual experience is prerequisite to the correct wiring of the cortex.
Source panels B and C.   Reprinted from Hubel DH, Wiesel TN: "Ferrier Lecture: Functional Architecture of Macaque Monkey Visual Cortex." *Proceedings of the Royal Society of London* [Series B: Biological Sciences] 198:1–59, 1977. Used with permission.

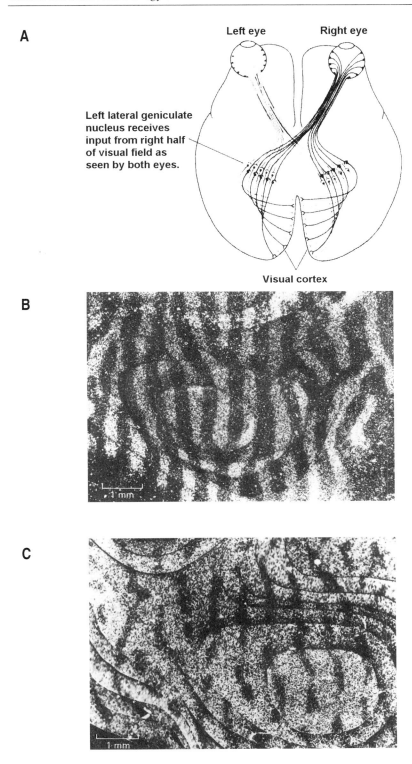

A

Left eye   Right eye

**Left lateral geniculate
nucleus receives
input from right half
of visual field as
seen by both eyes.**

Visual cortex

B

1 mm

C

1 mm

essential for survival of dopaminergic neurons. In Alzheimer's disease, the loss of cholinergic neurons may result from a NGF deficiency in regions that they innervate or perhaps aberrant handling of NGF once it is taken up by the basal forebrain neurons. Once molecular explanations can be integrated into detailed functional knowledge of neurons and the neuronal systems of which they are part, a unified picture of brain functioning and the underlying neuropathology may emerge.

REFERENCES

Alberts B, Bray D, Lewis J, et al: Molecular Biology of the Cell, 2nd Edition. New York, Garland, 1989

Axelrod J, Burch RM, Jelsema CL: Receptor-mediated activation of phospholipase A_2 via GTP-binding proteins: arachidonic acid and its metabolites as second messengers. Trends Neurosci 11:117–123, 1988

Baraban JM, Worley PF, Snyder SH: Second messenger systems and psychoactive drug action: focus on the phosphoinositide system and lithium. Am J Psychiatry 146:1251–1260, 1989

Barde Y-A: Trophic factors and neuronal survival. Neuron 2:1524–1534, 1989

Barondes SH: The biological approach to psychiatry: history and prospects. J Neurosci 10:1707–1710, 1990

Bekkers JM, Stevens CF: Presynaptic mechanism for long-term potentiation in the hippocampus. Nature 346:724–729, 1990

Berridge MJ, Irvine RF: Inositol phosphates and cell signaling. Nature 341:197–205, 1989

Berridge MJ, Downes CP, Hanley MR: Neural and developmental actions of lithium: a unifying hypothesis. Cell 59:411–419, 1989

Bliss TVP, Douglas RM, Errington ML, et al: Correlation between long-term potentiation and release of endogenous amino acids from dentate gyrus of anaesthetized rats. J Physiol (Lond) 377:391–408, 1986

Braha O, Dale N, Hochner B, et al: Second messengers involved in the two processes of presynaptic facilitation that contribute to sensitization and dishabituation in *Aplysia* sensory neurons. Proc Natl Acad Sci U S A 87:2040–2044, 1990

Brown TH, Kairiss EW, Keenan CL: Hebbian synapses: biophysical mechanisms and algorithms. Annu Rev Neurosci 13:475–511, 1990

Choi DW: Glutamate neurotoxicity and diseases of the nervous system. Neuron 1:623–634, 1988

Choi DW, Rothman SM: The role of glutamate neurotoxicity in hypoxic-ischemic neuronal death. Annu Rev Neurosci 13:171–182, 1990

Constantine-Paton M, Cline HT, Debski E: Patterned activity, synaptic convergence, and the NMDA receptor in developing visual pathways. Annu Rev Neurosci 13:129–154, 1990

Cooper JR, Bloom FE, Roth RH: The Biochemical Basis of Neuropharmacology, 5th Edition. New York, Oxford University Press, 1986

Dash PK, Hochner B, Kandel ER: Injection of the cAMP-responsive element into the nucleus of *Aplysia* sensory neurons blocks long-term facilitation. Nature 345:718–721, 1990

Goodman CS, Bastiani MJ, Doe CQ, et al: Cell recognition during development. Science 225:1271–1279, 1984

Hatten ME: Riding the glial monorail: a common mechanism for glial-guided neuronal migration in different regions of the developing mammalian brain. Trends Neurosci 13:179–84, 1990

Hawkins RD, Kandel ER: Is there a cell-biological alphabet for simple forms of learning? Psychol Rev 91:375–391, 1984

Hebb DO: The Organization of Behavior: A Neuropsychological Theory. New York, Wiley, 1949

Heffner CD, Lumsden AGS, O'Leary DDM: Target control of collateral extension and directional axon growth in the mammalian brain. Science 247:217–220, 1990

Hoffman RE: Computer simulations of neural information processing and the schizophrenia-mania dichotomy. Arch Gen Psychiatry 44:178–188, 1987

Hubel DH, Wiesel TN: Ferrier lecture: functional architecture of macaque monkey visual cortex. Proc R Soc Lond [Biol] 198:1–59, 1977

Hubel DH, Wiesel TN, LeVay S: Plasticity of ocular dominance columns in monkey striate cortex. Philos Trans R Soc Lond [Biol] 278:377–409, 1977

Huganir RL, Greengard P: Regulation of receptor function by protein phosphorylation. Trends Pharmacol Sci 8:472–477, 1987

Jessell TM: Adhesion molecules and the hierarchy of neural development. Neuron 1:3–13, 1988

Kandel ER: Genes, nerve cells, and the remembrance of things past. J Neuropsychiatry Clin Neurosci 1:103–125, 1989

Kandel ER, Schwartz JH: Principles of Neural Science, 2nd Edition. New York, Elsevier, 1985

Kater SB, Mattson MP, Guthrie PB: Calcium-induced neuronal degeneration: a normal growth cone regulating signal gone awry? Ann N Y Acad Sci 568:252–261, 1989

Keinänen K, Wisden W, Sommer B, et al: A family of AMPA-selective glutamate receptors. Science 249:556–560, 1990

Kennedy MB: Regulation of neuronal function by calcium. Trends Neurosci 11:417–420, 1989a

Kennedy MB: Regulation of synaptic transmission in the central nervous system: long-term potentiation. Cell 59:777–787, 1989b

Kleinschmidt A, Bear MF, Singer W: Blockade of NMDA receptors disrupts experience-dependent plasticity of kitten striate cortex. Science 238:355–358, 1987

Landis SC: Target regulation of neurotransmitter phenotype. Trends Neurosci 13:344–350, 1990

Lipton SA, Kater SB: Neurotransmitter regulation of neuronal outgrowth, plasticity and survival. Trends Neurosci 12:265–270, 1989

Livingstone M, Hubel D: Segregation of form, color, movement, and depth: anatomy, physiology, and perception. Science 240:740–749, 1988

Llinás R: The intrinsic electrophysiological properties of mammalian neurons: insights into central nervous system function. Science 242:1654–1664, 1988

Llinás R, Jahnsen H: Electrophysiology of mammalian thalamic neurones in vitro. Nature 297:406–408, 1982

Lynch MA, Errington ML, Bliss TVP: Nordihydroguaiaretic acid blocks the synaptic component of long-term potentiation and the associated increases in release of glutamate and arachidonate: an in vivo study in the dentate gyrus of the rat. Neuroscience 30:693–701, 1989

Malenka RC, Kauer JA, Perkel DJ, et al: The impact of postsynaptic calcium on synaptic transmission: its role in long-term potentiation. Trends Neurosci 12:444–450, 1989

Malinow R, Tsien RW: Presynaptic enhancement shown by whole-cell recordings of long-term potentiation in hippocampal slices. Nature 346:177–180, 1990

Malinow R, Schulman H, Tsien RW: Inhibition of postsynaptic PKC or CaMKII blocks induction but not expression of LTP. Science 245:862–866, 1989

Mattson MP, Kater SB: Excitatory and inhibitory neurotransmitters in the generation and degeneration of hippocampal neuroarchitecture. Brain Res 478:337–348, 1989

Mattson MP, Murrain M, Guthrie PB, et al: Fibroblast growth factor and glutamate: opposing roles in the generation and degeneration of hippocampal neuroarchitecture. J Neurosci 9:3728–3740, 1989

Miller KD, Keller JB, Stryker MP: Ocular dominance column development: analysis and simulation. Science 245:605–615, 1989

Morgan JI, Curran T: Stimulus-transcription coupling in neurons: role of cellular immediate-early genes. Trends Neurosci 12:459–462, 1989

Neer EJ, Clapham DE: Roles of G protein subunits in transmembrane signaling. Nature 333:129–134, 1988

Olney JW, Misra CH, deGubareff T: Cysteine-S-sulfate: brain damaging metabolite in sulfite oxidase deficiency. J Neuropathol Exp Neurol 34:167–177, 1975

Pardes H: Neuroscience and psychiatry: marriage or coexistence. Am J Psychiatry 143:1205–1212, 1986

Piomelli D, Greengard P: Lipoxygenase metabolites of arachidonic acid in neuronal transmembrane signaling. Trends Pharmacol Sci 11:367–373, 1990

Piomelli D, Volterra A, Dale N, et al: Lipoxygenase metabolites of arachidonic acid as second messengers for presynaptic inhibition of *Aplysia* sensory cells. Nature 328:38–43, 1987

Purves D: Body and Brain: A Trophic Theory of Neural Connections. Cambridge, MA, Harvard University Press, 1988

Purves D, Lichtman JW: Principles of Neural Development. Sunderland, MA, Sinauer, 1985

Rakic P: Mode of cell migration to the superficial layers of fetal monkey neocortex. J Comp Neurol 145:61–84, 1972

Reiter HO, Stryker MP: Neural plasticity without postsynaptic action potentials: less-active inputs become dominant when kitten visual cortical cells are pharmacologically inhibited. Proc Natl Acad Sci U S A 85: 3623–3627, 1988

Role LW, Schwartz JH: Cross-talk between signal transduction pathways. Trends Neurosci 12 (11):centerfold, 1989

Ross EM, Gilman AG: Pharmacodynamics: mechanisms of drug action and the relationship between drug concentration and effect, in The Pharmacological Basis of Therapeutics, 7th Edition. Edited by Gilman AG, Goodman LS, Rall TW, et al. New York, Macmillan, 1985, pp 35–48

Schofield PR, Shivers BD, Seeburg PH: The role of receptor subtype diversity in the CNS. Trends Neurosci 13:8–11, 1990

Sejnowski TJ, Koch C, Churchland PS: Computational neuroscience. Science 241:1299–1306, 1988

Servan-Schreiber D, Printz H, Cohen JD: A network model of catecholamine effects: gain, signal-to-noise ratio, and behavior. Science 249:892–895, 1990

Silver RA, Lamb AG, Bolsover SR: Elevated cytosolic calcium in the growth cone inhibits neurite elongation in neuroblastoma cells: correlation of behavioral states with cytosolic calcium concentration. J Neurosci 9:4007–4020, 1989

Sokoloff P, Giros B, Martres M-P, et al: Molecular cloning and characterization of a novel dopamine receptor (D_3) as a target for neuroleptics. Nature 347:146–151, 1990

Spencer PS, Ludolph A, Dwivedi MP, et al: Lathyrism: evidence for role of the neuroexcitatory amino acid BOAA. Lancet 2:1066–1067, 1986

Spencer PS, Nunn PB, Hugon J, et al: Guam amyotrophic lateral sclerosis-parkinsonism-dementia linked to a plant excitant neurotoxin. Science 237:517–522, 1987

Sweatt JD, Kandel ER: Persistent and transcriptionally dependent increase in protein phosphorylation in long-term facilitation of *Aplysia* sensory neurons. Nature 339:51–54, 1989

Takeichi M: Cadherin cell adhesion receptors as a morphogenetic regulator. Science 251:1451–1455, 1991

Tank DW, Sugimori M, Connor JA, et al: Spatially resolved calcium dynamics of mammalian Purkinje cells in cerebellar slice. Science 242:773–777, 1988

Tessier-Lavigne M, Placzek M, Lumsden AGS, et al: Chemotropic guidance of developing axons in the mammalian central nervous system. Nature 336:775–778, 1988

Weinberger DR: Implications of normal brain development for the pathogenesis of schizophrenia. Arch Gen Psychiatry 44:660–669, 1987

Wexler NS, Rose EA, Housman DE: Molecular approaches to hereditary diseases of the nervous system: Huntington's Disease as a paradigm. Annu Rev Neurosci 14:503–529, 1991

Williams JH, Errington ML, Lynch MA, et al: Arachidonic acid induces a long-term activity-dependent enhancement of synaptic transmission in the hippocampus. Nature 341:739–742, 1989

Young AB, Greenamyre JT, Hollingsworth Z, et al: NMDA receptor losses in putamen from patients with Huntington's Disease. Science 241:981–983, 1988

Chapter 2

Human Electrophysiology: Basic Cellular Mechanisms

Robert W. McCarley, M.D.

This chapter provides a brief review and update on fundamental mechanisms important for understanding neuronal activity and communication at the level of single cells. A more detailed account, with a different emphasis, appears in Chapter 1. There follows a brief note on evoked potential (EP) and electroencephalogram (EEG) analysis. These sections were primarily written for the reader with some knowledge of cellular neurophysiology who wishes a brief review of fundamental concepts and an update on recent advances.

INTRODUCTION TO NEUROPHYSIOLOGY

The *neuron* is a cell specialized for the use of electrical signaling for information transmission; it may be viewed as an evolutionary outgrowth of the need for more rapid transmission and more precise selection of target elements than was possible with humoral transmission (the release of chemical agents into blood or extracellular fluid). The reader is cautioned that the description in this section is a simplified account and one that is primarily based on mammalian systems; more complete accounts can be found in textbooks such as those by Kandel and Schwartz (1985) and Smith (1989).

All neurons have a *cell body (or soma)* and are distinguished from other body cells by the presence of dendrites and axons. The *dendrites* may be thought of as an extension of the "input zone" on the cell body, and their shape often appears tailored to their inputs, with the pyramidal cell dendritic structure being typical of many neurons in regularly layered structures of the brain such as the cerebral cortex, where there are distinct input zones. The more spherical dendritic tree found in brain stem reticular neurons tends to occur in structures without a distinct ordering of different input zones. Figure 2–1 illustrates these two examples of neuronal shape. The axon is a long extension of the neuron that forms the "output element" for transmitting the

This work was supported by grants from the Department of Veterans Affairs, Medical Research Service, and the National Institute of Mental Health (R37 MH39-683 and R01 MH40-799). This chapter was prepared as part of the author's employment with the federal government and, therefore, is in the public domain.

electrical activation of the soma to a target neuron; it may have numerous branches, called collaterals. Electrical signals traveling down the axon form a propagating wave of depolarization termed the *action potential*; this originates in the soma when the electrical potential on the membrane is sufficiently reduced (membrane depolarization). Thus understanding the mechanisms controlling soma membrane polarization is essential for understanding electrical signaling in the brain.

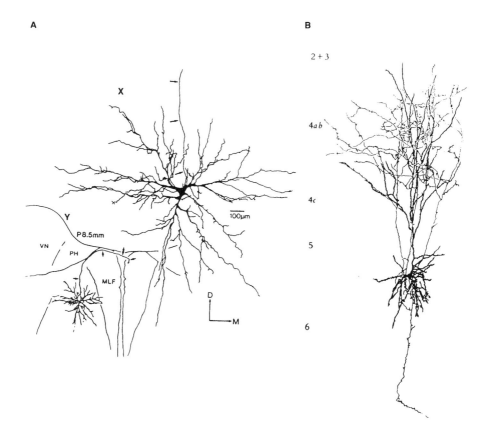

Figure 2–1. *Panel A:* Depiction of a giant neuron of the cat bulbar reticular formation, a region without regular spatial orientation of neurons and their dendrites. Note the extension of dendrites in all directions in the enlarged view of the neuron X; Y shows the axon (arrows) turning to enter the medial longitudinal fasciculus, a fiber bundle comprised of similar spinal cord-projecting neurons. The giant neurons of the brain stem reticular formation are among the largest in the nervous system and likely mediate quick reflex responses. *Panel B:* A pyramidal cell of the rhesus monkey primary visual cortex. The neocortex has many such regularly arranged, radially oriented neurons, with a characteristic apical dendrite orientation in layer 4 and the pyramidal cell body in layer 6. The axon of this neuron is shown leaving the cortex in its path to the lateral geniculate nucleus. It is a corticothalamic projection neuron and part of a feedback loop, because geniculocortical neurons send axons to the cortex that synapse on the dendrites of the illustrated neuron.
Sources. *Panel A* is a camera lucida drawing by A. Mitani in the author's laboratory; *Panel B* is adapted from Nauta and Feirtag 1986.

CONTROL OF NEURONAL MEMBRANE POLARIZATION

The cell *membrane* is a bilayer (double layer) of lipids that separates the interior of the cell from its environment. The cell membrane itself acts as a nonconducting capacitor with the cell interior electrically negative with respect to the outside. Most mammalian neurons, when not being stimulated, have a "resting" membrane polarization of about −70 millivolts (mV). By convention the membrane polarization level is always given in terms of the difference between the interior voltage and the exterior voltage, with the exterior voltage taken to be zero.

Not all of the cell membrane is a nonconductive lipid bilayer; incorporated in the membrane are specialized large protein molecules that form membrane-spanning channels that permit the passage of ions such as potassium ions (K⁺). These *ion channels* are usually selective in allowing the flow of only certain ions. The "resting potential" of the neuron arises because of the differences in distribution of electrically charged ions on the inside and outside of the neuronal membrane.

Most of the inside negativity of the resting membrane potential is due to K⁺. This negative membrane polarization can be thought of as occurring in the following way: K⁺ concentration is greater on the inside of the cell than on the outside, and thus K⁺ tends to flow down its concentration gradient, from the inside to the outside (Figure 2–2). That is, excess internal K⁺ concentration leads to flow of the K⁺ through a particular set of potassium channels to the outside of the membrane. Negatively charged

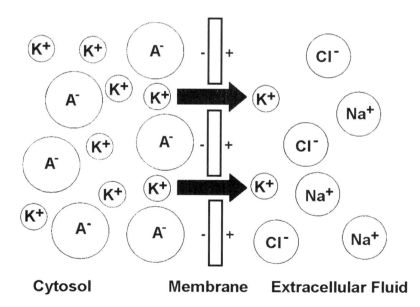

Cytosol   **Membrane**   **Extracellular Fluid**

Figure 2–2.   Schematic of generation of the resting membrane potential. The concentration gradient causes potassium ions (K⁺) to move out of the cell (*arrows*) until this force is balanced by a counteracting electrical potential difference, positive charges on the outside and negative charges on the inside of the membrane. Most of the potential is attributable to K⁺; contributions from other ions have been omitted for simplicity. A⁻ = anions (negatively charged ions; amino acids and proteins); Na⁺ = sodium ions; Cl⁻ = chloride ions.

proteins and amino acids (referred to here collectively as anions) on the inside of the cell are too large to pass through the ion channels, and thus there is a concentration of negative charges on the inside of the neuron and of positive charges on the outside of the neuron. The migration of K^+ from inside to outside continues until the buildup of electrical charge resulting from separation of K^+ and the anions (positive electrical charges on the outside and negative charges on the inside) is strong enough to balance exactly the driving force from the K^+ concentration difference. The membrane potential at which balance is achieved is called the K^+ equilibrium potential and is close to the membrane resting potential.

Sodium ions (Na^+) also contribute to the resting membrane potential, although much less than K^+ because of the lesser permeability of the membrane to Na^+, even though these ions are much more heavily concentrated on the outside than on the inside. The low interior concentration of Na^+ is maintained by an active (energy-consuming) pump that transports Na^+ to the outside and exchanges three Na^+ ions for two K^+ ions. In most neurons, chloride ions do not play a role in resting membrane potential generation because they are in electrical and concentration equilibrium. Calcium ions (Ca^{2+}) are important in many signaling processes but do not play a large role in the resting membrane potential because the permeability of the membrane is low to these ions at the resting potential level.

ACTION POTENTIAL GENERATION

The *action potential* consists of a membrane depolarization followed by a repolarization (Figure 2–3). During the depolarization the inside of the membrane loses its negative charge with respect to the outside and actually becomes slightly positive, about +10 to +30 mV relative to the outside of the neuronal membrane. This depolarization is followed by a repolarization, a return of the membrane potential to its resting level.

As noted above, the most important channel for the resting membrane potential is the potassium channel. This is called a *passive ion channel* because it is not voltage sensitive. The channels important for the action potential are *voltage-sensitive channels*, that is, their conductivity to ions varies with membrane potential voltage.

The sodium channel and Na^+ are of primary importance in the depolarization. The generation of the action potential proceeds in the following way. There is an initial small depolarization of the membrane potential that may be due to excitatory input from other neurons. As the membrane depolarizes the voltage sensitive sodium chan-

Figure 2–3.   *(at right) Panel A:* The time course of action potential voltage. *Panel B:* The time course of depolarizing inward sodium current (Na^+) and the repolarizing outward potassium current (K^+); currents are expressed in terms of the permeability (conductance) of the membrane for the two ions. Note the after-hyperpolarization following the action potential (*panel A*) is due to the persistence of the outward K^+ current.
Source panels A and B.   Adapted from Hodgkin and Huxley 1952; Darnell et al. 1990.
Panel C: Action potential traveling down an axon, flow is right to left. The depolarizing leading edge consists of inrushing sodium currents and the repolarizing trailing edge consists of outward, repolarizing potassium currents.
Source panel C.   Adapted from Smith 1989.

A   Depolarization (↑) and hyperpolarization (↓)

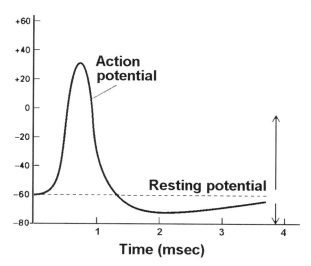

B   Changes in ion permeabilities

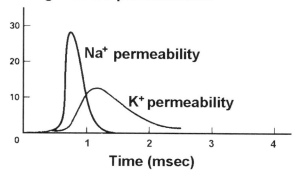

C

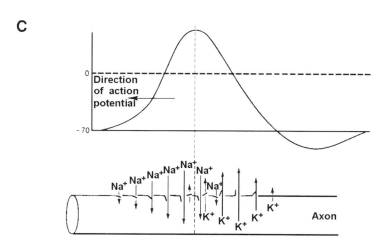

nels begin to open, and Na⁺ flows from the region of high concentration outside the neuron through the channels into the neuron. The inrush of positive charges tends to depolarize the neuron. As long as the initial depolarization is not too great and does not exceed a certain threshold, the membrane potential is restored to its resting level by an efflux of K⁺ through the channels described above. However, with stronger initial depolarization, the voltage-sensitive sodium channels allow more Na⁺ to enter the neuron, and sufficient Na⁺ enters so that the efflux of K⁺ cannot keep up with the rate of Na⁺ entry.

The more Na⁺ that enters the cell, the more the membrane is depolarized, the more Na⁺ is admitted by the voltage-sensitive Na⁺ channels, and so on. Thus there is a positive feedback resulting in an avalanche of Na⁺ entry. This leads to the membrane potential's becoming positive at the peak of the action potential. Schematically,

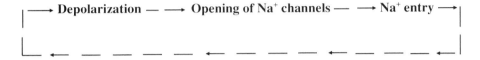

The membrane repolarization part of the action potential is due to two main factors:

1. As the membrane potential depolarizes, *voltage-sensitive potassium channels* slowly open. (This is a different potassium channel than the passive channel responsible for the membrane potential.) This delayed-opening potassium channel allows K⁺ to flow out of the neuron's interior to the outside, reducing the number of positive charges on the inside and thus tending to repolarize the membrane. (At the height of the action potential the cell interior is positive, and the driving forces on K⁺ flow are both this positive voltage and the internal concentration level.) The open potassium channels close as the membrane potential repolarizes.
2. The *voltage-dependent sodium channels* close as a result of the depolarization, a process known as inactivation.

NEUROTRANSMITTER RELEASE BY DEPOLARIZATION OF THE NERVE TERMINAL

Most neurons use electrical conduction (propagation of the action potential down the axon) as the first step in influencing target neurons. The second step is release of packets of neurotransmitters at the nerve terminal. The packets of neurotransmitter molecules are stored in the *presynaptic* terminal in structures called vesicles. When the membranes of the vesicles fuse with the exterior cell membrane, the contents of the vesicle (the neurotransmitters) are released and diffuse across the *synapse,* the small gap between nerve terminal and the target neuron. The release of neurotransmitters at the presynaptic terminal occurs because the action potential depolarizes the terminal and this depolarization opens *voltage-sensitive calcium channels.* Ca²⁺ entry into the terminal triggers the fusion of vesicles with the membrane of the terminal and neurotransmitter release into the synaptic gap between the presynaptic and postsynaptic neuron. The resulting alterations of membrane potential in the postsynaptic neuron are called *postsynaptic potentials (PSPs).*

ACTION OF NEUROTRANSMITTERS AT RECEPTORS

Neurotransmitters act on specialized membrane structures in the postsynaptic neuron called *receptors*. Receptor is a generalized term for the membrane sites that bind the neurotransmitter molecules. (In general cell biology, receptor is used even more generally to include all structures, including those on the interior of the cell, that preferentially bind a variety of molecules, including circulating hormones and even viruses.) Molecular biological techniques have led to structural identification of membrane receptor components and to physical models of how receptors act. In general, receptors are composed of proteins that coil in and out of the neuronal membrane and have specialized exterior portions for binding neurotransmitters. Receptors may be classified by their mode of action on the target neuron. The classification of signal elements (or messengers) in Table 2–1 illustrates some of the different modes of action. The fundamental notion is that the *first messengers,* the neurotransmitters, may cause the production of second or third messengers, which have additional actions on the target neuron, usually acting to prolong responses.

First Messengers: Neurotransmitters

Neurotransmitter-receptor binding may directly affect ion channels. The term for a substance that binds at a receptor is a *ligand,* and ion channels of this class are called *ligand-gated ion channels.* An example is the nicotinic receptor, in which binding of acetylcholine (the ligand) leads to a direct change in receptor conformation that allows passage of certain positively charged ions (cations), typically Na^+ and K^+. The molecular structure of this receptor is shown in Figure 2–4. As might be suspected from the direct coupling, this class of receptor is characterized by rapid opening of the ion channel and hence a quick responsiveness.

Depolarizing PSPs are called *excitatory PSPs (EPSPs)* because the neuron is brought closer to the threshold for discharge of an action potential. EPSPs result from a net increased internal positivity, which may arise either from an influx of positive ions or a decrease in an ongoing efflux of positive ions. *Inhibitory PSPs (IPSPs)* hyperpolarize the membrane, make the interior more negative, and thus move the membrane potential farther from action potential discharge threshold. IPSPs may result from an influx of negative ions or from an increased efflux of positive ions.

Second Messengers: cAMP and Intracellular Intermediaries

Neurotransmitter-receptor binding may **indirectly** affect ion channels and also cellular metabolism. In this class of receptor the binding of the neurotransmitter to the

Table 2–1.   Classification of signal elements (messengers)

Messenger type	Example	Site	Mode of action
First messengers	Neurotransmitters	Synapse	Gates ion channels
Second messengers	cAMP	Cytosol	Affects cell metabolism
Third messengers	c-fos	Nucleus	Regulates DNA transcription

Note.   cAMP = cyclic adenosine monophosphate; c-fos = fos proto-oncogene.

receptor induces a cascade of effects that culminates in effects on the ion channel and/or may induce changes in the cell metabolism. This action may occur via second messengers acting in the cytosol and/or through a *guanine nucleotide-binding protein (G protein)* in the cell membrane. Perhaps the best known example is the β_2-adrenergic receptor (Figure 2–5). At this receptor, binding of the neurotransmitter norepinephrine activates a G protein in the neuronal membrane; this G protein in turn regulates the activity of the catalytic subunit of the enzyme adenylate cy-

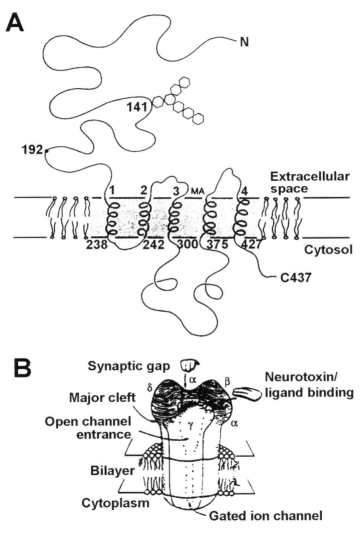

Figure 2–4. Nicotinic acetylcholine receptor. *Panel A:* Schematic of the human subunit of this receptor and its coils in and out of the cell membrane. The binding site for acetylcholine is near amino acid residue number 192. *Panel B:* Schematic of the entirety of this ligand-gated receptor. There are 5 subunits. Note the proximity to the gated ion channel of the unit containing the binding site for acetylcholine and other ligands.
Source. Adapted from Smith 1989.

clase, which in turn catalyzes the synthesis of *cyclic adenosine monophosphate (cAMP)*. (See the sketch of dynamics of G protein activation in Figure 2–5.)

The cAMP is the *second messenger,* acting in the cytosol of the neuron. The cAMP activates a cAMP-dependent protein kinase. The consequences of this activation depend on the substrate for the particular protein kinase that is activated. One consequence may be the phosphorylation of proteins constituting or closely associated with the ion channel, with consequent alterations in permeability (Figure 2–5). Other effects of the second messengers may include regulation of proteins involved in transmitter synthesis and release. Schematically,

Neurotransmitter-receptor binding
- → G protein activation
- → adenylate cyclase activation
- → second messenger production (such as cAMP)
- → protein kinase activation
- → phosphorylation of ion channel and/or metabolic effects

This particular schematic is for the G protein involved in *stimulation* of the second messenger system, G_s. Other effects may include *inhibition* through activation of another class of G proteins, G_i.

An example of β receptor effect is the reduction of the slow-onset hyperpolarization that follows an action potential in hippocampal pyramidal neurons and causes a "shutting down" or *accommodation* of repetitive discharges. This reduction of the after-hyperpolarization is mediated by the chain of events schematized above, with activation of the protein kinase A, which, in turn, modifies and reduces ion flow in the potassium channel responsible for the after-hyperpolarization (Nicoll 1988).

The *muscarinic acetylcholine receptor* also indirectly affects the ion channel—an action that is in contrast with the direct effects mediated by the nicotinic acetylcholine receptor. At least five subtypes of the muscarinic receptor are known. The M1 subtype is defined by its high affinity for the antagonist pirenzepine; at the M1 receptor acetylcholine binding leads to membrane G_i protein activation and inhibition of adenylate cyclase and cAMP production. Other receptor subtypes have a lower affinity for pirenzepine. The M2 receptor also works through a G protein coupled system but with a different mode of action on the ion channel than either the M1 or β_2-adrenergic receptor: the entire complex of acetylcholine/M2 receptor/G protein/guanosine triphosphate (GTP) interacts with a potassium ion channel to decrease the outward flow of K^+ and hence to depolarize the cell (Yatani et al. 1987).

Calcium as a second messenger: excitatory amino acid receptors, long-term potentiation, synaptic plasticity, and learning. The importance of intracellular calcium as a second messenger should be emphasized, and there are many examples of the important role of calcium in general cellular physiology. They include triggering secretion (insulin and digestive enzymes), contraction (muscle), and conversion of glycogen to glucose. Because of the importance of the phenomenon for psychiatry, the role of calcium in initiating *long-term potentiation (LTP)* is emphasized here (see also Cotman et al. 1989; Mayer and Miller 1990). (This is an area of intense current work, and some important questions about the mechanisms of LTP remain.)

Briefly, LTP can be viewed as an elementary form of "associative learning." Coupling of weak input with a strong input to hippocampal neurons leads to a "long-term potentiation" of the weak input, a potentiation that lasts days or even weeks. The role of increased intracellular calcium is thought to be critical.

Before discussing LTP further, it is useful to say a few words about the receptor that mediates it. This is one of the receptors for the amino acid glutamate (or aspartate); the glutamate/aspartate receptor types are collectively known as *excitatory amino acid (EAA)* receptors, because of their excitatory action.

The *N*-methyl-ᴅ-aspartate (NMDA) EAA receptor (Figure 2–6) is especially important in LTP because the ion channel associated with it is permeable to Ca^{2+}. Other types of EAA receptors are kainate receptors and α-amino-3-hydroxy-5-methyl-4-isoxazole propionic acid (AMPA) receptors (AMPA receptors are also called quisqualate receptors); kainate and AMPA receptors are collectively termed *non-NMDA receptors* and do not admit Ca^{2+} ions.

Opening of the NMDA ion channel allows Ca^{2+} to flow down the concentration gradient and enter the neuron; there is, however, a voltage dependency of the permeability of the NMDA channel to Ca^{2+}, due to a voltage-dependent blockade of the channel by magnesium. At membrane potentials near resting voltages, the blockade is nearly complete. However as the membrane becomes more depolarized the blockade lessens. This voltage dependence makes the necessity of pairing inputs with weak effects with stronger inputs to produce LTP understandable: the strong inputs depolarize the neuron via kainate and AMPA (non-NMDA) channels and this depolarization allows increased Ca^{2+} entry because of decreased magnesium blockade of the NMDA ion channel. Both the NMDA and non-NMDA receptors are ligand-gated, but the Ca^{2+} admitted by the NMDA receptor plays the role of a second messenger and is likely critical for the production of the long-term alterations underlying LTP. The secondary responses mediated by a rise in intracellular Ca^{2+} include changes in other second messengers, such as the stimulation of phospholipases to produce diacylglycerol, inositol triphosphate, and arachidonic acid—factors that may be important in the initiation and maintenance of LTP.

Yet another important EAA receptor type is the "metabotropic" EAA receptor; these receptors are not coupled to an ion channel, but rather act to cause a G protein stimulated release of Ca^{2+} from intracellular stores, an action mediated by inositol

Figure 2–5. *(at right)* β-Adrenergic receptor: G protein and cyclic adenosine monophosphate (cAMP) coupling. *Panel A:* Dynamics of collision-coupling of β-adrenergic receptor with G proteins. 1) and 2) The binding of norepinephrine to the receptor (R) activates it by altering its conformation (solid portions of the sketch represent component activation). 3) When the activated receptor comes into contact with G protein β and γ subunits it couples to them and causes a conformational change. 4) This conformational change frees the Gα subunit and causes the Gα subunit to release its guanosine diphosphate (GDP) in exchange for guanosine triphosphate (GTP). 5) The Gβ subunit now sticks to and activates the membrane bound adenylate cyclase (C), which in turn catalyzes the dephosphorylation of adenosine triphosphate (ATP) to cAMP, one of the most important second messengers. *Panel B:* Schematic of cAMP second messenger effects on ion channels. cAMP in the cytosol acts on the regulatory subunit (R) of a protein kinase (PK); this enables the catalytic subunits (C) to phosphorylate a channel protein and thereby change conformation and affect ion permeability. ADP = adenosine diphosphate. *Source.* Adapted from Smith 1989.

triphosphate. This receptor has recently been cloned and found to be structurally distinctive, with no sequence similarity to other G protein coupled receptors; it has extensive expression in hippocampus and cerebellum (Masu et al. 1991).

Calcium and growth and development of neurons.   Not only does intracellular Ca^{2+} appear to play an important role in adult synaptic plasticity, it is also important

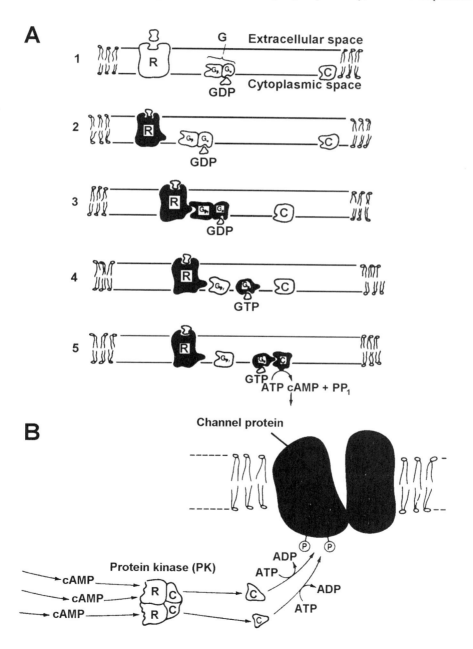

in neurotransmitter-mediated regulation of neuronal growth and development (Lipton and Kater 1989). Intracellular calcium concentrations have an inverted U functional relationship to neuronal growth; at lower levels increasing Ca^{2+} increases growth whereas at higher levels Ca^{2+} increases lead to destruction of neuronal processes. In the visual system (optic tectum) of amphibians, specificity of input from each eye is maintained by glutamate acting at NMDA receptors.

Calcium and excitotoxicity. An important area of current interest is the toxic effects of excessive EAA receptor stimulation, a phenomenon called *excitotoxicity,* which is likely responsible for much of the cellular damage that occurs following decreased oxygenation and/or decreased glucose supply to brain, such as occurs during stroke. The basic concept is that these conditions favor membrane depolarization

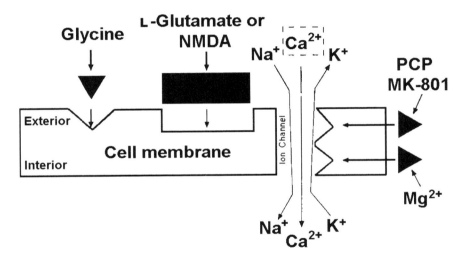

Figure 2–6. Schematic of the *N*-methyl-D-aspartate (NMDA) receptor-ion channel complex. The agonist for the receptor site is NMDA or L-glutamate. The attachment of the agonist to the receptor site (rectangle) leads to opening of the ion channel in the neuronal membrane. A key feature of the NMDA receptor ion channel, in contrast to other excitatory amino acid receptor channels, is that it allows the passage of calcium ions (Ca^{2+}, highlighted) from outside to inside the neuron (in addition to allowing the entry of sodium ions [Na^+] and the exit of potassium ions [K^+]). As described in the text, Ca^{2+} is important both in excitotoxicity and in long-term alterations of neuronal properties such as long-term potentiation. Both phencyclidine (PCP, "angel dust") and MK-8O1 are noncompetitive blockers of the ion channel. NMDA neurotransmission has a distinctive nonlinear property in that the effect of opening the NMDA channel is dependent on the degree of membrane polarization. At membrane polarization voltages typical of the cell at rest, about −70 mV, the magnesium ion (Mg^{2+}) blocks the channel nearly completely; however this blockage is voltage-dependent, becoming progressively less with membrane depolarization. This progressive decrease in Mg^{2+} blockage produces a positive feedback for NMDA neurotransmission. With opening of the ion channel, the membrane potential is depolarized by the inrush of Na^+ and Ca^{2+}. This depolarization reduces the Mg^{2+} channel blockage, with consequent admission of more Na^+ and Ca^{2+}, more membrane depolarization, less Mg^{2+} blockade, more depolarization, and so on. The glycine site is included in the schematic because this glycine receptor modulates the effect of NMDA.

and hence increased Ca^{2+} entry, with the increased intracellular Ca^{2+} being toxic to the neurons. Increased Ca^{2+} entry occurs both as a result of decreased magnesium blockade of NMDA receptors and/or through voltage-sensitive Ca^{2+} channels. Excitotoxicity may also be important in degenerative diseases, where there may be abnormal sensitivity to NMDA or some form of dysregulation of EAA channels. Such a mechanism has been proposed for Huntington's chorea (see Cotman et al. 1989). More recently a dysregulation of EAA channels has been hypothesized for schizophrenia (McCarley et al. 1991), with the important additional consideration that EAA receptor dysregulation may also interfere with normal neural development (see discussion above and in Chapter 1).

Third Messengers: c-fos and jun

Immediate early genes.   An important recent development has been the realization that neurotransmitters may activate mechanisms regulating the transcription of DNA, the genetic material. The induction of the *immediate early genes (IEGs)* such as "c-fos" and "jun" is one example of this mechanism. The term *fos* was first used to describe the oncogene encoded by the *F*inkel-Biskis-Jenkins murine *o*steogenic *s*arcoma virus. The normal cellular sequences from which the viral oncogene (v-fos) was derived are referred to as the *fos proto-oncogene* or *c-fos.*

In normal cells the level of the protein product of the c-fos gene, Fos, is highly regulated; many stimuli, some associated with cellular differentiation and some linked with neuronal excitation, lead to a transient induction of c-fos messenger RNA (mRNA). The name for the IEG jun was derived from the oncogene carried by the avian sarcoma virus ASV17; *ju-nana* is Japanese for 17. (For a discussion of stimulus-transcription coupling, see Morgan and Curran 1989, 1991.) Schematically,

Neurotransmitter-receptor binding
- → change in second messenger levels
- → induction of transcription of the genes c-fos and jun
- → c-fos and jun mRNAs present in cytoplasm for about 1–2 hours
- → translation of Fos and Jun proteins
- → possible alterations in posttranslational modification (e.g., phosphorylation) of Fos by stimuli
- → translocation to nucleus and formation of a Fos-Jun dimer (Fos has half life of about 2 hours)
- → Fos-Jun dimer complex binds to DNA regulatory element (AP-1 site)
- → increase in transcription of DNA
- → increase in production of a particular protein

This is an area of intense research and hence of great flux in defining both which neurotransmitters and stimuli lead to the IEG production and which proteins are regulated by this transcriptional control, a much more difficult question. Neurotransmitters-receptors reported to modulate c-fos expression include EAAs (especially NMDA, but also kainate), dopamine, opioids, cholecystokinin, progesterone, interleukin-1 (IL-1), and nicotine. Stimuli and conditions known to activate c-fos include heat shock, dehydration, electrical stimulation, seizures (especially in hippocampus), manipulation of internal calcium concentration, treadmill locomotion, and stimulation with light (see Morgan and Curran 1991). Although this list is long, it should not be assumed that all cellular activation leads to c-fos production and that c-fos production is nonspecific.

There appears to be a relatively specific production of c-fos in the hypothalamic suprachiasmatic nucleus (SCN). The SCN contains the basic mechanisms of the circadian clock, which regulates the circadian oscillations of many body systems including temperature and sleep. This clock may be reset to an earlier time (this kind of resetting is called phase advancing) in response to a light stimulus occurring just before the expected onset of light in the environment. Several groups of investigators have found that light stimuli applied at this time—but not at other circadian times that do not induce the same phase reset—have the capability of inducing c-fos. Although it has been hypothesized that the transcriptional regulation of DNA is important in resetting the circadian clock, this has not yet been proven.

The induction of IEGs may be very important for psychiatry because this process may mediate long-term alterations important for behavior. Obviously the key step to understanding the functional significance of IEG stimulation of transcription is knowing which protein is being transcribed; unfortunately this is also the most difficult step.

cAMP-inducible genes.   Stimulation of the second messenger cAMP by neurotransmitters may, as discussed above, control DNA transcription *indirectly* through induction of c-fos and other IEGs. There are also genes that are *directly* regulated by cAMP, including those for the neurotransmitter peptides somatostatin and vasointestinal peptide (VIP) (Montminy et al. 1990). This regulation is thought to be accomplished via cAMP-induced release of the active C subunit of protein kinase A; the C subunit moves to the nucleus where it phosphorylates a cAMP responsive element binding protein (CREB). The consequent conformational change in CREB allows it to interact with a target protein and stimulate gene production.

EVOKED POTENTIALS (EP) AND THE EEG

Recording of individual neurons, the ideal means of analyzing brain information transmission, can only be done in humans under very special circumstances, and much of our knowledge of human systems electrophysiology comes through recordings of EPs and the EEG. These techniques use large electrodes and do not record the activity of individual neurons but rather the summated activity of many neural elements. We here briefly outline the essential concepts relevant to EP and EEG generation, taking the EP first. EPs may be thought of as summations of the voltage alterations generated by populations of neural elements in response to a stimulus, typically an external sensory stimulus.

Most of the components of the EP arise from PSPs and not action potentials, which generally are too brief and too asynchronous to summate and produce an EP. (Some of the very short latency [<10 milliseconds] brain stem auditory EP components are derived from synchronous volleys of action potentials and are an important exception to this rule.)

Figure 2–7 illustrates a depolarizing PSP in the soma; this PSP is generated by the influx of positive ions. The influx of positive ions defines the soma as a current "sink" in this case because, by convention, current is composed of positive ion flow. In contrast, the apical dendrites act as a "source" of current flow. This current flow pattern defines a dipole, literally a "two pole" with the positive pole in the dendrites and the negative in the soma. In the case of a hyperpolarizing PSP in the soma, the dipole polarity would be reversed, with source (positive pole) in the soma and sink in the dendrites; it will be recalled that membrane hyperpolarization arises as the consequence of a net efflux of positive ions. In cerebral structures with a regular laminar structure such as the cortex and hippocampus, such a simple dipole model repeated over many constituent neurons provides a reasonable first approximation to how EPs are generated. Many investigators are currently exploring the use of modeling "equivalent dipoles" as a representation of the average amplitude and polarity within a cerebral region, such as the sensory receiving areas of the cortex.

Practical constraints to localizing the source of EPs include the use of scalp recordings and the consequent "smearing" of current flow as the boundaries between zones of different conductivities are traversed. For example, the brain and its extracellular fluid is a much better conductor than the scalp. Studies by Cohen, Cuffin, and associates (Cohen et al. 1990) have applied an experimental approach to the question of the accuracy of source localization possible with electrical signals. Using patients who had deep electrodes implanted to locate the seizure source before surgery, these investigators passed a low-level signal through two deep electrodes (a true dipole source!) and then examined how closely the signal source within the brain could be

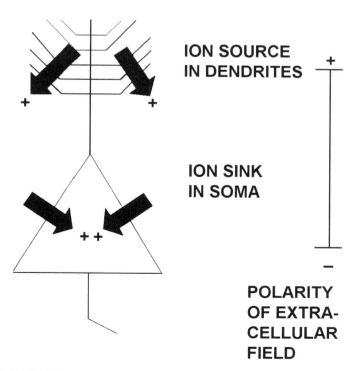

Figure 2–7. Dipole generated by soma depolarization in a pyramidal neuron. (See text for discussion.)

localized from scalp electrode recordings. Brain localization was found to be surprisingly good, being correct on the average to within about 1 cm.

Another rather surprising finding of this study was the failure of the magnetoencephalogram (MEG) to localize the source with any significantly greater accuracy than the EEG. The MEG is a recording of the magnetic field generated by neural activity and is analogous to the electrical field recorded by the EEG. There currently is considerable debate over whether the MEG will show greater localizing power than the EEG for EPs. The MEG is particularly useful in detecting generating dipoles that are tangentially oriented to the brain surface, but is not sensitive to radially oriented dipoles. The EEG is equally sensitive to tangential and radial dipoles. Finally, it is important to emphasize that the biological EP signals recorded from the scalp are of quite low level, often a few microvolts; thus signal averaging is typically used for EP recording to extract the signal from the ongoing EEG and from noise sources, such as muscle activity.

The EEG can be understood as the record of spontaneous voltage fluctuations, as "endogenously generated EPs," although the brain source of the recorded fluctuations is often difficult to pinpoint, with the important exceptions of large amplitude changes due to pathological synchronization of neural elements, such as spikes from seizure discharge. The EEG serves a very useful purpose in pinpointing changes in alertness and sleep stages by changes in its frequency content.

The *alpha rhythm* has a frequency range of 8–13 Hz, occurs during wakefulness, appears on eye closure, disappears with eye opening, and is best recorded over the occipital scalp region. Depth recordings in animals indicate alpha rhythm frequencies may also be present in visual thalamus (lateral geniculate body, pulvinar) and the cortical component appears to be generated in relatively small cortical areas that act as epicenters. Unfortunately, there are as yet almost no cellular studies bearing on the genesis of this rhythm, although interaction of corticocortical and thalamocortical neurons has been postulated (Steriade et al. 1990).

REFERENCES

Cohen D, Cuffin BN, Yunokuchi MS, et al: MEG versus EEG localization test using implanted sources in the human brain. Ann Neurol 28:811–817, 1990

Cotman CW, Bridges RJ, Taube JS, et al: The role of the NMDA receptor in central nervous system plasticity and pathology. Journal of NIH Research 1:65–74, 1989

Darnell J, Lodish H, Baltimore D: Molecular Cell Biology, 2nd Edition. New York, Scientific American Books, 1990

Hodgkin AL, Huxley AF: A quantitative description of membrane current and its application to conduction and excitation in nerve. J Physiol 117:500–544, 1952

Kandel E, Schwartz JH (eds): Principles of Neural Science. New York, Elsevier, 1985

Lipton SA, Kater SB: Neurotransmitter regulation of neuronal outgrowth, plasticity and survival. Trends Neurosci 12:265–270, 1989

McCarley RW, Faux SF, Shenton ME, et al: Event-related potentials in schizophrenia: their biological and clinical correlates and a new model of schizophrenic pathophysiology. Schiz Res 4:209–231, 1991

Masu M, Tanabe Y, Tsuchida K, et al: Sequence and expression of a metabotropic glutamate receptor. Nature 349:760–765, 1991

Mayer ML, Miller RJ: Excitatory amino acid receptors, second messengers and regulation of intracellular Ca^{2+} in mammalian neurons. Trends Pharmacol Sci 11:254–260, 1990

Montminy MR, Gonzalez GA, Yamamoto KK: Regulation of cAMP-inducible genes by CREB. Trends Neurosci 13:184–188, 1990

Morgan JI, Curran T: Stimulus-transcription coupling in neurons: role of cellular immediate-early genes. Trends Neurosci 12:459–462, 1989

Morgan TJ, Curran T: Stimulus-transcription coupling in the nervous system: involvement of the inducible proto-oncogenes fos and jun, in Annual Review of Neuroscience. Edited by Cowan WM, Shooter EM, Stevens CF, et al. Palo Alto, CA, Annual Reviews, 1991, pp 421–451

Nauta WJH, Feirtag M: Fundamental Neuroanatomy. New York, WH Freeman, 1986

Nicoll RA: The coupling of neurotransmitter receptors to ion channels in the brain. Science 241:545–551, 1988

Smith CUM: Elements of Molecular Neurobiology. New York, Wiley, 1989

Steriade M, Gloor P, Llinás RR, et al: Basic mechanisms of cerebral rhythmic activities. Electroencephalogr Clin Neurophysiol 76:481–508, 1990

Yatani A, Codina J, Brown AM, et al: Direct activation of mammalian atrial muscarinic potassium channels by GTP regulatory protein Gk. Science 235:207–211, 1987

Chapter 3

Functional Neuroanatomy From a Neuropsychological Perspective

Daniel Tranel, Ph.D.

Dysfunction of neuroanatomical systems in the human brain can lead to a wide variety of cognitive and behavioral manifestations, including changes in intellect, memory, language, perception, judgment and decision making, and personality. Recent advances in neuroanatomical analysis (H. Damasio and Damasio 1989) and neuropsychological measurement (see Chapter 5) have revealed a number of orderly relationships between neural and psychological systems. The precision of knowledge regarding such relationships has reached a level that was only hinted at in the work of several decades ago.

The discussion in this chapter, which focuses on the neuropsychological correlates of damage to a number of neuroanatomical regions, makes some assumptions that may restrict the range of application of the principles and conclusions reviewed. It is assumed that the human brain under consideration is endowed with conventional hemispheric dominance, that is, with speech and linguistic functions lateralized to the left hemisphere. The discussion also assumes normal acquisition and development of cognitive capacities.

The findings presented here are derived from research that has used the lesion method as the primary paradigm of scientific inquiry. This method (Anderson et al. 1990; H. Damasio and Damasio 1989) is centered on cognitive experimentation in adult humans with focal brain lesions. In general, such lesions are caused by cerebrovascular disease, surgical ablation of nonmalignant cerebral tumors, some viral infections of the central nervous system, traumatic brain injury, and degenerative disease. Dating back to the innovative formulations of Geschwind (1965), there has been a resurgence of interest in the lesion method. Much of this renewed popularity can be traced to the advent of modern neuroimaging techniques in the mid-1970s, beginning with computed tomography (CT) and continuing with the emergence of magnetic resonance imaging (MRI) in the early 1980s. These procedures have greatly increased the precision and reliability of neuroimaging definition and, together with increased sophistication of neuropsychological experimentation (Benton 1988), have allowed more powerful analysis of brain-behavior relationships and more detailed and elaborate theoretical specification (A. R. Damasio 1989).

This work was supported by National Institute of Neurological Disorders and Stroke Grant P01-NS19632. The author thanks Dr. Antonio Damasio for his unwavering encouragement and support, and Dr. Hanna Damasio for her kind assistance with the figures.

THE TEMPORAL LOBES

This section focuses on several major subdivisions within the temporal lobe: 1) the posterior portion of the superior temporal gyrus (area 22), which, on the left side, forms the heart of what is traditionally known as *Wernicke's area*; 2) the lateral aspect inferior to the superior temporal gyrus, which comprises the human inferior temporal (IT) region (for the purposes of this section, this region is extended posteriorly to include the occipitotemporal junction and anteriorly to include the temporal pole); and 3) the mesial aspect, especially the hippocampal system formed by the entorhinal cortex, amygdala, and hippocampus proper (Figure 3–1).

Lateral/Inferior Temporal Region

Posterior component.   As depicted in Figure 3–1, the posterior portion of the IT region comprises the posterior parts of the middle, inferior, and fourth temporal gyri, an area that corresponds primarily to cytoarchitectonic field 37. This discussion considers this region together with the posteriorly adjacent occipitotemporal junction, formed by the lower part of cytoarchitectonic fields 18 and 19 and the subjacent white matter. Lesions to posterior IT, especially bilateral ones, can produce unimodal, visually based disorders of recognition. When the lesions extend posteriorly into the inferior portion of the visual association cortices formed by areas 18 and 19, patients lose their ability to recognize visual stimuli at the level of unique identity. Because basic visual perception is unaltered, the presentation conforms to the classic notion of associative agnosia, that is, a normal percept stripped of its meaning (Teuber 1968). The best studied and most common form is agnosia for faces, known as *prosopagnosia* (Table 3–1).

Prosopagnosia is hallmarked by an inability to recognize the identity of previously known faces and an inability to learn new ones. The defect is severe, with patients losing the ability to recognize faces of family members, close friends, and even their own face in a mirror. However, it is confined to the visual channel; hearing the voice associated with an unrecognized face will elicit prompt and accurate recognition. For most persons with prosopagnosia, the ability to recognize facial expressions and to judge gender and estimate age from face information is well preserved (Tranel et al. 1988).

Full-blown "associative" prosopagnosia is nearly always associated with bilateral lesions to posterior IT and the inferior sector of fields 18 and 19 (Benton 1990; A. R. Damasio et al. 1982b, 1990b; Meadows 1974b). An MRI of a patient with this type of prosopagnosia is presented in Figure 3–2. Unilateral occipitotemporal lesions usually do not cause severe and lasting prosopagnosia, although such lesions may cause significant disturbances in face recognition. On the left, such lesions can produce a partial recognition defect termed *deep prosopagnosia* (A. R. Damasio et al. 1988), in which target faces are misidentified as someone who is very similar to the correct person in terms of gender, age, or activity (e.g., recognizing Magic Johnson as Michael Jordan).

In addition to disturbances of recognition of unique visual stimuli, lesions to IT can also produce impairments in the visual recognition of stimuli as members of a specific category. For example, when confronted with the picture of a fox or lion, patients may indicate that it is an "animal," but the specific type will elude them. Shown a robin, a patient might respond "bird." Such patients can only recognize the superordinate category to which the entity belongs, but not the subordinate, basic object level (as defined by Rosch et al. 1976). The impairment may not affect all types of entities equally, but instead may be related in a general sense to the conceptual-lexical category to which entities belong. For example, patients who have far greater

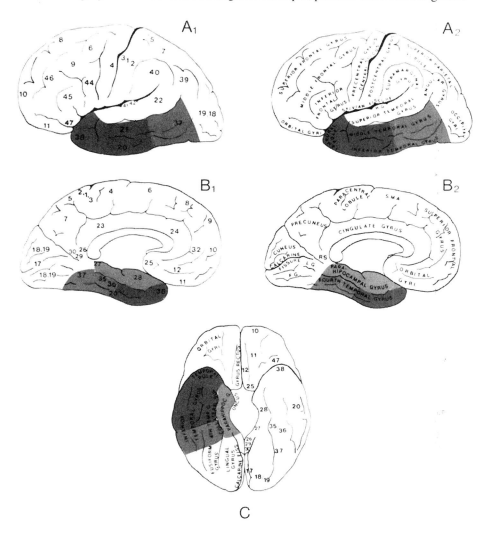

Figure 3–1. Three major subdivisions of the temporal lobe: posterior inferotemporal region (*shown in green*); anterior inferotemporal region (*shown in red*); mesial region (*shown in yellow*). Numbers corresponding to Brodmann's cytoarchitectonic areas are depicted on A_1, B_1, and the right side (left hemisphere) of C, and standard gyri names are shown on corresponding A_2, B_2, and the left side (right hemisphere) of C. Lateral (A_2 and A_2), mesial (B_1 and B_2, and inferior (C) views are represented. (Please refer to page 59 of *The American Psychiatric Press Textbook of Neuropsychiatry,* Second Edition, for the full-color figure.)

recognition impairment for natural entities such as animals or vegetables tend to have much less impairment for manmade entities such as tools and utensils (A. R. Damasio 1990; A. R. Damasio et al. 1990d; Warrington and McCarthy 1987; Warrington and Shallice 1984).

Anterior component.   The anterior component of the lateral/inferior temporal lobe (Figure 3–1) is formed by the anterior portion of the middle, inferior, and fourth temporal gyri (comprised by cytoarchitectonic fields 21 and 20), together with the tem-

Table 3–1.   Neuropsychological manifestations of temporal lobe lesions

	Hemispheric side of lesion		
Region	Left	Right	Bilateral
Lateral/inferior			
Posterior	"Deep" prosopagnosia; mild defects in category-level object recognition	Transient prosopagnosia; mild defects in category-level object recognition	Severe, permanent prosopagnosia; associative visual agnosia; severe defects in category-level object recognition
Anterior	Anomia; restricted naming impairments; defective proper naming	Anomia for facial expressions	Anomia; retrograde amnesia
Mesial	Anterograde amnesia for verbal material	Anterograde amnesia for nonverbal material	Severe anterograde amnesia for verbal and nonverbal material

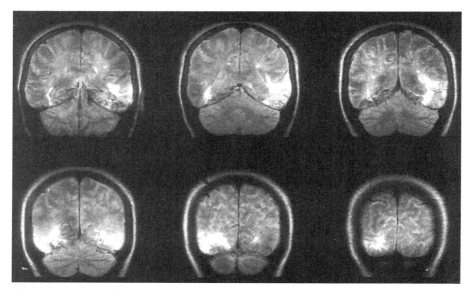

Figure 3–2.   T2-weighted magnetic resonance image (MRI) of a 67-year-old, right-handed woman, which shows bilateral occipitotemporal lesions (showing as white, or "bright" signal). In these coronal cuts, the left hemisphere is on the right, and the most anterior cut is in the upper left-hand corner of the figure. The woman developed severe, permanent prosopagnosia after sustaining these lesions.

poral pole (area 38). For many decades, the prevailing wisdom was that lesions to the left anterolateral temporal lobe do not cause memory defects or deficits in speech or language (Penfield and Roberts 1959). Even naming impairments were considered rare following anterior left temporal lesions. However, recent observations have made it clear that left anterolateral temporal lesions *do* cause naming deficits, although such defects may be restricted to certain conceptual-lexical categories (A. R. Damasio 1990; A. R. Damasio et al. 1990d; Tranel 1991a). The left anterolateral temporal region is also now understood to be a cortical area that subserves access to the reference lexicon (A. R. Damasio et al. 1990d; Graff-Radford et al. 1990a). Naming defects may be confined to certain conceptual-lexical categories; for example, patients may lose the ability to produce proper names, while preserving the capacity to produce common names (Semenza and Zettin 1989).

Neuropsychological correlates of damage to the right anterolateral temporal region are less well understood. In one case with this type of lesion (Rapcsak et al. 1989), the patient had a selective defect in naming facial expressions such as happiness, sadness, surprise, and fear. However, the patient did not have an impairment in recognition, even with regard to the emotional facial expressions that were not correctly named. Other observations have indicated that the right anterolateral temporal region may play a crucial role in retrograde episodic memory, that is, in the retrieval of entities and events that are highly specific and unique to an individual's autobiography.

Mesial Temporal Region

The mesial sector of the temporal lobe is formed by the parahippocampal gyrus (cytoarchitectonic areas 28 and 27), and by the adjoining hippocampal system including the amygdala, entorhinal cortex, and hippocampus proper (Figure 3–1). Since the landmark report by Scoville and Milner (1957) on patient H.M., who became severely amnesic after bilateral mesial temporal lobe resection for control of intractable seizures, the mesial aspect of the temporal lobes has been linked unequivocally to memory function.

More than three decades of research on H.M. (for summary, see Corkin 1984; Gabrieli et al. 1988; Sagar et al. 1990), and on similar patients, have demonstrated that the hippocampus is critical for the acquisition of new information (i.e., for anterograde memory). However, the hippocampus is not needed for the retrieval of old information (retrograde memory) (Milner 1972). Patient R.B. (Zola-Morgan et al. 1986), who had pathologically confirmed bilateral lesions limited to the CA_1 sector of the hippocampus, is another example of the marked anterograde amnesia that can occur following circumscribed bilateral hippocampal lesions. Patient Boswell (A. R. Damasio et al. 1985a), had bilateral damage to the entire mesial sector of the temporal lobes (hippocampus, amygdala, and entorhinal cortex), and also nonmesial damage (in areas 38, 20, 21, and 37). In the anterograde compartment, Boswell's memory profile is similar to that for H.M. and R.B.; however, on the retrograde side, unlike H.M. and R.B., Boswell also had severe impairment (A. R. Damasio et al. 1985a, 1987, 1989c; Haist et al. 1990).

With respect to amnesia associated with hippocampal damage, there is a consistent relationship between the side of the lesion and the type of learning impairment.

Specifically, damage to the left-hippocampal system produces an amnesic syndrome that affects verbal material but spares nonverbal material; conversely, damage to the right-hippocampal system affects nonverbal material but spares verbal material (Frisk and Milner 1990; Milner 1968, 1972; Smith and Milner 1989; Tranel 1991a). In addition, the hippocampal system does not appear to play a role in the learning of perceptuomotor skills, known as *nondeclarative memory*. Patient H.M., for example, can learn skills such as mirror drawing and mirror reading (Corkin 1965, 1968) even though he has no recall of the situation in which the learning of those skills took place.

The role of the amygdala in memory has been a source of controversy. Studies in nonhuman primates have yielded conflicting results, with some finding that the amygdala is critical for normal learning (Mishkin 1978; Murray 1990; Murray and Mishkin 1984, 1985, 1986), and others maintaining that the amygdala does not play a crucial role (Zola-Morgan et al. 1989). One human study found a memory defect associated with bilateral amygdala damage (Tranel and Hyman 1990).

THE OCCIPITAL LOBES

The neuroanatomical arrangement of structures in and near the occipital lobes is depicted in Figure 3–3. On the lateral aspect of the hemispheres, the occipital lobes comprise the visual association cortices in areas 18 and 19. These areas continue in the mesial aspect. The mesial sector also includes the primary visual cortices (area 17), formed by the cortex immediately above and below the calcarine fissure. To establish neuropsychological correlates of the occipital lobes, the region can be subdivided in the vertical plane at the level of the calcarine fissure so that dorsal (superior) and ventral (inferior) components can be designated. Neuropsychological manifestations of occipital lobe lesions are summarized in Table 3–2.

Dorsal Component

The dorsal component of the occipital lobes comprises the primary visual cortex superior to the calcarine fissure (area 17) and the superior portion of the visual association cortices (areas 18 and 19). For the purposes of this discussion, this region is considered in combination with the anteriorly adjacent parietal areas, including the posterior part of the superior parietal lobule (area 7) and the posterior part of the angular gyrus (area 39).

An intriguing presentation occurs when lesions involve the association cortices of areas 18 and 19. When such lesions encroach upon the adjacent parietal region comprised by areas 39 and 7, patients commonly develop a constellation of defects known as *Balint's syndrome*. Balint's syndrome is based on the presence of three components: visual disorientation (also known as *simultanagnosia*), ocular apraxia (also known as *psychic gaze paralysis*), and optic ataxia. The key constituent in the syndrome, however, is visual disorientation.

Visual disorientation.   Visual disorientation can be conceptualized as an inability to attend to more than a very limited sector of the visual field at any given moment. Patients report that they can see clearly in only a small part of the field, the rest being out of focus and in a sort of "fog." The sector of clear vision, moreover, is unstable and may shift without warning in any direction, so that patients experience a literal "jumping about" of their visual perception. Such patients are incapable of constructing a spatially coherent visual field and cannot follow trajectories of stimuli or place stimuli in their proper locations in space. Perception of motion is often impaired. For example, patients may fail to recognize a familiar gait or stride or to understand pan-

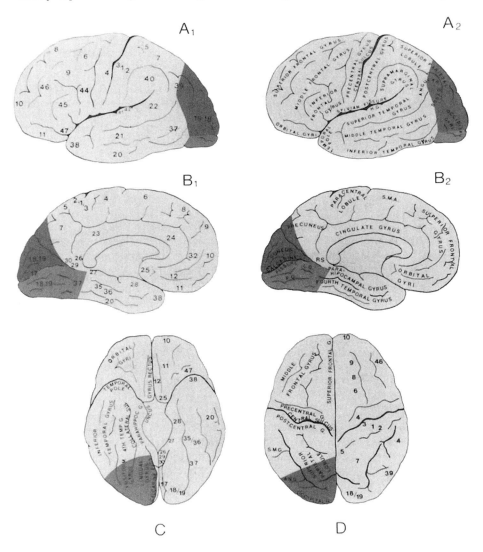

Figure 3–3. Two major subdivisions of the occipital lobe: dorsal (superior) component (*shown in red*); ventral (inferior) component (*shown in green*). Numbers corresponding to Brodmann's cytoarchitectonic areas are depicted on A_1, B_1, and the right side (left hemisphere) of C and D, and standard gyri names are shown on corresponding A_2, B_2, and the left side (right hemisphere) of C and D. Lateral (A_1 and A_2), mesial (B_1 and B_2), inferior (C), and superior (D) views are represented. (Please refer to page 65 of *The American Psychiatric Press Textbook of Neuropsychiatry*, Second Edition, for the full-color figure.)

Table 3–2.   Neuropsychological manifestations of occipital lobe lesions

Region	Hemispheric side of lesion		
	Left	**Right**	**Bilateral**
Dorsal	Partial or mild Balint's syndrome	Partial or mild Balint's syndrome	Balint's syndrome (visual disorientation, ocular apraxia, optic ataxia); defective motion perception; astereopsis
Ventral	Right hemiachrom-atopsia; "pure" alexia	Left hemiachromatopsia; apperceptive visual agnosia (especially when dorsal sector of right occipital cortices is also damaged); defective facial imagery	Full-field achromatopsia; associative visual agnosia; prosopagnosia

tomime (A. R. Damasio et al. 1989b, 1990a). Patients with visual disorientation can perceive color and shape normally, as long as objects are appreciated within a clear sector of the visual field.

Ocular apraxia.   Ocular apraxia is a deficit of visual scanning that consists of an inability to direct gaze voluntarily toward a stimulus located in peripheral vision and to bring it into central vision. Patients fail to direct saccades toward stimuli that have appeared in the panorama of their visual fields, or they produce saccades that are inaccurate and miss the target.

Optic ataxia.   Optic ataxia is a disturbance of visually guided reaching behavior. Patients are not able to point accurately at a target under visual guidance (e.g., they cannot point precisely to the examiner's fingertip or to items such as a cup or coin). However, pointing to targets on their own body does not pose a problem as this can be accomplished on the basis of somatosensory information. As alluded to above, the full Balint's syndrome is generally associated with bilateral occipitoparietal lesions, although unilateral lesions can also produce the syndrome, especially when they are on the right. When lesions are confined to the superior occipital cortices without extension into the parietal region, visual disorientation is likely to occur without associated ocular apraxia or optic ataxia. The defects in motion perception that are frequent in patients with Balint's syndrome are probably related to damage in the lower-parietal/lateral-occipital region (area 39). Many patients with Balint's syndrome have an impairment of stereopsis (the process of recovery of depth from visual information dependent on binocular visual interaction), although complete astereopsis is seen only in the setting of bilateral lesions (Rizzo 1989; Rizzo and Hurtig 1987).

Ventral Component

The ventral component of the occipital lobes comprises the primary visual cortex immediately below the calcarine fissure (area 17) and the inferior portion of the visual association cortices (areas 18 and 19). The latter component corresponds to the lingual and fusiform gyri (Figure 3–3; *C*). The following discussion treats this region together with the posterior part of area 37, that is, the occipitotemporal junction.

Acquired achromatopsia. Acquired (or "central") achromatopsia is a disorder of color perception involving all or part of the visual field, with preservation of form vision, caused by damage to the inferior visual association cortex and/or its subjacent white matter (A. R. Damasio 1985; A. R. Damasio et al. 1980; Meadows 1974a). Patients lose color vision in a quadrant, a hemifield, or the entire visual field. If the loss is partial, patients may complain that colors appear "washed out" or "dirty"; if it is entire, all forms are seen in shades of black and white. However, perception of form, per se, is unaltered, and depth and motion perception are also normal.

The "purest" form of the disorder is a left hemiachromatopsia associated with a unilateral right occipitotemporal lesion, unaccompanied by other neuropsychological defects. A comparable lesion on the left will produce right hemiachromatopsia, but most of those patients also typically have alexia (see below). Bilateral occipitotemporal lesions may cause full-field achromatopsia, and such patients frequently also manifest associative visual agnosia (especially prosopagnosia).

In a study reported by A. R. Damasio et al. (1989a), achromatopsia was associated with lesions to the middle third of the lingual gyrus and with infracalcarine lesions that damaged the white matter immediately behind the posterior tip of the lateral ventricle. These findings are consistent with data from positron-emission tomography (PET) studies suggesting a similar "color center" (Corbetta et al. 1990; Lueck et al. 1989) and with the extensive research on nonhuman primates indicating separate cellular channels within area 17 dedicated to the processing of color, form, and motion (Hubel and Livingstone 1987; Livingstone and Hubel 1984, 1987, 1988).

Apperceptive visual agnosia. Apperceptive agnosia was originally attributed to the disturbed integration of otherwise normally perceived components of a stimulus (Lissauer 1890), and in general the concept has persisted as a useful designation for recognition defects in which there is a substantial perceptual component. A common form of apperceptive agnosia occurs in the visual modality, with right-sided lesions involving both the inferior and superior sectors of the posterior visual association cortices (Figure 3–4). Patients with apperceptive visual agnosia have difficulty perceiving all parts of a visual array simultaneously and in generating the image of a whole entity, given a part. When shown a part of a house, or a car, the patient will be unable to imagine the whole object and thus fail to recognize the stimulus. A related defect is the inability to assemble parts of a model into a meaningful ensemble (e.g., the patient may be unable to assemble various face parts to form a spatially correct whole) (A. R. Damasio et al. 1990b; Davidoff and Donnelly 1990).

Acquired alexia. Lesions that disconnect both visual association cortices from the dominant, language-related temporoparietal cortices can produce a complete or partial impairment in reading, a condition known as *acquired* (or "pure") *alexia*. Acquired alexia can be caused by a single lesion in the region behind, beneath, and under the occipital horn of the left lateral ventricle, by damaging pathways en route from the callosum and pathways en route from the left visual association cortex (A. R. Damasio and Damasio 1983). Another setting is the combination of a lesion in the corpus callosum, which disconnects right-to-left visual information transfer, and a lesion in the left occipital lobe, which disconnects left visual association cortex from left language cortex (Geschwind 1965; Greenblatt 1983). Such lesions are likely to produce a right hemianopia, a frequent but not invariable (Greenblatt 1973) accompaniment of pure alexia.

The "purity" of the condition stems from the fact that patients with these lesions do not develop disturbances in writing or other aspects of speech and language operation. Thus, this type of alexia is distinct from the types of reading defects common

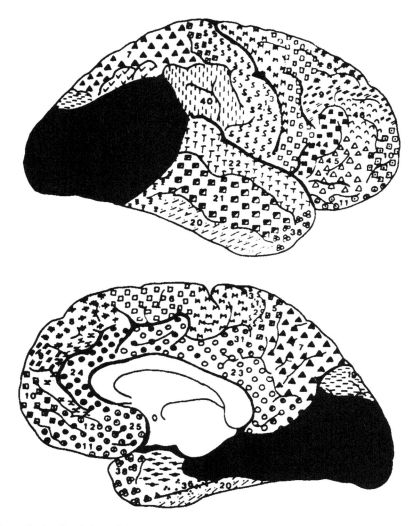

Figure 3–4.   Depiction of the lesion of a 68-year-old, right-handed man who suffered an infarction that destroyed right posterior parietal and occipital cortices. Note that the lesion (marked in black) includes visual association cortices both above and below the calcarine fissure. The man had apperceptive prosopagnosia.

in aphasic patients (Benson 1979; Benson et al. 1971). In this sense, pure alexia can be construed as a disturbance of visual pattern recognition. Pure alexia is also known as *alexia without agraphia,* or *pure word blindness.*

THE PARIETAL LOBES

On the lateral aspect of the cerebral hemisphere, the parietal lobes comprise a large expanse of cortex that is bounded by the central (Rolandic) sulcus anteriorly, the fissure of Sylvius inferiorly, and the occipital cortices posteriorly (Figure 3–5). It is important to maintain a clear distinction between the right and left hemispheres, as many correlates of the parietal region are highly lateralized. In the discussion below, no strict distinction is made between neighboring regions because many of the neuropsychological manifestations considered here (Table 3–3) are connected to regions that are both in and near the parietal cortices.

Temporoparietal Junction

In the left hemisphere, an area of cortex formed by the posterior part of the superior temporal gyrus (posterior area 22) constitutes the core of a region known as *Wernicke's area* (Figure 3–5). The posterior part of the inferior parietal lobule (including parts of the angular [area 39] and supramarginal [area 40] gyri) is usually included as part of "greater Wernicke's area." This region is firmly linked to a constellation of speech and language functions, whose disruption constitutes the syndrome known as *Wernicke's aphasia* (Benson 1989).

The syndrome is hallmarked by fluent, paraphasic speech production; impaired repetition; and defective aural comprehension. Patients can produce speech without hesitation, and the phrase length and melodic contour of utterances are normal; however, there are frequent errors in the choice of individual words used to express an idea (paraphasias). The comprehension defect frequently involves both aural and written forms of language (Figure 3–6).

In the right hemisphere, lesions in the region of the temporoparietal junction may impair the processing of music and other spectral auditory information. One intriguing neuropsychological correlate of this region is the ability to recognize familiar voices. Van Lancker and colleagues (Van Lancker and Kreiman 1988; Van Lancker et al. 1988) have reported that lesions to the right parietal cortices disrupt this function, even though auditory acuity is fundamentally unaltered, a condition the authors termed *phonagnosia.*

Bilateral lesions to the posterior part of the superior temporal gyrus lead to the syndrome of auditory agnosia, in which the patient is unable to recognize both speech and nonspeech sounds (Vignolo 1982). Almost always caused by stroke, this condition involves the sudden and complete inability to identify the meaning of verbal and nonverbal auditory signals (e.g., spoken words, familiar environmental sounds such as a telephone ringing or a knock on the door).

Inferior Parietal Lobule

The inferior parietal lobule comprises the supramarginal (area 40) and angular gyri (area 39) (Figure 3–5). On the left side, lesions to the supramarginal gyrus and the

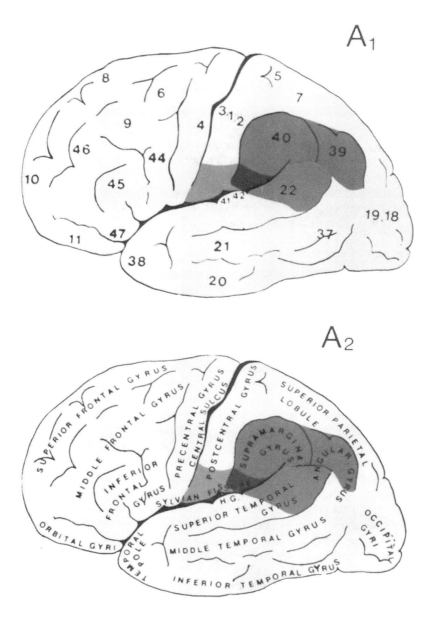

Figure 3–5. Subdivisions of the parietal lobe and nearby regions. The temporoparietal junction, formed by the posterior part of the superior temporal gyrus (area 22), is shown in red. The inferior parietal lobule (shown in green) is formed by the angular (area 39) and supramarginal (area 40) gyri. The parietal operculum is formed by the inferior aspect of the postcentral gyrus (shown in yellow) and a bit of the anteroinferior aspect of the supramarginal gyrus (shown in overlapping yellow and green). Numbers corresponding to Brodmann's cytoarchitectonic areas are depicted on A_1, and standard gyri names are shown on the corresponding A_2. The figures depict a lateral view. (Please refer to page 71 of *The American Psychiatric Press Textbook of Neuropsychiatry,* Second Edition, for the full-color figure.)

neighboring parietal operculum (the area of cortex formed by the most inferior portion of the postcentral gyrus), and/or the underlying white matter, cause a speech and language disturbance known as *conduction aphasia* (Benson et al. 1973). Conduction aphasia has also been reported with lesions that damage the primary auditory cortex (areas 41 and 42) and extend into the insular cortex and underlying white matter (H. Damasio and Damasio 1980).

The core feature of conduction aphasia is a marked defect in verbatim repetition. Speech production is fluent but is dominated by phonemic paraphasic errors, and comprehension may be mildly compromised. Naming is defective and dominated by phonemic errors. Another distinctive feature of this conduction is that patients cannot write to dictation but are able to write spontaneously with minimal error and to copy.

Table 3–3. Neuropsychological manifestations of parietal lobe lesions

Region	Hemispheric side of lesion		
	Left	Right	Bilateral
Temporoparietal junction (including posterior part of superior temporal gyrus)	Wernicke's aphasia	Amusia; defective music recognition; "phonagnosia"	Auditory agnosia
Inferior parietal lobule	Conduction aphasia; tactile agnosia	Neglect; anosognosia; anosodiaphoria; tactile agnosia	?

Note. ? = Neuropsychological correlates of such a lesion pattern are not well established.

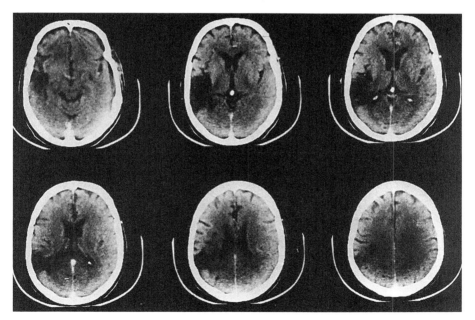

Figure 3–6. Computed tomography (CT) scan of a 56-year-old, right-handed man who developed Wernicke's aphasia following a left middle cerebral artery infarction. The lesion (area of low density) is centered squarely in Wernicke's area, including the posterior superior temporal gyrus (*top row*) and part of the inferior parietal lobule (*bottom row*).

On the right side, the most consistent and striking neuropsychological correlates of lesions to the inferior parietal lobule are *neglect* and *anosognosia*. Neglect, associated especially with temporoparietal lesions that include the angular (area 39) and supramarginal (area 40) gyri (Heilman et al. 1983), refers to a condition whereby the patient fails to attend to stimuli in the contralateral hemispace. In the visual modality, for example, the patient will not attend to the left hemifield and will fail to report stimuli from that side even when it can be demonstrated that there is no impairment of form vision (hemianopia). In principle, neglect can occur in relationship to any sensory modality, but in practice the visual and auditory varieties are most common.

Anosognosia is another frequent correlate of damage to the right inferior parietal lobule. This term was originally applied to patients who denied that a paretic limb was in fact paretic or that it even belonged to them (Babinski 1914). Denial of sensory loss and cognitive disturbance have also been included under the concept of anosognosia (Anderson and Tranel 1989). Anosognosia can be operationally defined as a significant discrepancy between the patient's report of his or her disabilities and the objective evidence regarding his or her level of functioning.

A related term is *anosodiaphoria,* which refers to the condition in which patients appear unconcerned with, or minimize the significance of, neurological deficits. It is common for patients to manifest anosognosia early in the course of illness and for this to gradually evolve into anosodiaphoria. In both conditions, common neuropsychological correlates are defects in visuospatial and visuoconstructional abilities and left hemispatial neglect (Benton 1985; Benton and Tranel 1993).

Tactile agnosia has been described in connection with lesions to the inferior parietal lobule and nearby posterior/superior temporal cortices on either the right or left side (Caselli 1991). Patients lose the ability to recognize objects presented via the tactile modality, even when basic aspects of somatosensory function are normal or near normal. This condition differs from prosopagnosia in that it involves a disruption of recognition at the basic object level, rather than at the level of unique identity (Tranel 1991b). Thus patients with tactile agnosia cannot recognize stimuli such as keys, pencils, and eating utensils when those items are presented in the somatosensory modality.

THE FRONTAL LOBES

The frontal lobes can be divided into several distinct anatomical regions (Figure 3–7), each of which has a number of relatively specific neuropsychological manifestations (Table 3–4).

Frontal Operculum

The frontal operculum is formed by areas 44, 45, and 47 (Figure 3–7). On the left side, the heart of this region (areas 44 and 45) is known as *Broca's area.* The region is dedicated to a set of speech and language functions whose disruption produces a distinctive pattern of aphasia termed *Broca's aphasia.* Patients with Broca's aphasia have nonfluent speech (short utterances, long response latencies, flat melodic contour) and agrammatism. Paraphasias are common, a defect in repetition is invariably present, and most patients have defective naming and impaired

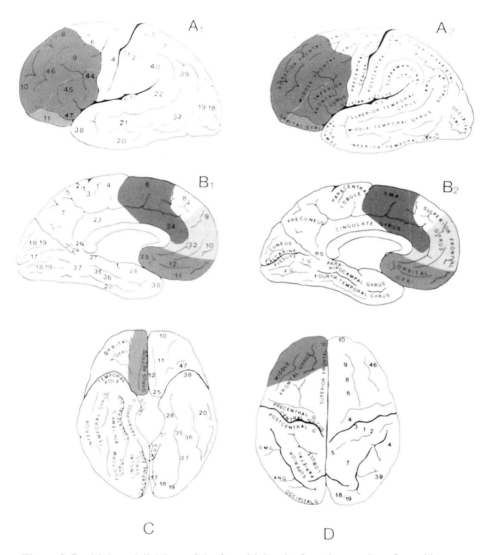

Figure 3–7. Major subdivisions of the frontal lobe: the frontal operculum, formed by areas 44, 45, and 47 (*shown in red*); the superior mesial region, formed by the mesial aspect of area 6 and the anterior part of the cingulate gyrus (area 24) (*shown in green*); the inferior mesial region, formed by the basal forebrain and the orbital cortices (areas 11, 12, and 25) (*shown in dark yellow*); and the lateral prefrontal region, formed by the lateral aspects of areas 8, 9, 46, and 10 (*shown in purple*). The ventromedial frontal lobe is comprised by the orbital region (*shown in dark yellow*) and the lower mesial (area 32 and the mesial aspect of areas 10 and 9) cortices (*shown in light yellow*). Numbers corresponding to Brodmann's cytoarchitectonic areas are depicted on A_1, B_1, and the right side (left hemisphere) of C and the right side (right hemisphere) of D, and standard gyri names are shown on corresponding A_2, B_2, and the left side of C and D. Lateral (A_1 and A_2), mesial (B_1 and B_2), inferior (C), and superior (D) views are represented. (Please refer to page 77 of *The American Psychiatric Press Textbook of Neuropsychiatry,* Second Edition, for the full-color figure.)

Table 3–4. Neuropsychological manifestations of frontal lobe lesions

Region	Hemispheric side of lesion	
	Left	**Right**
Frontal operculum	Broca's aphasia	"Expressive" aprosodia
Superior mesial region	Akinetic mutism[a]	Akinetic mutism[a]
Inferior mesial region		
Basal forebrain	Anterograde and retrograde amnesia with confabulation; worse for verbal stimuli	Anterograde and retrograde amnesia with confabulation; worse for nonverbal stimuli
Orbital	Defective social conduct; "acquired" sociopathy[a]	Defective social conduct; "acquired" sociopathy[a]
Lateral prefrontal region	Impaired verbal intellect; defective recency and frequency judgments for verbal material; defective verbal fluency; impaired "executive functions"	Impaired nonverbal intellect; defective recency and frequency judgments for nonverbal material; defective design fluency; impaired "executive functions"

[a]Condition is similar for left-sided and right-sided lesions; bilateral lesions produce a more severe version of the same condition.

writing. By contrast, language comprehension is relatively preserved. A CT of a typical person with Broca's aphasia is illustrated in Figure 3–8.

Lesions in structures anterior, superior, and deep to Broca's area, but sparing most or all of areas 44 and 45, will commonly produce transcortical motor aphasia (Rubens 1976), which resembles Broca's aphasia except that a repetition defect is absent. In the right hemisphere, lesions to the frontal operculum have been linked to defects in paralinguistic communication, but propositional speech and language are not affected (Ross 1981). Specifically, patients may lose the ability to implement normal patterns of prosody and gesturing; their communication is characterized by flat, monotone speech, loss of spontaneous gesturing, and impaired ability to repeat affective contours (e.g., to implement emotional tones in speech, such as happiness or sadness).

Superior Mesial Region

The superior mesial aspect of the frontal lobes comprises a set of structures that are critical for the initiation of movement and emotional expression. The supplementary motor area (the mesial aspect of area 6) and anterior cingulate (area 24) cortices are especially important (Figure 3–7). Lesions in this region produce a syndrome of *akinetic mutism* (A. R. Damasio and Van Hoesen 1983), in which the patient makes no effort to communicate, either verbally or by gesture, and maintains an empty, noncommunicative facial expression. Movements are limited to tracking of moving targets with the eyes and body and arm movements connected with daily necessities such as eating, pulling up bedclothes, and going to the bathroom. There does not appear to be a significant difference in the profile of akinetic mutism as a function of side of lesion; left- and right-sided lesions lead to more or less equivalent defects.

Inferior Mesial Region

Inferiorly, the mesial aspect of the frontal lobes can be subdivided into the orbital region (areas 11 and 12) and the basal forebrain, which forms the most posterior extension of the inferior mesial region (Figure 3–7). The neuropsychological correlates of these regions are quite different.

Basal forebrain. The basal forebrain comprises a set of bilateral paramidline gray nuclei that includes the septal nuclei, the diagonal band of Broca, the nucleus accumbens, and the substantia innominata. Lesions to this area, commonly caused by the rupture of aneurysms located in the anterior communicating artery or in the anterior cerebral artery, cause a distinctive neuropsychological syndrome in which memory defects figure most prominently (Alexander and Freedman 1983; A. R. Damasio et al. 1985b; A. R. Damasio et al. 1989c).

The amnesic profile of basal forebrain patients has several intriguing features. It is characterized by an impairment in the integration of modal stimuli, so that patients are able to learn and recall separate aspects of entities and events, but cannot associate these into an integrated memory. Another frequent manifestation in basal forebrain patients is the proclivity for confabulation. The fabrications have a dreamlike quality and occur spontaneously (i.e., they are not prompted by the need to fill gaps of missing

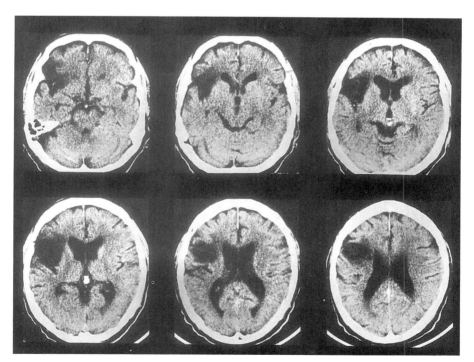

Figure 3–8.   Computed tomography (CT) scan of a 76-year-old, right-handed man who developed Broca's aphasia after a left frontal infarction. The lesion, showing as a well-defined area of low density, is squarely in the heart of "Broca's area" (i.e., the frontal opercular region formed by areas 44 and 45).

information in attempting to respond to an examiner's questions). The memory defects of basal forebrain patients can persist well into the phase of recovery, so that even after many years patients will continue to manifest learning and recall deficits and a tendency to confabulate.

Orbital region.   The orbital and lower mesial frontal cortices (including cytoarchitectonic fields 11, 12, 25, 32, and the mesial aspect of fields 10 and 9; see Figure 3–7) form the ventromedial frontal lobe, and a number of important neuropsychological correlates have been established for this region. Patients with ventromedial damage, provided the lesion does not extend into the basal forebrain, do not generally develop memory disturbances. In fact, such patients are remarkably free of conventional neuropsychological defects. Patient E.V.R., initially described by Eslinger and Damasio (1985), is prototypical (Figure 3–9). Findings from E.V.R., together with observations of several other similar patients (Ackerly and Benton 1948; Brickner 1934, 1936; Hebb and Penfield 1940), have revealed that ventromedial frontal damage causes a severe disruption of social conduct, including defects in planning, judgment, and decision making, although there may be little or nothing deficient in formal neuropsychological testing (Stuss and Benson 1986). E.V.R., for example, retained superior intellectual and memory capacities following bilateral frontal lobe resection for removal of an orbitofrontal meningioma; however, his social conduct after surgery was marked by numerous instances of inappropriate behavior, disastrous judgment,

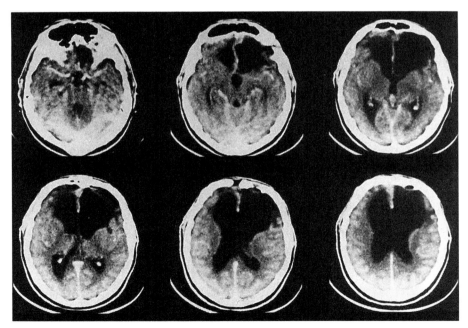

Figure 3–9.   Computed tomography (CT) scan of a 44-year-old, right-handed man who underwent resection of a large orbitofrontal meningioma. The lesion, showing as an area of low density, comprises bilateral destruction of the orbital and lower mesial frontal cortices. The basal forebrain is spared. The man developed severe changes in personality but did not manifest defects in conventional neuropsychological procedures.

and impaired interpersonal relationships. The importance of these developments in patient E.V.R. is underscored by the fact that he had been virtually flawless in these domains before his brain damage; he had been a model citizen, with a sound marriage and good standing in his community and in his profession.

Other patients have been described in whom a severe defect in social conduct followed bilateral ventromedial frontal lobe lesions (Anderson et al. 1988; A. R. Damasio et al. 1989d). As in patient E.V.R., these patients maintained normal or near-normal levels of performance in most areas of neuropsychological functioning, including intellect, memory, perception, and language, and none suffered from a social conduct disorder before the onset of brain damage. One theory posits that the social conduct disorder arises because these patients have lost the ability to activate somatic states (i.e., " feeling" states) that were learned in connection with reward and punishment. When confronted with social stimulus configurations, they cannot access critical guideposts that would normally assist in selection of appropriate and advantageous responses. Preliminary testing of this theory has revealed that ventromedial damaged patients have defective autonomic responses to socially charged stimuli (A. R. Damasio et al. 1990c).

Lateral Prefrontal Region

The dorsolateral aspect of the frontal lobes comprises a vast expanse of cortex that occupies cytoarchitectonic areas 8, 9, 46, and 10 (Figure 3–7). The functions of the lateral prefrontal region exclusive of the frontal operculum and other language-related structures discussed above are not well understood. Presumably, this region is involved in higher-order integrative and executive control functions; damage to this sector has been linked to intellectual deficits (see Stuss and Benson 1986). Another manifestation is memory impairment that affects judgments of recency and frequency of events, but not the content of the events.

The dorsolateral frontal cortices have been linked to the verbal regulation of behavior (Luria 1969). Verbal fluency, as measured by the ability to generate word lists under certain stimulus constraints, is notably impaired in many patients with dorsolateral lesions, especially when lesions are bilateral or on the left side (Benton 1968). Unilateral right dorsolateral lesions may impair fluency in the nonverbal domain. Finally, deficits on laboratory tests of "executive function," measuring ability to form, maintain, and change cognitive sets, as well as the tendency to perseverate (e.g., the Wisconsin Card Sorting Test), are usually maximal with dorsolateral lesions, although by no means specific (Anderson et al. 1991; Milner 1963).

SUBCORTICAL STRUCTURES

Two sets of subcortical structures are discussed here: the basal ganglia and the thalamus. A summary of neuropsychological manifestations of damage to these structures is presented in Table 3–5.

Basal Ganglia

The basal ganglia are a set of deep gray nuclear structures, the putamen and caudate. On the left side, lesions to these structures produce a speech and language disturbance that involves a mixture of manifestations not easily classified according to standard aphasia nomenclature; hence, the pattern is known as *atypical aphasia* (A. R. Damasio et al. 1982a; Naeser et al. 1982).This aphasia is characterized by speech that is usually fluent but paraphasic and dysarthric; auditory comprehension is typically poor, and in some cases repetition is impaired. Patients with basal ganglia lesions and aphasia tend to show very good recovery (H. Damasio et al. 1984). An MRI of a patient with a basal ganglia lesion and atypical aphasia is shown in Figure 3–10.

Thalamus

Disturbances of speech and language have been linked to damage in the dominant thalamus (Mohr et al. 1975). This language disorder tends to be primarily a deficit at the semantic level, with prominent word-finding impairment, defective confrontation naming, and semantic paraphasias. This pattern has a number of resemblances to the transcortical aphasias; it has been linked to damage in anterior thalamic nuclei (Graff-Radford and Damasio 1984; Graff-Radford et al. 1985).

Another well-studied neuropsychological correlate of thalamic lesions is memory impairment. In the setting of chronic alcoholism and the development of

Table 3–5.   Neuropsychological manifestations of subcortical lesions

Basal ganglia	Atypical aphasia (left-sided lesions); dysarthria; aprosodia
Thalamus	Thalamic aphasia (left-sided lesions); anterograde amnesia with confabulation; retrograde amnesia with temporal gradient; impairments in "executive functions"; attention/concentration defects

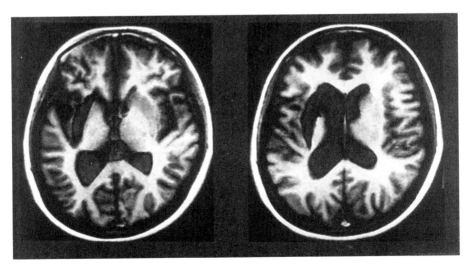

Figure 3–10.   T1-weighted magnetic resonance image (MRI) of a 35-year-old, right-handed woman who sustained a subcortical hemorrhage. The lesion, showing as an area of black on these transverse cuts, involves the left basal ganglia, including the head and body of the caudate nucleus, and part of the putamen. The woman had a characteristic "basal ganglia" type aphasia, with marked dysarthria and mixed linguistic impairments.

Korsakoff's syndrome, such lesions typically involve the dorsomedial nucleus of the thalamus along with other diencephalic structures, such as the mammillary bodies. The amnesic profile associated with such lesions has been extensively investigated (Butters 1984; Victor et al. 1989). In general, such patients develop a severe antero-grade amnesia that covers all forms of declarable information; however, similar to patients such as H.M. and Boswell, learning of perceptuomotor skills is spared. A distinctive feature of patients with Korsakoff's syndrome is their tendency to confab-ulate when asked direct questions regarding recent memory (Victor et al. 1989).

Thalamic lesions occurring as a consequence of stroke can also produce signifi-cant amnesia (Graff-Radford et al. 1985). Memory impairment is most severe when the lesions are anterior and bilateral (Graff-Radford et al. 1990b). Such lesions, which may interfere with hippocampal-related neural systems (e.g., the mammillothalamic tract) and with amygdala-related systems (e.g., the ventroamygdalofugal pathway), produce an amnesic profile characterized by severe anterograde amnesia which spares nondeclarative learning, and a retrograde defect which is temporally graded. Posterior thalamic lesions, even when bilateral, are not associated with significant or lasting amnesia (Graff-Radford et al. 1990b).

CONCLUSIONS

Understanding the salient neuropsychological correlates of variously placed cere-bral lesions is of obvious importance for the accurate diagnosis and effective man-agement of patients who suffer brain injury. Another consideration, of no less importance, is the relevance of such understanding for the development of theoret-ical formulations regarding brain-behavior relationships (A. R. Damasio 1989). As our understanding advances, it becomes increasingly important to appreciate the significance of both sides of the brain-behavior equation and to realize that no ap-proach that emphasizes one side to the exclusion of the other can be ultimately successful.

REFERENCES

Ackerly SS, Benton AL: Report of a case of bilateral frontal lobe defect. Research Publication of the Association for Research in Nervous and Mental Disease 27:479–504, 1948

Alexander MP, Freedman M: Amnesia after anterior communicating artery rupture. Neurology 33 (suppl 2):104, 1983

Anderson SW, Tranel D: Awareness of disease states following cerebral infarction, dementia, and head trauma: standardized assessment. The Clinical Neuropsychologist 3:327–339, 1989

Anderson SW, Damasio H, Tranel D, et al: Neuropsychological correlates of bilateral frontal lobe lesions in humans. Society for Neuroscience Abstracts 14:1288, 1988

Anderson SW, Damasio H, Tranel D: Neuropsychological impairments associated with lesions caused by tumor or stroke. Arch Neurol 47:397–405, 1990

Anderson SW, Damasio H, Jones RD, et al: Wisconsin Card Sorting Test performance as a measure of frontal lobe damage. J Clin Exp Neuropsychol 13:909–922, 1991

Babinski J: Contribution a l'etude des troubles mentaux dans l'hemiplegie organique cerebrale (agnosognosie). Rev Neurol 27:845–847, 1914

Benson DF: Aphasia, Alexia, and Agraphia. London, Churchill Livingstone, 1979

Benson DF: Classical syndromes of aphasia, in Handbook of Neuropsychology, Vol 1. Edited by Boller F, Grafman J. Amsterdam, Elsevier, 1989, pp 267–280

Benson DF, Brown J, Tomlinson EB: Varieties of alexia. Neurology 21:951–957, 1971

Benson DF, Sheremata WA, Bouchard R, et al: Conduction aphasia: a clinicopathological study. Arch Neurol 28:339–346, 1973

Benton AL: Differential behavioral effects in frontal lobe disease. Neuropsychologia 6:53–60, 1968

Benton AL: Visuoperceptual, visuospatial, and visuoconstructive disorders, in Clinical Neuropsychology, 2nd Edition. Edited by Heilman KM, Valenstein E. New York, Oxford University Press, 1985, pp 151–186

Benton AL: Neuropsychology: Past, present, and future, in Handbook of Neuropsychology, Vol 1. Edited by Boller F, Grafman J. Amsterdam, Elsevier, 1988, pp 1–27

Benton AL: Facial recognition 1990. Cortex 26:491–499, 1990

Benton AL, Tranel D: Visuoperceptual, visuospatial, and visuoconstructive disorders, in Clinical Neuropsychology, 3rd Edition. Edited by Heilman KM, Valenstein E. New York, Oxford University Press, 1993

Brickner RM: An interpretation of frontal lobe function based upon the study of a case of partial bilateral frontal lobectomy. Research Publication of the Association for Research in Nervous and Mental Disease 13:259–351, 1934

Brickner RM: The Intellectual Functions of the Frontal Lobes: Study Based Upon Observation of a Man After Partial Bilateral Frontal Lobectomy. New York, Macmillan, 1936

Butters N: Alcoholic Korsakoff's syndrome: an update. Semin Neurol 4:226–244, 1984

Caselli RJ: Rediscovering tactile agnosia. Mayo Clin Proc 66:129–142, 1991

Corbetta M, Miezin FM, Dobmeyer S, et al: Attentional modulation of neural processing of shape, color, and velocity in humans. Science 248:1556–1559, 1990

Corkin S: Tactually guided maze learning in man: effects of unilateral cortical excisions and bilateral hippocampal lesions. Neuropsychologia 3:339–351, 1965

Corkin S: Acquisition of motor skill after bilateral medial temporal-lobe excision. Neuropsychologia 6:255–264, 1968

Corkin S: Lasting consequences of bilateral medial temporal lobectomy: clinical course and experimental findings in HM. Semin Neurol 4:249–259, 1984

Damasio AR: Disorders of complex visual processing: agnosias, achromatopsia, Balint's syndrome, and related difficulties of orientation and construction, in Principles of Behavioral Neurology. Edited by Mesulam M-M. Philadelphia, PA, FA Davis, 1985, pp 259–288

Damasio AR: Time-locked multiregional retroactivation: a systems-level proposal for the neural substrates of recall and recognition. Cognition 33:25–62, 1989

Damasio AR: Category-related recognition defects as a clue to the neural substrates of knowledge. Trends Neurosci 13:95–98, 1990

Damasio AR, Damasio H: Anatomical basis of pure alexia. Neurology 33:1573–1583, 1983

Damasio AR, Van Hoesen GW: Emotional disturbances associated with focal lesions of the limbic frontal lobe, in Neuropsychology of Human Emotion. Edited by Heilman KM, Satz P. New York, Guilford, 1983, pp 85–110

Damasio AR, Yamada T, Damasio H, et al: Central achromatopsia: behavioral, anatomical, and physiologic aspects. Neurology 30:1064–1071, 1980

Damasio AR, Damasio H, Rizzo M, et al: Aphasia with lesions in the basal ganglia and internal capsule. Arch Neurol 39:15–20, 1982a

Damasio AR, Damasio H, Van Hoesen GW: Prosopagnosia: anatomic basis and behavioral mechanisms. Neurology 32:331–341, 1982b

Damasio AR, Eslinger P, Damasio H, et al: Multimodal amnesic syndrome following bilateral temporal and basal forebrain damage. Arch Neurol 42:252–259, 1985a

Damasio AR, Graff-Radford NR, Eslinger PJ, et al: Amnesia following basal forebrain lesions. Arch Neurol 42:263–271, 1985b

Damasio AR, Damasio H, Tranel D, et al: Additional neural and cognitive evidence in patient DRB. Society for Neuroscience Abstracts 13:1452, 1987

Damasio AR, Tranel D, Damasio H: "Deep" prosopagnosia: a new form of acquired face recognition defect caused by left hemisphere damage. Neurology 38 (suppl 1):172, 1988

Damasio AR, Damasio H, Tranel D, et al: Effects of selective visual cortex lesions in humans. Paper presented at the 12th annual meeting of the European Neurological Association and 21st annual meeting of the European Brain and Behaviour Society, Turin, Italy, September 1989a

Damasio AR, Tranel D, Damasio H: Disorders of visual recognition, in Handbook of Neuropsychology, Vol 2. Edited by Boller F, Grafman J. Amsterdam, Elsevier, 1989b, pp 317–332

Damasio AR, Tranel D, Damasio H: Amnesia caused by herpes simplex encephalitis, infarctions in basal forebrain, Alzheimer's disease, and anoxia, in Handbook of Neuropsychology, Vol 3. Edited by Boller F, Grafman J. Amsterdam, Elsevier, 1989c, pp 149–166

Damasio AR, Tranel D, Damasio H: Recognition of complex social configurations is impaired by frontal lobe lesions. J Clin Exp Neuropsychol 11:55, 1989d

Damasio AR, Damasio H, Tranel D: Impairments of visual recognition as clues to the processes of categorization and memory, in Signal and Sense: Local and Global Order in Perceptual Maps. Edited by Edelman GM, Gall WE, Cowan WM. New York, Wiley-Liss, 1990a, pp 451–473

Damasio AR, Tranel D, Damasio H: Face agnosia and the neural substrates of memory. Ann Rev Neurosci 13:89–109, 1990b

Damasio AR, Tranel D, Damasio H: Individuals with sociopathic behavior caused by frontal damage fail to respond autonomically to social stimuli. Behav Brain Res 41:81–94, 1990c

Damasio AR, Damasio H, Tranel D, et al: Neural regionalization of knowledge access: preliminary evidence, in Cold Spring Harbor Symposia on Qualitative Biology, Vol LV. Cold Spring Harbor, NY, Cold Spring Harbor Laboratory Press, 1990d, pp 1039–1047

Damasio H: Neuroimaging contributions to the understanding of aphasia, in Handbook of Neuropsychology, Vol 2. Edited by Boller F, Grafman J. Amsterdam, Elsevier, 1989, pp 3–46

Damasio H, Damasio AR: The anatomical basis of conduction aphasia. Brain 103:337–350, 1980

Damasio H, Damasio AR: Lesion Analysis in Neuropsychology. New York, Oxford University Press, 1989

Damasio H, Eslinger P, Adams HP: Aphasia following basal ganglia lesions: new evidence. Semin Neurol 4:151–161, 1984

Davidoff JB, Donnelly N: Object superiority: a comparison of complete and part probes. Acta Psychol 73(3):225–243, 1990

Eslinger PJ, Damasio AR: Severe disturbance of higher cognition after bilateral frontal lobe ablation: patient EVR. Neurology 35:1731–1741, 1985

Frisk V, Milner B: The relationship of working memory to the immediate recall of stories following unilateral temporal or frontal lobectomy. Neuropsychologia 28:121–135, 1990

Gabrieli JDE, Cohen NJ, Corkin S: The impaired learning of semantic knowledge following bilateral medial temporal-lobe resection. Brain Cogn 7:157–177, 1988

Geschwind N: Disconnexion syndromes in animals and man. Brain 88:237–294, 585–644, 1965

Graff-Radford NR, Damasio H: Disturbances of speech and language associated with thalamic dysfunction. Semin Neurol 4:162–168, 1984

Graff-Radford NR, Damasio H, Yamada T, et al: Nonhemorrhagic thalamic infarctions: clinical, neurophysiological and electrophysiological findings in four anatomical groups defined by CT. Brain 108:485–516, 1985

Graff-Radford NR, Damasio AR, Hyman BT, et al: Progressive aphasia in a patient with Pick's disease: a neuropsychological, radiologic, and anatomic study. Neurology 40:620–626, 1990a

Graff-Radford NR, Tranel D, Van Hoesen GW, et al: Diencephalic amnesia. Brain 113:1–25, 1990b

Greenblatt SH: Alexia without agraphia or hemianopia: anatomical analysis of an autopsied case. Brain 96:307–316, 1973

Greenblatt SH: Localization of lesions in alexia, in Localization in Neuropsychology. Edited by Kertesz A. New York, Academic, 1983, pp 323–356

Haist F, Squire LR, Damasio AR: Extensive retrograde amnesia in two severely amnesic patients on tests of familiarity and name completion ability. Society for Neuroscience Abstracts 16:287, 1990

Hebb DO, Penfield W: Human behavior after extensive bilateral removals from the frontal lobes. Archives of Neurology and Psychiatry 44:421–438, 1940

Heilman KM, Valenstein E, Watson RT: Localization of neglect, in Localization in Neuropsychology. Edited by Kertesz A. New York, Academic, 1983, pp 471–492

Hubel DH, Livingstone MS: Segregation of form, color, and stereopsis in primate area 18. J Neurosci 7:3378–3415, 1987

Lissauer H: Ein Fall von Seelenblindheit nebst einem Beitrag zur Theorie derselben. Arch Psychiatr Nervenkr 21:22–70, 1890

Livingstone MS, Hubel DH: Anatomy and physiology of a color system in the primate visual cortex. J Neurosci 4:309–356, 1984

Livingstone MS, Hubel DH: Psychological evidence for separate channels for the perception of form, color, movement, and depth. J Neurosci 7:3416–3468, 1987

Livingstone MS, Hubel DH: Segregation of form, color, movement, and depth: anatomy, physiology, and perception. Science 240:740–749, 1988

Lueck CJ, Zeki S, Friston KJ, et al: The color centre in the cerebral cortex of man. Nature 340:386–389, 1989

Luria AR: Frontal lobe syndromes, in Handbook of Clinical Neurology, Vol 2. Edited by Vinken PG, Bruyn GW. North Holland, Amsterdam, 1969, pp 725–757

Meadows JC: Disturbed perception of colors associated with localized cerebral lesions. Brain 97:615–632, 1974a

Meadows JC: The anatomical basis of prosopagnosia. J Neurol Neurosurg Psychiatry 37:489–501, 1974b

Milner B: Effects of different brain lesions on card sorting: the role of the frontal lobes. Arch Neurol 9:90–100, 1963

Milner B: Visual recognition and recall after right temporal-lobe excision in man. Neuropsychologia 6:191–209, 1968

Milner B: Disorders of learning and memory after temporal lobe lesions in man. Clin Neurosurg 19:421–446, 1972

Mishkin M: Memory in monkeys severely impaired by combined but not separate removal of amygdala and hippocampus. Nature 273:297–298, 1978

Mohr JP, Watters WC, Duncan GW: Thalamic hemorrhage and aphasia. Brain Lang 2:3–17, 1975

Murray EA: Representational memory in nonhuman primates, in Neurobiology of Comparative Cognition. Edited by Kesner RP, Olton DS. Hillsdale, NJ, Lawrence Erlbaum Associates, 1990, pp 127–155

Murray EA, Mishkin M: Severe tactual as well as visual memory deficits follow combined removal of the amygdala and hippocampus in monkeys. J Neurosci 4:2565–2580, 1984

Murray EA, Mishkin M: Amygdalectomy impairs crossmodal association in monkeys. Science 228:604–606, 1985

Murray EA, Mishkin M: Visual recognition in monkeys following rhinal cortical ablations combined with either amygdalectomy or hippocampectomy. J Neurosci 6:1991–2003, 1986

Naeser MA, Alexander MP, Helm-Estabrooks N, et al: Aphasia with predominantly subcortical lesion sites. Arch Neurol 39:2–14, 1982

Penfield W, Roberts L: Speech and Brain Mechanisms. Princeton, NJ, Princeton University Press, 1959

Rapcsak SZ, Kaszniak AW, Rubens AB: Anomia for facial expressions: evidence for a category specific visual-verbal disconnection syndrome. Neuropsychologia 27:1031–1041, 1989

Rizzo M: Astereopsis, in Handbook of Neuropsychology, Vol 2. Edited by Boller F, Grafman J. Amsterdam, Elsevier, 1989, pp 415–427

Rizzo M, Hurtig R: Looking but not seeing: attention, perception, and eye movements in simultanagnosia. Neurology 37:1642–1648, 1987

Rosch E, Mervis CB, Gray WD, et al: Basic objects in natural categories. Cognitive Psychology 8:382–439, 1976

Ross ED: The aprosodias: functional-anatomic organization of the affective components of language in the right hemisphere. Arch Neurol 38:561–569, 1981

Rubens AB: Transcortical motor aphasia, in Studies in Neurolinguistics, Vol 1. Edited by Whitaker H, Whitaker HA. New York, Academic, 1976, pp 293–303

Sagar HJ, Gabrieli JDE, Sullivan EV, et al: Recency and frequency discrimination in the amnesic patient HM. Brain 113:581–602, 1990

Scoville WB, Milner B: Loss of recent memory after bilateral hippocampal lesions. J Neurol Neurosurg Psychiatry 20:11–21, 1957

Semenza C, Zettin M: Evidence from aphasia for the role of proper names as pure referring expressions. Nature 342:678–679, 1989

Smith ML, Milner B: Right hippocampal impairment in the recall of spatial location: encoding deficit or rapid forgetting? Neuropsychologia 27:71–81, 1989

Stuss DT, Benson DF: The Frontal Lobes. New York, Raven, 1986

Teuber H-L: Alteration of perception and memory in man: reflections on methods, in Analysis of Behavioral Change. Edited by Weiskrantz L. New York, Harper & Row, 1968

Tranel D: Dissociated verbal and nonverbal retrieval and learning following left anterior temporal damage. Brain Cogn 15:187–200, 1991a

Tranel D: What has been rediscovered in "Rediscovering tactile agnosia"? Mayo Clin Proc 66:210–214, 1991b

Tranel D, Hyman BT: Neuropsychological correlates of bilateral amygdala damage. Arch Neurol 47:349–355, 1990

Tranel D, Damasio AR, Damasio H: Intact recognition of facial expression, gender, and age in patients with impaired recognition of face identity. Neurology 38:690–696, 1988

Van Lancker D, Kreiman J: Unfamiliar voice discrimination and familiar voice recognition are independent and unordered abilities. Neuropsychologia 25:829–834, 1988

Van Lancker D, Cummings J, Kreiman J, et al: Phonagnosia: a dissociation between familiar and unfamiliar voices. Cortex 24:195–209, 1988

Victor M, Adams RD, Collins GH: The Wernicke-Korsakoff Syndrome and Related Neurologic Disorders Due to Alcoholism and Malnutrition, 2nd Edition. Philadelphia, PA, FA Davis, 1989

Vignolo LA: Auditory agnosia. Philos Trans R Soc Lond [Biol] 298:49–57, 1982

Warrington EK, McCarthy RA: Categories of knowledge: further fractionations and an attempted integration. Brain 110:1273–1296, 1987

Warrington EK, Shallice T: Category specific semantic impairments. Brain 107:829–854, 1984

Zola-Morgan S, Squire LR, Amaral DG: Human amnesia and the medial temporal region: enduring memory impairment following a bilateral lesions limited to field CA1 of the hippocampus. J Neurosci 6:2950–2967, 1986

Zola-Morgan S, Squire LR, Amaral DG, et al: Lesions of perirhinal and parahippocampal cortex that spare the amygdala and hippocampal formation produce severe memory impairment. J Neurosci 9:4355–4370, 1989

Section II

Neuropsychiatric Assessment

Chapter 4

Bedside Neuropsychiatry: Eliciting the Clinical Phenomena of Neuropsychiatric Illness

Fred Ovsiew, M.D.

This chapter is designed to provide the neuropsychiatric clinician with a scheme for gathering data at the bedside. To this end, in this chapter I review the tools offered by history taking and examination for discovering the contribution of cerebral dysfunction to psychological abnormality.

TAKING THE HISTORY

Obtaining a history is an active process on the part of the interviewer, who must have in mind a matrix to be filled in with information. Discovering that the patient is unable to give an adequate account of his or her life and illness should prompt, first, a search for other informants, and, second, a search for an explanation of the incapacity.

Birth history.   The neuropsychiatric history begins even before birth. Maternal illness in pregnancy and the process of labor and delivery must be reviewed with an eye to untoward events associated with fetal maldevelopment. The neuropsychiatrist must inquire about maternal illness, bleeding, and substance abuse during pregnancy; the course of labor; and fetal distress at birth and in the immediate postnatal period. Such complications are associated with neurological signs at birth, though these signs may be subtle and not apparent on the ordinary examination of the newborn (Prechtl 1967).

Developmental history.   At times the historian can gather information from the first few seconds of extrauterine life, for example when Apgar scores are available in hospital records. More commonly, the examiner must rely on parental recollection of milestones: the age at which the child crawled, walked, spoke words, spoke sentences, went to school, and so on. Parents may be able to compare the patient with a "control" sibling. The infant's temperament may give clues to persisting traits. School performance is an important marker of both the intellectual and the social competence of

The author thanks Jeffrey Cummings, M.D., and Philip Gorelick, M.D., for their helpful critiques and Professor W. Alwyn Lishman for his critique and for his examples and encouragement.

the child, and often it is the only information available about premorbid intellectual level. Childhood illness, including febrile convulsions, head injury, and central nervous system infection, is sometimes the precursor of adult neuropsychiatric disorder.

Handedness.   At the bedside, the simplest and most obvious indicator of cerebral dominance is handedness. Numerous questionnaires are available, though their psychometric properties leave something to be desired (Bryden 1977). Fortunately, a few simple inquiries yield information that has an excellent correlation with behavioral observation. Asking the patient which hand he or she uses to write, throw, draw, and use a scissors or toothbrush (Bryden 1977) serves well to establish handedness. With some nonverbal patients (e.g., severely mentally retarded patients), throwing a ball or a crumpled piece of paper to the patient allows a simple examination for handedness.

History of ictal events.   Many sorts of spells or attacks occur in neuropsychiatric patients, and taking the history of a paroxysmal event has certain requirements regardless of the nature of the event. Ounsted et al. (1987) have argued that attacks of many types—ranging from a sneeze through orgasm to the epileptic seizure—share characteristics because they represent the nervous system's "going absolute." The clinician must be concerned with the phases of the paroxysm, starting with a prodrome, then the aura, then the remainder of the ictus (the aura being the onset or core of the ictus), and finally the aftermath. For any attack disorder, it must be determined how frequent and stereotyped the events are. Rapidity of onset and offset; disturbance of consciousness or of language; the occurrence of autochthonous sensations, ideas, and emotions and of lateralized motor dysfunction; the purposefulness and coordination of actions; memory for the spell; and the duration of the recovery period must be ascertained.

I begin the seizure inquiry by asking if the patient has just one sort of spell or more than one. This reduces confusion for the patient who has both partial and generalized seizures, and many patients with pseudoseizures will say in nearly so many words that they have epileptic spells and then the other sort that happens when they are upset. Adverse mood changes commonly occur on the days preceding a seizure (Blanchet and Frommer 1986), but remarkably little is understood of the mechanism of such prodromes to seizures.

History of head injury.   The length of the anterograde amnesia—from the moment of trauma to the recovery of the capacity for consecutive memory—can be learned either from the patient or from hospital records. The patient can say what the last memories before the accident are; from last memory to injury is the period of retrograde amnesia. The length of these intervals and the duration of coma are correlated with the severity of brain damage (Lishman 1987). Usually posttraumatic amnesia is the best indicator. The nature of the trauma, including its psychosocial setting, should be learned; the most important fact about a head injury can be the reckless behavior that produced it.

Alcohol and drug use.   The substance abuse history must be taken from all patients. Questions about vocational, family, and medical impairment attributable to abuse; shame and guilt over abuse and efforts to control it; morning or secret drinking; blackouts; and other issues help the clinician identify pathological behavior in this sphere.

History of mild cognitive impairment.   One commonly encounters patients with mild, chronic, stable, global cognitive disturbance who do not meet the diagnostic criteria for dementia; the most frequent condition giving rise to this state is traumatic brain injury. Lezak (1978) stressed the patients' experience of perplexity, distractibility, and fatigue in mild and severe brain injury. In my experience, some cognitive symptoms reported by patients are so characteristic as to be diagnostic of organic illness. Other features, such as the tendency to emotional lability and irritability, are characteristic of but not specific to organic states. The loss of the capacity for divided attention is highly characteristic of mild cerebral disease. Distractibility is heightened, and automatic tasks begin to require attention and effort. These symptoms were described and demonstrated many years ago (Brodal 1973; Chapman and Wolff 1958); but in our passion for localization, some of them, being dependent on the bulk of disease in the hemispheres but independent of its location, have been forgotten.

Appetitive functions.   Appetitive functions refer to sleep, eating, and sexual interest and performance. Disturbed sleep is common among patients with mental disorders of any origin, as well as in the general population. In a search for clues to organic factors, the clinician inquires about the pattern of disturbance: the early waking of depressive illness, nighttime wakenings related to pain or nocturnal myoclonus, the excessive daytime sleepiness of narcolepsy and sleep apnea, sleep attacks in narcolepsy, and the periodic excessive somnolence of the Kleine-Levin syndrome and related disorders. Loss of dreaming has been reported in association with cerebral disease (Greenberg and Farah 1986).

Patterns of abnormal eating behavior can be recognized beyond the anorexia of depressive illness and anorexia nervosa: the hyperphagia of hypothalamic disease, in which food exerts an irresistible attraction; the mouthing and eating of nonfood objects in bilateral amygdaline disease (the Klüver-Bucy syndrome); and the impulsive stuffing of food into the mouth in frontal disease.

The details of abnormal sexual performance can usually be elicited without great difficulty, and its nature can be related to the known physiology of sexual function (Boller and Frank 1982). Sexual interest (libido) is, in my view, more difficult to elucidate. Hyposexuality does seem to be a recognizable feature of epilepsy, although its mechanism is still subject to controversy (Toone et al. 1989). A change in a person's habitual sexual interests, either quantitative or qualitative, occurring de novo in adult life, may bespeak organic disease (Miller et al. 1986).

Aggression.   Patterns of aggressive behavior in brain disease have been described and related to the locus of injury (Ovsiew and Yudofsky 1993), and epileptic violence has been clearly described (Fenwick 1989). Features of aggressive behavior such as its onset and offset; the patient's mental state and especially clarity of consciousness during the violent period; his (and it is usually males in question) capacity for planned, coordinated, and well-organized action as displayed in the act; his regret or otherwise afterward; and any associated symptoms may yield clues to the contribution of cerebral dysfunction to the behavior.

Personality change.   Persisting alterations in or exaggerations of personality traits, if not related to an abnormal affective state or psychosis, may be important indicators of the development of cerebral disease. A particular set of changes in personality traits is said to be distinctive in temporal lobe epilepsy. These include the development of mystical or religious interests, a shorter temper, and hyposexuality. Whether these traits are related to epilepsy, to the temporal lobe injury underlying epilepsy, or merely to psychopathology remains controversial (Bear et al. 1989).

Occupational history.   The relationship of occupational hazards to illness is an entire medical specialty, and an outline for the elicitation of relevant information has been prepared (Occupational and Environmental Health Committee of the American Lung Association of San Diego and Imperial Counties 1983). Exposures to heavy metals or volatile hydrocarbons and repeated blows to the head in boxers are examples of occupational causes of neuropsychiatric illness. Apart from etiological information, the clinician needs to know about the patient's work in order to gauge premorbid capacities and to assess disability.

Family history.   Genetic contributors to many neuropsychiatric illnesses are well delineated (e.g., in Huntington's disease); in others the contribution is probable but the mechanism less clear (e.g., in Tourette's syndrome). In epilepsy, there appears to be genetic transmission of a seizure threshold, so that even with a known cerebral insult the family history of epilepsy influences whether seizures occur (Engel 1989). Inquiring about the family history of neuropsychiatric illness relative by relative, even constructing a family tree with the assistance of collateral informants, reveals more relevant information than probes such as "Is there any mental illness in the family?"

EXAMINING THE PATIENT

The British neurologist Henry Miller (1975) referred to psychiatry as "neurology without physical signs." Geoffrey Lloyd (1983) called psychosomatics "medicine without signs." Neuropsychiatry can be considered "psychiatry with signs." The neuropsychiatric examination seeks signs of cerebral dysfunction. Sometimes clinicians attempt to elicit not signs of brain disease but so-called positive signs of nonorganic states. Vibratory sensation that shows lateralized deficit on the sternum is an example. These signs are of limited use, not because they are uncommon in hysteria, but because suggestibility is common in organic mental states as well (Gould et al. 1986). This discussion focuses on the scientific basis for inference from the clinician's observations in the examination room to encourage the thoughtful use of probes guided by specific hypotheses about brain dysfunction.

General Appearance

Asymmetry.   Abnormal development of a hemisphere may be betrayed by slight differences in the size of the thumbs or thumbnails. Occasionally this can be a lateralizing sign in epilepsy.

Minor physical anomalies.   Table 4–1 lists minor physical anomalies that are stable through childhood and presumably into adulthood. They may occur in subjects with no neuropsychiatric illness; no individual anomaly, except perhaps head circumference (Steg and Rapoport 1975), has a correlation with psychopathology. The deviation can be confidently traced to the first 4 months of fetal life, and a correlation with both paternal psychopathology and obstetric complications suggests that either genetic or traumatic factors can give rise to the disturbance of gestation (Firestone and Peters 1983). Presumably the relationship of the anomalies to the brain disorder lies in a subtle disturbance of cerebral development occurring at the same period of gestation. Such abnormalities have been shown to correlate with the presence of schizophrenia, especially with early onset of illness and poor premorbid functioning (Green et al. 1989; Gualtieri et al. 1982); autism (Gualtieri et al. 1982; Steg and Rapoport 1975); impulsive, hyperactive, and aggressive behavior in male children (Fogel et al. 1985; Gualtieri et al. 1982) and perhaps inhibitedness in female children (Fogel et al. 1985); and recidivistic criminal violence (Kandel et al. 1989).

Olfaction

Abnormalities of the sense of smell are not infrequent among neuropsychiatric patients and can be of functional importance and diagnostic significance. Hyposmia or anosmia can be detected in Alzheimer's disease, Parkinson's disease, normal aging, schizophrenia, multiple sclerosis, subfrontal tumor, and traumatic brain injury (Eslinger et al. 1982; Harrison and Pearson 1989; Pinching 1977). The most common cause of hyposmia, however, is local disease of the nasal mucosa, and the examiner must exclude this before regarding a finding as neuropsychiatrically significant.

The Eyes

Pupils, corneas, and irises.   The dilated pupils of anticholinergic toxicity may be a clue to the cause of delirium, the small pupils of opiate intoxication to substance abuse. Argyll Robertson pupils—bilaterally small, irregular, and reactive to accommodation but not light—are still a characteristic accompaniment of neurosyphilis in the antibiotic era (Luxon et al. 1979).

A Kayser-Fleischer ring is invariably present when Wilson's disease affects the brain, with the possible rare exception of the patient with coexisting bilateral annulus senilis (Scheinberg et al. 1986). This brownish-green discoloration of the cornea begins at the limbus, at 12 o'clock then 6 o'clock, spreading from each location medially

---

Table 4–1.   Minor physical anomalies

Head	High palate
Head circumference outside the normal range (normal male: 21"–23"; normal female: 20.5"–22.5")	Furrowed tongue
	Hands and feet
Fine "electric" hair (won't comb down)	Curved fifth finger (clinodactyly)
More than one hair whorl	Single palmar crease (as is seen in Down's syndrome)
Abnormal epicanthic folds of the eyes	
Hypertelorism or hypotelorism	Wide gap between the first and second toes
Low-set ears (entirely below plane of the pupils)	Partial syndactyly of the toes
Malformed or asymmetric ears	Third toe longer than second toe

and laterally until a complete ring is formed. Because a Kayser-Fleischer ring can be difficult to discern in patients with dark irises, slit-lamp examination should supplement bedside inspection (Marsden 1987; Walshe 1986).

Visual fields.   When lesions disrupt the white matter of the temporal lobe, a congruent homonymous upper quadrantanopsia or even a full homonymous hemianopsia can result from involvement of Meyer's loop, the portion of the optic radiation that dips into the temporal lobe (Falconer and Wilson 1958). Delirium from posterior cerebral or right middle cerebral artery infarction also has been described, with hemianopsia as a regular accompaniment (Devinsky et al. 1988).

Blinking.   The normal response to regular 1-per-second tapping on the glabella (with the examiner behind the patient so that the striking finger is not within the patient's visual field) is blinking to the first few taps, then habituation and no blinking. Karson (1988) suggested considering "about 20" blinks per minute as a normal spontaneous blink rate. The rate of spontaneous blinking seems to be under dopaminergic control (Karson 1983). This is shown by the clinical finding that blink rate is low in parkinsonism and increases with effective levodopa (L-dopa) treatment (Karson et al. 1984) and by the laboratory finding that blink rate is inversely correlated with monoamine oxidase level (Freed et al. 1980).

Stevens (1978) drew attention to abnormalities of blinking in schizophrenic patients (and reminded us that Kraepelin, among other early investigators, had already commented on them). She found high spontaneous rates of blinking, paroxysms of rapid rhythmic blinking during episodes of abnormal behavior, and abnormal responses to glabellar tap. On glabellar tap, Stevens's patients either failed to blink, produced a shower of blinks, or failed to habituate. Although her patients were drug free, few were neuroleptic naive, so she could not distinguish between an abnormality intrinsic to schizophrenia and a tardive dyskinesia.

Eye movements.   In the same report, Stevens (1978) called attention to early observations by Kraepelin and others of abnormal eye movements in psychotic patients. She noted gaze abnormalities, abnormality in eye contact with the examiner (e.g., fixed staring or no eye contact), impaired convergence movements, and irregular smooth pursuit movements (the sort of movements generated when the patient follows the examiner's finger with the eyes).

Elucidating the abnormalities of eye movement in neuropsychiatric patients requires the separate examination of voluntary eye movements without fixation ("look to the left"), generation of saccades to a target ("look at my finger, now at my fist"), and smooth pursuit movement ("follow my finger"). Early failure of vertical saccades, with intact function of the lower motor neuron, is the hallmark of progressive supranuclear palsy. The finding is of impaired voluntary eye movements, but the patient is still able to generate full upgaze and downgaze when fixing the eyes on a still target while the examiner moves the patient's head up and down (the doll's eye maneuver). Slowed or hypometric saccades are a feature of Huntington's disease. An internuclear ophthalmoplegia may reveal an illness marked by vague sensory symptoms to be multiple sclerosis. Palsies of eye movement in a confused patient may indicate Wernicke's encephalopathy. In head-eye synkinesia, the patient automatically moves the head along with the eyes in shifting gaze. This sign has been demonstrated in schizophrenia (Kolada and Pitman 1983) and is seen in dementia.

Apraxia of gaze is, like other apraxias, a failure of voluntary movement with the preserved capacity for spontaneous movement, in this case horizontal or vertical gaze. It is a feature of Balint's syndrome (De Renzi 1985). So-called apraxia of eye opening is probably an extrapyramidal disorder of lid movement (Lepore and Duvoisin 1985). The status of apraxia of eye closure is more complicated; in at least some cases, a supranuclear motor disorder affects other bulbar musculature and the designation *apraxia* is inappropriate (Ross Russell 1980). In some cases, there is a link to impersistence (discussed below) (Fisher 1956).

Facial Movement

Dissociated facial paresis.   The presence of a double dissociation in the realm of facial movement demonstrates that emotional movements and volitional ones are separately organized (Monrad-Krohn 1924). A paresis seen in movements to command ("show me your teeth") is sometimes overcome in spontaneous smiling; this indicates disease in pyramidal pathways. The inverse phenomenon—normal movement to command but asymmetry of spontaneous emotional movements—is seen with disease in thalamus (Bogousslavsky et al. 1988), temporal lobe (Remillard et al. 1977); striatum and internal capsule (Trosch et al. 1990); and premotor cortex (Laplane et al. 1976). Damasio and Maurer (1978) reported the occurrence of this sign in autism and argued that it indicated disease in limbic regions.

Facial expression.   The "omega sign" and Verraguth's folds are long-recognized facial signs of depressive illness (Figure 4–1) (Greden et al. 1985). Many brain diseases can be recognized by characteristic facial appearances (e.g., Wilson's disease and myotonic dystrophy).

Speech

Dysarthria.   In pyramidal disorders, the speech output is slow, strained, and slurred in articulation. Often accompanying the speech disorder are the other features of pseudobulbar palsy, including dysphagia, drooling, and a disturbance of the expression of emotions. Usually the causative lesions are bilateral, although the onset of the disorder may be after an acute unilateral lesion, the lesion of the opposite hemisphere having preexisted the new lesion. Unilateral lesions of the left motor cortex and frontal operculum can cause dysarthria (discussed below). Bulbar, or flaccid, dysarthria is marked by breathiness and nasality, with impaired articulation present as well. Signs of lower motor neuron involvement can be found in the bulbar musculature. The lesion is in the lower brain stem. Scanning speech is a characteristic sign of disease of the cerebellum and its connections; the speech output is irregular in rate with equalization of the stress on the syllables. In extrapyramidal disorders and in depression, speech is hypophonic and monotonous, often tailing off with longer phrases.

Stuttering.   Stuttering, or stammering, of the developmental sort has been studied extensively, but its cause is unknown. Acquired stuttering is less common and differs from the developmental variety by its occurrence on any syllable in a word (not just initial syllables) and on grammatical words as well as substantives. Anxiety and the secondary signs of a struggle to speak (e.g., grimacing), common in developmental stuttering, are absent in the acquired form (Ludlow et al. 1987).

Dysprosody. Monrad-Krohn (1947) described dysprosody or "altered melody of language" in a patient with a war-time missile injury of the left frontotemporal region. She showed aphasic troubles, mild right-sided signs, and slight personality change. Most strikingly, her speech pattern had changed, so that she sounded like a German when she spoke her native Norwegian. Later, other researchers (Tucker et al. 1977; Ross and Mesulam 1979) reported cases in which right-hemisphere lesions led to loss of the affective elements of speech. Ross (1981) schematized these syndromes—the "aprosodias"—as mirror images of left-hemisphere aphasic syndromes.

The examiner confronted with a patient who has a disturbance of prosody in spontaneous speech looks for dysarthria and aphasia. The examiner must listen for prosodic elements; ask the patient to produce statements in various emotional tones

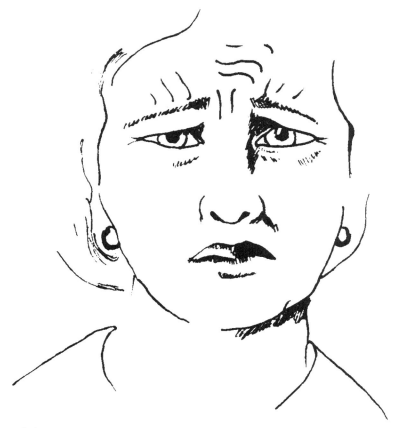

Figure 4–1. The omega sign is the o-shaped pattern of wrinkles between and above the eyebrows. Verraguth's folds are the wrinkles sloping medially above the eyebrows.
Source. Adapted from Greden et al. 1985. Used with permission.

(e.g., anger, sadness, surprise, and joy); produce such emotional phrasings himself or herself, using a neutral sentence ("I am going to the store") while turning away from the patient, and ask the patient to identify the emotion; and ask the patient to reproduce an emotional phrasing the examiner has generated. It can be seen that this duplicates the structure of the examination for disorders of propositional language.

Echolalia.   In this phenomenon, another person's speech is repeated by the patient in an automatic fashion, that is, without communicative intent or effect. Sometimes the patient repeats only the last portion of what he hears, beginning with a natural break in the utterance. Grammatical corrections may be made, if the examiner deliberately utters a grammatically incorrect sentence. The patient may make pronoun reversals (e.g., "I" for "you"), altering the sentence in a grammatically appropriate way, or may automatically complete a well-known phrase uttered by the examiner. "Roses are red," says the examiner; "roses are red, violets are blue," responds the patient. Speaking to the patient in a foreign language can elicit obviously automatic echolalic speech (Lecours et al. 1983).

The anatomic and psychopathological associations of echolalia have been reviewed (Ford 1989). Its occurrence in transcortical aphasia marks the intactness of primary language areas in the frontal and temporal lobes, with syntax thus unimpaired but disconnected from control by other cerebral functions. Autism, Tourette's syndrome, and disorders of the startle reaction are other underlying disorders. Echolalia also can be seen in catatonic states. It also occurs as a normal phenomenon in the learning of language in infancy (Lecours et al. 1983).

Palilalia.   This phenomenon is the automatic repetition of the patient's own final word or phrase, the voice trailing off in volume and festinant in rate. It can occur separately from echolalia or other disturbances of speech. It seems to be related to bilateral disease of the basal ganglia (Boller et al. 1973), although general paresis and epilepsy with a supplementary motor area focus have been implicated as well (Critchley 1927; Geschwind 1964).

Mutism.   The first step in examining an alert patient who does not speak is to discover whether the disorder is due to elementary sensorimotor abnormalities involving the apparatus of speech. These local disturbances can be recognized by examining phonation, articulation, and nonspeech movements of the relevant musculature (e.g., swallowing and coughing). If an elementary disorder is not at fault, the examination proceeds to a search for specific disturbances of verbal communication. It is necessary to determine whether the patient makes any spontaneous attempt at communication through means other than speech (e.g., gesturing, writing, arranging block letters, or using sign-language).

A wide variety of disorders can produce mutism. Some patients with lesions restricted to the lower primary motor cortex and the adjacent frontal operculum have a disorder that begins with mutism then recovers through severe dysarthria without agrammatism (Schiff et al. 1983). Lesions involving additional surrounding territory may produce language impairment proper (Alexander 1989). In transcortical motor aphasia there is a prominent disturbance of spontaneous speech, occasionally beginning as mutism (Alexander 1989).

Abnormalities of Movement

Weakness.   Caplan et al. (1990) described the features of a nonpyramidal hemimotor syndrome with caudate lesions. Patients show clumsiness and decreased spontaneous use of the affected limbs; associated movements are decreased as well. What appears on initial testing to be paresis proves to be a slow development of full strength; if coaxed and given time, the patient shows mild weakness at worst. Freund and Hummelsheim (1985) explored the motor consequences of lesions of the premotor cortex. They observed a decrease in spontaneous use of the arm and attributed it to a failure of postural fixation; when supported, the arm showed at worst mild slowing of finger movements. The defect in elevation and abduction of the arm was best demonstrated by asking the patient to swing the arms in a windmill movement. Movement rapidly decomposed when such coordination was required. Pyramidal signs (e.g., increased tendon jerks, Babinski reflex, and spasticity) may be absent in patients with these findings. Stressed gait (e.g., walking heel-to-toe or on the outer aspects of the feet) may reveal a mild asymmetry in patients without other signs.

Akinesia.   Akinesia has several aspects: delay in the initiation of movement, slowness in the execution of movement, and special difficulty with complex movements (Marsden 1986). The disturbance is conveniently examined by requiring the patient to perform a repeated action, such as tapping thumb to forefinger, or two actions at once. A decrement in amplitude or freezing in the midst of the act is observed. When established, akinesia is unmistakable in the patient's visage and demeanor, and in the way he or she sits motionlessly and has trouble rising from the chair.

Agitation.   *Agitation* refers to an increased amount of motor activity accompanying a dysphoric mood. Agitation is an important finding in confusional states, but not by any means a universal one. The term *delirium* is reserved by some for a confusional state (or "acute organic reaction") in which agitation and abnormal perceptual experiences are prominent. Why certain etiologies of confusion (e.g., alcohol withdrawal, hypoxemia, the postictal twilight state, and infarction in the territory of the posterior cerebral artery) commonly produce agitation and others do not is virtually unstudied. A hypothesis about preferential involvement of limbic brain regions is irresistible but entirely speculative.

Akathisia.   Motor restlessness accompanied by an urge to move but not by abnormal mood is referred to as *akathisia*. The difficulty of eliciting the account of subjective restlessness from a psychotic patient is well known, but it is important for the clinician to distinguish akathisia from anxious or psychotic agitation (Ball 1985). Complaints specifically referable to the legs are far more characteristic of akathisia than of anxiety (Braude et al. 1983). In addition, the objective manifestations of akathisia are characteristic (Gibb and Lees 1986). Although by derivation akathisia refers to an inability to sit, its manifestations are most prominent when the patient attempts to stand still. When required to do so, the patient shifts weight from foot to foot, producing a "marching in place" appearance. Seated, the patient may shuffle or tap the feet or repeatedly cross the legs. When the disorder is severe, the recumbent patient may show myoclonic jerks or a coarse tremor of the legs.

Hypertonus.   Three forms of increased muscle tone concern the neuropsychiatrist: spasticity, rigidity, and paratonia. In spasticity, tone is increased in flexors in the upper extremity, extensors in the lower, but not in the antagonists. The hypertonus shows the characteristic of an increase in resistance followed by an immediate decrease (the clasp-knife phenomenon) and is dependent on the velocity of the passive movement. This is the typical hemiplegic pattern of hemisphere stroke. In rigidity, tone is increased in agonists and antagonists throughout the range of motion, thus the term *lead-pipe* rigidity; the increase is not velocity dependent. This is the characteristic hypertonus of extrapyramidal disease. In paratonia, or *Gegenhalten,* increased tone is erratic and dependent on the intensity of the imposed movement (i.e., oppositional). This pattern of hypertonus is characteristically related to extensive brain dysfunction.

Dystonia.   Dystonia refers to "sustained muscle contractions, frequently causing twisting and repetitive movements, or abnormal postures" (Fahn et al. 1987, p. 335). The contractions may be generalized or focal. Typically the dystonic arm hyperpronates, with a flexed wrist and extended fingers; the dystonic lower extremity shows an inverted foot with plantar flexion. A number of syndromes of focal dystonia are well recognized, such as torticollis, writer's cramp, and blepharospasm with jaw and mouth movements (Meige syndrome). A dystonic pattern of particular interest is oculogyric crisis, in which there is forced deviation of the eyes sometimes accompanied by forced thinking or other psychological disturbance (Owens 1990). It is characteristic of dystonic movements to worsen with voluntary action and to be evoked only by very specific action patterns. Especially in an early stage or mild form of the illness, this can produce apparently bizarre symptoms, such as a patient who cannot walk because of twisting feet and legs but who is able to run. Adding to the oddness is the frequent capacity of the patient to reduce the involuntary movement by using sensory tricks (*le geste antagoniste*). Dystonia, including oculogyric crisis, can occur as an acute or tardive effect of dopamine blockade (Owens 1990).

Tremor.   All tremors are rhythmic, regular, oscillating movements around a joint. Three major forms of tremor are distinguished. In rest tremor, the movement is present distally when the limb is supported and relaxed; action reduces the intensity of the tremor. The frequency is usually low, about 4–8 cycles/second. This is the well-known tremor of parkinsonism. Because the amplitude of the tremor diminishes with action, rest tremor is usually less disabling than it might appear. In postural tremor, the outstretched limb oscillates. At times this can be better visualized by placing a piece of paper over the outstretched hand. Several forms of postural tremor have been distinguished, of varying frequencies and amplitudes. Postural tremor is produced by anxiety, certain drugs (e.g., caffeine, lithium, steroids, and adrenergic agonists for asthma), and the disease hereditary essential tremor. A coarse, irregular, rapid postural tremor is frequently seen in metabolic encephalopathy (Plum and Posner 1980). In intention tremor, the active limb oscillates more prominently as the limb approaches its target during goal-directed movements. This is seen in disease of the cerebellum and its connections. If physical maneuvers produce a change of tremor frequency (as opposed to amplitude), as when the tremulous extremity adopts the frequency of a repetitive action (e.g., finger tapping of the opposite extremity), hysteria should be suspected (Koller et al. 1989).

Chorea. Choreatic movements are "brief, random, sudden, rapid, arrhythmic, involuntary movements" (Padberg and Bruyn 1986, p. 549), which dance over the patient's body. The patient may incorporate these movements into purposeful ones, in an effort to hide the chorea when it is mild. As with dystonia, chorea may become more evident when elicited by gait or other activity. Predominantly proximal movements, large in amplitude and violent in force, are called *ballistic.*

Late-onset abnormal movements due to antipsychotic drugs—tardive dyskinesia—are usually choreatic and predominantly involve oral and facial musculature. Occasionally the movements are somewhat asymmetric (Altshuler et al. 1988). In the setting of psychosis, the clinician must not assume that chorea is tardive dyskinesia but must consider a differential diagnosis of diseases that can produce both chorea and psychosis (e.g., Wilson's disease, systemic lupus erythematosus, Huntington's disease, and Fahr's syndrome) (Hyde et al. 1991).

Myoclonus. This term refers to a complex set of abnormal movements that share suddenness as a key characteristic (Hallett and Ravits 1986). Myoclonus does not show the continuous, dancelike flow of movement that characterizes chorea. When myoclonus is rhythmic, it differs from tremor in having an interval between individual movements, a "square wave" rather than a "sine wave." The distinction of myoclonus from tic is partly based on subjective features: the individual with a tic reports a wish to move, a sense of relief after the movement, and the ability to delay the movement (albeit at the cost of increasing subjective tension). Also, tics can be more complex and stereotyped than myoclonic jerks. Some myoclonus is stimulus sensitive; stimulation such as a tap with the reflex hammer evokes a myoclonic jerk. Other forms of myoclonus are evoked by action, notably postanoxic myoclonus responsive to serotonin agonists. Myclonus can be the only pointer to noncompulsive status epilepticus as the cause of a confusional state (Tomson et al. 1992).

Tic. Tics are sudden jerks, sometimes simple (such as a blink or a grunt) but sometimes as complex as a well-organized voluntary movement (such as repeatedly touching an object or speaking a word) (Jankovic 1987). In addition to the subjective features noted above, tics differ from many other abnormal movements in persisting during sleep.

Stereotypy and mannerism. Lees (1988) offered the following definition of stereotypy: "purposeless, rhythmic, repetitive movements carried out at the expense of all other motor activity for long periods of time" (p. 258). In schizophrenia, a delusional idea associated with such abnormal movements can sometimes, but not always, be elicited (Jones 1965). Similar abnormal movements are seen in autism and in congenital blindness and severe mental retardation, but not in blindness or brain damage that is acquired late (Ridley and Baker 1982). Amphetamine intoxication is a well-recognized cause of stereotypy. Manneristic movements are purposeful movements carried out in a bizarre way, which at times make the diagnosis of schizophrenia evident from across a room.

Asterixis. Repeated momentary loss of postural tone produces a flapping movement of the outstretched hands (asterixis) originally described in the context of liver failure.

It has subsequently been recognized to occur in many or all states of metabolic encephalopathy and in all muscle groups. Young and Shahani (1986) recommended eliciting it by asking the patient to dorsiflex the index fingers for 30 seconds while the hands and arms are outstretched, with the patient watching to ensure maximum voluntary contraction. Bilateral asterixis is a very valuable sign because it points unmistakably to a toxic-metabolic confusional state. Rarely, asterixis is unilateral and reflects a lesion of contralateral thalamic, parietal, or medial frontal structures (Young and Shahani 1986).

Catatonia.   Catatonia can be defined broadly as abnormality of movement or muscle tone associated with psychosis (Fisher 1989a) or more narrowly as "at least one motor sign (catalepsy, posturing, or waxy flexibility) in combination with at least one sign of psycho-social withdrawal or excitement and/or bizarre repetitious movement (mutism, negativism, impulsiveness, grimacing, stereotypies, mannerisms, command automatism, echopraxia/echolalia or verbigeration)" (Barnes et al. 1986, p. 991).

Primitive Reflexes

The localizing value and clinical significance of primitive reflexes, such as the grasp, suck, snout, and palmomental, is incompletely understood. Landau (1989) stated that all primitive reflexes indicate widespread cerebral dysfunction with relative sparing of the primary motor cortex. Brodal (1981), however, linked the grasp reflex quite specifically with disease of the contralateral supplementary motor area. To consider them all equally as frontal release reflexes would seem to go beyond the available evidence. Some less familiar reflexes, such as the nucho-cephalic (Jenkyn et al. 1975), avoidance (Denny-Brown 1958), and self-grasping (Ropper 1982), may prove to be relatively specific and of localizing value. But overall these reflexes have probably been given too much weight in the neuropsychiatric examination, and some, such as the snout and palmomental, are useless when taken alone.

"Soft Signs"

"Soft signs" refers to a variegated set of findings taken to demonstrate impairment in sensorimotor integration and motor control (Heinrichs and Buchanan 1988). A sign presumably related to high-level integration of sensation is graphesthesia: the examiner traces numbers on the patient's hand, and the patient must read the numbers with eyes closed. Many indicators of defective control of complex motor activity have been proposed (Manschreck 1983). The bedside examiner can seek mild clumsiness by asking the patient to tap the hand or foot or perform other rapid alternating movements; motor inhibition by looking for mirror movements, discussed above; and motor control on tests of perseveration and reciprocal action programs, discussed below.

Signs of Callosal Disconnection

The history often discloses features typical of disconnection, including dissociative phenomena (e.g., between what the patient is saying and what the left hand is doing). Most remarkably the patient reports behavioral conflict between the hands or merely a sense that the left hand behaves in an alien fashion. On examination, the patient shows an inability to name odors presented to the right nostril. In visual field testing, a hemianopsia appears to be present in each hemifield alternately, opposite to the hand the patient uses to point to stimuli (e.g., when the patient uses the left hand, he or she responds only to stimuli in the left hemifield).

An apraxia of the left hand can be shown by the usual testing maneuvers. Because verbal information processed in the left hemisphere cannot be transferred to the right and because the right hemisphere has limited capacity to understand spoken commands, the patient is not able to produce appropriate responses with the left hand to spoken commands. Similarly, writing with the left hand is impossible (Geschwind and Kaplan 1962). For reciprocal reasons, the right hand shows a constructional disorder.

The patient has an anomia for unseen objects felt with the left hand. If the examiner places one of the patient's hands (again unseen) into a given posture, the patient is unable to match the posture with the other hand. Similarly the patient cannot touch with the left thumb the finger of the left hand corresponding to the finger of the right hand touched by the examiner, and vice versa.

Orientation

Although the neuropsychology of disorientation is not well elucidated (Daniel et al. 1987), it is possible for a patient to be unable to give the date or place because of an impairment in attention, memory, language, or content of thought. The neuropsychiatrist probes these mechanisms by the use of more specific tasks in order to arrive at a diagnosis. Delirious disorientation has been distinguished from delusional disorientation in Jacksonian terms by Levin (1956), who pointed out that the delirious patient mistakes the unfamiliar for the familiar—reducing the novel to the automatic—as when he reports that the hospital is a factory where he formerly worked. By contrast the schizophrenic patient mistakes the familiar for the unfamiliar, as when he locates himself on Mars.

Attention

Deficits occur in the capacity to maintain attention to external stimuli (vigilance), the capacity to attend consistently to internal stimuli (concentration), and the capacity to shift attention from one stimulus to another. Vigilance can be assessed by the patient's capacity to perform a continuous performance task; a bedside version, the "A" test, has been developed (Strub and Black 1988). The patient is presented with a string of letters, one per second, and is required to signal at each occurrence of the letter A. A single error of omission or of commission is considered abnormal. Concentration can be assessed by the patient's capacity to recite the numbers from 20 to 1. A pathognomonic error is to begin to give the ordinary forward order: "20, 19, 18, 17, 18. . . . " This amounts to a failure to inhibit the intrusion of the more familiar set.

Digit span is a classical psychological test of attention, easily performed at the bedside. The examiner recites strings of numbers, slowly, clearly, and without phrasing into chunks. The patient is required to repeat them immediately. Subsequently, the patient can be asked to repeat strings of digits after reversing them mentally. The normal forward digit span is usually considered to be a minimum of five. The backward digit span may depend on visuospatial processing and attention (Black 1986).

Neglect.   The patient who pays no attention to the left side of the body and the left side of space is one of the most dramatic phenomena in neuropsychiatry (Heilman et al. 1985). The bedside clinician can readily identify such patients; they entirely ignore one half of space, leaving their left arm out of the sleeve of their gown, the left side of their breakfast uneaten, and so on. Milder degrees of neglect can be recognized using a line bisection task (patients must place an *X* at the midpoint of a line drawn by the examiner) or a cancellation task (in which patients cross out letters or other items for which they must search on a page) (Figure 4–2). Mesulam (1981) constructed a useful network theory in which parietal cortex, frontal cortex, and cingulate cortex interact to allow attention to the opposite side of space; lesions produce distinguishable contralateral sensory neglect, directional hypokinesia, and reduction in motivational value respectively.

Hypermetamorphosis.   Wernicke (Klüver and Bucy 1939) coined the term *hypermetamorphosis* to refer to an excessive and automatic attention to environmental stim-

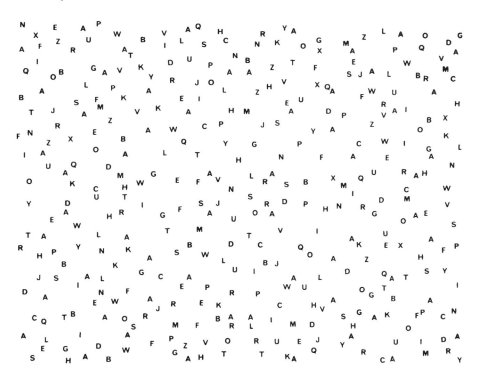

Figure 4–2.   Mesulam's letter-cancellation task. The patient must spot all the examples of a given letter in the random array and cross them out.
Source.   Reprinted from Mesulam M-M: *Principles of Behavioral Neurology.* Philadelphia, PA, FA Davis, 1985. Used with permission.

uli. For example, a patient may carry on a running commentary about elements of the environment: "You're wearing a tie, there's a picture on the wall."

Memory

The ordinary bedside testing of verbal memory can be done briefly and validly, as Kopelman (1986) has shown. Not all tests are of equal power, however. Recall of paragraph-length material after a 45-minute delay may be ideal, but recall of a name and address after several minutes is simple and satisfactory (Katzman et al. 1983; Kopelman 1986). Similar testing of figural memory at the bedside is also easily done. For example, Weintraub and Mesulam's three-words/three-shapes test (1985) compares verbal and figural memory side-by-side in a quick and simple fashion. I sometimes ask patients to recall the three directions I just pointed (using more complex directions, such as off at a diagonal, rather than up or down). Whether remote memory can be validly assessed at the bedside is uncertain since the examiner may not be able to construct probes to which he or she knows the correct responses (e.g., "To what elementary school did you go?"). For ordinary bedside purposes, a rough estimate of normal or abnormal remote memory may be all we can attain.

Language and Praxis

Aphasia.   There are six main areas of language function that the clinician examines. (See Chapter 12 for a more complete discussion of language disorders.)

1. *Spontaneous speech.* The clinician has ample opportunity to hear the patient speak during the routine clinical interview. Nonetheless, it is essential to listen for a period with an ear to language abnormalities. One listens first for fluency, which refers to several characteristics of speech: its melody, its effortfulness, its rate, and the length of phrases (normal being three to five words). Second, one listens for errors, both of syntax and of word-choice (lexicon). Agrammatism, emptiness, and paraphasic errors can be noted.
2. *Repetition.* It is important to test repetition by offering the patient phrases of increasing length and grammatical complexity. For example, one may start with single words, continue with simple phrases, then invert the phrases into questions, and then make up phrases of grammatical "function" words ("no ifs, ands, or buts" has become traditional).
3. *Naming.* One has already listened for paraphasic errors in the course of the patient's spontaneous speech. Ordinarily more detailed testing by confrontation naming can be simply performed using items at hand (e.g., a watch and its parts, parts of the body, items of clothing). Naming is dependent on the frequency of the target word in the vocabulary, so testing must use less frequently named items to detect mild but clinically meaningful deficits. The examiner should be aware that occasionally patients have extraordinary domain-specific dissociations in naming ability; for example, the ability to name vegetables may be intact but the ability to name animals devastated (Humphreys and Riddoch 1987).

4. *Comprehension.* Test comprehension by asking yes-no questions of progressive difficulty (e.g., "Am I wearing a hat?"; "Is there a tree in the room?"; "Does lunch come before dinner?"; or "Is ice cream hotter than coffee?") Motor responses should not be required (point to the ceiling and so on). Patients with anterior aphasia often have mild disorders of comprehension of syntactically complex material. This can be observed by asking patients to interpret sentences using the passive voice and similarly difficult constructions (e.g., "The lion was killed by the tiger. Which animal was dead?")

5. *Reading.* Reading comprehension can conveniently be tested by offering the same stimuli as were used orally. Alexia can be present with no other abnormality of language (alexia without agraphia).

6. *Writing.* This is most conveniently tested by asking the patient to write spontaneously a short paragraph about his illness or being in the hospital. Because agraphia is a constant accompaniment of aphasic syndromes, the writing sample is a good screening test of language function (always assuming premorbid literacy), and may reveal visuopractic problems as well. It is a particularly nice test in revealing confusional states; Chédru and Geschwind (1972a, 1972b) showed that writing is highly sensitive to disturbance in this setting. Similarly, agraphic errors can be seen in writing samples of patients with Alzheimer's disease earlier in the course than aphasic errors in spontaneous speech (Faber-Langendoen et al. 1988; Horner et al. 1988).

Ideomotor apraxia. An incapacity to perform skilled movements in the absence of elementary sensory or motor dysfunction that explains the defect is known as *apraxia.* Limb-kinetic apraxia amounts to a nonpyramidal clumsiness (Freund and Hummelsheim 1985). Ideational apraxia is revealed by requiring the patient to perform learned movements to command. For oral apraxia, suitable tests are "Show me how you would blow out a match" or "How do you lick a postage stamp?" For limb apraxia, the patient should demonstrate waving goodbye, thumbing a ride, using a hammer or comb or toothbrush, and the like.

Visuospatial Function

Copying a Greek cross, intersecting pentagons, a figure from the Bender-Gestalt test, or the figures in Mesulam's three-shapes test, or drawing a clock face serves as a suitable screen for disorders of visuospatial function. More subtle abnormality may be sought using the Rey Complex Figure (see Chapter 5). Copying performance is impaired by both left- and right-sided lesions, although differently. Having the patient change color of ink several times during the copying process reveals the steps taken to produce it (Milberg et al. 1986). The difference between a piecemeal approach (the patient slavishly copies element by element) and a gestalt approach (the patient grasps the major structures) can be noted, with the former suggestive of right-sided disease. If vision is impaired, it is possible to test related functions by topographic skills; "If I go from Chicago to New York, is the Atlantic Ocean in front of me, behind me, to my left or right?" is a sample probe, although such skills are not universal in the general population, and caution must be used in interpreting the results. Patients who lack other obvious deficits but with delusional intensity mistake their location have been described under the terms "redu-plicative paramnesia" (Pick 1903), "disorientation for place" (Fisher 1982), and "délire spatial" (spatial delusion) (Vighetto et al. 1985).

The Form of Thought

Thought disorder.   Thought disorder in functional psychosis has been the subject of much study, and descriptive terms for its features—poverty of speech, pressure of speech, derailment, tangentiality, incoherence, and so on—have been carefully de-fined (Andreasen 1979). Cutting and Murphy (1988) usefully differentiated between an intrinsic thinking disturbance (including loose associations, concreteness, over-inclusiveness, and illogicality); a disorder of the expression of thought (including disturbed pragmatics of language); and a deficit in real-world knowledge (which can produce odd conversational interchange). They argued that the distinctive pattern of schizophrenic thought is suggestive of right-hemisphere dysfunction. Many authors have noted the similarity between the negative features of thought disorder and the characteristics of the frontal lobe syndrome. Cutting (1987) contrasted the positive features of thought disorder in schizophrenia with the thinking process of delirious patients. The latter were prominently illogical or slowed and impoverished in output; more distinctively, the delirious patients gave occasional irrelevant replies amid com-petent responses. Levin (1956) discussed this contrast as well. The form of thought in mentally retarded and dementia patients has not been well described.

Confabulation.   The confabulating patient fabricates material in response to the examiner's queries and may tell tales spontaneously as well. Severe or elaborate con-fabulation betokens disease outside memory systems, particularly the failure of self-monitoring characteristic of frontal disease. Akin to confabulation is a phenomenon Geschwind (1982) called "wild paraphasia." He offered the example of a patient who names an iv pole a Christmas tree decoration. Here again the failure lies not within language systems but in the cerebral apparatus for self-monitoring.

The narrative process in the interview setting.   It is said that in psychiatry the en-tire interview is the examination. What conclusions can the neuropsychiatrist draw from the way the patient tells his story? This subject has come under study with regard to patients with right-hemisphere disease (Van Lancker and Kempler 1987; Wapner et al. 1981). Despite the adequacy of their lexical and syntactic performance, such patients have deficits in the capacity to tell a story, recognize the point of a joke, or understand metaphor and idiom. Words and sentences are normal, but paragraphs are not. Wapner et al. (1981) offered a qualitative description of the discourse of right-hemisphere patients: they rarely give "I don't know" responses, rather they contrive some answer even if implausible; they fail to draw appropriate inferences, especially from emotional data, so that incongruity is not recognized; and sense of humor is impaired.

The Content of Thought

The nature of psychotic ideation and experience does not readily differentiate or-ganic psychoses from "functional" psychoses. Johnstone et al. (1988) and Feinstein and Ron (1990) showed that "first-rank" symptoms of schizophrenia occur in psychoses accompanying diagnosable brain disease, as Schneider (1974) must have recognized when he indicated that they held pathognomonic significance in a non-organic psychosis. As a rule, psychotic states related to deep brain lesions (e.g., in basal ganglion disease) resemble idiopathic schizophrenia more closely than those seen with cortical disease (Cummings 1985). Disorders of identification such as Capgras's and Fregoli's syndromes may suggest right-hemisphere dysfunction (Joseph et al. 1990).

With increasing cognitive impairment, the complexity of delusions is reduced (Burns et al. 1990; Cummings 1985). Often the delusional ideas in dementia have an ad hoc quality: a purse is misplaced, and the delusion arises that someone is stealing personal items. Delusions or hallucinations in Alzheimer's disease may be a marker of a more severe or rapidly progressive process (Lopez et al. 1991). When delusions or hallucinations occur in a patient with dementia, the clinician must exclude a supervening toxic-metabolic encephalopathy. Cutting (1987) pointed out that themes of "imminent misadventure to others" and "bizarre happenings in the immediate vicinity" characterize the delusions in delirium as opposed to those in acute schizophrenic psychosis.

Visual hallucinations have correctly been taken as suggestive of organic states, especially if auditory hallucinations are absent, but visual hallucinations also are common in idiopathic schizophrenia (Bracha et al. 1989). Visual hallucinations without other psychopathology, usually in the presence of ocular disease with visual loss, are also common, especially among the elderly (Gold and Rabins 1989); visual hallucinations in a hemifield blind from cerebral disease are well known and not necessarily associated with other psychopathology. Vivid, elaborate, and well-formed visual hallucinations, often crepuscular (so-called peduncular hallucinosis), may occur with disease in the upper brain stem (Caplan 1980). Hallucinations in the other sensory modalities may have specific regional associations (e.g., olfactory hallucinations with temporal lobe pathology). Some of the abnormal experiences that are well known in temporal lobe epilepsy–the elaborate mental state described by Hughlings-Jackson, including déjà vu, jamais vu, metamorphopsia, and the like (see Gloor et al. 1982)— may occur in affective disorders as well (Silberman et al. 1985).

Emotion and Its Display

The assessment of emotion and its modulation are performed by the clinician as a natural part of the observation of the patient during the examination. In addition, the examiner asks questions about the patient's emotional experience. There is no substitute for extended and sensitive conversation.

Pathological laughter and crying are defined not only by the lack of congruent inner experience but also by the elicitation of the behavior by nonemotional stimuli (such as waving a hand before the patient's face) and by the all-or-none character of the response (Poeck 1985). One must distinguish this sign—usually representing lesions of the descending tracts modulating brain stem centers—from the affective dyscontrol, with lability and shallowness, that occurs in frontal disease or dementia. This latter finding, also called *emotionalism,* was studied by House et al. (1989), who took its defining characteristics to be an increase in the amount of tearfulness (or, more rarely, laughter) and the sudden, unexpected, and uncontrollable quality of the tears. They found it to be common, associated with cognitive impairment, and related to left frontal and temporal lesions; but it was not dissociated from the patient's emotional experience or situation.

Apathy is the absence or quantitative reduction of affect. It differs from depression; even the slowed, unexpressive depressed patient reports unpleasant emotional experience if carefully questioned. Euphoria, a persistent and unreasonable sense of well-being without the elevated mental and motor rate of a manic state, is often alluded to in connection with multiple sclerosis, almost always signaling substantial cognitive impairment.

The Initiation and Organization of Action

Perseveration. Perseveration refers to the continuation into present activity of elements of previous actions. Luria (1965) devised a number of bedside tasks to probe the programming of action and to reveal perseveration. In the simplest of motor tasks, the patient is asked to form alternately a ring and a fist with his hand. In the most characteristic form of abnormality, the patient perseverates on one position or the other, even while correctly saying aloud "ring—fist—ring—fist." This is the disconnection of action from verbal mediation that Luria regarded as the essence of frontal dysfunction (Luria and Homskaya 1963). A similar task, but one of greater difficulty, is to alternate from fist to edge of hand to palm, or the patient can be asked to alternate repeatedly from outstretched left fist and right palm to right fist and left palm.

Other ways to elicit perseveration include obtaining a writing sample, or asking the patient to produce repeated sequences of two crosses and a circle or three triangles and two squares. Yet others have used tasks of reciprocal action programs. For example, the patient is asked to point with one finger when the examiner points with two, and vice versa. I sometimes ask the patient to tap once when I tap twice, and vice versa; I do this immediately after employing a go/no-go tapping task (see below), thus complicating the demand for the use of a new response strategy. Continuous perseveration, in Sandson and Albert's terminology (1987), entails continuation or prolongation of response without cessation. This may be tested by asking the patient to produce repeated loops or the letters *m* and *n* (in cursive script).

Perseveration can be seen in disease of a wide variety of brain regions, but when related to disease outside frontal regions it is characteristically limited to a specific modality of processing or response. For example, a patient with disease in temporoparietal language areas may make recurrent perseverative errors on language testing. Sandson and Albert (1987) claimed that continuous perseveration is related to nondominant hemisphere disease. Fisher (1989b) pointed out that perseverative activity in a broad sense is one of the important general principles of cerebral dysfunction; it occurs in confusional states, dementia, ideational apraxia, and transient global amnesia—whenever the brain is working sufficiently poorly in generating effective new action programs.

Disinhibition. The loss of the capacity for planful action leaves the patient with organic cerebral disease prey to impulses. For the most part, the clinician learns about such deficits from the history. Usually, but not always, the structuring effect of the interview and examination prevents display of impulsive behavior. In my opinion, the sort of question often used to examine "judgment" ("What would you do if you found a stamped, addressed envelope in the street?") is not useful. A simple bedside test to demonstrate this defect is a tapping task in which the patient is instructed to tap for one stimulus and to refrain for another: "When I tap once I want you to tap twice; when I tap twice you do nothing at all." After a practice trial, a single error of commission represents a failure. Leimkuhler and Mesulam (1985) showed the test's validity as a sign of medial frontal dysfunction in one case.

Ideational apraxia.   Rarely, focal lesions produce ideational apraxia, but far more often it occurs in association with confusional states or severe dementia and represents a global disorder of the organization of behavior. The phenomenon is the incapacity to carry out a sequential or ordered set of actions toward a unitary goal. For example, the patient may be able to carry out the individual acts involved in preparing a letter to be sent—folding it, placing it in the envelope, sealing the envelope—but not be able to do them in the proper order to produce a useful result.

Abulia.   Adams and Fisher (Fisher 1984) resurrected the old term *abulia* to describe the slowness and loss of spontaneity in cerebral disease, of which the extreme case is akinetic mutism. Whereas apathy is in the emotional sphere, abulia is in the sphere of action: a pathological absence. In its less severe form, the phenomena include slowness, delays before response, laconic speech, and a reduction in initiative and effort, perhaps with the patient performing only one of a series of requested actions. Fisher (1968) used the term *intermittent interruption of behavior* to describe a transient but repeated lack of response of this sort. At times even severe abulia can be overcome by stimuli that elicit automatic responses.

Generating lists of words by categories—"Name all the animals you can think of, or all the items one might buy in a supermarket"—requires sustained attention to a task and the ability to organize an effective search of memory as well as intact language and, of course, a certain amount of real-world knowledge. Quantitative scoring—the BDAE data suggest 12 animals in 1 minute as a cutoff for normal performance (Goodglass and Kaplan 1983)—is only part of the story. The examiner also must assess the strategy the patient applies. Normally, a patient names all the animals that come to mind from one class, say barnyard animals, then switches to another class, say jungle animals. The patient with a disorder of spontaneity and flexible attention has trouble picking a productive strategy and switching it when necessary.

Impersistence.   Fisher (1956) described the incapacity of certain patients to sustain activities they were capable of beginning. The patient with impersistence peeks when asked to do tasks requiring the eyes to be closed or gaze to be averted. Maintaining eyelid closure, tongue protrusion, mouth opening, and lateral gaze to the left may be the tasks most sensitive to this incapacity. In most but not all studies, impersistence has been a pointer to right-hemisphere disease (De Renzi et al. 1986; Jenkyn et al. 1977; Kertesz et al. 1985).

Utilization behavior.   Lhermitte et al. (1986) described new signs in frontal disease. In imitation behavior, the patient imitates the gestures and behavior of the examiner even if asked to stop. This is taken to be a deliberate, not an automatic or reflex, response; patients explain that they feel they have to imitate. The authors differentiated this phenomenon from echopraxia, which is taken to be automatic.

The frontal lobes provide a capacity for individual autonomy; with dysfunction of the frontal system, a state of environmental dependency is produced. As this worsens, not only is there imitation of social behavior but also a similar pseudovoluntary use of objects in the physical environment, known as "utilization behavior." For example, seeing a pitcher and a glass, the patient pours and drinks water as if it were required of him. Echopraxia has been described in a variety of conditions, including Tourette's syndrome, schizophrenia, and dementia (Lees 1985). Unfortunately, the descriptions of the patient's understanding of what they are doing may not be sufficient to be sure that echopraxia differs from what Lhermitte et al. (1986) described as imitation behavior.

Awareness of deficit.   The patient who lacks awareness of a deficit obvious to everyone else is a common phenomenon in neuropsychiatry, one with important implications for treatment. The striking state of anosognosia in right-parietal lesions with denial of a left hemiparesis is well recognized, but the phenomenon has a much wider reach. A range of states occurs, from minimization of the gravity of the deficit to denial of its impact to bizarre denial of ownership of the affected body part. For example, psychotic patients regularly are unaware of the pathological nature of their perceptions and beliefs and resent attempts to intervene (Amador et al. 1991). It is common for the patient with Alzheimer's disease to lack awareness of the reason his or her spouse is bringing him or her to see the doctor. It is not unusual for a patient to be unaware of a hemianopsia, but he or she may recognize it when it is pointed out. The possible mechanisms of these states have been reviewed extensively (Levine 1990; McGlynn and Schacter 1989). The bedside examiner should repeatedly explore with the patient his understanding of the nature of his symptoms.

Psychological Management in the Neuropsychiatric Examination

In neuropsychiatry—as in all of medicine—the diagnostic evaluation is also part of the psychological treatment. The interest shown by the examiner, the rapport formed with the patient and the family, and the laying on of hands all form the basis of subsequent treatment and must be attended to from the beginning of the consultation.A common difficulty for beginners is how to introduce the formal cognitive inquiry. Most of the time patients report symptoms that can lead naturally—that is, naturally from the patient's point of view—to a cognitive examination. For example, a patient with depressive symptoms may report trouble concentrating. If the examiner then says, "Let me ask you some questions to check your concentration," the patient is likely to collaborate without feeling offended. At this point nearly any tasks can be introduced.

At what point in the interview should this be done? If the initial few minutes of the patient's talk gives reason to suspect substantial cognitive difficulty, one may wish to do at least some of the testing promptly. Not all of the cognitive examination needs to be done at once, although many examiners prefer to do so. Fatigue is an important factor in the cognitive performance of many patients, and long examinations may not elicit their best performances. Caplan (1978) pointed out that variability in performance is characteristic of patients with cerebral lesions and that perseveration may lead to drastic declines as tasks proceed. For this reason short snatches of probing may yield new perspectives on a patient's capacities as well as avoid the catastrophic reaction that ensues when a patient's capacities are exceeded.

CONCLUSIONS

The complete examination is a figment. No practical examination can include all possible elements, and if it did it would be mindless. The expert clinician is con-

---

Table 4–2. Screening tests for cognitive impairment

Mini-Mental State Exam

Maximum
score

5	What is the (year)(season)(date)(day)(month)?
5	Where are we: (state)(county)(town)(hospital)(floor)?
3	Name three objects: 1 second to say each. Then ask the patient all three after you have said them. Give 1 point for each correct answer. Then repeat them until he learns all three. Count trials and record.
5	Serial 7s. 1 point for each correct. Stop after five answers. Alternatively spell *world* backward.
3	Ask for the three objects repeated above. Give 1 point for each correct.
2	Name a pencil and a watch.
1	Repeat the following: "No ifs, ands, or buts."
3	Follow a 3-stage command: "Take a paper in your right hand, fold it in half, and put it on the floor."
1	Read and obey the following: "CLOSE YOUR EYES."
1	Write a sentence.
1	Copy a design: intersecting pentagons each side about 1 inch

---

Orientation-Memory-Concentration Test

Items		Maximum error	Score	Weight	
1	What year is it now?	1	___	× 4 =	___
2	What month is it now?	1	___	× 3 =	___
Memory phrase	Repeat this phrase after me: John Brown, 42 Market St., Chicago				
3	About what time is it (within 1 hour)?	1	___	× 3 =	___
4	Count backwards from *20* to *1*.	2	___	× 2 =	___
5	Say the months in reverse order.	2	___	× 2 =	___
6	Repeat the memory phrase.	5	___	× 2 =	___

Sources. Mini-Mental State Exam reprinted from Folstein MF, Folstein SE, McHugh PR: "Mini-Mental State: A Practical Method for Grading the Cognitive State of Patients for the Clinician." *Journal of Psychiatric Research* 12:189–198, 1975. Used with permission.
Orientation-Memory-Concentration Test reprinted from Katzman R, Brown T, Fuld P, et al: "Validation of a Short Orientation-Memory-Concentration Test of Cognitive Impairment." *American Journal of Psychiatry* 140:734–739, 1983. Used with permission.

stantly generating hypotheses and constructing an examination to confirm or refute them (Caplan 1990). The diagnostician as historian is constantly aiming at writing the patient's biography: how did *this* person arrive at *this* predicament at *this* time? Diagnosis in neuropsychiatry does not mean the search only for etiology, nor only for localization, nor only for functional capacity. It means the construction of a pathophysiological and psychopathological formulation from cause to effect, from etiologic factor to symptomatic complaint or performance. The formulation of a pathogenetic mechanism that leads from cause—in genetic endowment, perinatal injury, acquired illness, or environmental provision—to effect—the symptoms and signs we have reviewed—is a paragraph, not a phrase, and provides a rational framework for intervention in each of these domains.

Systematic assessment of major areas of functioning, whether there are pointers to abnormality or not, is essential. For example, every patient should be screened for cognitive abnormality. Several investigators have developed brief screening tests of cognitive functioning. Some of these, including the Mini-Mental State Exam (Folstein et al. 1975) (Table 4–2), were reviewed by Nelson et al. (1986). Katzman et al. (1983) offered a particularly simple and well-validated screening examination for dementia (Table 4–2). Batteries such as these are most useful for the recognition of diffuse intellectual decline, such as in Alzheimer's disease. They provide repeatable, quantifiable measures that can be noted in the patient's record.

As this chapter has shown, many areas not included in such cognitive screening approaches are relevant to the recognition of cerebral disease in patients with psychopathology. Historical indicators, focal areas of cognitive dysfunction, physical signs, and the patient's behavior and discourse taken as a whole can be reviewed for clues to pathogenesis. In the cognitive examination, not only the quantitative but also the qualitative aspects of performance—the nature of errors, the choice of strategies are revealing. With growing expertise, the examiner can go beyond screening and toward formulation as discussed above.

REFERENCES

Alexander MP: Frontal lobes and language. Brain Lang 37:656–691, 1989

Altshuler LL, Cummings JL, Bartzokis G, et al: Lateral asymmetries of tardive dyskinesia in schizophrenia. Biol Psychiatry 24:83–86, 1988

Amador XF, Strauss DH, Yale SA, et al: Awareness of illness in schizophrenia. Schizophr Bull 17:113–132, 1991

Andreasen NC: Thought, language, and communication disorders. Arch Gen Psychiatry 36:1315–1321, 1979

Ball R: Drug-induced akathisia: a review. J R Soc Med 78:748–752, 1985

Barnes MP, Saunders M, Walls TJ: The syndrome of Karl Ludwig Kahlbaum. J Neurol Neurosurg Psychiatry 49:991–996, 1986

Bear D, Hermann B, Fogel B: Interictal behavior syndrome in temporal lobe epilepsy: the views of three experts. Journal of Neuropsychiatry and Clinical Neurosciences 1:308–318, 1989

Black FW: Digit repetition in brain-damaged adults: clinical and theoretical implications. J Clin Psychol 42:770–782, 1986

Blanchet P, Frommer GP: Mood change preceeding epileptic seizures. J Nerv Ment Dis 174:471–476, 1986

Bogousslavsky J, Regli F, Uske A: Thalamic infarcts: clinical syndromes, etiology, and prognosis. Neurology 38:837–848, 1988

Boller F, Frank E: Sexual Dysfunction in Neurological Disorders: Diagnosis, Management, and Rehabilitation. New York, Raven, 1982

Boller F, Boller M, Denes G, et al: Familial palilalia. Neurology 23:1117–1125, 1973

Bracha HS, Wolkowitz OM, Lohr JB, et al: High prevalence of visual hallucination in research subjects with chronic schizophrenia. Am J Psychiatry 146:526–528, 1989

Braude WM, Barnes TRE, Gore SM: Clinical characteristics of akathisia: a systematic investigation of acute psychiatric inpatient admissions. Br J Psychiatry 143:139–150, 1983

Brodal A: Self-observations and neuro-anatomical considerations after a stroke. Brain 96:675–694, 1973

Brodal A: Neurological Anatomy in Relation to Clinical Medicine, 3rd Edition. New York, Oxford University Press, 1981

Bryden MP: Measuring handedness with questionnaires. Neuropsychologia 15:617–624, 1977

Burns A, Jacoby R, Levy R: Psychiatric phenomena in Alzheimer's disease, I: disorders of thought content. Br J Psychiatry 157:72–76, 1990

Caplan LR: Variability of perceptual function: the sensory cortex as a "categorizer" and "deducer." Brain Lang 6:1–13, 1978

Caplan LR: "Top of the basilar" syndrome. Neurology 30:72–79, 1980

Caplan LR: The Effective Clinical Neurologist. Cambridge, Blackwell, 1990

Caplan LR, Schmahmann JD, Kase CS, et al: Caudate infarcts. Arch Neurol 47:133–143, 1990

Chapman L, Wolff HG: Disease of the neopallium and impairment of the highest integrative functions. Med Clin North Am 42:677–689, 1958

Chédru F, Geschwind N: Disorders of higher cortical functions in acute confusional states. Cortex 8:395–411, 1972a

Chédru F, Geschwind N: Writing disturbances in acute confusional states. Neuropsychologia 10:343–353, 1972b

Critchley M: On palilalia. Journal of Neurology and Psychopathology 8:23–31, 1927

Cummings JL: Organic delusions: phenomenology, anatomical correlations, and review. Br J Psychiatry 146:184–197, 1985

Cutting J: The phenomenology of acute organic psychosis: comparison with acute schizophrenia. Br J Psychiatry 151:324–332, 1987

Cutting J, Murphy D: Schizophrenic thought disorder: a psychological and organic interpretation. Br J Psychiatry 152:310–319, 1988

Damasio AR, Maurer RG: A neurological model for childhood autism. Arch Neurol 35:777–786, 1978

Daniel WF, Crovitz HF, Weiner RD: Neuropsychological aspects of disorientation. Cortex 23:169–187, 1987

De Renzi E: Disorders of spatial orientation, in Handbook of Clinical Neurology, Vol 45: Clinical Neuropsychology. Edited by Frederiks JAM. Amsterdam, Elsevier, 1985, pp 405–422

De Renzi E, Gentilini M, Bazolli M: Eyelid movement disorders and motor impersistence in acute hemisphere disease. Neurology 36:414–418, 1986

Denny-Brown D: The nature of apraxia. J Nerv Ment Dis 126:9–32, 1958

Devinsky O, Bear D, Volpe BT: Confusional states following posterior cerebral artery infarction. Arch Neurol 45:160–163, 1988

Engel J: Seizures and Epilepsy. Philadelphia, PA, FA Davis, 1989

Eslinger PJ, Damasio AR, Van Hoesen GW: Olfactory dysfunction in man: anatomical and behavioral aspects. Brain and Cognition 1:259–285, 1982

Faber-Langendoen K, Morris JC, Knesevich JW, et al: Aphasia in senile dementia of the Alzheimer type. Neurology 23:365–370, 1988

Fahn S, Marsden CD, Calne DB: Classification and investigation of dystonia, in Movement Disorders, 2nd Edition. Edited by Marsden CD, Fahn S. London, Butterworths, 1987, pp 332–358

Falconer MA, Wilson JL: Visual field changes following anterior temporal lobectomy: their significance in relation to "Meyer's loop" of the optic radiation. Brain 81:1–14, 1958

Feinstein A, Ron MA: Psychosis associated with demonstrable brain disease. Psychol Med 20:793–803, 1990

Fenwick P: The nature and management of aggression in epilepsy. Journal of Neuropsychiatry and Clinical Neuroscience 1:418–425, 1989

Firestone P, Peters S: Minor physical anomalies and behavior in children: a review. J Autism Dev Disord 13:411–425, 1983

Fisher CM: Intermittent interruption of behavior. Transactions of the American Neurological Association 93:209–210, 1968

Fisher CM: Disorientation for place. Arch Neurol 39:33–36, 1982

Fisher CM: Abulia minor vs agitated behavior. Clin Neurosurg 31:9–31, 1984

Fisher CM: "Catatonia" due to disulfiram toxicity. Arch Neurol 46:798–804, 1989a

Fisher CM: Neurologic fragments, II: remarks on anosognosia, confabulation, memory, and other topics; and an appendix on self-observation. Neurology 39:127–132, 1989b

Fisher M: Left hemiplegia and motor impersistence. J Nerv Ment Dis 123:201–218, 1956

Fogel CA, Mednick SA, Michelsen N: Hyperactive behavior and minor physical anomalies. Acta Psychiatr Scand 72:551–556, 1985

Folstein MF, Folstein SE, McHugh PR: Mini-Mental State: a practical method for grading the cognitive state of patients for the clinician. J Psychiatr Res 12:189–198, 1975

Ford RA: The psychopathology of echophenomena. Psychol Med 19:627–635, 1989

Freed WJ, Kleinman JE, Karson CN, et al:. Eye-blink rates and platelet monoamine oxidase activity in chronic schizophrenic patients. Biol Psychiatry 15:329–332, 1980

Freund H-J, Hummelsheim H: Lesions of premotor cortex in man. Brain 108:697–733, 1985

Geschwind N: Non-aphasic disorders of speech. Int J Neurol 4:207–214, 1964

Geschwind N: Disorders of attention: a frontier in neuropsychology. Philos Trans R Soc Lond [Biol] 298:173–185, 1982

Geschwind N, Kaplan E: A human cerebral deconnection syndrome: a preliminary report. Neurology 12:675–685, 1962

Gibb WRG, Lees AJ: The clinical phenomenon of akathisia. J Neurol Neurosurg Psychiatry 49:861–866, 1986

Gloor P, Olivier A, Quesny LF, et al: The role of the limbic system in experiential phenomena of temporal lobe epilepsy. Ann Neurol 12:129–140, 1982

Gold K, Rabins PV: Isolated visual hallucinations and the Charles Bonnet syndrome: a review of the literature and presentation of six cases. Compr Psychiatry 30:90–98, 1989

Goodglass H, Kaplan E: The Assessment of Aphasia and Related Disorders, 2nd Edition. Philadelphia, PA, Lea & Febiger, 1983

Gould R, Miller BL, Goldber MA, et al: The validity of hysterical signs and symptoms. J Nerv Ment Dis 174:593–597, 1986

Greden JF, Genero N, Price HL: Agitation-increased electromyogram activity in the corrugator muscle region: a possible explanation of the "omega sign"? Am J Psychiatry 142:348–351, 1985

Green MF, Satz P, Gaier DJ, et al: Minor physical anomalies in schizophrenia. Schizophr Bull 15:91–99, 1989

Greenberg MS, Farah MJ: The laterality of dreaming. Brain Cogn 5:307–321, 1986

Gualtieri CT, Adams A, Shen CD, et al: Minor physical anomalies in alcoholic and schizophrenic adults and hyperactive and autistic children. Am J Psychiatry 139:640–643, 1982

Hallett M, Ravits J: Involuntary movements, in Diseases of the Nervous System: Clinical Neurobiology. Edited by Asbury AK, McKhann GM, McDonald WI. Philadelphia, PA, WB Saunders, 1986, pp 452–460

Harrison PJ, Pearson RCA: Olfaction and psychiatry. Br J Psychiatry 155:822–828, 1989

Heilman KM, Watson RT, Valenstein E: Neglect and related disorders, in Clinical Neuropsychology, 2nd Edition. Edited by Heilman KM, Valenstein E. New York, Oxford University Press, 1985, pp 243–293

Heinrichs DW, Buchanan RW: Significance and meaning of neurological signs in schizophrenia. Am J Psychiatry 145:11–18, 1988

Horner J, Heyman A, Dawson D, et al: The relationship of agraphia to the severity of dementia in Alzheimer's disease. Arch Neurol 45:760–763, 1988

House A, Dennis M, Molyneux A, et al: Emotionalism after stroke. BMJ 298:991–994, 1989

Humphreys GW, Riddoch MJ: On telling your fruit from your vegetables: a consideration of category-specific deficits after brain damage. Trends Neurosci 10:145–148, 1987

Hyde TM, Hotson JR, Kleinman JE: Differential diagnosis of choreiform tardive dyskinesia. Journal of Neuropsychiatry and Clinical Neurosciences 3:255–268, 1991

Jankovic J: The neurology of tics, in Movement Disorders, 2nd Edition. Edited by Marsden CD, Rahn S. London, Butterworths, 1987, pp 383–405

Jenkyn LR, Walsh DB, Walsh BT, et al: The nuchocephalic reflex. J Neurol Neurosurg Psychiatry 38:561–566, 1975

Jenkyn LR, Walsh DB, Culver CM, et al: Clinical signs in diffuse cerebral dysfunction. J Neurol Neurosurg Psychiatry 40:956–966, 1977

Johnstone EC, Cooling NJ, Frith CD, et al: Phenomenology of organic and functional psychoses and the overlap between them. Br J Psychiatry 153:770–776, 1988

Jones IH: Observations on schizophrenic stereotypes. Compr Psychiatry 6:323–335, 1965

Joseph AB, O'Leary DH, Wheeler HG: Bilateral atrophy of the frontal and temporal lobes in schizophrenic patients with Capgras syndrome: a case-control study using computed tomography. J Clin Psychiatry 51:322–325, 1990

Kandel E, Brennan PA, Mednick SA, et al: Minor physical anomalies and recidivistic adult criminal behavior. Acta Psychiatr Scand 79:103–107, 1989

Karson CN: Spontaneous eye-blink rates and dopaminergic systems. Brain 106:643–653, 1983

Karson CN: Physiology of normal and abnormal blinking, in Advances in Neurology, Vol 49: Facial Dyskinesias. Edited by Jankovic J, Tolosa E. New York, Raven, 1988, pp 25–37

Karson CN, Burns RS, LeWitt PA, et al: Blink rates and disorders of movement. Neurology 34:677–678, 1984

Katzman R, Brown T, Fuld P, et al: Validation of a short orientation-memory-concentration test of cognitive impairment. Am J Psychiatry 140:734–739, 1983

Kertesz A, Nicholson I, Cancelliere A, et al: Motor impersistence: a right-hemisphere syndrome. Neurology 35:662–666, 1985

Klüver H, Bucy PC: Preliminary analysis of functions of the temporal lobes in monkeys. Archive of Neurology and Psychiatry 42:979–1000, 1939

Kolada SJ, Pitman RK: Eye-head synkinesia in schizophrenic adults during a repetitive visual search task. Biol Psychiatry 18:675–684, 1983

Koller W, Lang A, Vetere-Overfield B, et al: Psychogenic tremors. Neurol 39:1094–1099, 1989

Kopelman MD: Clinical tests of memory. Br J Psychiatry 148:517–525, 1986

Landau WM: Reflex dementia: disinhibited primitive thinking. Neurology 39:133–137, 1989

Laplane D, Orgogozo JM, Meininger V, et al: Paralysie faciale avec dissociation automatic-volontaire inverse par lesion frontale: son origine corticale: ses relations avec l'A.M.S. Rev Neurol 132:725–734, 1976

Lecours AR, Lhermitte F, Bryans B: Aphasiology. London, Balliere Tindall, 1983

Lees AJ: Tics and Related Disorders. Edinburgh, Churchill Livingstone, 1985

Lees AJ: Facial mannerisms and tics, in Facial Dyskineasias (Advances in Neurology Series, Vol 49). New York, Raven, 1988, pp 255–261

Leimkuhler ME, Mesulam M-M: Reversible go–no go deficits in a case of frontal lobe tumor. Ann Neurol 18:617–619, 1985

Lepore FE, Duvoisin RC: "Apraxia" of eyelid opening: an involuntary levator inhibition. Neurology 35:423–427, 1985

Levin M: Thinking disturbances in delirium. Archives of Neurology and Psychiatry 75:62–66, 1956

Levine DN: Unawareness of visual and sensorimotor defects: a hypothesis. Brain Cogn 13:233–281, 1990

Lezak MD: Subtle sequelae of brain damage: perplexity, distractibility, and fatigue. Am J Phys Med 57:9–15, 1978

Lhermitte F, Pillon B, Serdaru M: Human autonomy and the frontal lobes, I: imitation and utilization behavior: a neuropsychological study of 75 patients. Ann Neurol 19:326–334, 1986

Lishman WA: Organic Psychiatry: The Psychological Consequences of Cerebral Disorder, 2nd Edition. Oxford, Blackwell, 1987

Lloyd G: Medicine without signs. BMJ 287:539–542, 1983

Lopez OL, Becker JT, Brenner RP, et al: Alzheimer's disease with delusions and hallucinations: neuropsychological and electroencephalographic correlates. Neurology 41:906–912, 1991

Ludlow CL, Rosenberg J, Salazar A, et al: Site of penetrating brain lesions causing chronic acquired stuttering. Ann Neurol 22:60–66, 1987

Luria AR: Two kinds of motor perseveration in massive injury of the frontal lobes. Brain 88:1–10, 1965

Luria AR, Homskaya ED: Le trouble du role régulateur du langage au cours des lésions du lobe frontal. Neuropsychologia 1:9–26, 1963

Luxon L, Lees AJ, Greenwood RJ: Neurosyphilis today. Lancet 1:90–93, 1979

McGlynn SM, Schacter DL: Unawareness of deficits in neuropsychological syndromes. J Clin Exp Neuropsychol 11:143–205, 1989

Manschreck TC: Psychopathology of motor behavior in schizophrenia. Progress in Experimental Personality Research 12:53–99, 1983

Marsden CD: Basal ganglia and motor dysfunction, in Diseases of the Nervous System: Clinical Neurobiology. Edited by Asbury AK, McKhann GM, McDonald WI. Philadelphia, PA, WB Saunders, 1986, pp 394–400

Marsden CD: Wilson's disease. Q J Med 65:959–966, 1987

Mesulam M-M: A cortical network for directed attention and unilateral neglect. Ann Neurol 10:309–325, 1981

Mesulam M-M: Principles of Behavioral Neurology. Philadelphia, PA, FA Davis, 1985

Milberg WP, Hebben N, Kaplan E: The Boston Process Approach to neuropsychological assessment, in Neuropsychological Assessment of Neuropsychiatric Disorders. Edited by Grant I, Adams KM. New York, Oxford University Press, 1986, pp 65–86

Miller BL, Cummings JL, McIntyre H, et al: Hypersexuality or altered sexual preference following brain injury. J Neurol Neurosurg Psychiatry 49:867–873, 1986

Miller H: Psychiatry—medicine or magic? in Contemporary Psychiatry: Selected Reviews from the British Journal of Hospital Medicine. Edited by Silverstone T, Barraclough B. Ashford, England, Headley, 1975, pp 462–466

Monrad-Krohn GH: On the dissociation of voluntary and emotional innervation in facial paresis of central origin. Brain 47:22–35, 1924

Monrad-Krohn GH: Dysprosody or altered "melody of language." Brain 70:405–415, 1947

Nelson A, Fogel BS, Faust D: Bedside cognitive screening instruments: a critical assessment. J Nerv Ment Dis 174:73–83, 1986

Occupational and Environmental Health Committee of the American Lung Association of San Diego and Imperial Counties: Taking the occupational history. Ann Intern Med 99:641–651, 1983

Ounsted C, Lindsay J, Richards P: Temporal Lobe Epilepsy 1948–1986: A Biographical Study. Oxford, Blackwell Scientific, 1987

Ovsiew F, Yudofsky SC: Agression: a neuropsychiatric perspective, in Rage, Power, and Aggression. Edited by Glick RA, Roose SP. New Haven, CT, Yale University Press, 1993, pp 213–230

Owens DGC: Dystonia: a potential psychiatric pitfall. Br J Psychiatry 156:620–634, 1990

Padberg GW, Bruyn GW: Choreadifferential diagnosis, in Handbook of Clinical Neurology, Vol 5: Extrapyramidal Disorders. Edited by Vinken PJ, Bruyn GW, Klawans HL. Amsterdam, Elsevier, 1986, pp 549–564

Pick A: Clinical studies, III: on reduplicative paramnesia. Brain 26:260–267, 1903

Pinching AJ: Clinical testing of olfaction reassessed. Brain 100:377–388, 1977

Plum F, Posner JB: The Diagnosis of Stupor and Coma, 3rd Edition. Philadelphia, PA, FA Davis, 1980

Poeck K: Pathological laughter and crying, in Handbook of Clinical Neurology, Vol 45: Clinical Neuropsychology. Edited by Frederiks JAM. Amsterdam, Elsevier, 1985, pp 219–225

Prechtl HFR: Neurological sequelae of prenatal and perinatal complications. BMJ 4:763–767, 1967

Remillard GM, Andermann F, Rhi-Sausi A, et al: Facial asymmetry in patients with temporal lobe epilepsy: a clinical sign useful in the lateralization of temporal epileptogenic foci. Neurology 27:109–114, 1977

Ridley RM, Baker HF: Stereotypy in monkeys and humans. Psychol Med 12:61–72, 1982

Ropper AH: Self-grasping: a focal neurological sign. Ann Neurol 12:575–577, 1982

Ross ED: The aprosodias: functional-anatomic organization of the affective components of language in the right hemisphere. Arch Neurol 38:561–569, 1981

Ross ED, Mesulam M-M: Dominant language functions of the right hemisphere? Arch Neurol 36:144–148, 1979

Ross Russell RW: Supranuclear palsy of eyelid closure. Brain 103:71–82, 1980

Sandson J, Albert ML: Perseveration in behavioral neurology. Neurology 37:1736–1741, 1987

Scheinberg IH, Sternlieb I, Walshe JM: Wilson's disease and Kayser-Fleischer rings. Ann Neurol 19:613–614, 1986

Schiff HB, Alexander MP, Naeser MA, et al: Aphemia: clinical-anatomic correlations. Arch Neurol 40:720–727, 1983

Schneider K: Primary and secondary symptoms in schizophrenia, in Themes and Variations in European Psychiatry: An Anthology. Edited by Hirsch SR, Shepherd M. Bristol, England, John Wright & Sons, 1974, pp 40–44

Silberman EK, Post RM, Nurnberger J, et al: Transient sensory, cognitive and affective phenomena in affective illness: a comparison with complex partial epilepsy. Br J Psychiatry 146:81–89, 1985

Steg JP, Rapoport JL: Minor physical anomalies in normal, neurotic, learning disabled, and severely disturbed children. Journal of Autism and Childhood Schizophrenia 5:299–307, 1975

Stevens JR: Eye blink and schizophrenia: psychosis or tardive dyskinesia. Am J Psychiatry 135:223–226, 1978

Strub RL, Black FW: The bedside mental status examination, in Handbook of Neuropsychology, Vol I. Edited by Boller F, Grafman J. Amsterdam, Elsevier, 1988, pp 29–46

Tomson T, Lindbum U, Nilsson BY: Nonconvulsive status epilepticus in adults: thirty-two consecutive patients from a general hospital population. Epilepsia 33:829–835, 1992

Toone BK, Edeh J, Nanjee MN, et al: Hyposexuality and epilepsy: a community survey of hormonal and behavioural changes in male epileptics. Psychol Med 19:937–943, 1989

Trosch RM, Sze G, Brass LM, et al: Emotional facial paresis with striatocapsular infarction. J Neurol Sci 98:195–201, 1990

Tucker DM, Watson RT, Heilman KM: Discrimination and evocation of affectively intoned speech in patients with right parietal disease. Neurology 27:947–950, 1977

Van Lancker DR, Kempler D: Comprehension of familiar phrases by left- but not by right-hemisphere damaged patients. Brain Lang 32:265–277, 1987

Vighetto A, Henry E, Garde P, et al: Le délire spatial: une manifestation des lésions de l'hémisphàre mineur. Rev Neurol 141:476–481, 1985

Walshe JM: Wilson's disease, in Handbook of Clinical Neurology, Vol 49: Extrapyramidal Disorders. Edited by Vinken PJ, Bruyn GW, Klawans HL. Amsterdam, Elsevier, 1986, pp 223–238

Wapner W, Hamby S, Gardner H: The role of the right hemisphere in the apprehension of complex linguistic materials. Brain Lang 14:15–33, 1981

Weintraub S, Mesulam M-M: Mental state assessment of young and elderly adults in behavioral neurology, in Principles of Behavioral Neurology. Edited by Mesulam M-M. Philadelphia, PA, FA Davis, 1985, pp 71–123

Young RR, Shahani BT: Asterixis: one type of negative myoclonus, in Myoclonus (Advances in Neurology Series, Vol 43). Edited by Fahn S. New York, Raven, 1986, pp 137–156

Chapter 5

The Neuropsychological Evaluation

Diane B. Howieson, Ph.D.
Muriel D. Lezak, Ph.D.

Neuropsychological evaluations have been used since the 1940s for the diagnosis of acquired or congenital problems presumed to be a result of brain disease or trauma (Hebb 1942; Teuber 1948). The neuropsychologist assesses brain function inferred from an individual's cognitive, sensory, motor, emotional, or social behavior. During the early history of neuropsychology, these assessments were often the most direct measure of brain integrity in persons without localizing neurological signs and symptoms and with problems confined to higher mental functions. Neuropsychological measures still are useful diagnostic indicators of brain dysfunction for many conditions and will remain the major diagnostic modality for some (Eisenberg and Levin 1989; Jernigan and Hesselink 1987; Mapov 1988). Diagnosis of brain damage has become increasingly accurate in recent decades as a result of improved visualization of brain structure by computed tomography (CT), magnetic resonance imaging (MRI), and angiography (Theodore 1988). These developments have allowed a shift in the focus of neuropsychological assessment from the diagnosis of possible brain damage to a better understanding of specific brain-behavior relationships and of the psychosocial consequences of brain damage.

WHEN A NEUROPSYCHOLOGICAL EVALUATION IS INDICATED

Patients referred to a neuropsychologist for assessment may be classified into one of three groups. The first and probably largest group consists of patients with known brain damage. The more common brain disorders are cerebrovascular disorders, head injury, hydrocephalus, Alzheimer's disease, Parkinson's disease, multiple sclerosis, Huntington's chorea, tumors, seizures, and infections. A neuropsychological evaluation can be useful in defining the nature and severity of resulting functional problems. The assessment provides information about the patient's cognition, personality characteristics, social behavior, emotional status, and adjustment to limitations. The individual's potential for independent living and productive activity can be derived from these data. Information about the patient's behavioral strengths and weaknesses can be used for treatment planning, vocational training, competency determination, and counseling for both patients and their families (Acker 1989).

The second group of patients referred to a neuropsychologist consists of persons with a known risk factor for brain damage in whom a change in behavior might be the result of such disease or injury to the brain. In these cases a neuropsychological evaluation might be used both to provide evidence of brain dysfunction and to describe the nature and severity of problems. Many medical conditions can affect brain function (Tarter et al. 1988). It can be disrupted by systemic illnesses: endocrinopathies; metabolic and electrolyte disturbances; diseases of the kidney, liver, and pancreas; nutritional deficiencies; toxins; and conditions producing decreased blood supply to the brain (e.g., trauma, vascular disorders, cardiac disease, pulmonary disease, anemia, carbon monoxide, and complications of anesthesia or surgery). Age and health habits must also be taken into consideration when evaluating a person's behavioral alterations because they affect the probability of cerebral disorder (Dubois et al. 1990; Kolb 1989). In addition, many medicines can disrupt cognition through their subtle effects on alertness, attention, and memory (Cope 1988; Schmidt 1986).

In the last group, brain disease or trauma often is suspected based on the observation of a change in a person's behavior without an identifiable etiology; that is, the patient has no known risk factors for brain damage, and this diagnosis is considered on the basis of exclusion of other diagnoses. Frequently psychiatrists are asked to evaluate an adult with no previous psychiatric history who has had an uncharacteristic change in behavior or personality and for whom no obvious sources of current emotional distress can be identified. The list of differential diagnoses is long and may include a wide variety of brain disorders that range from metabolic disturbance, vitamin deficiency, endocrine disorder, and heavy metal poisoning to neoplasm, infection, and multiple small strokes. The psychiatric literature contains numerous examples of individuals who were being treated for psychiatric illness before it was discovered that they had brain disease, such as a frontal lobe tumor (Berg 1988; Kasztiak et al. 1985).

The most common application of the neuropsychological evaluation of adults without obvious risk factors for brain damage is in the early detection of progressive dementia, such as dementia of the Alzheimer type (Huff et al. 1987; LaRue and Jarvik 1987). Most persons have symptoms associated with dementia for at least 1 year before they see a health care provider because the problems initially are minor and easily attributed to factors such as aging or recent emotional stress. The progression of these symptoms is insidious, and people have "good" as well as "bad" days during the early course of this illness. Neuropsychological assessment is useful in evaluating whether problems noted by the family or the individual are age related, attributable to other factors such as depression, or suggestive of an early dementing illness. During the past decade, human immunodeficiency virus (HIV) infection and the complications of drug abuse have been added as conditions that can produce an insidious dementia in younger persons (Van Gorp et al. 1989).

Another condition that produces no clinical clues for brain damage except for a change in behavior is the so-called silent stroke. Without obvious sensory, motor, or speech problems, a stroke may go undetected yet produce a persistent change in behavior or abilities. A series of small strokes can produce an insidious dementia. Environmental toxins comprise another class of hidden conditions that present general patterns of neuropsychological impairment (Freed and Kandel 1988; Weiss 1983).

Neuropsychological signs and symptoms that are possible indicators of a pathological brain process are presented in Table 5–1. Positive neuropsychological diagnoses are much more likely to be made when risk factors for brain dysfunction exist or signs and symptoms of brain dysfunction are observed than when neuropsychological diagnoses are considered solely on the basis of exclusion of other diagnoses.

One of the greatest challenges for a neuropsychologist is to assess whether psychiatric patients have evidence of an underlying brain disorder. Many psychiatric patients without neurological disease have cognitive disruption and behavioral or emotional aberrations that also occur in patients with brain damage (Frith and Done

Table 5–1. Neuropsychological signs and symptoms that are possible indicators of a pathological brain process

Functional class	Symptoms and signs
Speech and language	Dysarthria Dysfluency Marked change in amount of speech output Paraphasias Word-finding problems
Academic skills	Alterations in reading, writing frequent letter or number reversals, calculating, and number abilities
Thinking	Perseveration of speech Simplified or confused mental racking reasoning and concept formation
Motor	Weakness or clumsiness particularly if lateralized Impaired fine motor coordination (e.g., changes in handwriting) Apraxias Perseveration of action components
Memory[a]	Impaired recent memory for verbal or visuospatial material or both Disorientation
Perception	Diplopia or visual field alterations Inattention (usually left-sided) Somatosensory alterations (particularly if lateralized) Inability to recognize familiar stimuli (agnosia)
Visuospatial abilities	Diminished ability to perform manual skills (e.g., mechanical repairs and sewing) Spatial disorientation Left-right disorientation Impaired spatial judgment (e.g., distances angulation)
Emotions[b]	Diminished emotional control with temper outburst and antisocial behavior Diminished empathy or interest in interpersonal relationships Affective changes Irritability without evident precipitating factors Personality change
Comportment[b]	Altered appetites and appetitive activities Altered grooming habits (excessive fastidiousness and carelessness) Hyper- or hypoactivity Social inappropriateness

[a]Many emotionally disturbed persons complain of memory deficits, which most typically reflect the person's self-preoccupation, distractibility, or anxiety rather than a dysfunctional brain. Thus memory complaints in themselves do not necessarily warrant neuropsychological evaluation.

[b]Some of these changes are most likely to be neuropsychologically relevant in the absence of depression, although they can also be mistaken for depression.

1988; Taylor and Abrams 1987). Anxiety and depression often impair concentration and memory and may also slow thinking (Mayes 1988; Stromgren 1977). Numerous studies (Heaton et al. 1978; Lenzer 1980) have shown that neuropsychological test scores alone often fail to discriminate between patients with schizophrenia and those with brain damage. Although neuropsychological assessment provides a measure of the type and degree of cognitive disorder, it often cannot specify the etiology of the disturbance. In the absence of known or suspected brain injury, a patient with known psychiatric illness and nonspecific cognitive impairment is most likely experiencing cognitive disruption on the basis of the psychiatric illness. On the other hand, an adult patient previously functioning well and with no history of psychiatric illness or recent stress would be suspect for brain disease.

THE ROLE OF THE REFERRING PSYCHIATRIST

The referring psychiatrist has the tasks of selecting patients who might benefit from an evaluation, preparing them, and formulating referral questions that best define the needed neuropsychological information. A valid evaluation depends on obtaining the patient's best performance. It usually is impossible to obtain satisfactory evaluations of patients who are uncooperative, fatigued, actively psychotic, seriously depressed, or highly anxious. For example, seriously depressed patients may resemble patients with mild dementia by their poor performance on cognitive tests, and the evaluation may underestimate the individual's full potential (Marcopulos 1989). Whenever possible such patients should be referred after there has been clinical improvement, when the results may be more representative of the patient's true ability.

Preparation of the patient for the evaluation is important to obtain the patient's cooperation and alleviate unnecessary anxiety. The patient should understand the nature and purpose of the evaluation. How the evaluation is designed depends on whether the patient is a candidate for psychotherapy or, for example, requesting evaluation for a personal injury lawsuit. The more explicit the referral question is, the more likely it is that the evaluation will provide useful information.

THE ASSESSMENT PROCESS

Interview and observation are the chief means by which neuropsychological evaluations are conducted. The main purposes of the interview are to elicit the patient's and family's complaints, understand the circumstances in which these problems occur, and evaluate the patient's attitude toward these problems. Understanding the range of the patient's complaints, as well as which ones the patient views as most troublesome, contributes to the framework on which the assessment and recommendations are based.

Patients with certain neuropsychological conditions lack awareness of their problems or diminish the significance of them. Many patients with right-hemisphere stroke, Alzheimer's disease, and frontal lobe damage are unaware of or unable to appreciate the problems resulting from their brain injury. Conversely, patients, families, or caregivers sometimes attribute problems to brain damage when a careful history suggests otherwise.

The interview provides an opportunity to observe the patient's appearance, speech, motor abilities, and to evaluate affect, appropriateness of behavior, orientation, insight, and judgment. The interview can provide information about the patient's premorbid intellectual ability and personality, occupational and school background, social situation, and ability to use leisure time.

The tests used by neuropsychologists are standardized observation tools that provide normative data that can aid in interpreting clinical observations. Various assessment approaches are available, all of which have in common the goals of determining whether the patient shows evidence of brain dysfunction and of identifying the nature of any problems detected. The two main approaches are individually tailored examinations and fixed assessment procedures.

The former approach, often referred to as *hypothesis testing,* involves obtaining information about the patient's medical and psychological background and his or her activities. Hypotheses regarding neuropsychological deficits are generated and tested (Kaplan 1988). Obtaining as much information as possible before the assessment procedure begins allows for the efficient generation of specific hypotheses. Moreover, hypothesis testing continues throughout the assessment. When a problem is observed on a particular test, new hypotheses are generated or old ones are modified. Typically, the examination focuses on problem areas while briefly screening those areas that appear to be relatively intact. When detailed information about residual competencies is required (e.g., in developing a remediation program), the focus may be expanded to assess areas of strength.

A second approach to neuropsychological testing involves using a fixed battery of tests that examine the same range of cognitive and behavioral functioning in every individual (Boll 1981; Reitan and Wolfson 1985). Fixed battery examinations frequently last from 6 to 8 hours. The advantage of fixed batteries is that the patient has a fairly broad-based examination. The consistency of the administration procedures and wide range of data make batteries useful for research purposes.

Cognitive performance is only one aspect of an assessment. A full evaluation of the individual assesses emotional and social characteristics as well. Many patients with brain injury have changes in personality, mood, or ability to control emotional states (Lishman 1987). In some cases these changes may be secondary to cognitive impairment. Right-hemisphere stroke patients may show impaired processing of emotional material and complex social situations, which leads to interpersonal problems (Lezak 1979). Although the history and observers' reports will inform the examiner of changes in these characteristics, current emotional status and personality can also be evaluated by standard psychological tests. Performance by brain-injured populations on some of these tests have shown patterned alternations of personality and emotional status (Lezak et al. 1990; Robinson et al. 1984).

NEUROPSYCHOLOGICAL TESTING

An important component of neuropsychological evaluations is psychological testing in which an individual's cognitive, and often emotional, status and executive functioning are assessed. (For a relatively complete review of available tests see Lezak, in press.) Neuropsychological assessment differs from psychological assessment in its basic assumptions. The latter compares the individual's responses with normative data from a sample of people from the population at large taking the same test (Anastasi 1988). The neuropsychological assessment of adults relies on comparisons between the patient's present level of functioning and the known or estimated level of premorbid functioning (Lezak 1986).

Most tests of abilities are designed with the expectation that only very few persons will obtain a perfect score and that most scores will cluster in a middle range. For these tests, scores are reported as a continuous variable. The scores of many persons taking the test can be plotted as a distribution curve. Most scores on tests of complex learned behaviors fall into a characteristic bell-shaped curve called a *normal distribution curve*. The statistical descriptors of the curve are the "mean" or average of all scores, the degree of spread of scores about the mean expressed as the "standard deviation," and the "range" or highest to lowest scores obtained.

An individual's score is compared with the normative data, often by calculating a standard or *z* score, which describes the individual's performance in terms of standard deviations from the mean. Using this calculation, scores within ±0.6 standard deviations are considered average because 50% of the normative sample scored within this range. Moreover, *z* scores are used to describe the probability that a deviant response occurs by chance or because of an impairment. A performance in the below-average direction that is greater than 2 standard deviations from the mean usually is described as "impaired" because 97.8% of the normative sample taking the test achieved better scores.

Some test makers recommend "cutoff" scores to evaluate certain test performances. The cutoff scores represent those exceeded by most neuropsychologically intact persons; scores below the cutoff point are typically achieved by persons suffering impairment in the relevant abilities. Cutoff scores usually are derived on the basis of the distribution of scores of a healthy control sample. The threshold for "normal" is typically set at 1.5 standard deviations below the mean to include the top 95% of the control sample. Cutoff scores work best on tests of abilities normally expected in all adults, such as basic language or motor skills.

Some psychological tests detect subtle deficits better than others. Tests of concentration and new learning are more sensitive than many other cognitive tests at reflecting brain damage because a wide variety of brain disorders can easily disrupt performance on them. However, other factors such as depression, anxiety, medicine side effects, and low energy level due to systemic illness may also disrupt cognition on these sensitive tests. Therefore, they are sensitive to cognitive disruption but not specific to one type of cognitive disturbance, such as brain damage. The specificity of a test in indicating a disorder depends on the overlap in distribution of scores between persons who are intact and those who have the disorder (Figure 5–1). The less overlap there is, the more diagnostic the test result will be. Many neuropsychological tests offer a tradeoff between sensitivity and specificity.

Indications of brain dysfunction come from qualitative features of the patient's performance as well as from test scores (Pankratz and Taplin 1982; Walsh 1985). There are many reasons for failing a test, and a poor score does not tell the means to the end. Some features of behavioral disturbance show up best in the manner in which the patient approaches the testing situation or behaves with the examiner. Patients with brain injury are prone to problems with short attention span, distractibility, impulsiveness, poor self-monitoring, disorganization, irritability, perplexity, and suspiciousness. A sensitive and knowledgeable examiner can distinguish these factors from simple cognitive incompetence.

Interpretation Principles and Cautions

The interpretation of test data is based on performance expectations for each individual patient, which require that deviations from expectation be evaluated in terms of known deficit patterns (Lezak 1983, 1986). Most people perform within a statistically definable range on cognitive tests, and this range of performance levels is considered to be characteristic of them. Deviations below this expected range raise the question of an impairment.

The assumptions of deficit measurement are valid in most cases, although outliers do exist who show an unusual variability on cognitive tasks (Matarazzo and Prifitera 1989). Multiple measures on similar tasks increase the reliability of findings. If someone has a deviant score on a task, performance on other tasks requiring the same skills will show whether the deviant finding persists across tasks. If so, the finding is considered reliable.

Interpretation of test performances also must take into account demographic variables. When estimating the premorbid ability levels necessary for making individual

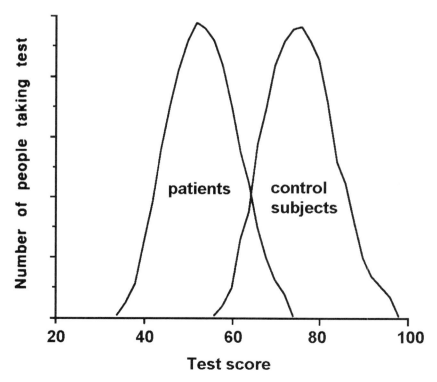

Figure 5–1.   Distribution of hypothetical test scores by a control group and a patient group. In this case, scores between 56 and 74 occurred in both groups. The smaller the area of overlapping curves, the higher the test specificity.

comparisons, the examiner must consider the patient's educational and occupational background, sex, and race along with his or her level of test performance. The more severely impaired a patient is, the more unlikely it is that performance will reach premorbid levels on any of the tests, thus increasing the examiner's reliance on demographic and historical data (Crawford et al. 1989; Karzmark et al. 1985). Some tests, such as recognition vocabulary and fund of information, are fairly resistant to disruption by brain damage and may offer the best estimates of premorbid ability (Baddeley et al. 1988; Crawford et al. 1988).

For meaningful interpretations of neuropsychological test performance, examiners must rely on many tests and search for a response pattern that makes neuropsychological sense. Because there are few pathognomonic findings in neuropsychology, or most other branches of medical sciences for that matter (Sox et al. 1988), response patterns can often suggest several diagnoses. For example, a performance pattern including slowed thinking and mild impairment of concentration and memory is a nonspecific finding associated with several conditions: very mild dementia, a mild post concussion syndrome, mild toxic encephalopathy, multiple sclerosis, depression, or fatigue, to name a few. Other patterns may be highly specific for certain conditions. The findings of left-sided neglect and visuospatial impairment are highly suggestive of brain dysfunction and specifically occur with right-hemisphere damage. For many neuropsychological conditions, typical patterns of deficits are known, and the examiner evaluates the patient's performances in light of these known patterns for a possible match.

The Major Test Categories

Intellectual ability. The most commonly used sets of tests of general intellectual function of adults are contained in one or another version of the Wechsler Adult Intelligence Scale (WAIS) (Wechsler 1944, 1955, 1981). These batteries of brief tests, often referred to as *subtests,* provide scores on various cognitive tasks covering a range of skills. Each version was originally developed as an "intelligence" test to predict academic and vocational performance of neurologically intact adults by giving an "IQ" score: an intelligence quotient score based on the mean performance. The battery of 11 tests was designed to assess relatively distinct areas of cognition, such as arithmetic, abstract thinking, and visuospatial organization, and thus are differentially sensitive to dysfunction of various areas of the brain. Therefore, the WAIS is often used to screen for specific areas of cognitive deficits. When given to neuropsychologically impaired persons, the summary IQ scores can be very misleading because they will be affected by specific cognitive deficits yet in themselves provide no clue to the nature of contributing brain disorder(s) (Lezak 1988).

In some cases neuropsychologists have used discrepancies between summed scores on the Verbal Scale of the WAIS (i.e., Verbal IQ) and summed scores on the Performance Scale (i.e., Performance IQ) to indicate a specific area of cognitive deficit. The procedure has developed because left-hemisphere lesions tend to produce a relatively depressed Verbal IQ score, whereas both right-hemisphere lesions and diffuse damage (as in dementing conditions) produce a depressed Performance IQ score. Since even this amount of summation can mask important data it is important to use and interpret these tests discretely.

The equivalent tests for assessing children are the Wechsler Intelligence Scale for Children-Revised (WISC-R; Wechsler 1974) and the newly revised Wechsler Intelligence Scale for Children–Third Edition (WISC-III; Wechsler 1991). They contain subtests similar to the WAIS, but appropriate for children 6–16 years old.

Language.   Lesions to the hemisphere dominant for speech and language, which is the left hemisphere in 95%–97% of right-handers and 60%–70% of left-handers (Strauss and Goldsmith 1987), can produce any of a variety of disorders of symbol formulation and use (i.e., the aphasias). Although many aphasiologists argue against attempting to classify all patients into one of the standard aphasia syndromes because of individual differences, aphasic patients tend to be grouped according to whether the main disorder is in language comprehension (receptive aphasia), expression (expressive aphasia), repetition (conduction aphasia), or naming (anomic aphasia). Many comprehensive language assessment tests are available. Comprehensive aphasia test batteries are best administered by speech pathologists or other clinicians with special training in this field. These batteries usually include measures of spontaneous speech, speech comprehension, repetition, naming, reading, and writing.

Attention and mental tracking.   A frequent consequence of brain injury is slowed thinking and impaired ability for focused behavior (Gronwall and Sampson 1974). In addition, damage to the brain stem or diffuse damage involving the cerebral hemispheres can produce various attentional deficits. Many neuropsychological assessments include measures of these abilities. The Wechsler scales contain several. The Digit Span subtest measures attention span or short-term memory for numbers by assessing forward digit repetition. The task also measures backward digit repetition, which is a more demanding task requiring concentration and mental tracking. It is not uncommon for patients with brain damage, even those who are severely impaired, to perform poorly only on the backward repetition portion of this test.

Another commonly used measure of concentration and mental tracking is the Trail Making Test (Armitage 1946). In part A of this test, the patient is asked to draw rapidly and accurately a line connecting in sequence a random display of numbered circles on a page. The level of difficulty is increased in part B by having the patient again sequence a random display of circles, this time containing both numbers and letters, requiring the patient to go from *1* to *A* to *2* to *B* to *3*, and so forth (Figure 5–2). It examines concentration, visual scanning, and flexibility in shifting cognitive sets. This test is among those that are most sensitive to the presence of brain injury (Crockett et al. 1988; van Zomeren and Brouwer 1990).

In cases of subtle brain injury, assessment sensitivity can be increased by selecting a more difficult measure of concentration and mental tracking, such as the Paced Auditory Serial Addition Test (PASAT; Gronwall 1977). The patient is required to add consecutive pairs of numbers rapidly under an interference condition. As numbers are presented at a fixed rate, the patient must always add the last two numbers presented and ignore the number that represents the last summation. For example, if the numbers "*3-5-2-7*" are presented, the patient must respond "*8*" after the number *5*, and then "*7*" after the number *2*, and then "*9*." It is a difficult task because of the strong tendency to add the last number presented to the last summation.

Memory.   Memory is another cognitive function often impaired by brain injury. Many diffuse brain injuries produce general impairments in abilities for learning and retention. Many focal brain injuries also produce memory impairments, with left-hemisphere lesions most likely to produce primarily verbal memory deficits, whereas visuospatial memory impairments tend to be associated with right-hemisphere lesions (Milner 1978; Ojemann and Dodrill 1985). Memory impairment often is a prominent feature of herpes encephalitis, hypoxia, closed head injury, and neurological degenerative diseases such as multiple sclerosis and early stages of Alzheimer's disease (Kapur 1988; Mayes 1988). Conditions that produce amnesic syndromes in which memory impairment is paramount include Huntington's chorea, Korsakoff's syndrome, and some anoxic conditions (Butters et al. 1976; Parkin et al. 1987).

In most cases of brain injury, memory for information learned before the injury is relatively preserved compared with new learning. For this reason many patients

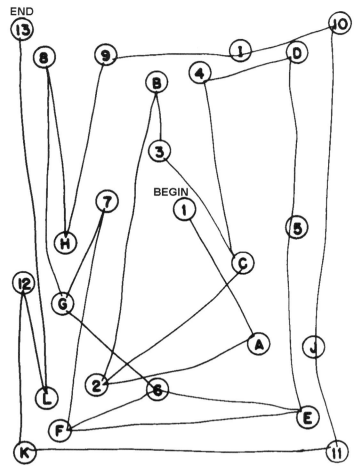

Figure 5–2.   Trail Making Test (Armitage 1946) part B performance by a 61-year-old man with normal-pressure hydrocephalus. Two type of errors are demonstrated: erroneous sequencing (1 → A → 2 → C) and failure to alternate between numbers and letters (D → 5 → E → F).

with memory impairment perform relatively well on tests of fund of information or recall of remote events. However, amnesic disorders can produce a retrograde amnesia extending back weeks, months, or years before the onset of the injury. The retrograde amnesia of Huntington's chorea or Korsakoff's syndrome can extend decades (Butters and Miliotis 1985; Cermak 1982).

The Wechsler Memory Scale-Revised (WMS-R; Wechsler 1987) is the most commonly used set of tests of new learning and retention in the United States. This battery is composed of subtests measuring free recall or recognition of both verbal and visuospatial material. Also, the WMS-R includes measures of recall of personal information and attention, concentration, and mental tracking. Other memory tests frequently used include word-list learning tasks, such as the Rey Auditory Verbal Learning Test (Rey 1964) or the California Verbal Learning Test (Delis et al. 1986) and visuospatial tasks, such as the Rey Complex Figure Test (Baser and Ruff 1987).

Perception.   Perception arising from any of the sensory modalities can be affected by brain disease. Perceptional inattention (sometimes called *neglect*) is one of the major perceptual syndromes because of its frequency in association with focal brain damage (Bisiach and Vallar 1988; Posner 1988). This phenomenon involves diminished or absent awareness of stimuli in one side of personal space by a patient with an intact sensory system. Unilateral inattention is often most prominent after acute-onset brain injury such as stroke. Most commonly seen is left-sided inattention associated with right-hemisphere stroke.

Several techniques can be used to elicit unilateral inattention. Visual inattention can be assessed using a Line Bisection Test (Schenkenberg et al. 1980), in which the patient is asked to bisect a series of lines on a page, or to cross out a designated symbol distributed among other similar symbols on a page (Bisiach and Vallar 1988; Gauthier et al. 1985). The most commonly used forms of perceptual tests assess perceptual discrimination among similar stimuli. These visual tests may include discrimination of geometric forms, angulation, color, faces, or familiar objects (Lezak 1983; McCarthy and Warrington 1990; Newcombe and Ratcliff 1989). Some perceptual tasks examine ability for perceptual synthesis. The Hooper Visual Organization Test (Hooper 1958) presents line drawings of familiar objects in fragmented, disarranged pieces and asks for the name of each object. Many of these tests also can be administered in tactile versions (Craig 1985; Varney 1986). Frequently used tactile tests include form recognition and letter or number recognition (Reitan and Wolfson 1985).

Another important area of perceptual assessment is recognition of familiar visual stimuli. Although the syndromes are rare and often occur independently of one another, a brain injury can produce an inability to recognize visually familiar objects (visual object agnosia) or faces (prosopagnosia) (Benson 1989; Damasio et al. 1989). Recognition assessment typically involves asking the patient to give the name of real objects or of representations of objects, sometimes in a masked or distorted form. The WAIS includes a perceptual task in which the patient is asked to identify missing features of line drawings of familiar objects.

Praxis.   Many aphasic patients have at least one form of apraxia. Their inability to perform the required sequence of motor activities is not based on motor weakness. Rather, the deficit is in planning and carrying out the required activities (Jason 1990).

Tests of praxis measure the patient's ability to reproduce learned movements of the face or limbs. These learned movements can include the use of objects (usually in pantomime), gestures, or sequences of movements demonstrated by the examiner (Christensen 1979).

Constructional ability.   Although constructional problems were once considered a form of apraxia, analysis has shown that the underlying deficits involve impaired appreciation of one or more aspects of spatial relationships, including distortions in perspective, angulation, size, and distance judgment or difficulty appreciating or integrating details. Therefore, unlike apraxia, the problem is not an inability to draw lines or assemble constructions, but rather misperceptions and misjudgments involving spatial relationship or the fine-grained characteristics of a percept. Lesions of the posterior cerebral cortex cause the greatest difficulty with constructions, with right-hemisphere lesions producing greater deficits than left-hemisphere lesions. Neuropsychological assessments may include any of a number of measures of visuospatial processing. Patients may be asked to copy geometric designs, such as the Rey Complex Figure (Rey 1964) presented in Figure 5–3. The WAIS battery includes constructional tasks involving reconstructing designs with blocks and assembling puzzle pieces (Wechsler 1944, 1955, 1981).

Conceptual functions.   Conceptual dysfunction tends to occur with serious brain injury regardless of site. Most neuropsychological tests require intactness of simple conceptual functioning. For example, reasoning skills are required for the successful performance of most WAIS tests: Comprehension assesses commonsense verbal reasoning and interpretation of proverbs, Picture Completion requires perceptual reasoning, Similarities measures ability to make verbal abstractions by asking for similarities between objects or concepts, Arithmetic involves arithmetic problem solving, Picture Arrangement examines sequential reasoning for thematic pictures, and Block Design and Object Assembly test visuospatial analysis and problem solving of block designs and puzzles.

A   **B**

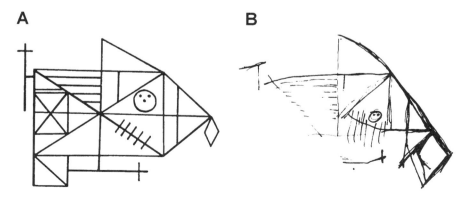

Figure 5–3.   Rey Complex Figure (*panel A*) and copy (*panel B*) by a 42-year-old, right-handed man who had a right frontoparietal stroke 4 days before this examination. The copy shows the patient's neglect of the left and lower portions of the figure, a strong perseverative tendency, as well as visuospatial fragmentation.

Other commonly used tests of concept formation include the Category Test (Halstead 1947) and the Wisconsin Card Sorting (WCS) Test (Berg 1948). These tests measure concept formation, hypothesis testing, problem solving, and flexibility of thinking. The Category Test presents patterns of stimuli and requires the patient to figure out a principle or concept that is true for each item within a set based on feedback about the correctness of each response. The WCS and the Category Test both require the patient to figure out a principle that is true for items within a set. The examiner changes the correct principle as the test proceeds without warning the patient. Therefore, the patient must realize that a shift in principles has occurred and act accordingly.

Executive functions. Executive functions include abilities to formulate a goal, make plans, and effectively carry out goal-directed plans and to monitor and self-correct spontaneously and reliably (Lezak 1982). These are difficult tasks for many patients with frontal lobe or diffuse brain injuries. Yet they are essential for most adult responsible and socially appropriate conduct. Tasks that best assess executive functions are tests of planning and/or open-ended tests that permit the patient to decide when the task is complete. One type of test that requires planning is a maze. The patient must plan an exit to the maze, which involves foresight to minimize trial-and-error behavior. Other tasks that rely heavily on planning for successful completion are multistep tasks requiring decision making or priority setting. Few neuropsychological tests are designed specifically to assess this aspect of behavior, yet many complex tasks depend on this analysis.

Inertia presents one of the most difficult assessment problems for neuropsychologists because there are few open-ended tests that measure initiation or ability to carry out purposeful behavior. By their very nature, most tests are structured and require little initiation by the patient (Lezak 1982). Examples of less structured tests include the Tinker Toy Test, in which patients decide what to build and how to design it (Bayless et al. 1989), and free drawing tests, in which patients are requested to draw a bicycle or house. Because there are few rules, patients must choose their level of productivity.

Motor functions. Neuropsychological tests can supplement the neurological examination of motor functions by providing standardized measures of motor activities. Normative data have been acquired for commonly measured functions such as grip strength and finger tapping (Bornstein 1985). More complex tests of fine motor coordination include tests that require patients to rapidly place pegs in holes, such as the Grooved Pegboard Test (Baser and Ruff 1987) and the Purdue Pegboard Test (Purdue Research Foundation 1948).

Personality and emotional status. Numerous questionnaires have been developed to measure symptoms of physical and emotional distress of patients with neurological or medical problems (Lezak 1989). Many tests originally devised as measures of psychological distress or psychiatric illness have been used with brain-injured persons. The revised version of the Symptom Check List-90 (SCL-90-R; Derogatis 1983) is a self-report of symptoms associated with psychiatric disorders when they occur at high-frequency levels. The Minnesota Multiphasic Personality Inventory (MMPI;

Hathaway and McKinley 1951; Welsh and Dahlstrom 1956) has been used extensively with brain-injured patients (Chelune et al. 1986; Mueller and Girace 1988). The revised version—MMPI-2 (Butcher and Pope 1990; Butcher et al. 1989)—contains the same basic clinical scales with deletions of a small percentage of the items and new normative data.

In general, persons with brain damage tend to have elevated MMPI profiles, which may reflect the relatively frequent incidence of emotional disturbance in these patients (Filskov and Leli 1981), their accurate reporting of symptoms and deficits (Lezak 1983), or their compromised ability to read or understand the test questions. Elevations in the Hypochondriasis (Hs), Hysteria (Hy), and Schizophrenia (Sc) scales are common because many "neurological" symptoms appear on these scales (Alfano et al. 1990). The interpretation of MMPI data for persons with brain damage must take into account the contributions of neurological symptoms, emotional reactions to brain injury, and premorbid personality.

Many attempts have been made to use the MMPI to differentiate diagnoses of psychiatric and neurological illness. Results generally have been unsatisfactory, probably because of the extreme variety of brain injury and their associated problems (Alfano et al. 1990; Gass et al. 1990; Mueller and Girace 1988). The MMPI also has been an inefficient instrument for localizing cerebral lesions (Lezak 1983).

Special Assessment Tools

Batteries.   Many examiners use a preferred battery of tests, such as the WAIS (described earlier) in evaluating patients. Of the commercial batteries designed for neuropsychological evaluations, by far the most popular in the United States is the Halstead-Reitan Neuropsychological Test Battery. This battery was designed to assess frontal lobe disorders by W. C. Halstead (1947) and revised by R. Reitan (1969), who recommended this battery as a diagnostic test for all kinds of brain damage. The tests include the Category Test (described above); the Tactual Performance Test, a tactile visuospatial performance and memory test; the Rhythm Test, a nonverbal auditory perception test; Speech Sounds Perception Test, a phoneme discrimination test; the Finger Tapping Test, a motor speed test; the Trail Making Test (described above); a shortened version of Wepman's Aphasia Screening Test, which Wepman later rejected as inadequate (Snow 1987); a sensory examination; and a measure of grip strength. Most examiners administer this battery with one of the forms of the WAIS, WMS, and MMPI.

Examinations designed to address specific diagnostic questions are available. Several dementia examinations have been devised. The Mattis Dementia Rating Scale (Mattis 1988) contains items assessing attention, initiation and/or perseveration, construction, conceptualization, and memory and is useful in distinguishing dementia from cognitive decline associated with aging.

Screening tests.   Many clinicians would like to have a brief, reliable screening examination with good sensitivity for brain damage that is of unknown etiology or only suspected. However, brief examinations are often too restricted in range or too simple to be sensitive to subtle or circumscribed areas of dysfunction. The commonly used Mini-Mental State Exam (MMSE; Folstein et al. 1975) contains only 11 simple tasks.

It is useful for examining patients with global confusion or poor memory. However, many patients with brain injury, such as those with stroke, mild to moderate head injury, and even early dementia, perform adequately on this examination. (Auerbach and Faibish 1989; Naugle and Kauczak 1989).

As screening examinations become lengthier and contain more difficult items their usefulness improves. An example of an expanded examination that has proven useful for screening is the Neurobehavioral Cognitive Status Examination (NCSE; Kiernan et al. 1987; Schwamm et al. 1987). This examination takes approximately 30 minutes and contains reasonably difficult items of attention; language comprehension, repetition, and naming; constructional ability; memory; calculations; reasoning; and judgment, which together make it fairly sensitive (Figure 5–4). As a screening examination, the NCSE does not substitute for a thorough neuropsychological examination. It may be used to acquire information to decide whether further evaluation is warranted.

Competency. A cognitive competency determination usually is based on a specialized interview in which the ability to handle financial matters and/or make decisions regarding well-being is assessed by asking patients about their personal situation. The patients' understanding of their personal needs is more relevant to a competency de-

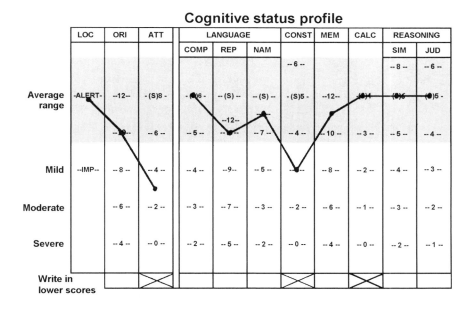

Figure 5–4. The Neurobehavioral Cognitive Status Examination (NCSE) performance profile of a 42-year-old alcoholic man, showing mild deficits on attention and constructional tasks. LOC = level of consciousness; ORI = orientation; ATT = attention; COMP = comprehension; REP = repetition; NAM = naming; CONST = construction; MEM = memory; CALC = calculations; SIM = similarities; JUD = judgment; (S) = screening item; IMP = impaired.

Source. Reprinted from Northern California Neurobehavioral Group: *Test Booklet for the Neurobehavioral Cognitive Status Examination.* Fairfax, CA, 1988. Copyright 1988, The Northern California Neurobehavioral Group, Inc. Used with permission.

termination than a score on a formal test. Nevertheless, the Cognitive Competency Test (Wang et al. 1987) is a useful component of a competency examination of patients with brain injury because it evaluates cognitive skills required to maintain safe and independent living. The test samples a wide range of cognitive skills varying from overlearned, basic living skills (e.g., counting change) to memory, abstract problem solving, and safety judgment.

TREATMENT AND PLANNING

Examination findings provide information about an individual's strengths and weaknesses necessary for formulating treatment interventions. Clinical interventions vary according to each individual's specific needs. Many patients with brain damage have primary or secondary emotional problems for which psychotherapy or counseling may seem advisable. However, patients with brain damage frequently have problems that compromise their capacity to use such treatment. Foremost among these problems are cognitive rigidity, which may limit the patient's adaptability, and defective learning, which may restrict his or her ability to acquire new attitudes, understanding, or interpersonal skills. Evaluation findings are also frequently used for consideration of a person's ability for independence in society and for estimating educational or vocational potential.

CONCLUSIONS

The field of neuropsychology is enriched by the diversity of areas of expertise of those interested in the study of brain-behavior relationships. Professionals in this field come from backgrounds in psychology, psychiatry, neurology, neurosurgery, and language pathology to name only a few. In psychology alone professionals come from backgrounds in clinical, cognitive, developmental, and physiological psychology.

Professionals qualified to provide clinical evaluations have both expertise in brain-behaviors relationships and skills in diagnostic assessment and counseling (Bornstein 1988a, 1988b). There are a growing number of qualified neuropsychologists and a recently established recognition of proficiency in this subspecialty area by the American Board of Professional Psychology's award of Diploma in Clinical Neuropsychology (Bieliauskas and Matthews 1987).

REFERENCES

Acker MB: A review of the ecological validity of neuropsychological tests, in The Neuropsychology of Everyday Life: Assessment and Basic Competencies. Edited by Tupper DE, Cicerone KD. Boston, Kluver Academic, 1989, pp 19–55

Alfano DP, Finlayson AJ, Stearns GM, et al: The MMPI and neurologic dysfunction: profile configuration and analysis. Clinical Neuropsychologist 4:69–79, 1990

Anastasi A: Psychological Testing, 6th Edition. New York, Macmillan, 1988

Armitage SG: An analysis of certain psychological tests used for the evaluation of brain injury. Psychological Monographs (No 277) 60:1–48, 1946

Auerbach VS, Faibish GM: Mini-Mental State Examination: diagnostic limitations in a hospital setting (abstract). J Clin Exp Neuropsychol 11:75, 1989

Baddeley A, Emslie H, Nimmo-Smith I: Estimating premorbid intelligence (abstract). J Clin Exp Neuropsychol 10:326, 1988

Baser CA, Ruff RM: Construct validity of the San Diego Neuropsychological Test Battery. Archives of Clinical Neuropsychology 2:13–32, 1987

Bayless JD, Varney NR, Roberts RJ: Tinker Toy Test performance and vocational outcome in patients with closed head injuries. J Clin Exp Neuropsychol 11:913–917, 1989

Benson DF: Disorders of visual gnosis, in Neuropsychology of Visual Perception. Edited by Brown JW. New York, IRBN, 1989, pp 59–76

Berg EA: A simple objective test for measuring flexibility in thinking. J Gen Psychol 39:15–22, 1948

Berg RA: Cancer, in Medical Neuropsychology. Edited by Tarter RE, Van Thiel DH, Edwards KL. New York, Plenum, 1988, pp 265–290

Bieliauskas LA, Matthews CG: American Board of Clinical Neuropsychology: Policies and Procedures. The Clinical Neuropsychologist 1:21–28, 1987

Bisiach E, Vallar G: Hemineglect in humans, in Handbook of Neuropsychology, Vol 1. Edited by Boller F, Grafman J, Rizzolatti G, et al. Amsterdam, Elsevier, 1988, pp 195–222

Boll TJ: The Halstead-Reitan Neuropsychology Battery, in Handbook of Clinical Neuropsychology. Edited by Filskov SB, Boll TJ. New York, Wiley-Intersciences, 1981, pp 577–607

Bornstein RA: Normative data on selected neuropsychological measures from a nonclinical sample. J Clin Psychol 41:651–659, 1985

Bornstein RA: Entry into clinical neuropsychology: graduate, undergraduate, and beyond. Clinical Neuropsychologist 2:213–220, 1988a

Bornstein RA: Reports of the Division 40 Task Force on Education, Accreditation, and Credentialing. Clinical Neuropsychologist 2:25–29, 1988b

Butcher JN, Pope KS: MMPI-2: a practical guide to clinical, psychometric, and ethical issues. Independent Practitioner 10:20–25, 1990

Butcher JN, Dahlstrom WG, Graham JR, et al: Minnesota Multiphasic Personality Inventory (MMPI-2): Manual for Administration and Scoring. Minneapolis, MN, University of Minnesota Press, 1989

Butters J, Miliotis P: Amnesic disorders, in Clinical Neuropsychology, 2nd Edition. Edited by Heilman KM, Valenstein E. New York, Oxford University Press, 1985, pp 403–451

Butters N, Tarlow S, Cermak LS, et al: A comparison of the information processing deficits of patients with Huntington's chorea and Korsakoff's syndrome. Cortex 12:134–144, 1976

Cermak LS (ed): Human Memory and Amnesia. Hillsdale, NJ, Laurence Erlbaum Associates, 1982

Chelune GJ, Ferguson W, Moehle K: The role of standard cognitive and personality tests in neuropsychological assessment, in Clinical Application of Neuropsychological Test Batteries. Edited by Incagnoli T, Goldstein G, Golden CJ. New York, Plenum, 1986, pp 75–119

Christensen A-L: Luria's Neuropsychological Investigation: Test Manual, 2nd Edition. Copenhagen, Munksgaard, 1979

Cope DN: Neuropharmacology and brain damage, in Neuropsychological Rehabilitation. Edited by Christensen A-L, Uzzell B. Boston, MA, Kluver Academic, 1988, pp 19–38

Craig JC: Tactile pattern perception and its perturbations. J Acoust Soc Am 77:238–246, 1985

Crawford JR, Parker DM, Besson JAO: Estimation of premorbid intelligence in organic conditions. Br J Psychiatry 153:178–181, 1988

Crawford JR, Stewart LE, Cochrane RHB, et al: Estimating premorbid IQ from demographic variables: regression equations derived from a UK sample. Br J Clin Psychol 280:275–278, 1989

Crockett D, Tallman K, Hurwitz T, et al: Neuropsychological performance in psychiatric patients with or without documented brain dysfunction. Int J Neurosci 41:71–79, 1988

Damasio AR, Tranel D, Damasio H: Disorders of visual recognition, in Handbook of Neuropsychology, Vol 2. Edited by Boller F, Grafman J. Amsterdam, Elsevier, 1989, pp 317–332

Delis DC, Kramer JH, Kaplan E, et al: California Verbal Learning Test. San Antonio, TX, Psychological Corporation, 1986

Derogatis LR: Symptom Checklist-90, Revised (SCL-90-R). Towson, MD, Clinical Psychometric Research, 1983

Dubois B, Pillon B, Sternic N, et al: Age-induced cognitive deficit in Parksinson's disease. Neurology 40:38–41, 1990

Eisenberg HM, Levin HS: Computed tomography and magnetic resonance imaging in mild to moderate head injury, in Mild Head Injury. Edited by Levin HS, Eisenberg HM, Benton AL. New York, Oxford University Press, 1989, pp 133–141

Filskov SB, Leli DA: Assessment of the individual in neuropsychological practice, in Handbook of Clinical Neuropsychology. Edited by Filskov SB, Boll TJ. New York, Wiley, 1981, pp 545–576

Folstein MF, Folstein SE, McHugh PR: Mini-Mental State: A practical method for grading the cognitive state of patients for the clinician. J Psychiatr Res 12:189–198, 1975

Freed DM, Kandel E: Long-term occupational exposure and the diagnosis of dementia. Neurotoxicology 9:391–400, 1988

Frith CD, Done DJ: Towards a neuropsychology of schizophrenia. Br J Psychiatry 153:437–443, 1988

Gass CS, Russell EW, Hamilton RA: Accuracy of MMPI-based inferences regarding memory and concentration in closed-head-trauma patients. Psychological Assessment: A Journal of Consulting and Clinical Psychology 2:175–178, 1990

Gauthier L, Gauthier S, Joanette Y: Visual neglect in left, right, and bilateral Parkinsonians (abstract). J Clin Exp Neuropsychol 7:145, 1985

Gronwall DMA: Paced Auditory Serial-Addition Task: a measure of recovery from concussion. Percept Mot Skills 44:367–373, 1977

Gronwall DMA, Sampson H: The psychological effects of concussion. Auckland, New Zealand, University Press, 1974

Halstead WC: Brain and Intelligence. Chicago, IL, University of Chicago Press, 1947

Hathaway SR, McKinley JC: The Minnesota Multiphasic Personality Inventory Manual (Revised). New York, Psychological Corporation, 1951

Heaton RK, Baade LE, Johnson KL: Neuropsychological test results associated with psychiatric disorders in adults. Psychol Bull 85:141–162, 1978

Hebb DO: The effect of early and late brain injury upon test scores, and the nature of normal adult intelligence. Proceedings of the American Philosophical Society 85:275–292, 1942

Hooper HE: The Hooper Visual Organization Test. Los Angeles, CA, Western Psychological Services, 1958

Huff FJ, Growdon JH, Corkin S, et al: Age at onset and rate of progression of Alzheimer's disease. J Am Geriatr Soc 35:27–30, 1987

Jason GW: Disorders of motor function following cortical lesions: review and theoretical considerations, in Cerebral Control of Speech and Limb Movements. Edited by Hammond GR. Amsterdam, Elsevier, 1990, pp 141–168

Jernigan TL, Hesselink JR: Human brain-imaging: basic principles and applications in psychiatry, in Psychiatry, Vol 3. Edited by Michels R, Cavenar JO. Philadelphia, PA, JB Lippincott, 1987, Chapter 51, pp 1–9

Kaplan E: A process approach to neuropsychological assessment, in Clinical Neuropsychological and Brain Function: Research, Measurement, and Practice. Edited by Boll T, Bryant BK. Washington, DC, American Psychological Association, 1988, pp 125–167

Kapur N: Memory Disorders in Clinical Practice. London, Butterworths, 1988

Karzmark P, Heaton RK, Grant I, et al: Use of demographic variables to predict full scale IQ: A replication and extension. J Clin Exp Neuropsychol 7:412–420, 1985

Kaszniak AW, Sadeh M, Stern LZ: Differentiating depression from organic brain syndromes in older age, in Depression in the Elderly: An Interdisciplinary Approach. Edited by Chaisson-Stewart GM. New York, Wiley, 1985, pp 161–189

Kiernan RJ, Mueller J, Langston JW, et al: The Neurobehavioral Cognitive Status Examination: a brief but differentiated approach to cognitive assessment. Ann Intern Med 107:481–485, 1987

Kolb B: Preoperative events and brain damage: a commentary, in Preoperative Events: Their Effects on Behavior Following Brain Damage. Edited by Schulkin J. New York, Erlbaum, 1989, pp 305–311

LaRue A, Jarvik LR: Cognitive function and prediction of dementia in old age. Int J Aging Hum Dev 25:79–89, 1987

Lenzer I: Halstead-Reitan Test Battery: problem of differential diagnosis. Percept Mot Skills 50:611–630, 1980

Lezak MD: Behavioral concomitants of configurational disorganization. Paper presented at the seventh annual meeting of the International Neuropsychological Society, New York, February 1979

Lezak MD: The problem of assessing executive functions. International Journal of Psychology 17:281–297, 1982

Lezak MD: Neuropsychological Assessment, 2nd Edition. New York, Oxford University Press, 1983

Lezak MD: An individualized approach to neuropsychological assessment, in Clinical Neuropsychology. Edited by Logue PE, Schear JM. Springfield, IL, CC Thomas, 1986, pp 29–49

Lezak MD: IQ: R.I.P. J Clin Exp Neuropsychol 10:351–361, 1988

Lezak MD: Assessment of psychosocial dysfunctions resulting from head trauma, in Assessment of the Behavioral Consequences of Head Trauma, Vol 7: Frontiers of Clinical Neuroscience. Edited by Lezak MD. New York, Alan R Liss, 1989, pp 113–144

Lezak MD: Neuropsychological Assessment, 3rd Edition. New York, Oxford University Press (in press)

Lezak MD, Witham R, Bourdette D: Emotional impact of cognitive inefficiencies in multiple sclerosis (abstract). J Clin Exp Neuropsychol 12:50, 1990

Lishman WA: Organic Psychiatry, 2nd Edition. Oxford, England, Blackwell Scientific, 1987

McCarthy RA, Warrington EK: Cognitive Neuropsychology: A Clinical Introduction. San Diego, CA, Academic Press, 1990

Mapov RL: Testing to detect brain damage; an alternative to what may no longer be useful. J Clin Exp Neuropsychol 10:271–278, 1988

Marcopulos BA: Pseudodementia, dementia, and depression: test differentiation, in Testing Older Adults: A Reference Guide for Geropsychological Assessments. Edited by Hunt T, Lindley CJ. Austin, TX, Pro-ed, 1989, pp 70–91

Matarazzo JD, Prifitera A: Subtest scatter and premorbid intelligence: lessons from the WAIS-R standardization sample. J Consult Clin Psychol 1:186–191, 1989

Mattis S: Dementia Rating Scale (DRS) Manual. Odessa, FL, Psychological Assessment Resources, 1988

Mayes AR: Human Organic Memory Disorders. New York, Cambridge University Press, 1988

Milner B: Clues to the cerebral organization of memory, in Cerebral Correlates of Conscious Experience (INSERM Symposium No. 6). Edited by Buser PA, Rougeul-Buser A. Amsterdam, Elsevier/North Holland Biomedical, 1978, pp 139–153

Mueller SR, Girace M: Use and misuse of the MMPI, a reconsideration. Psychol Rep 63:483–491, 1988

Naugle RI, Kauczak K: Limitations of the Mini-Mental State Examination. Cleve Clin J Med 56:277–281, 1989

Newcombe F, Ratcliff G: Disorders of visuospatial analysis, in Handbook of Neuropsychology, Vol 2. Edited by Boller F, Grafman J. Amsterdam, Elsevier, 1989, pp 333–356

Northern California Neurobehavioral Group: Test Booklet for the Neurobehavioral Cognitive Status Examination. Fairfax, CA, 1988

Ojemann GA, Dodrill CB: Verbal memory deficits after left temporal lobectomy for epilepsy. J Neurosurg 62:101–107, 1985

Pankratz LD, Taplin JD: Issues in psychological assessment, in Critical Issues, Developments, and Trends in Professional Psychology. Edited by McNamara JR, Barclay AG. New York, Praeger, 1982, pp 115–151

Parkin AJ, Miller J, Vincent R: Multiple neuropsychological deficits due to anoxic encephalopathy: a case study. Cortex 23:655–665, 1987

Posner MI: Structures and functions of selective attention, in Clinical Neuropsychology and Brain Function: Research, Measurement, and Practice. Edited by Boll T, Bryan BK. Washington, DC, American Psychological Association, 1988, pp 169–202

Purdue Research Foundation. Examiner's Manual for the Purdue Pegboard. Chicago, IL, Science Research Associates, 1948

Reitan RM: Manual for the Administration of Neuropsychological Test Batteries for Adults and Children. Indianapolis, IN, Author, 1969

Reitan RM, Wolfson D: The Halstead-Reitan Neuropsychological Test Battery: Theory and Clinical Interpretation. Tucson, AZ, Neuropsychology Press, 1985

Rey A: L'examen clinique en psychologie. Paris, Presses Universitaires de France, 1964

Robinson RG, Kubos KL, Starr LB, et al: Mood disorders in stroke patients. Importance of location of lesion. Brain 107:81–93, 1984

Schenkenberg T, Bradford DC, Ajax ET: Line bisection and unilateral visual neglect in patients with neurologic impairment. Neurology 30:509–517, 1980

Schmidt D: Toxicity of anti-epileptic drugs, in Recent Advances in Epilepsy (No 3). Edited by Pedley TA, Meldrum. New York, Churchill Livingstone, 1986, pp 211–232

Schwamm LH, Van Dyke C, Kiernan RJ, et al: The Neurobehavioral Cognitive Status Examination: comparison with the Cognitive Capacity Screening Examination and the Mini-Mental State Examination in a neurosurgical population. Ann Intern Med 107:486–491, 1987

Snow WG: Aphasia Screening Test performance in patients with lateralized brain damage. J Clin Psychol 43:266–271, 1987

Sox HC, Blatt MA, Higgins MC, et al: Medical Decision Making. Boston, MA, Butterworths, 1988

Strauss E, Goldsmith SM: Lateral preferences and performance on non-verbal laterality tests in a normal population. Cortex 23:495–503, 1987

Stromgren LS: The influence of depression on memory. Acta Psychiatr Scand 56:109–128, 1977

Tarter RE, Van Thiel DH, Edwards KL: Medical Neuropsychology. New York, Plenum, 1988

Taylor MA, Abrams R: Cognitive impairment patterns in schizophrenia and affective disorder. J Neurol Neurosurg Psychiatry 50:895–899, 1987

Teuber H-L: Neuropsychology, in Recent Advances in Diagnostic Psychological Testing. Edited by Harrower MR. Springfield, IL, CC Thomas, 1948, pp 30–52

Theodore WH: Clinical neuroimaging, in Frontiers of Neuroscience, Vol 4. Edited by Theodore WH. New York, Alan R Liss, 1988

Van Gorp WG, Miller EN, Satz P, et al: Neuropsychological performance in HIV-1 immunocompromised patients. J Clin Exp Neuropsychol 11:763–773, 1989 van Zomeren AH, Brouwer WH: Assessment of attention, in Principles and Practice of Neuropsychological Assessment. Edited by Crawford J, McKinlay W, Parker D. London, Taylor & Francis, 1990

Varney NR: Somesthesis, in Experimental Techniques in Human Neuropsychology. Edited by Hannay HJ. New York, Oxford University Press, 1986, pp 212–237

Walsh KW: Understanding Brain Damage. Edinburgh, Churchill Livingstone, 1985

Wang PL, Ennis KE, Copland SL: CCT: Cognitive Competency Test Manual. Toronto, Ontario, Department of Psychology, Mount Sinai Hospital, 1987

Wechsler D: The Measurement of Adult Intelligence, 3rd Edition. Baltimore, MA, Williams & Wilkins, 1944

Wechsler D: WAIS Manual. New York, Psychological Corporation, 1955

Wechsler D: WISC-R Manual: Wechsler Intelligence Scale for Children-Revised. New York, Psychological Corporation, 1974

Wechsler D: WAIS-R Manual. New York, Psychological Corporation, 1981

Wechsler D: Wechsler Memory Scale-Revised Manual. San Antonio, TX, Psychological Corporation, 1987

Wechsler D: WISC-III Manual: Wechsler Intelligence Scale for Children-Third Edition. New York, Psychological Corporation, 1991

Weiss B: Behavioral toxicology and environmental health science. Am Psychol 38:1174–1187, 1983

Welsh GS, Dahlstrom WG (eds): Basic Readings on the MMPI in Psychology and Medicine. Minneapolis, MN, University of Minnesota Press, 1956

Chapter 6

Electrodiagnostic Techniques in Neuropsychiatry

Thomas C. Neylan, M.D.
Charles F. Reynolds III, M.D.
David J. Kupfer, M.D.

Computed tomography (CT) and magnetic resonance imaging (MRI) have overshadowed electrodiagnostic techniques in clinical neuropsychiatry. However, as Niedermeyer (1990) suggested, clinicians must avoid overreliance on brain morphology for diagnosis. Electrophysiological techniques are powerful and perhaps underutilized for measuring brain dysfunction that might otherwise be missed with CT or MRI. They complement imaging techniques by providing a noninvasive measure of physiology.

ELECTROENCEPHALOGRAPHY

Theoretical Overview of EEG

The electrical signal detected by the electroencephalograph is the final summation of a multitude of potentials generated by the cerebral cortex. The structural organization of the cerebral cortex can be conceptualized as a mosaic of vertical columns with apical dendrites oriented toward the surface and axons projecting to deeper structures (Fenton 1989). Thus the signal detected by the scalp electrode is predominated by the excitatory and inhibitory postsynaptic potentials on dendrites and neuronal cell bodies, and not the deeper axon action potentials (Goff et al. 1978; Goldensohn 1979). The superficial cortical layers are influenced by projections from the thalamus, which in turn receive input from the reticular activating system. Thus the cortical electroencephalography (EEG) is regulated by brain stem structures controlling arousal and sleep. For example, during waking, the brisk tonic activity of the reticular activating system leads to the desynchronization of the cortical EEG.

Although brain potentials may range in frequency from 0.1 to 1,000 Hz (Niedermeyer 1990; Rodin et al. 1971), the EEG has an upper frequency range of

This work was supported in part by Grants MH 00295 (to CFR: RSA), MH37869 (to CFR), MH30915 (to DJK), and AG06836 (to CFR).

approximately 70 Hz. This range is subdivided into frequency bands defined as beta (Hz > 13), alpha (8–13 Hz), theta (4–7 Hz), and delta (≤ 3 Hz) (Figure 6–1). Frequencies such as the alpha rhythm are better detected than higher frequencies, which are highly asynchronous and attenuated by transmission through the skull and scalp (Cooper et al. 1965).

Overview of Clinical EEG

The routine EEG is performed when the subject is awake and at rest. Activation procedures such as hyperventilation and photic stimulation may be used to elicit abnormal activity. Sleep deprivation can increase the sensitivity for detecting epileptiform activity. The electrode placement generally follows the standard 10–20 montage (Jasper 1958). Special leads electrodes such as nasopharyngeal or ethmoid electrodes may be used to increase sensitivity or further enhance localization of abnormal discharges.

The most prevalent method of analysis of the EEG in the clinical setting remains visual analysis by the electroencephalographer. The record is first examined for focal abnormalities, epileptiform activity, paroxysmal activity, asymmetries, and artifact. Then the background activity is quantified with respect to frequency and amplitude. It is perhaps this aspect of EEG analysis that holds the most promise in electrophysiological research in neuropsychiatry. Because there are no specific waveforms seen in neuropsychiatric disorders, electrophysiological differentiation of patients from control subjects may be obtainable only by demonstrating a quantitative difference between the two groups (Shagass 1977).

The EEG is a nonspecific indicator of cerebral function. Any pathophysiological insult to the central nervous system can result in alterations in electrophysiology. Thus with few exceptions (Table 6–1), the EEG does little in providing a precise diagnosis. EEG abnormalities are most pronounced with acute injuries of the outer cortex. Disorders that affect deep brain structures or result in a chronic indolent loss of neurons may show little to no EEG changes (Fenton 1989).

Epilepsy and Epileptiform Activity

The most important use of EEG continues to be in the diagnosis of seizure disorders. No other brain abnormality has an electrophysiological pattern as distinctive as epilepsy (Duffy 1988). Spikes, defined as a potential with a duration of less than 70 milliseconds (msec); sharp waves (70–200 msec); and polyspikes, frequently followed by a slow wave, are often seen interictally in epilepsy patients (Aminoff 1986; Goodin and Aminoff 1984). The study of the behavioral consequences of epilepsy has a rich history (Reynolds 1989) and is discussed in detail in Chapter 15 of this volume.

Epileptiform activity is found in 1%–10% of the nonepileptic general population (Zivin and Marsan 1968). It is occasionally seen in nonepileptic patients who are on antidepressant or antipsychotic medications (Fenton 1989). More frequently, nonepileptic patients may have paroxysmal EEG activity during sedative-hypnotic withdrawal states. This illustrates the importance of the clinical maxim: "Treat the patient, not the EEG."

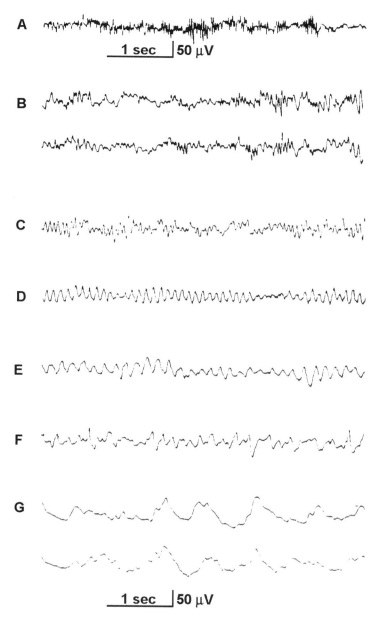

Figure 6–1. The electroencephalographic frequencies. *A,* fast activity, around 30–35 per second: fast beta range. *B,* mixed activity with beta waves in the 20–25 per second range. *C,* mixed activity with beta waves in the 14–18 per second range. *D,* alpha rhythm, 9 per second. *E,* theta rhythm 5–6 per second. *F,* mixed delta and theta activity, mainly in the 2.5–5 per second range. *G,* predominant delta activity, mostly in the 1–1.5 per second range.
Source. Reprinted from Niedermeyer E: "Introduction to Electroencephalography," in *The Epilepsies: Diagnosis and Management.* Baltimore, MD, Urban & Schwarzenberg, 1990, pp. 35–49. Used with permission.

Aging, Dementia, and Delirium

The background alpha rhythm changes very little with normal aging (Visser 1985) and is extremely useful in longitudinal studies. A drop of 1 Hz over a short period of time may indicate a significant encephalopathic process, even though the alpha rhythm remains in the normal range (Pro and Wells 1977). The EEG is useful in the study and diagnosis of cognitive disorders. For example, EEG slowing has been found to be correlated with the severity of dementia (Fenton 1986) and the number of senile plaques (Deisenhammer and Jellinger 1974) in Alzheimer's disease. Similarly, the severity of delirium has been found to be correlated with EEG abnormalities (Romano and Engel 1944). The EEG is a valuable tool in hospital psychiatry because it can help distinguish a mild delirium from major depression.

Schizophrenia

Abnormal EEGs have been described in up to 80% of schizophrenic patients, although studies with adequate control subjects have reported a much lower rate (McKenna et al. 1985). Studies (Nasrallah 1986) have documented EEG asymmetries, particularly in the left hemisphere. Although an abnormal EEG may be a predictor for drug resistance to neuroleptic medications (Itil 1982), its principal clinical use in schizophrenia is as a screening tool for gross neuropathology or seizure disorder.

Table 6–1. Electroencephalographic (EEG) findings in a sample of neuropsychiatric disorders

Disorder	EEG findings
Epilepsy	Focal and generalized spikes, sharp waves, polyspikes, and spike-wave complexes
Delirium	Generalized slowing and irregular high-voltage delta activity
Encephalitis	Background slowing, diffuse epileptiform activity, and periodic lateralized epileptiform discharges (PLEDs)
Barbiturate or benzo-diazepine intoxication	Background slowing and diffuse superimposed beta activity
Tumor or infarction	Focal slowing at border of infarction or tumor and necrotic tissue is electrically silent
Aging	Generalized slowing of alpha rhythm, diffuse theta and delta activity, decline of low-voltage beta activity, and focal delta activity in temporal areas
Dementia	Accelerated development of EEG changes of normal aging, paroxysmal bifrontal delta activity, and asymmetry between hemispheres
Creutzfeldt-Jakob disease and subacute sclerosing panencephalitis	Periodic complexes
Uremic or hepatic encephalopathy	Triphasic waves

Source. Adapted from Fenton 1989.

Screening EEGs

The routine use of screening EEGs in psychiatric patients remains controversial because it is unclear how significant the abnormal EEG is in redirecting treatment choices. A retrospective study of 698 psychiatric inpatients (Warner et al. 1990) found that a screening EEG altered the clinical diagnosis in only 1.7% of cases.

Quantitative EEG

Spectral analysis uses the *fast Fourier transform* method to analyze the relative predominance or power of any EEG frequency band (Press et al. 1986). The correlation between the spectra of contralateral or adjacent leads provides a measure of EEG coherence. Analysis of EEG spectra and coherence can distinguish patients with Alzheimer's disease from those with multi-infarct dementia, as well as from control subjects (Leuchter and Walter 1989).

Brain Mapping

Brain mapping combines the qualitative analysis of EEG data with a spatial dimension in the form of topographical mapping (Duffy et al. 1979). Brain mapping devices can analyze the EEG frequency content and assign it a visual analogue, such as color. Electrophysiological data from multiple subjects can be summarized into a consolidated group map, which can be used to visually and statistically compare various patient groups with control subjects (Rosse et al. 1987). For example, several studies (Guenther et al. 1986; Morihisa et al. 1983) have shown that schizophrenic patients have more delta activity, particularly over the frontal cortex, compared with control subjects. Preliminary findings with dementia have shown a significant difference in power between presenile-onset and senile-onset patients, whereas little difference was seen between young and old control subjects (Gueguen et al. 1989). An American Psychiatric Association task force report (American Psychiatric Association 1991) concluded that quantitative EEG had its greatest utility in disorders with slow-wave abnormalities.

MAGNETOENCEPHALOGRAPHY

Magnetoencephalography (MEG) is the recording of the magnetic fields generated by intraneuronal electric current. The "right-hand rule" of electromagnetism is that magnetic fields occur at right angles to the direction of current flow. Thus the MEG signal can be conceptualized as the magnetic counterpart to the EEG or evoked potential (EP) signal (Reeve et al. 1989). MEG naturally complements EEG and has potential advantages in localization and a broader range in frequency resolution (Rose et al. 1987). Perhaps its greatest promise is to accurately detect the neuronal sources of known EEG and EP signals (Reeve et al. 1989; Reite et al. 1989). The models that link magnetic topography to the source of the electromagnetic activity remain to be validated. The principal disadvantage of MEG is that the magnetometer must contend with a low signal-to-noise ratio necessitating the use of expensive shielding from ambient magnetic noise.

POLYSOMNOGRAPHY

Overview of What Polysomnography Measures

Normal sleep consists of recurring 70- to 120-minute cycles of non-rapid-eye-movement (NREM) and REM sleep characterized polysomnographically by the EEG, the electrooculogram (EOG), and the electromyogram (EMG) (Rechtschaffen and Kales 1968). Typically, sleep progresses from wakefulness through the 4 stages of NREM sleep until the onset of the first REM period. The length of the first NREM period is referred to as *REM latency*—an important variable in diagnosing narcolepsy and in research studies of major depression.

During wakefulness, the EEG is characterized by low-voltage fast activity consisting of a mix of alpha (8–13 Hz) and beta (>13 Hz) frequencies. Stage 1 of NREM sleep is a transitional stage between wakefulness and sleep during which the predominant alpha rhythm disappears, giving way to the slower theta (4–7 Hz) frequencies. Tonic EMG activity decreases, and the eyes move in a slow rolling pattern. Stage 2 is characterized by a background theta rhythm and the episodic appearance of sleep spindles (brief bursts of 12–14 Hz activity) and K complexes (a K complex is a single high-amplitude, slow-frequency electronegative wave followed by a single electropositive wave). Muscle tone remains diminished and eye movements are rare (Figure 6–2). Stages 3 and 4, also called slow-wave or delta sleep, are defined as epochs of sleep consisting of more than 20% and 50%, respectively, of high-amplitude activity in the delta band (0.5–3.0 Hz). Muscle tone is nearly atonic and eye movements are absent (Figure 6–3). REM sleep is characterized by a low-amplitude, mixed frequency EEG, rapid eye movements, and absent muscle tone (Figure 6–4).

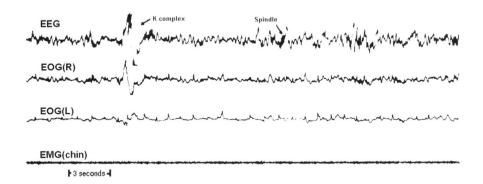

Figure 6–2. Stage 2 non-rapid-eye-movement (NREM) sleep in a 32-year-old man. The electroencephalogram (EEG) shows characteristic phasic events: K complexes and spindles. Slow eye movements have disappeared from the right (R) and left (L) electrooculograms (EOGs), which now reflect largely brain rather than eye potentials. The chin electromyogram (EMG) is lower than in wakefulness, but not atonic as in rapid-eye-movement (REM) sleep. As stage 2 deepens, the incidence of delta activity (0.5–3 Hz) gradually increases until the subject is considered to be in slow-wave sleep (stages 3 and 4).

Source. Reprinted from Reynolds CF, Kupfer DJ: "Sleep Disorders," in *American Psychiatric Press Textbook of Psychiatry.* Edited by Talbott JA, Hales RE, Yudofsky SC. Washington, DC, American Psychiatric Press, 1988, pp. 737–752. Used with permission.

A thorough polysomnographic study provides data on sleep continuity, sleep architecture, REM physiology, sleep-related respiratory impairment, oxygen desaturation, cardiac arrhythmias, and periodic movements. Additional measures may include nocturnal penile tumescence, temperature, and infrared video monitoring.

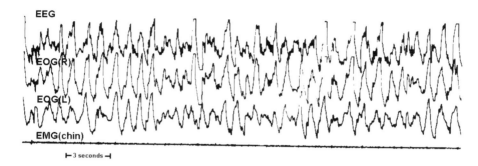

Figure 6–3. Stage 4 non-rapid-eye-movement (NREM) sleep (slow-wave sleep) in a 31-year-old man. The electroencephalogram (EEG) shows at least a 50% incidence of high-amplitude delta activity (75–200µV, 0.5–3 Hz). Similar activity is also "seen" by the right (R) and left (L) electrooculogram (EOG) electrodes. The chin electromyogram (EMG) shows very little tonic activity. Arousal thresholds are greatest now. Stage 3 is basically similar, but with lower overall incidence of delta activity (20%–50% of the epoch).

Source. Reprinted from Reynolds CF, Kupfer DJ: "Sleep Disorders," in *American Psychiatric Press Textbook of Psychiatry.* Edited by Talbott JA, Hales RE, Yudofsky SC. Washington, DC, American Psychiatric Press, 1988, pp. 737–752. Used with permission.

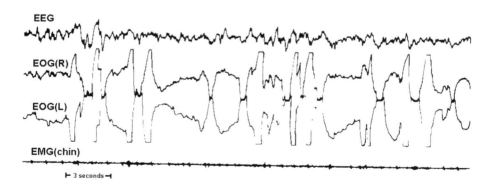

Figure 6–4. Rapid-eye-movement (REM) sleep in a 32-year-old man. The electroencephalogram (EEG) shows low-voltage, desynchronized (i.e., variable frequency) activity, similar to wakefulness (hence the frequent designation of REM sleep as "paradoxical" sleep), whereas the right (R) and left (L) electrooculograms (EOGs) show the highly characteristic binocularly conjugate rapid eye movements and the chin electromyogram (EMG) reflects inhibition of muscle tone.

Source. Reprinted from Reynolds CF, Kupfer DJ: "Sleep Disorders," in *American Psychiatric Press Textbook of Psychiatry.* Edited by Talbott JA, Hales RE, Yudofsky SC. Washington, DC, American Psychiatric Press, 1988, pp. 737–752. Used with permission.

Polysomnography remains the principal diagnostic tool used in the field of sleep medicine.

Polysomnography in Evaluation of Chronic Insomnia

The routine use of polysomnography in the evaluation of chronic insomnia is controversial. For practical, economic, and scientific reasons the pro forma use of polysomnography is not warranted. However, polysomnography yields important diagnostic information in 49%–65% of chronic insomnia patients that was not discernible from a thorough clinical assessment (Jacobs et al. 1988). It is not clear if the additional information yielded by polysomnography favorably alters clinical outcome (Regestein 1988); field studies examining this question are currently under way.

Polysomnography in the Evaluation of Hypersomnia

Approximately 4%–5% of the general population complain of excessive sleepiness (Bixler et al. 1979). Hypersomnolence is clinically more alarming than insomnia because of the higher degree of psychosocial impairment, as well as the high rate of automobile and occupational accidents (Guilleminault and Carskadon 1977; Roth et al. 1989). The routine use of polysomnography in the evaluation of hypersomnolent patients is well justified given the high incidence of sleep apnea and narcolepsy in this group (Coleman et al. 1982).

The Multiple Sleep Latency Test (MSLT; Carskadon et al. 1986) is the most objective and valid measure of excessive sleepiness. In the MSLT, the patient is given the opportunity to fall asleep in a darkened room for five 20-minute periods in 2-hour intervals across the patient's usual period of wakefulness. An average sleep latency of less than 5 minutes indicates a pathological degree of sleepiness (Carskadon et al. 1981). The detection of sleep-onset REM periods in the MSLT has become a cornerstone in the diagnosis of narcolepsy (Mitler 1982).

EVOKED POTENTIALS

Evoked potentials (EPs) are measured by the technique of signal averaging, in which electrophysiologic responses to repeated stimulation are superimposed by computer analysis. Signal averaging enhances the stimulus-specific response, or EP, and causes the background activity to average to zero (Knight 1985).

Signal averaging quickly led to the characterization of the somatosensory, visual, and brain stem auditory EPs. These potentials have well-defined positive and negative peaks and occur within the first 50 msec after the stimulus. They represent the electrical activity of the primary neural pathway from sensory receptor to the cortex (Rosse et al. 1987) and are useful for determining that the neuroanatomy of the sensory pathways is intact. Structural damage (e.g., as may result from multiple sclerosis) or functional impairment will result in abnormal primary sensory EPs.

The middle (50–250 msec) and late (250–500 msec) potentials are of particular interest in neuropsychiatry because they represent higher cognitive processes. Cognitions take place in milliseconds and often manifest electrophysiologically in high-frequency cortical activity (Knight 1985). Multiple middle and late potentials are studied in neuropsychiatry; several are named for the experimental condition that elicits the response (e.g., the contingent negative variation and selective attention effect), while others are named for their electrophysiological characteristics, such as the P300 (positive wave 300 msec).

The contingent negative variation (CNV), often referred to as the *readiness potential,* is a negative potential that occurs after a warning stimulus alerts the subject that a second stimulus demanding a response is forthcoming (Fenwick 1989). It represents a preparation or priming of the cortex to facilitate an expected activity.

The P300 potential has received the greatest attention in neuropsychiatric electrophysiology. It is elicited when a subject correctly identifies a rare stimulus presented sequentially with other nontarget stimuli. Multiple studies have found that schizophrenic patients have abnormal P300 potentials. The most consistent finding is a reduction in amplitude (Figure 6–5). Pfefferbaum et al. (1989) found that P300 abnormalities were evident in both medicated patients and drug-free patients and were associated with negative symptoms. EP studies of information processing using the P300 response have shown that schizophrenic patients have difficulties in screening out distracting stimuli, suggesting that these patients have impaired sensorimotor gating or filtering of internal and external stimuli (Grillon et al. 1990; Braff and Geyer 1990).

Middle and late EPs may provide important insights to the physiology of attention, categorization, and filtering of sensory stimuli. However, unlike earlier peaks, they are more prone to experimental artifact. Motivation, level of consciousness, medications, sensory acuity, and movement artifact all can confound the data (Rosse et al. 1989). Studies currently under way are examining EP patterns in genetic studies of first-degree relatives of patients with neuropsychiatric disorders.

ELECTRODERMAL ACTIVITY

The conductance of electricity through skin is dependent on sweat gland activity, which in turn is controlled by the sympathetic nervous system (Rosse et al. 1987). Measuring skin conductance therefore provides an indirect measure of arousal. Raine et al. (1990) found that low arousal, as measured by electrodermal activity, predicted future criminal behavior. This supports a theory that criminality is associated with decreased central and autonomic arousal (Eysenck 1977).

CONCLUSIONS

Neuropsychiatric electrophysiology continues to be a powerful clinical and research tool. It remains one of the few noninvasive probes of brain function. Future advances in this field will likely come from computer quantitative analysis of EEG, polysomnographic, or EP data obtained from well-defined clinical populations and well-selected control groups. The clinical applicability of quantitative EEG and EP techniques holds much promise, but has yet to be firmly established.

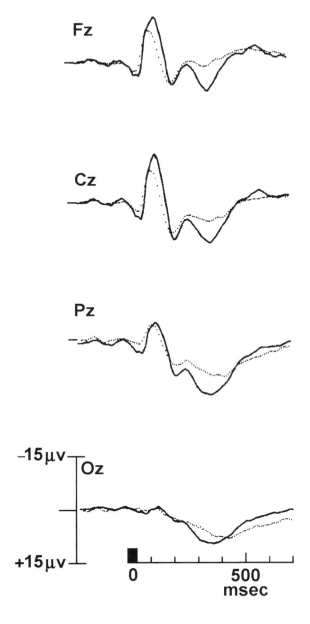

Figure 6–5. Event-related potentials (ERPs) of a group of 19 control subjects (*solid line*) overlaid with a group of 26 outpatients with schizophrenia. The data represent the grand mean ERP at midline electrodes in response to an infrequent auditory tone that the subject counts silently. Positivity is drawn downward. Thus P300 is the large positive wave appearing at approximately 300 milliseconds (msec) and is significantly larger in the control subjects than in the patients. P300 is most prominent at the midline parietal (Pz) electrode. Fz = midline frontal; Cz = central midline; Oz = midline occiptal.

Source. From S. R. Steinhauer, Department of Veterans Affairs Medical Center; University of Pittsburgh School of Medicine, Pittsburgh, Pennsylvania.

REFERENCES

American Psychiatric Association Task Force on Quantitative Electrophysiologic Assessment: Quantitative electroencephalography: a report on the present state of computerized EEG techniques. Am J Psychiatry 148: 961–964, 1991

Aminoff MJ: Electroencephalography: general principles and clinical applications, in Electrodiagnosis in Clinical Neurology. Edited by Aminoff MJ. New York, Churchill Livingstone, 1986, pp 21–75

Bixler EO, Kales A, Soldatos CR, et al: Prevalence of sleep disorders in the Los Angeles metropolitan area. Am J Psychiatry 136:1257–1262, 1979

Braff DL, Geyer MA: Sensorimotor gating and schizophrenia. Arch Gen Psychiatry 47:181–188, 1990

Carskadon MA, Harvey K, Dement WC: Sleep loss in young adolescents. Sleep 4:299–312, 1981

Carskadon MA, Dement WC, Mitler MM, et al: Guidelines for the Multiple Sleep Latency Test (MSLT): a standard measure of sleepiness. Sleep 9:519–524, 1986

Coleman RM, Roffwarg HP, Kennedy SJ, et al: Sleep-wake disorders based on a polysomnographic diagnosis: a national cooperative study. JAMA 247:997–1003, 1982

Cooper R, Winter AL, Crow HJ, et al: Comparison of subcortical, cortical and scalp activity using chronically indwelling electrodes in man. Electroencephalogr Clin Neurophysiol 18:217–228, 1965

Deisenhammer E, Jellinger K: EEG in senile dementia. Electroencephalogr Clin Neurophysiol 36:91, 1974

Duffy FH: Issues facing the clinical use of brain electrical activity mapping, in Functional Brain Imaging. Edited by Pfurtscheller G, Lopes da Silva FH. Toronto, Ontario, Hans Huber, 1988, pp 149–160

Duffy FH, Burchfiel IL, Lombroso CT: Brain electrical activity mapping (BEAM): a method for extending the clinical utility of EEG and evoked potential data. Ann Neurol 5:309–332, 1979

Eysenck HJ: Crime and Personality. St Albans, England, Paladin Frogmore, 1977

Fenton GW: The electrophysiology of Alzheimer's disease. Br Med Bull 42:29–33, 1986

Fenton GW: The EEG in neuropsychiatry, in The Bridge Between Neurology and Psychiatry. Edited by Reynolds EH, Trimble MR. Edinburgh, Churchill Livingstone, 1989, pp 302–333

Fenwick P: The significance of a seizure, in The Bridge Between Neurology and Psychiatry. Edited by Reynolds EH, Trimble MR. Edinburgh, Churchill Livingstone, 1989, pp 247–262

Goff WR, Allison T, Vaughan HG: The functional neuroanatomy of event-related potentials, in Event-Related Brain Potentials in Man. Edited by Callaway E, Tueting P, Koslow SH. New York, Academic Press, 1978, pp 1–79

Goldensohn ES: Neurophysiologic substrates of EEG activity, in Current Practice of Electroencephalography. New York, Raven, 1979, pp 421–439

Goodin DS, Aminoff MJ: Does the interictal EEG have a role in the diagnosis of epilepsy? Lancet 1:837, 1984

Grillon C, Courchesne E, Ameli R, et al: Increased distractibility in schizophrenic patients. Arch Gen Psychiatry 47:171–179, 1990

Gueguen B, Etevenon P, Plancon D, et al: EEG mapping in pathological aging and dementia: utility for diagnosis and therapeutic evaluation, in Topographic Brain Mapping of EEG and Evoked Potentials. Edited by Maurer Berlin, Springer-Verlag, 1989, pp 219–225

Guenther W, Breitling D, Banquet JP, et al: EEG mapping of left hemisphere dysfunction during motor performance in schizophrenia. Biol Psychiatry 21:249–262, 1986

Guilleminault C, Carskadon M: Relationship between sleep disorders and daytime complaints, in Sleep 1976. Edited by Koeller WP, Oevin PW. Basel, Karger, 1977, pp 95–100

Itil TM: The use of electroencephalography in the practice of psychiatry. Psychosomatics 23:799–813, 1982

Jacobs EA, Reynolds CF, Kupfer DJ, et al: The role of polysomnography in the differential diagnosis of chronic insomnia. Am J Psychiatry 145:346–349, 1988

Jasper HH: The ten-twenty electrode system of the International Federation. Electroencephalogr Clin Neurophysiol 10:371–375, 1958

Knight RT: Electrophysiology in behavioral neurology, in Principles of Behavioral Neurology. Edited by Mesulam M-M. Philadelphia, PA, FA Davis, 1985, pp 327–346

Leuchter AF, Walter DO: Diagnosis and assessment of dementia using functional brain imaging. International Psychogeriatrics 1:63–72, 1989

McKenna PJ, Kane JM, Parrish K: Psychotic syndromes in epilepsy. Am J Psychiatry 142:895–904, 1985

Mitler MM: The multiple sleep latency test as an evaluation for excessive somnolence, in Disorders of Sleeping and Waking: Indications and Techniques. Edited by Guilleminault C. Menlo Park, CA, Addison-Wesley, 1982, pp 145–153

Morihisa JM, Duffy FH, Wyatt RJ: Brain electrical activity mapping in schizophrenic patients. Arch Gen Psychiatry 40:719–728, 1983

Nasrallah HA: Is schizophrenia a left hemisphere disease? in Can Schizophrenia Be Localized in the Brain? Edited by Andreasen NC. Washington, DC, American Psychiatric Press, 1986, pp 55–74

Niedermeyer E: Introduction to electroencephalography, in The Epilepsies: Diagnosis and Management. Baltimore, MD, Urban & Schwarzenberg, 1990, pp 35–49

Pfefferbaum A, Ford JM, White PM, et al: P3 in schizophrenia is affected by stimulus modality, response requirements, medication status, and negative symptoms. Arch Gen Psychiatry 46:1035–1044, 1989

Press WH, Flannery BP, Teukolsky SA, et al: Numerical Recipes: The Art of Scientific Computing. New York, Cambridge University Press, 1986

Pro JD, Wells CE: The use of the electroencephalogram in the diagnosis of delirium. Diseases of the Nervous System 38:804–808, 1977

Raine A, Venables PH, Williams M: Relationships between central and autonomic measures of arousal at age 15 years and criminality at age 24 years. Arch Gen Psychiatry 47:1003–1007, 1990

Rechtschaffen A, Kales A: A Manual of Standardized Terminology, Techniques, and Scoring System for Sleep Stages of Human Subjects. Bethesda, MD, U.S. Department of Health, Education, and Welfare, Public Health Service, 1968

Reeve A, Rose DF, Weinberger DR: Magnetoencephalography: applications in psychiatry. Arch Gen Psychiatry 46:573–576, 1989

Regestein QR: Polysomnography in the diagnosis of chronic insomnia. Am J Psychiatry 145:1483, 1988

Reite M, Teale P, Goldstein L, et al: Late auditory magnetic sources may differ in the left hemisphere of schizophrenic patients. Arch Gen Psychiatry 46:565–572, 1989

Reynolds EH: Epilepsy and mental illness, in The Bridge Between Neurology and Psychiatry. Edited by Reynolds EH, Trimble MR. Edinburgh, Churchill Livingstone, 1989, pp 231–246

Reynolds CF, Kupfer DJ: Sleep disorders, in American Psychiatric Press Textbook of Psychiatry. Edited by Talbott JA, Hales RE, Yudofsky SC. Washington, DC, American Psychiatric Press, 1988, pp 737–752

Rodin E, Onuma T, Wasson S, et al: Neurophysiological mechanism involved in grand mal seizures induced by metrazol and megimide. Electroencephalogr Clin Neurophysiol 30:62–72, 1971

Romano J, Engel CL: Delirium, I: electroencephalographic data. Archives of Neurology and Psychiatry 51:356–377, 1944

Rose DF, Smith PD, Sato S: Magnetoencephalography and epilepsy research. Science 238:329–335, 1987

Rosse RB, Owen CM, Morihisa JM: Brain imaging and laboratory testing in neuropsychiatry, in The American Psychiatric Press Textbook of Neuropsychiatry. Edited by Hales RE, Yudofsky SC. Washington, DC, American Psychiatric Press, 1987, pp 17–39

Rosse RB, Warden DL, Morihisa IM: Applied Electrophysiology, in Comprehensive Textbook of Psychiatry, 5th Edition. Edited by Kaplan HI, Sadock BJ. Baltimore, MD, Williams & Wilkins, 1989, pp 74–85

Roth T, Roehrs T, Carskadon M, et al: Daytime sleepiness and alertness, in Principles and Practices of Sleep Medicine. Edited by Kryger MH, Roth T, Dement WC. Philadelphia, PA, WB Saunders, 1989, pp 14–23

Shagass C: Twisted thoughts, twisted brain waves? in Psychopathology and Brain Dysfunction. Edited by Shagass C, Gershon S, Friedhoff AJ. New York, Raven, 1977, pp 353–378

Visser SL: EEG and evoked potentials in the diagnosis of dementia, in Senile Dementia of the Alzheimer Type. Edited by Traber J, Gispen WH. Berlin, Springer, 1985, pp 102–116

Warner MD, Boutros NN, Peabody CA: Usefulness of screening EEGs in a psychiatric inpatient population. J Clin Psychiatry 51:363–364, 1990

Zivin L, Marsan CA: Incidence and prognostic significance of "epileptiform" activity in the EEG of nonepileptic subjects. Brain 91:751–779, 1968

Chapter 7

Brain Imaging in Neuropsychiatry

David G. Daniel, M.D.
Jeffrey R. Zigun, M.D.
Daniel R. Weinberger, M.D.

Increasingly incisive imaging techniques have revolutionized clinical research and practice in neuropsychiatry by providing noninvasive methods of direct study of the anatomy, physiology, and biochemistry of the living brain. Already, convincing findings have emerged suggesting that these techniques are indeed capable of associating disorders of behavior and cognition with identifiable neurobiological pathology. Clinically they currently are most useful for ruling out nonpsychiatric etiologies of behavioral disorders including space occupying lesions, vascular disease, and degenerative processes. At this time, there are no brain imaging findings that are pathognomonic or even strongly suggestive of a diagnosis of any primary psychiatric disorder.

Use of in vivo structural brain imaging techniques in neuropsychiatric research has advanced through pneumoencephalography (Jacobi and Winkler 1927) to computed tomography (CT) (Johnstone et al. 1976) and most recently to magnetic resonance imaging (MRI). The latter provides the best resolution of any currently available in vivo technology for examining brain structure or function. Neurofunctional imaging systems used relatively widely in psychiatric research range from relatively inexpensive and labor-unintensive devices designed for two-dimensional measurement of regional cerebral blood flow (rCBF) and electrical activity (electroencephalography [EEG]) to progressively more sophisticated tomographic techniques such as single photon emission computed tomography (SPECT) and positron-emission tomography (PET).

IN VIVO STRUCTURAL BRAIN IMAGING

The methods of the two primary techniques of obtaining structural brain images (CT and MRI) are threefold: 1) a device is used to pass energy through (CT) or excite nuclei (MRI) in tissue, 2) a detector device measures energy which passes through (CT) or is given off by tissue (MRI), and 3) a computer model is used to reconstruct a three-dimensional image of the tissue in the form of slices.

CT Scanning

Like classical radiological procedures, CT scanning exploits the fact that tissues of differing electron density differentially absorb X rays. Transaxially oriented slices (i.e., the plane oriented perpendicularly to the longitudinal axis) are generated by having a collimated X-ray source rotate around and pass thin beams of radiation through the body while detectors are arrayed to detect nonabsorbed X rays on the opposite side. A computer then applies a mathematical algorithm to create slices from multiple linear X-ray projections (Fullerton and Potter 1988). Image enhancement can be obtained with electron dense iodinated contrast materials to provide greater distinction of lesions that involve abnormal vascular structures or a disruption of the blood-brain barrier.

MRI Scanning

MRI is a nonradiological technique that exploits electromagnetic phenomena in biological tissues to generate images (Keller 1990). Atoms with unpaired nucleons, that is having an odd number of protons or neutrons (e.g., hydrogen, 1; carbon, 13; fluorine, 19; sodium, 23; and phosphorus, 31), exhibit net magnetization and behave as infinitesimally small dipoles. In the natural state, the random distribution of dipoles in tissue results in no net magnetic direction. MRI scanners use a strong magnetic field (0.15–2.0 teslas) to artificially align the magnetic dipoles so that one net direction is created. After the dipoles are aligned in the magnet, they are briefly exposed to short-wave radio frequencies. For each type of atom at a given magnetic field strength there is a unique radio frequency (the Larmour frequency) at which nuclei absorb energy and move to an excited state. The nuclei are then allowed to relax back to their original aligned state in the magnetic field. During relaxation, absorbed excitation energy is released in the form of radio wave signals, which are then measured and computer processed to create an image. It is the "resonance" of the magnetic nuclei going from relaxed to excited state and then back to the relaxed state that gives MRI its name.

Traditionally, MRI images are described as T1, T2, or proton density weighted. The degree to which a scan depicts attributes of one of these variables is determined by the timing and strength of the radio frequency excitation (pulse sequences). "T1 relaxation time" is the constant describing the time after excitation when 63% of magnetization returns to the longitudinal axis (in the direction of the externally applied field). T1- and proton-density-weighted scans are best at defining anatomy and showing gray/white matter differences, whereas T2-weighted scans are best at revealing subtle pathological changes. In T1- and proton-density-weighted MRI scans, cerebrospinal fluid (CSF) appears black and parenchyma appears gray or white. In T2-weighted scans, CSF appears white. T2-weighted scans are the ones associated with the "unidentified bright objects" (UBOs) described in more detail below.

Gadolinium DTPA was the first MRI contrast-enhancing agent approved for use in the United States (Niendorf et al. 1990). Because this agent does not normally cross the blood-brain barrier, only pathological changes that disrupt the barrier will lead to tissue enhancement.

Research Findings

Organic mental disorders.   Thus far, no pathognomonic anatomic changes detectable in vivo have been identified for any psychiatric disorders except those secondary to vascular disease, neoplasms, or specific neurological diseases such as multiple sclerosis (MS). Neurodegenerative disorders such as Alzheimer's disease typically show pronounced generalized atrophy and ventriculomegaly. In Pick's disease the atrophy may be relatively more severe in the frontal and anterior temporal lobes. Multiple small infarcts are associated with one of the two most common dementias, multi-infarct dementia. T2-weighted MRI scans are superior to CT in depicting such infarctions, which may be subtle (Erkinjuntti et al. 1987). Attempts to correlate measures of ventricular size, atrophy, tissue density, and signal hyperintensity on MRI with cognitive deficits in organic mental disorders appear promising but have, to date, yielded less robust relationships than expected (Bondareff et al. 1988).

Before the advent of CT scanning there was no radiological technique to indicate the presence of ischemic cerebrovascular disease. On a CT scan, ischemic parenchymal change is noticeable as a decrease in tissue density, usually after a 5- to 10-day delay. T2-weighted MRI scanning has the advantage of showing ischemic changes within hours of an event. In CT scanning of intracerebral hemorrhage, extravasated blood is seen acutely as a collection of increased density that then resolves to become isodense with surrounding brain tissue and eventually hypodense. MRI scans, especially with gadolinium contrast, can also depict bleeding early in the evolution of pathological events, although it may not differentiate hemorrhage from edema as clearly as CT scanning can.

For tumor detection the order of increasing sensitivity is unenhanced CT, enhanced CT, T2-weighted MRI, and gadolinium-contrasted MRI. T2-weighted images depict edematous pathological changes by highlighting areas in which water leaks out of normal tissue. Therefore, differentiating tumor and edema can be difficult in some cases with T2-weighted MRI images. Gadolinium enhancement for MRI is especially helpful for extraaxial tumors (meningioma and neuroma). Metastatic lesions with punctate disruptions of the blood-brain barrier are more noticeable with contrast-enhanced CT or MRI. In seizure disorders due to mass lesions (e.g., vascular malformations or tumors), CT or MRI scanning provides additional information about the size and location of pathology. Discrete structural lesions or increased intensity on T2-weighted MRI scans that reflect sclerotic changes is seen in many of these patients (Jack et al. 1990).

Structural imaging findings are consistent with postmortem neuropathology in some movement disorders with prominent psychiatric manifestations. In Huntington's disease bilateral atrophy of the head of the caudate nucleus and associated loss of the normal shape of the frontal horns of the lateral ventricles are common findings, particularly later in the course of the disorder. In contrast no consistently replicated findings have been associated with tardive dyskinesia, which also presents with choreiform movements. In Parkinson's disease, MRI often reveals narrowing of the pars compacta of the substantia nigra (Braffman et al. 1988). MRI is also useful in detecting and monitoring iron and copper deposition in hemochromatosis and Wilson's disease, respectively. In hemiballismus the MRI may detect contralateral infarction of the subthalamic nucleus.

MRI has significantly contributed to the diagnosis and monitoring of MS (Kelly et al. 1983). Before the advent of MRI, laboratory evaluation focused on CSF studies and sensory-evoked potentials. Although CT scans occasionally show hypodense old demyelinated plaques, T2-weighted MRI scans reveal not only clinically expected lesions but also previously unrecognized small areas of demyelination that may or may not evolve into plaques (Figure 7–1).

Schizophrenia.   Within several years of the development of CT scanning, the first report of brain changes in schizophrenia was published (Johnstone et al. 1976). Over the course of the last 15 years, hundreds of studies have been conducted. The following observations have been made about changes in the brains of patients with schizophrenia compared with those of control subjects (Zigun and Weinberger 1992):

- Enlargement of the lateral ventricles
- Enlargement of the third ventricle
- Dilatation of cortical sulci
- Thinning of cerebellar folia
- Reversal of normal cerebral asymmetries
- Changes in brain density
- Changes in corpus callosum size and shape
- Changes in thalamic size
- Changes in temporal lobe structures

Of these observations, lateral and third ventricular enlargement, dilatation of cortical sulci, and changes in temporal lobe structures have been consistently replicated. The others are less clearly demonstrated.

Increased size of the lateral ventricles was the first and most consistently noted brain change in patients with schizophrenia. It is important to appreciate that the

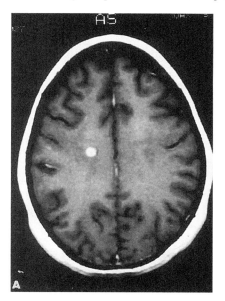 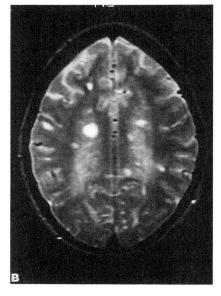

Figure 7–1.   T1-weighted (*panel A*) and T2-weighted (*panel B*) magnetic resonance imaging (MRI) transaxial views of the same subject illustrating demyelination secondary to multiple sclerosis. T1-weighted scans are superior for defining anatomy and differentiating gray and white matter, whereas T2-weighted scans better illustrate subtle pathological changes.

"ventriculomegaly" described in the neuropsychiatric literature is smaller than the amount of ventricular enlargement indicated when a neuroradiologist makes a clinical diagnosis. Decreases in the size of the hippocampus have been reported by several groups including a study with monozygotic twins discordant for schizophrenia (Suddath et al. 1990). There have also been reports of increases in the size of the temporal horns and decreases in the volume of temporal lobe tissue (Bogerts et al. 1990; Johnstone et al. 1989; Suddath et al. 1990).

Despite the information these findings have contributed to our understanding of pathological processes in schizophrenia, they do not represent criteria by which a diagnosis can be made. The great variation in the size of brain structures in control subjects is such that although more schizophrenic patients than control subjects may have larger ventricles, there are many such patients with ventricles smaller than those of control subjects. In a review (Daniel et al. 1991) of all English-language studies in which individual data points of ventricle-to-brain ratio in schizophrenic patients were published, the distribution of schizophrenic patients was found to overlap with that of control subjects (although shifted upward toward the abnormal end). This finding appears to be true for the other structural differences described as well.

Mood disorders.   Studies of structural changes in patients with unipolar depression have almost as many negative as positive reports using CT or MRI. Findings of enlarged ventricles in depressed patients are also complicated by a correlation with length of illness, which is not the case with schizophrenic patients. Further, unlike the first-break studies in the schizophrenia literature, there have not been findings of changes in patients on first presentation for depression compared with age-matched control subjects (Iacono et al. 1988). As with studies of unipolar patients, some reports have claimed an increase in ventricular size in bipolar patients compared with control subjects, whereas others have not (Dewan et al. 1988).

MRI studies have indicated a greater incidence of T2-weighted, high-intensity (i.e., bright areas on the scan) lesions in affective disorders. Although these lesions suggest that structural changes are present in some patients with mood disorders, they are not a consistent or specific finding. In fact, high-signal, white matter lesions (so-called UBOs) occur in older control subjects with no apparent neuropsychiatric compromise.

Other psychiatric disorders.   In some patients with eating disorders, abnormalities are visible on CT and MRI scans that usually resolve with symptom amelioration. Patients with bulimia nervosa have been reported to have enlarged ventricles at normal weights (Dolan et al. 1988), although this was not found in other studies (Lankenau et al. 1985). The implications of these findings are not clear.

Chronic alcohol abuse is another psychiatric disorder frequently associated with brain changes seen on CT and MRI scans. The primary changes seen are cortical and cerebellar atrophy and in many cases ventricular enlargement. In many such patients, these changes are partially reversible with abstinence. Several studies (see Besson 1990) have used measures of T1 and T2 characteristics to establish tissue effects of acute and chronic alcohol intake. Although increased relaxation times have been noted, it is not yet clear how to interpret these findings.

Clinical Indications for Structural Brain Imaging in Neuropsychiatry

Although promising research findings related to pathophysiology of mental illness have been obtained with CT and MRI scanning, clinical applications are limited. In effect, the use of CT or MRI scanning in diagnosis of psychiatric disorders is to assist in ruling out neurological disorders with psychiatric manifestations. At this time, no primary psychiatric disorder can be diagnosed solely by neuroanatomic imaging. Certain findings may support diagnosis of selected organic mental disorders but are rarely pathognomonic. A summary of indications for CT and MRI in evaluating psychiatric symptoms include

1. Dementia or other clinically significant, unexplained cognitive deterioration
2. Movement disorder of uncertain etiology, including tardive dyskinesia
3. First episode of psychosis (not associated with conclusive precipitant, such as intoxication or delirium) regardless of age
4. First episode of major affective disorder over age 40 years
5. Anorexia nervosa
6. Any psychiatric syndrome accompanied by unexplained neurological deficits
7. Any patient with psychotic or major affective disorder with an atypical or resistant response to standard pharmacotherapy (Weinberger 1984)

Clearly, structural imaging has provided the most benefit in portraying vascular abnormalities, infarcts, and tumors. In cases involving localizing neurological signs and symptoms, these modalities will provide rapid confirmation of pathology as well as assist in differential diagnosis. For seizure patients, with or without EEG changes, MRI also provides a means of establishing a locus of pathology and may assist in neurosurgical treatment.

Although CT and MRI scans are frequently ordered for patients suffering from dementia, the ability to distinguish pathological states is limited. Although not diagnostic, structural changes such as preferential involvement of the frontal and temporal cortex may suggest Pick's disease, especially when supported by neuropsychological findings of localized deficits. Multiple high-signal lesions suggest multi-infarct dementia and not Alzheimer's disease.

Structural imaging has much to offer for MS patients, in terms of both confirmation of diagnosis and the ability to monitor the progression of disease (and possibly the effects of treatment). Unfortunately, in the differential diagnosis of movement disorders, MRI and CT are less helpful. For example, they cannot currently differentiate Parkinson's disease from related syndromes (e.g., progressive supranuclear palsy or other types of Parkinson's syndrome). Anatomic imaging is helpful in identifying patients with parkinsonian symptoms due to some other pathological process (e.g., stroke, toxic exposure, or tumor) versus idiopathic forms. Though the demonstration of caudate atrophy may be of some help in the diagnosis of Huntington's disease, it is not always detectable early in the progression of the disorder.

CT Versus MRI Scanning

The choice of scanning modality involves a variety of considerations including availability, the type of pathology suspected, risks, and cost. MRI scanning has an advantage of higher resolution and distinction of gray-white definition as well as multiple angles for viewing. It also is superior for imaging almost all forms of brain pathology. It may, however, fail to differentiate hemorrhages, tumors and abscesses, or any of these from edema. CT scanning is the tomographic imaging modality of choice for studying the skull or spine and in instances of calcified lesions because MRI scans do not depict bone.

Neither procedure has much inherent risk in selected patients. CT scanning involves the use of ionizing radiation (usually 3–5 rads), although no increased risk of carcinogenicity has been definitively associated with this degree of radiation exposure. If pregnancy is an issue, MRI is clearly preferable. The iodinated contrast agents used in CT pose a slight risk for patients with iodine sensitivity. MRI alone has no known physical side effects for scanners below 2 teslas (the only scanners available clinically at this writing). Contraindications to MRI include patients with internal metal devices such as cardiac and neural pacemakers, cochlear and ocular implants, and shrapnel or surgical clips near brain or blood vessels. It is often possible to image a patient with MRI (even a patient with clips) when these foreign bodies are not paramagnetic, and in selected cases even when they are. Gadolinium contrast agents carry minimal side effects that are usually transient. CT scanners involve less claustrophobia and allow easier monitoring and access to the patient than most MRI scanners.

Although CT scans are less expensive currently, unless contraindications exist, the lack of ionizing radiation and the fact that little if any pathology is missed make MRI scanning the modality of choice at this time. A reading of "normal" on an MRI scan using appropriate pulse sequences effectively rules out clinically significant space-occupying structural brain lesions.

IN VIVO PHYSIOLOGICAL BRAIN IMAGING

All currently used physiological brain imaging techniques have three factors in common: 1) introduction into the body of a radioactive compound (a "tracer") that traces a neurobiological process and produces gamma rays ("photons"), 2) an extracranial device for counting and localizing the origin of the photon emissions, and 3) models for reconstruction of an image of the anatomic distribution and relative activity of the underlying physiological or neurochemical process being traced from the extracranial measurements of radiation.

The most common functional imaging parameters currently studied in neuropsychiatry are the local cerebral metabolic rate of glucose (LCMRglu), rCBF, and the density and binding affinity of neuroreceptors. Evidence suggestive of disordered neurotransmitter activity in many psychiatric disorders has generated enormous interest in quantification of receptor binding in vivo. This is accomplished by PET or SPECT measurement of the location of an injected radioactively labeled specific receptor ligand. Also, there is growing interest in quantification of the activity of enzymes, synthesis of proteins using labeled amino acids, and the metabolism of neurotransmitters.

The metabolic rate of glucose (currently the most widely measured parameter of cerebral function) reflects the extent to which regions of the brain are working or failing to work, but doesn't explain the etiology of the dysfunction. The metabolic rate of the primary cerebral energy substrate (glucose) is ascertained either by tagging a glucose analog (deoxyglucose) with the positron-emitting radionuclide fluorine-18 or by tagging glucose itself with carbon-11. Distribution of these compounds as measured by PET camera systems provides superb spatial resolution and anatomic detail. Radio-tagged deoxyglucose compounds are ideal for studying metabolism because physiologically they behave identically to glucose until they have entered the cell.

Two-Dimensional rCBF Measurement

The nontomographic two-dimensional (2-D) rCBF technique has been the most extensively used in vivo neurophysiological research technique in psychiatry other than EEG, but it is being rapidly supplanted by tomographic techniques such as PET and SPECT. SPECT and PET, although moderately and extremely more expensive and labor intensive, respectively, offer substantial advantages including 1) three-dimensional imaging, 2) improved resolution, and 3) the capacity to radioactively label a number of biologically important compounds.

PET

PET is the most sophisticated and expensive and has the highest resolution of any in vivo functional imaging technique. Although transverse section imaging with photons was described in 1962, the first positron computed tomograph was not developed until 1975 (Phelps et al. 1982). Currently, PET is limited to relatively few academic centers because the half-life of the radionuclides used to label tracers is so brief that a local cyclotron is required. A PET image is reconstructed in the following way. A positron-emitting radionuclide label is attached to a molecule of biological interest and is injected into the body. An emitted positron travels approximately 1–2 mm before colliding with an electron, resulting in an "annihilation reaction" in which two gamma rays are emitted at 180° from each other. A high degree of spatial resolution (2–6 mm) is attained using a fixed ring of extracranial detectors individually coded to photomultiplier tubes. The detectors are programmed to detect emissions that are paired at 180°. The resulting "rays," which characterize a line on which the annihilation reaction occurred, are mathematically reconstructed into the images of the distribution of the tracer.

SPECT

Unlike PET, SPECT uses single photon emitting radionuclides as tracers rather than relying on positron emitters to produce pairs of photons. Theoretically, this offers an advantage in resolution because no information about the location of the tracer is sacrificed by the distance the positron must travel before the annihilation reaction. However, with current technology, coincidence detection with PET and the considerably higher photon energy of the emissions lead to superior resolution compared with SPECT (less than 5 mm and 8 mm in-plane resolution, for PET and SPECT, respectively). SPECT has the potential for relatively widespread use compared with the limited distribution of PET scanning systems. This is primarily because single photon emitting compounds have relatively long physical half-lives and thus can be manufactured in one site and transported to distant sites, saving the costs of a cyclotron and extensive radiopharmaceutical staff associated with PET.

Research Findings

Organic mental disorders.   Despite the rapid proliferation of functional imaging research in the past decade, relatively few findings in neuropsychiatry have been independently verified. The most replicated findings are in disorders with relatively well-defined neuropathological or electrophysiological correlates, such as some forms of dementia and epilepsy. Both SPECT and PET have shown preliminary indications of adjunctive utility in the differential diagnosis of dementias (Figure 7–2). The decreased brain activity associated with cognitive deficits in dementia may be manifest in many ways, including decrements in rCBF, glucose metabolism, and neurotransmitter activity.

The patterns of distribution of these deficits appear to vary by illness. In Alzheimer's disease, extensive symmetrical parietal cortical deficits in uptake of the SPECT rCBF tracer iodine-123 IMP have been consistently observed (Cohen et al.

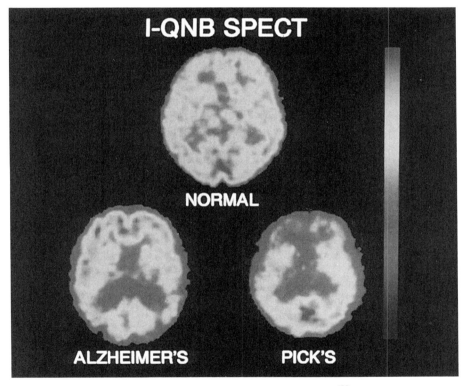

Figure 7–2.   Iodine-123-labeled 3-quinuclidinyl-4-iodobenzilate ([^{123}I]QNB [I-QNB; *in figure*]) single photon emission computed tomography (SPECT) scans of a control subject (normal) and patients with clinical diagnoses of Alzheimer's disease and Pick's disease. [^{123}I]QNB labels muscarinic acetylcholine receptors. The color scale is keyed to percentage receptor occupancy with warmer colors corresponding to greater relative receptor occupancy. Note the relatively posterior temporoparietal pattern of defects in the patient with Alzheimer's disease and the predominantly frontal anterior temporal pattern of defects in the patient with Pick's disease. (Please refer to page 179 of *The American Psychiatric Press Textbook of Neuropsychiatry,* Second Edition, for the full-color figure.)

1986; Jagust et al. 1987; Johnson et al. 1987; Mueller et al. 1986) and appear to correlate with cognitive deficits. Among patients with Alzheimer's disease, the [^{18}F]fluorodeoxyglucose (FDG) PET method has shown cerebral glucose metabolism to be globally reduced compared with that of age-matched control subjects. The deficits are typically most pronounced in the parietal cortex, followed by the temporal and to a lesser extent frontal cortices (Hoffman et al. 1989) and, unlike age-related findings in control subjects, persist after correction for cerebral atrophy and volume. Hypometabolic findings seem to be most pronounced in presenile-onset cases (Small et al. 1989) and correlate with cognitive deficits.

In vivo imaging of muscarinic acetylcholine receptors may also be useful in the differential diagnosis of dementia with early indications using SPECT suggestive of relative diminished density of muscarinic acetylcholine receptors in the posterior temporal-inferior parietal area (Weinberger et al. 1991). In Pick's disease and clinically related frontal dementia syndromes, deficits in rCBF, glucose metabolism, and muscarinic acetylcholine receptor density are suggestive of a lesion that is proportionately more anteriorly located than that seen in Alzheimer's disease. These findings mirror the characteristic pattern of cerebral atrophy. Multi-infarct dementia typically produces an irregular topographic pattern of rCBF and metabolic deficits. Although disparate functional imaging findings have been reported in depressive disorders (Chabrol et al. 1986; Sackeim et al. 1990; Silfverskiöld 1989), the so-called pseudodementia sometimes associated with major depression is not associated with a consistent pattern of metabolic or rCBF deficits. In Huntington's disease diminished caudate glucose metabolism is characteristic, but cortical metabolism is only slightly diminished, even in early cases.

In Parkinson's disease, progressive supranuclear palsy, and striatal-nigral degeneration, neuropathological findings are predominantly subcortical with relative sparing of the cortex, yet the most prominent functional imaging finding is hypometabolism of the frontal cortex, possibly because of loss of normal afferent activity. Sporadic reports of parkinsonian patients with dementia having metabolic or rCBF deficits similar to the parietotemporal pattern seen in Alzheimer's disease may reflect comorbidity of the two disorders. Seizure disorders have been associated with a number of rCBF and metabolic patterns both ictally and interictally that may aid in localization of focal abnormalities (Figure 7–3) even when the EEG findings are inconclusive (Theodore et al. 1983). In the ictal state, rCBF and metabolism are increased at the site from which the seizure originates and then propagate outward. Interictally the seizure focus usually shows deficits in rCBF and metabolism. These findings help in localization of epileptogenic foci for surgical excision and alleviate the need for implantation of depth electrodes.

Schizophrenia.   The most commonly examined issues in PET studies of schizophrenia to date are 1) global, anteroposterior, and lateralizing patterns of cerebral rCBF and metabolism and 2) dopamine, subtype 2 (D_2), receptor affinity and density.

Studies of rCBF and glucose metabolic patterns in schizophrenia have provided inconsistent findings in large part because of variations in patient experience and state. However, when imaging is performed during performance of a cognitive task that activates the prefrontal cortex of normal controls, deficits in prefrontal cortex rCBF and metabolism in schizophrenic patients are identified much more consistently. For

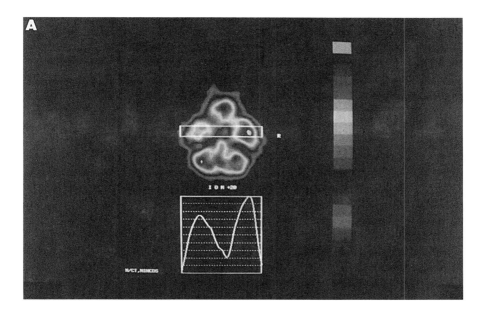

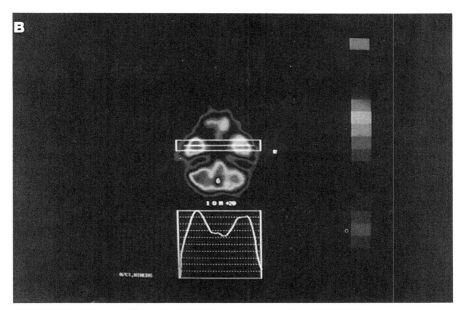

Figure 7–3.   Interictal [^{18}F]fluorodeoxyglucose (FDG) positron-emission tomography (PET) scan illustrating a hypometabolic area of 23% in the left temporal region of a patient with partial complex seizures confirmed by midtemporal epileptiform discharges seen on electroencephalography (*panel A*). In contrast, an ictal PET scan from the same patient illustrates hypermetabolic activity of 9% in the left temporal region (*panel B*). The color scale is keyed to the glucose utilization rate with the warmer colors indicating relatively higher rates of glucose utilization. *Source.*   Courtesy of W. H. Theodore and associates, National Institute of Neurological Diseases and Strokes, Bethesda, Maryland. (Please refer to page 180 of *The American Psychiatric Press Textbook of Neuropsychiatry,* Second Edition, for the full-color figure.)

example, in a recent study of 10 pairs of monozygotic twin pairs discordant for schizophrenia (Berman et al. 1992), the ill twin demonstrated less PFC rCBF activation than the well twin in 10 of 10 cases, suggesting that metabolic hypofrontality in schizophrenia is at least partially nongenetic in origin and is a consistent finding when interindividual variation is properly controlled for.

The dopamine hypothesis of the pathophysiology of schizophrenia has generated considerable interest in the measurement of dopamine receptor density (B_{max}) and affinity (K_d) in schizophrenia, particularly in patients not previously exposed to the potentially receptor-altering activity of neuroleptics. Although Wong et al. (1986) found two- to threefold higher dopamine receptor density in the caudate of a group of drug-naive patients with schizophrenia, such changes were not detected in several other reports (Farde et al. 1990; Herold et al. 1985; Martinot et al. 1990).

Mood disorders.   There are few consistent independently verified findings in mood disorders, both due to the modest number of investigations and variation in methodology. One PET finding in mood disorders that has been independently replicated is reduced, generalized global metabolism, possibly greatest in the left frontal cortex (Baxter et al. 1989; Martinot et al. 1990). The cyclic nature of most affective disorders permits each subject to serve as his or her own control for possible differentiation of the pathophysiology of euthymic, depressive, and manic states.

Other psychiatric disorders.   Anticipatory anxiety and lactate-induced panic are robustly associated with bilateral increases in activity of the anterior temporal poles (Nordahl et al. 1990; Reiman et al. 1986, 1989a, 1989b). In obsessive-compulsive disorder, findings of elevated metabolism in both the caudate nucleus (Baxter et al. 1988; Swedo et al. 1989) and frontal orbital cortex (Baxter et al. 1988; Nordahl et al. 1989; Swedo et al. 1989) may explain why surgical procedures that disconnect the prefrontal cortex from the caudate (i.e., leukotomy) sometimes are clinically effective for these patients.

CONCLUSIONS

Dramatic technologies for the noninvasive study of the anatomy and biochemistry of the living human brain now exist. Currently, the primary clinical usefulness of available imaging techniques is to rule out nonpsychiatric etiologies of behavioral and cognitive disorders. This is accomplished with MRI and CT. At present there is no accepted clinical indication for performing either a 2-D rCBF, SPECT, or PET scan on the brain. Although rCBF and cerebral glucose metabolism findings in epilepsy, Alzheimer's disease, and Huntington's disease are as close to clinically useful findings as have yet emerged, the frequency of false positives and false negatives has not yet been firmly established.

REFERENCES

Baxter LR, Swartz JM, Mazziotta JC: Cerebral glucose metabolic rates in nondepressed patients with obsessive-compulsive disorder. Am J Psychiatry 145:1560–1563, 1988

Baxter LR, Swartz JM, Phelps ME, et al: Reduction of prefrontal cortex glucose metabolism common in three types of depression. Arch Gen Psychiatry 46:243–250, 1989

Berman KF, Torrey EF, Daniel DG, et al: Regional cerebral blood flow in monozygotic twins discordant and concordant for schizophrenia. Arch Gen Psychiatry 49:927–934, 1992

Besson JAO: Magnetic resonance imaging and its applications in neuropsychiatry. Br J Pscyhiatry 157 (suppl 9):25–37, 1990

Bogerts B, Ashtari M, DeGreef G, et al: Reduced temporal limbic structure volumes on magnetic resonance images in first episode schizophrenia. Psychiatry Res 35:1–3, 1990

Bondareff W, Raval J, Colletti PM, et al: Quantative magnetic resonance imaging (MRI) and severity of dementia in Alzheimer's disease. Am J Psychiatry 145:853–858, 1988

Braffman BH, Grossman RI, Goldberg HI, et al: MR imaging of Parkinson's disease with spin-echo and gradient-echo sequences. American Journal of Neuroradiology 9:1093–1099, 1988

Chabrol H, Barrere M, Gwell A, et al: Hyperfrontality of cerebral blood flow in depressed adolescents. Am J Psychiatry 143:263–264, 1986

Cohen MB, Graham LS, Lake R, et al: Diagnosis of Alzheimer's disease and multiple infarct dementia by tomographic imaging of iodine-123 IMP. J Nucl Med 27:769–774, 1986

Daniel DG, Goldberg TE, Gibbons R, et al: Lack of a bimodal distribution of ventricular size in schizophrenia: a Gaussian mixture analysis of 1056 cases and controls. Biol Psychiatry 30:887–903, 1991

Dewan MJ, Haldipur CV, Lane EE, et al: Bipolar affective disorder, I: comprehensive quantitative computed tomography. Acta Psychiatr Scand 77:670–676, 1988

Dolan RJ, Mitchell J, Wakeling A: Structural brain changes in patients with anorexia nervosa. Psychol Med 18:349–353, 1988

Erkinjuntti T, Ketonen L, Sulkava R, et al: Do white matter changes on MRI and CT differentiate vascular dementia from Alzheimer's disease. J Neurol Neurosurg Psychiatry 50:37–42, 1987

Farde L, Wiesel F-A, Stone-Elander S, et al: D2 dopamine receptors in neuroleptic-naive schizophrenic patients: a positron emission tomography study with [C11] raclopride. Arch Gen Psychiatry 47:213–219, 1990

Fullerton GD, Potter JL: Computed tomography, in Textbook of Diagnostic Imaging. Edited by Putman CE, Ravin CE. Philadelphia, PA, WB Saunders, 1988, pp 47–60

Herold S, Leenders KL, Turton DR, et al: Dopamine receptor binding in schizophrenic patients as measured with [C11] methylspiperone and PET. J Cereb Blood Flow Metab 5 (suppl 1):S191–S192, 1985

Hoffman JM, Guze BH, Baxter LR, et al: 18F Fluorodeoxyglucose (FDG) and positron emission tomography (PET) in aging and dementia. Eur Neurol 29 (suppl 3):16–24, 1989

Iacono WG, Smith GN, Moreau M, et al: Ventricular and sulcal size at the onset of psychosis. Am J Psychiatry 145:820–824, 1988

Jack CR, Sharbrough FW, Twomey CK, et al: Temporal lobe seizures: lateralization with MR volume measurements of the hippocampal formation. Radiology 175:423–429, 1990

Jacobi W, Winkler H: Encephalographische studien an chronisch schizophrenen. Archiv für Psychiatrie und Nervenkrankheiten 81:299–332, 1927

Jagust WJ, Buddinger TF, Reed BR: Diagnosis of dementia with single photon emission computed tomography. Arch Neurol 44:258–262, 1987

Johnson KA, Mueller St, Walshe TM, et al: Cerebral perfusion imaging in Alzheimer's disease: use of single photon emission computed tomography and iofetamine hydrochloride I-123. Arch Neurol 44:165–168, 1987

Johnstone EC, Crow TJ, Frith CD, et al: Cererbral ventricular size and cognitive impairment in chronic schizophrenia. Lancet 2:924–926, 1976

Johnstone EC, Owens DGC, Crow TJ, et al: Temporal lobe structure as determined by nuclear magnetic resonance in schizophrenia and bipolar affective disorder. Journal of Neurology, Neurosurgery, and Psychiatry 52:736–741, 1989

Keller PJ: Basic Principles of Magnetic Resonance Imaging. Milwaukee, WI, General Electric, 1990

Kelly GR, Jackson JA, Leake DR, et al: CT versus NMR imaging of multiple sclerosis. American Journal of Neuroradiology 4:1136, 1983

Lankenau H, Swigar ME, Bhimani S, et al: Cranial CT scans in eating disorder patients and controls. Compr Psychiatry 26:136–147, 1985

Martinot J-L, Peron-Magnan P, Huret JD, et al: Striatal D2 dopaminergic receptors assessed with positron emission tomography [76Br] bromospiperone in untreated schizophrenic patients. Am J Psychiatry 147:44–50, 1990

Mueller SP, Johnson KA, Hamil D, et al: Assessment of I-123 IMP SPECT in mild/moderate Alzheimer's disease. J Nucl Med 27:889, 1986

Niendorf HP, Dinger JC, Haustein J, et al: Tolerance of Gd-DTPA: clinical experience, in Contrast Media in MRI. Edited by Dinger JC, Bydder G, Bucheler E, et al. Berlin, Medicom, 1990, pp 31–39

Nordahl TE, Benkelfat C, Semple WE, et al: Cerebral glucose metabolic rates in obsessive-compulsive disorder. Neuropsychopharmacology 2:23–28, 1989

Nordahl TE, Semple WE, Gross M, et al: Cerebral glucose metabolic differences in patients with panic disorder. Neuropsychopharmacology 3:261–272, 1990

Phelps ME, Mazziotta JC, Huang S-C: Study of cerebral function with positron computed tomography. J Cereb Blood Flow Metab 2:113–162, 1982

Reiman EM, Faichle ME, Robins E, et al: The application of positron emission tomography to the study of panic disorder. Am J Psychiatry 143:469–477, 1986

Reiman EM, Fusselman MJ, Fox PT, et al: Neuroanatomical correlates of anticipatory anxiety. Science 243:1071–1074, 1989a

Reiman EM, Raichle ME, Robins E, et al: Neuroanatomical correlates of lactate-induced anxiety attack. Arch Gen Psychiatry 46:493–500, 1989b

Sackeim HA, Prohovnik I, Moeller JR, et al: Regional cerebral blood flow in mood disorders, I: comparison of major depressives and normal controls at rest. Arch Gen Psychiatry 47:60–70, 1990

Silfverskiöld P, Risberg J: Regional cerebral blood flow in depression and mania. Arch Gen Psychiatry 46:253–259, 1989

Small GW, Kuhl DE, Riege WH, et al: Cerebral glucose metabolic patterns in Alzheimer's disease: effect of gender and age at dementia onset. Arch Gen Psychiatry 46:527–532, 1989

Suddath RL, Christison GW, Torrey EF, et al: Anatomical abnormalities in the brains of monozygotic twins discordant for schizophrenia. N Engl J Med 322:789–794, 1990

Swedo SE, Schapiro MB, Grady CL, et al: Cerebral glucose metabolism in childhood onset obsessive-compulsive disorder. Arch Gen Psychiatry 46:518–523, 1989

Theodore WH, Newmark ME, Sato S, et al: [18F]Fluorodeoxyglucose positron emission tomography in refractory partial seizures. Ann Neurol 14:429–437, 1983

Weinberger DR: Brain disease and psychiatric illness: when should a psychiatrist order a CAT scan? Am J Psychiatry 141:1521–1527, 1984

Weinberger DR, Gibson R, Coppola R, et al: The distribution of cerebral muscarinic acetylcholine receptors in vivo in patients with dementia: a controlled study with I-123 QNB and SPECT. Arch Neurol 48:169–176, 1991

Wong DF, Wagner HN, Tone LE, et al: Positron emission tomography reveals elevated D2 dopamine receptors in drug naive schizophrenics. Science 234:1558–1562, 1986

Zigun JR, Weinberger DRW: In vivo studies of brain morphology in schizophrenia, in New Biological Vistas on Schizophrenia. Edited by Lindenmayerand J-P, Stanley RK. New York, Brunner/Mazel, 1992, pp 57–81

Chapter 8

Epidemiology and Genetics of Neuropsychiatric Disorders

Dolores Malaspina, M.D.
H. Matthew Quitkin, A.B.
Charles A. Kaufmann, M.D.

From the time of Hippocrates, clinicians have suspected roles for both exogenous and endogenous factors in the etiology of disease (Lyons and Petrucelli 1987). During the past century, the powerful techniques of epidemiology and genetics have enabled us to identify specific environmental and hereditary contributions to illness.

EPIDEMIOLOGICAL STUDIES

Epidemiology is based on the fundamental assumption that factors causal to human disease can be identified through the systematic examination of different populations, or of subgroups within a population, in different places or at different times (Hennekens and Buring 1987). Epidemiological research may be viewed as directed at a series of questions: What is the frequency of a disorder? Are there subgroups in which the disorder is more frequent? What specific risk factors are associated with the disorder? Are these risk factors consistently and specifically related to the disorder? Does exposure to these factors precede the development of disease? A variety of epidemiological strategies have been developed to address these questions.

Measures of Disease Frequency

Measures of disease frequency serve as the basis for formulating and testing etiologic hypotheses because they permit a comparison of frequencies between different populations or among individuals within a population with particular exposures or characteristics. The two measures of disease frequency used most often are prevalence and incidence. Prevalence refers to the number of existing cases of a disease at a given point in time, as a proportion of the total population. Incidence

The authors express their thanks to Megan Harris. This work was supported in part by a National Institute of Mental Health Schizophrenia Academic Award KO7MH00824 (to DM), a Physician Scientist Award K11MH00682 (to CAK), a Stanley Scholar Award (to HMQ), and by the W.M. Keck Foundation.

refers to the number of new cases of a disease during a given period of time, as a proportion of the total population at risk. The two measures are interrelated: prevalence of a disease depends on both its incidence and duration. One can compare two populations with and without a factor suspected of contributing to the development of disease through the calculation of the ratio of disease frequency in the two populations; this is known as the *relative risk*.

Descriptive Studies

Correlational studies of populations and descriptive studies of single individuals or groups of individuals also contribute to formulating etiologic hypotheses by demonstrating a statistical association between exposure to specific risk factors and occurrence of disease. Hypotheses regarding risk factors may emerge from studying various characteristics of affected individuals (e.g., gender, age, and birth cohort), their place of residence, or the timing of their exposure. Descriptive studies, however, cannot be used to test etiologic hypotheses: they lack adequate comparison groups, making it difficult to determine the specificity of exposure to the disease, and they are cross-sectional, making it difficult to determine the temporal relationship between an exposure and the development of disease.

Analytic Studies

Etiologic hypotheses may be tested through various analytic strategies. These include case-control studies that compare exposure to a risk factor in individuals with a disease ("cases") with that in appropriate control subjects, as well as cohort studies that (retrospectively or prospectively) follow up groups of exposed individuals for development of disease.

Genetic Studies

Genetic research may be considered the subset of epidemiological research concerned with the contribution of inherited factors to the development of disease. It, too, may be conceptualized as directed at a series of questions: Is the disorder familial? Is it inherited? What is being inherited in the disorder (i.e., what constitutes predisposition to the disorder and what are the earliest manifestations of such predisposition)? What additional ("epigenetic") variables increase or decrease the chances of genetically predisposed individuals developing the disorder? How is the disorder inherited? Where, and what, are the abnormal genes conferring genetic risk? What are the molecular, and ultimately the pathological, consequences of these abnormal genes? Various genetic strategies have been developed to address these questions.

Family, twin, and adoption studies.   Family studies are a specific type of relative risk study. They can demonstrate an elevated risk for an illness in first-degree relatives of an affected individual compared with that in the general population (Table 8–1), but cannot distinguish if this elevated risk is due primarily to shared genetic or environmental factors. Other strategies, including twin and adoption studies, can further resolve the genetic contribution to the etiology of a disorder.

Although exposed to the same familial environment, monozygotic (MZ) and dizygotic (DZ) twin pairs differ in their genetic endowment (sharing 100% and 50% of their genes, respectively). When genetic factors are important in etiology, the MZ and DZ co-twins of probands will differ in their risk for the disorder. One can measure the heritability of a disorder by comparing the relative concordance rates for MZ and DZ twins.

Adoption studies are particularly useful in research of psychiatric disorders, for which cultural vertical transmission might allow for familial clustering of behaviors. Four types of adoption studies have been applied: 1) the adoptee study, which compares offspring separated from their affected mothers at birth with the adopted-away offspring of control mothers; 2) the cross-fostering study, which contrasts rates of illness among adoptees with biological parents without illness, reared by both affected and unaffected adoptive parents; 3) the adoptee's family study, in which biological relatives of affected adoptees are matched to the biological relatives of control adoptees, and their rates of illness are compared; and 4) the study of MZ twins reared apart.

High-risk studies. The high-risk approach represents a form of cohort study. Individuals at genetic risk for a disorder (e.g., those with affected parents) are followed prospectively, from early in life through the period of maximum risk for the disorder (Watt et al. 1984). This strategy permits the identification of features that are of primary pathogenic significance to the disorder, in contrast to those that are secondary to the illness or to its treatment. Moreover, by contrasting characteristics of at-risk individuals who go on to develop the disorder with characteristics of those who do not, this strategy allows for the identification of additional genetic and environmental influences that contribute to disease expression.

Table 8–1. Relative risk for neuropsychiatric disorders

Disease	Population prevalence per 100,000	Morbid risk in first-degree relatives (%)	Relative risk
Gerstmann-Sträussler syndrome	0.01	50	5,000,000
Acute intermittent porphyria	2	50	25,000
Metachromatic leukodystrophy	2.5	25–50	20,000
Myotonic dystrophy	5.5	50	9,090
Narcolepsy	10–100	30–50	5,000
Huntington's disease	19	50	2,630
Lesch-Nyhan syndrome	10	25	2,500
Wilson's disease	10	25	2,500
Pick's disease	24	17	708
Tourette's syndrome	28.7	3.6	125
Parkinson's disease	133	8.3	62.4
Bipolar disorder	500	8	16
Schizophrenia	900	12.8	14.2
Dyslexia	5,000–10,000	45	9.0
Epilepsy	1,700	4.1	2.4
Alzheimer's disease	7,700	14.4	1.90

Identifying the mode of inheritance. Even when family, twin, and adoption studies suggest a role for genetic factors, they say nothing of what, or even how many, genes are involved. Single-gene mutations produce more than 3,000 "monogenic" disorders, many of which affect mental functioning (McKusick 1983). These are inherited in a Mendelian dominant, recessive, or sex-linked manner. Nonetheless, any one monogenic disorder is rare, and common diseases are likely to be "polygenic," representing the combined small effects of many genes. Polygenic models have viewed diseases such as diabetes, atherosclerosis, or cleft lip (palate) as quasicontinuous or threshold characteristics (Reich et al. 1975). Even with genetic liability, environmental influences may be necessary for an illness to be expressed. Monogenic and polygenic transmission can be viewed as limiting cases of a general multifactorial transmission model that provides for the joint effects of a single major gene (or a few major genes), polygenic background, environmental influences (both intergenerational cultural factors and sporadic factors), and their interaction on inheritance.

Sophisticated research strategies, such as segregation analysis and pedigree analysis, allow direct comparison of monogenic and polygenic models. Segregation analysis compares the distribution of illness observed in family members to that predicted by a given genetic hypothesis and provides estimates of gene frequency and penetrance. Its power is limited because it treats each family as a separate observation but assumes the same genetic disorder is present in all families (Kidd 1981). Pedigree analysis examines more relationships within a given pedigree, identifying affected individuals over several generations. It is less likely to result in a Type II error, failing to support a particular genetic model because of etiologic heterogeneity, but more likely to result in a Type I error, because an individual pedigree may manifest an idiosyncratic form of the disorder (Elston and Stewart 1971; Goldin et al. 1981). Examination of multiplex sibships in which two or more sibs are affected represents a compromise approach between segregation and pedigree analysis (Anderson et al. 1981; Morton and Mi 1968).

Linkage analyses. Linkage studies are used to find the chromosomal locations of genes (or loci) involved in transmitting a disorder. They are based on establishing, within pedigrees, the coinheritance of the disorder with identifiable genetic markers of known chromosomal location. Mendel's second law (the law of independent assortment) (Cavalli-Sforza and Bodmer 1971) implies that the disease gene, and hence the disorder, will not be consistently coinherited with a marker allele derived from a different chromosome. Moreover, even if the disease and marker alleles originally lie on the same parental chromosome (i.e., are "syntenic"), they may become separated during gametogenesis through the process of "recombination" or "crossing-over," wherein genetic material on homologous chromosomes is exchanged (Figure 8–1). These rearranged chromosomes are ultimately passed on to the offspring. The probability of a disease and marker allele recombining depends on their distance from one another. If disease and marker alleles lie nearby one another, crossing-over will only rarely occur and parental gametes will be overrepresented. The disease and marker loci are then said to be "linked."

Linkage analysis depends on the ability to distinguish marker alleles inherited from one parent from those inherited from the other. To do this consistently, marker loci must be polymorphic, that is, they must harbor a number of allelic variants. A variety of polymorphic markers now exist, including restriction fragment length poly-morphisms (RFLPs) (Botstein et al. 1980) (Figure 8–2), minisatellite sequences (Jeff-erys et al. 1985), variable number tandem repeat (VNTR) sequences (Nakamura et al. 1987), and CA repeat sequences (Weber and May 1989).

Linkage analyses may be conveniently grouped into those involving anonymous markers, favored locus markers, and candidate genes. Anonymous markers, usually derived from noncoding DNA sequences, demonstrate significant polymorphism. When systematically drawn from throughout the genome, they may confirm linkage

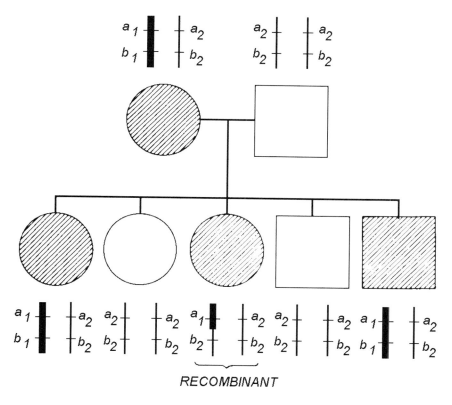

RECOMBINANT

Figure 8–1. Genetic linkage and recombination. Depicted is a hypothetical family (circles = females; squares = males) segregating for an autosomal dominant disease. The disease locus A (containing either the defective allele [a_1] or its normal counterpart [a_2]) lies close to a polymor-phic marker locus B (containing marker alleles b_1 and b_2). The mother is affected with the dis-ease (closed symbol) and is heterozygous at both the disease and marker loci. The father is unaffected (open symbol) and is homozygous at both loci. Because the disease and marker loci are genetically linked (i.e., they lie nearby one another), crossing-over rarely occurs between them. Most children who inherit the disease allele (a_1) will also receive the b_1 allele from their mother. Occasionally, a recombination event will occur in the mother, and she will transfer a chromosome bearing the b_2 marker allele along with the disease allele (as has occurred in the daughter labelled "recombinant").

Source. Reprinted from Rieder RO, Kaufmann CA: "Genetics," in *American Psychiatric Press Textbook of Psychiatry.* Edited by Talbott JA, Hales RE, Yudofsky SC. Washington, DC, American Psychiatric Press, 1988, pp. 33–65. Used with permission.

between a disorder and specific chromosomal regions. Conversely, they may reject linkage to these regions, thereby contributing to an "exclusion map" for the disorder. Markers from several regions may be examined concurrently; such a simultaneous search of the genome may detect multiple loci contributing to the disorder under epistasis. A major disadvantage of the anonymous marker approach is that it is undirected: at least 150 different markers must be examined to ensure that one lies within 10 cM of a major disease locus.

The favored locus approach narrows the search for linkage by examining markers derived from specific regions: portions of chromosomes involved in cytogenetic abnormalities associated with the disorder. Chromosomal translocations and deletions have provided important leads for linkage analyses of several neuropsychiatric disorders, including muscular dystrophy of the Duchenne type, Alzheimer's disease (AD), schizophrenia, and bipolar disorder.

Candidate genes offer the most focused approach. Hypothesis-dependent candidate genes (those nominated by neurobiological clues to disease pathogenesis) and hypothesis-independent candidate genes (those put forward without regard to pathogenic hypotheses) may be explored. An etiologic role for the candidate gene or nearby regions of the genome can be excluded with as little as one or a few recombinants. A disadvantage of the candidate gene approach is that these markers are not very polymorphic, as they are necessarily derived from coding regions of the genome. Moreover, this approach is so focused that it provides only limited information for an exclusion map.

The application of linkage analysis to complex disorders presents certain challenges. These may include 1) an unknown mode of inheritance; 2) incomplete penetrance, wherein additional environmental factors may be necessary for the final expression of even genetic forms of the disorder; 3) epistasis, where the disorder may

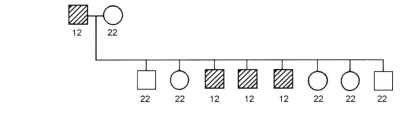

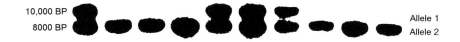

Figure 8–2. Coinheritance of a disease and a restriction fragment length polymorphism (RFLP). Depicted is a hypothetical family segregating an autosomal dominant disease (circles = females; squares = males; closed symbols = affected with the disease; open symbols = unaffected). There is an RFLP at the marker locus, resulting in two alleles, designated 1 (10,000 base pairs [bp]) and 2 (8,000 bp). The affected father and three affected sons all carry one copy of each allele. The unaffected mother and offspring have two copies of the normal allele. *Source.* Adapted from Gilliam et al. 1989.

result from the interaction of several major genes; 4) variable expression, in which a single form of the disorder may have several phenotypic expressions; 5) diagnostic instability, such that a subject's affection status may change over time; and 6) etiologic heterogeneity, under which an ordinarily genetic syndrome may have sporadic (environmentally produced) forms, known as *phenocopies,* as well as a variety of genetic forms resulting from disruption in a number of different genes, a condition known as "nonallelic heterogeneity." Clinical and statistical approaches to the linkage analysis of complex disorders exist for offsetting these uncertainties (Kaufmann and Malaspina 1991).

Molecular approaches. Once linkage analysis has implicated a particular chromosomal region in the etiology of a disorder, various molecular genetic approaches exist for identifying the disease gene and its pathological consequences. Thus markers in linkage disequilibrium with, and thus in close proximity to, the disease gene may be identified. Genetic markers flanking the disease gene may also be recognized, thereby defining the minimal genetic region containing the disease gene. Overlapping cytogenetic anomalies producing the disease may then narrow this minimal genetic region. When the region has been narrowed to less than 10^6 base pairs (bp) of DNA, physical cloning strategies may be invoked, including pulse-field gel electrophoresis, yeast artificial chromosomes, and chromosome walking, hopping, and jumping. Ultimately, "open-reading frames" of DNA, corresponding to the genes themselves, may be found (e.g., through the recognition of so-called CpG islands that bound them).

Physiologically important genes may then be distinguished by phylogenetic conservation, and those relevant to disease pathogenesis may be recognized through appropriate anatomic distribution of their corresponding messenger RNAs (mRNAs). Specific molecular abnormalities (e.g., insertions, deletions, and base substitutions) within the disease gene may then be discovered using single-strand conformational changes seen on denaturing gels, through the appearance of novel restriction endonuclease cleavage sites, or by direct DNA sequencing. The pathological consequences of the disease mutation may be determined by introducing the normal or disease gene into appropriate in vitro and in vivo model systems (Kimura et al. 1989; Rich et al. 1990).

SELECTED NEUROPSYCHIATRIC DISEASES

In the following sections, we discuss epidemiological and genetic studies of selected neuropsychiatric illnesses. For didactic purposes, we have chosen disorders affecting diverse functions of the nervous system and displaying diverse degrees of heritability, modes of inheritance, and molecular mechanisms.

Huntington's Disease

HD is a disorder characterized by progressive dementia and chorea. Age at onset is usually between 25 and 50 years: earlier presentation is often associated with a severe course and premonitory psychiatric disturbances. The dementia of HD is remarkable for poor cognitive ability generally; a lack of language disorder or other focal cortical deficits suggests subcortical pathology (Lishman 1987). Choreic movements consist of randomly timed and irregularly distributed jerks, grimaces, and twitches. In cases of very early onset, chorea may be replaced by akinesia and rigidity (the so-called Westphal variant). Psychiatric symptoms may include a change in personality, paranoia, psychosis, or depression.

Computed tomography (CT) scans of HD patients show dilated ventricles and atrophy of the caudate nucleus, with loss of the convex bulging of the nucleus into the frontal horn of the lateral ventricle. Neuropathological examination reveals significant damage to the caudate nucleus, putamen, and globus pallidus, in a pattern consistent with the destruction of glutamate-receptive neurons. This suggests an excitotoxic model for cell loss in the disease (Coyle and Schwarcz 1976).

Epidemiological studies.   The prevalence of HD was 19/100,000 among persons in Minnesota dying after the age of 40 (Heston and Mastri 1977).

Family studies.   The age at onset of HD is variable and appears to depend on the parental origin of the disease gene. Thus many early-onset cases inherit the HD gene from their father (and may demonstrate "anticipation," i.e., a significantly earlier age at onset than their father [Ridley et al. 1988]), whereas many late-onset cases inherit the gene from their mother. This "parental origin effect" has been attributed to maternally inherited extrachromosomal factors. It may also be explained by genomic imprinting, whereby a gene is differentially methylated (and therefore expressed) depending on whether it passed through the maternal or paternal germline (Reik 1988).

High-risk studies.   The amplitude of the somatosensory-evoked potential was diminished in 22 individuals at (50%) risk for HD compared with 22 hospitalized neurotic patients (Josiassen et al. 1988). Attempts to differentiate individuals who may go on to develop HD with oculomotor screening tests have proven less successful (Collewijn et al. 1988). The availability of DNA markers linked to the HD gene (see below) has allowed a comparison of asymptomatic individuals at high (96%) and low (4%) risk for having inherited the disease gene.

Mode of inheritance.   An autosomal dominant mode of inheritance for HD is suggested by family studies: affected individuals usually have an affected parent. Conversely, approximately one-half of the offspring of affected parents are themselves affected. Formal testing of this mode of inheritance by segregation analysis is complicated: the variable age at onset that characterizes the disease prevents unambiguous identification of gene carriers. Elston et al. (1980) performed a segregation analysis on data from 11 HD families comprising 430 individuals and one large seven-generation kindred of 559 individuals. Age at onset was assumed to be normally distributed. A dominant mode of inheritance fit both data sets; both Mendelian recessive and environmental hypotheses were rejected.

Linkage analysis.   The gene underlying HD was assigned to the short arm of chromosome 4 by demonstrating close linkage to the anonymous DNA marker D4S10 in a large Venezuelan kindred and a smaller American kindred (Gusella et al. 1983). Extension of these findings to pedigrees from throughout the world provided strong evidence against nonallelic heterogeneity in this disorder (Haines et al. 1986). Variability in phenotypic expression appears to characterize HD families linked to D4S10. Phenotypic variations within families may represent unlinked autosomal modifying loci that influence HD gene expression; variations across families may represent different allelic genes at the HD locus.

Molecular approaches.   The HD gene maps 4 cM distal to the D4S10 (G8) marker in the terminal 4p16.3 subband of chromosome 4. D4S10 and a novel marker, D4S90 (D5), lying even more distal on chromosome 4, may flank the HD gene (Youngman et al. 1989). Linkage disequilibrium between the HD gene and markers D4S95 and D4S98 also suggests that the gene lies proximal to D4S90 (Snell et al. 1989). It is currently estimated that the 2–3 megabase (Mb) region surrounding the HD locus contains 50 or more candidate genes: novel cloning strategies, such as "exon trapping" (Duyk et al. 1990) promise to reveal the identity of these candidates quickly. Two such candidates, 385 and IT7, corresponding to mRNAs expressed in the brain, have been identified recently: studies are currently under way to establish whether differences in the size and/or abundance of their respective transcripts characterize postmortem brain material from HD patients (Thompson et al. 1990).

Although the HD gene has yet to be isolated, the availability of several new highly polymorphic multiallele RFLPs in the vicinity of the HD gene allow for preclinical diagnosis (MacDonald et al. 1989). In one study (Misra et al. 1988), 37% of adults at high risk for HD had appropriate pedigree structures for presymptomatic testing; it was estimated that fetal exclusion tests could be performed in approximately 80% of at-risk pregnancies. The availability of markers linked to the HD locus allow for the study of nonfamilial, as well as familial, HD. Thus genotyping of the entirely asymptomatic extended family of an individual with typical HD (onset at age 36) revealed that several healthy siblings shared one or the other or both of the patient's haplotypes; this is consistent with the patient harboring a new mutation (Wolff et al. 1989).

Parkinson's Disease

Parkinson's disease (PD) is a progressive movement disorder characterized by tremor, rigidity, bradykinesia, and postural changes. It may be associated with a variety of psychiatric syndromes including cognitive and affective disturbances, personality changes, and psychosis (Lishman 1987).

Structural brain imaging in patients with PD has revealed ventricular enlargement and cortical atrophy greater than that seen in age-matched control subjects (Sroka et al. 1981). Neuropathological changes primarily include a loss of pigmented (dopaminergic) neurons in the zona compacta of the substantia nigra. Other neurons, such as those in the locus coeruleus and nucleus basalis of Meynert, may also be affected.

Epidemiological studies.   The prevalence of PD has been estimated as 133/100,000; the average age at onset is 63 years (Bekkelund et al. 1989). The incidence of the disorder has been reported as 11/100,000 person years (Hofman et al. 1989a). Studies of temporal trends in incidence in the nonindustrialized community of Rochester, Minnesota (Schoenberg 1987), suggested virtually no change over the previous 35 years.

In the United States, death rates for PD suggest that race (white greater than black), sex (male greater than female), and geography (north greater than south) are independent risk factors for the disease, perhaps reflecting an etiologic role for some environmental agent (Kurtzke and Goldberg 1988). In a cross-sectional survey in Israel (Goldsmith et al. 1990), spatial clustering of PD was found in three adjacent kibbutzim (prevalence 2.2%) and was felt to represent a common environmental factor (such as agricultural chemicals or drinking water).

In North America and Europe, early-onset PD appears to be associated with rural residence, perhaps reflecting exposure to pesticides, well water, or wood pulp (Tanner 1989). 1-Methyl-4-phenyl-1,2,3,6-tetrahydropyridine (MPTP) represents an environmental neurotoxin known to cause PD in man and primates (Marsden and Jenner 1987). Other studies have suggested increased risk with exposure to high blood mercury levels and decreased risk with early-life vitamin E intake (Golbe et al. 1990a; Ngim and Devathasan 1989).

Family studies.   Since the time of Gowers (1903), the observation that patients with PD frequently have affected relatives has suggested a role for genetic factors in the disease. Martin et al. (1973) examined aggregation of illness among the first-, second-, and third-degree relatives of patients with PD compared with the relatives of spouse control subjects; 26.8% of probands and 14.8% of control subjects reported at least one affected relative. The greatest risk was for the relatives of young probands (8.3% of the sibs of probands aged 35–44 were affected versus 1.4% of the sibs of probands aged 65–74). That younger-onset probands have a more familiar form of PD, however, has not been universally found (Marttila and Rinne 1988), and young and older forms of the disorder may not be clinically or pathologically distinguished. Young-onset PD should be distinguished from juvenile PD (onset before age 21), which is invariably familial (Quinn et al. 1987; Yokochi et al. 1984). PD may be three times more common among the relatives of AD probands than among control subjects, suggesting etiological overlap between these disorders (Hofman et al. 1989b).

Twin studies.   MZ concordance rates are only slightly higher than DZ rates for both narrowly defined PD and broadly defined PD (including typical PD, possible PD, atypical PD, and isolated dementia, the latter added to allow for cases of diffuse Lewy body disease, which may only present with dementia and which bears an uncertain etiologic relation to PD) (Johnson et al. 1990; Ward et al. 1983). Similarly, the prevalence of PD in twins is similar to that in the general population (Marttila et al. 1988).

Mode of inheritance.   PD may prove to be etiologically heterogeneous. Apparent autosomal dominant inheritance with reduced penetrance is found in some families (Farrer et al. 1989; Golbe et al. 1990b), although the presence of atypical features, such as cerebellar signs, has suggested that some of these families may be segregating olivopontocerebellar atrophy. Autosomal recessive inheritance may characterize juvenile-onset PD (Yamamura et al. 1973). Furthermore, maternal inheritance, suggesting a mitochondrial gene, may characterize others (Johnson et al. 1990). Martin et al. (1973) suggested a multifactorial polygenic mode of inheritance: this model is consistent with the observation that the risk for an individual to develop familial PD increases with the number of affected individuals in his or her family.

Alzheimer's Disease

AD accounts for about 70% of dementia. It usually begins after age 45, with a progressive clinical course leading to death. It is a clinical diagnosis of exclusion and can be detected with certainty only at autopsy. Many of the present epidemiological studies have been based only on presumed clinical diagnosis.

Personality changes usually precede neurological findings in AD. As the illness progresses, Babinski reflex, rigid limbs, frontal release findings, and seizures can appear. Laboratory examination is uninformative, and neuroimaging may reveal only cortical atrophy and ventriculomegaly. Degeneration is marked in the hippocampal formation of the temporal lobe and in the temporo-parieto-occipital association cortex. Primary motor and sensory areas are relatively spared.

The specific pathological phenomena are neurofibrillary tangles, senile plaques, and granulovacuolar degeneration. Subcortical structures are also affected. There is a loss of acetylcholinergic neurotransmitter cells from the nucleus basalis of Meynert (Whitehouse et al. 1981) that project widely to the cerebral cortex, hippocampus, and limbic formation. This loss of cholinergic axons underlies the cognitive deficits of AD (Coyle et al. 1983), and the decrement of the enzyme choline acetyltransferase (EC 2.3.1.6) correlates with the extent of dementia. It has recently been theorized that the neuronal degeneration in AD triggers compensatory mechanisms promoting neuronal growth and leading to further plaque formation and pathological changes (Crutcher et al. 1991).

AD is considered to be a disease process and not the normal process of brain aging. Age at onset of less than 60 years distinguishes presenile from senile dementia, although this is debatable. The neuropathology is the same, although population studies suggest that the presenile group has more language dysfunction and a more rapid clinical course (Seltzer and Sherwin 1983).

Epidemiological studies.   Approximately 10% of the population over age 65 and 45% of those over 85 are affected with AD. Theories implicated in its etiology include genetic mechanisms, viral infection, metal intoxication (notably aluminum), head trauma, and others. A review of the published prevalence of dementia found that the actual rates differed across studies and by methodology but that the rate doubled every 5.1 years. AD is said to be more common among women, whereas multi-infarct dementia is more common among men (Jorm et al. 1987).

Family studies.   Epidemiological studies reveal an increased prevalence of dementia in the family members of AD patients. The estimates of increased risk are variable and may be small: 10%–14.4% for parents and 3.8%–13.9% for siblings (Amaducci et al. 1986; Heston and Mastri 1977; Heyman et al. 1983).

Life table studies that adjust for non-AD deaths find the risk of AD may be as high as 50% in family members by age 90 and only 10% in control subjects (Huff et al. 1988; Mohs et al. 1987). These analyses support a common autosomal gene for AD with an age-dependent penetrance. However, Farrer et al. (1989), who also factored in diagnostic uncertainties, found a risk of only 24% to first-degree relatives by age 93 and of 16% to control subjects by age 90.

These and other estimates of the increase in AD risk to family members vary widely (St. George-Hyslop et al. 1989). Family studies are hindered by the late age at onset, because individuals can die from other conditions or develop a dementia from a different etiology. The increased family prevalence of AD may occur predominantly in the early-onset group (Heston 1981), although such cases just may be more easily ascertained and both early- and late-onset cases often occur within a single family. The relative contribution of genetic and environmental factors to the development of AD is unknown.

Twin studies.   A large twin study of AD is currently under way, but only a small number of twin studies have been published (Embry and Bruyland 1985; Nee et al. 1987). The concordance rates, thus far, are similar in MZ and DZ pairs (about 40%) with some pairs having quite disparate ages at onset. These twin studies support a large environmental influence on the etiology of AD.

Linkage analysis.   The occurrence of neuropathological changes indicative of AD in individuals with Down's syndrome directed a search for an AD locus on chromosome 21. This chromosome also contains the locus for the amyloid precursor protein (APP), the precursor of amyloid, itself a major constituent of the senile plaques of AD. St. George-Hyslop et al. (1987) first reported evidence for an AD gene linked to the pericentromeric region of chromosome 21 (Figure 8–3). The AD locus on chromosome 21 appears to be close to, but not colocalized with, the APP locus in some families (Tanzi et al. 1987). Yet, Hardy and associates (Goate et al. 1991) identified a mutation in the APP gene that cosegregated with AD in two unrelated chromosome 21–linked, early-onset families. This supports, but does not prove, a role for this abnormality and amyloid deposition in at least some families with AD. The positive linkage represented only a portion of families with familial AD, implying genetic heterogeneity. Although no second locus has been confirmed for AD, an association of familial AD with the apolipoprotein (APO) C2 allele on chromosome 19 has been described (Schellenberg et al. 1987), as well as linkage to two chromosome 19 markers (BCL3 and ATP1AC) (Pericak-Vance et al. 1990).

Molecular approaches.   As noted, the APP gene, coding for the precursor to β-amyloid, has been considered as a candidate gene for familial AD. It has been unclear if the amyloid deposition characteristic of AD is a secondary response to neuronal degeneration or of primary pathogenic significance. Although it is not abnormal in all AD patients, the cloning and characterization of APP may allow the identification of other abnormal genes (Schellenberg et al. 1989). These genes may participate in coding or controlling mechanisms for APP or other proteins involved in AD.

Schizophrenia

Schizophrenia refers to a group of serious psychiatric disorders characterized by "positive" (psychotic) symptoms, "negative" (deficit) symptoms, early onset, and a chronic deteriorating course. It is a common and particularly crippling syndrome:

the lifetime morbid risk for schizophrenia is 0.9% (Gottesman and Shields 1982). Most patients are initially affected in young adulthood; 50% go on to experience some disability throughout their lives, and an additional 25% never recover and require lifelong care.

The genetic contribution to schizophrenia was recognized by early investigators, such as Bleuler (1911), who noted that relatives of patients were often tainted by hereditary mental disease. Other nonaffective psychoses, schizoaffective disorder, and schizotypal and paranoid personality disorders also aggregate in the biological relatives of schizophrenic probands (Baron et al. 1983; Kendler and Gruenberg 1984). It is not clear, however, what inherited factor predisposes to schizophrenia. In addition to the so-called schizophrenia spectrum disorders, other candidates include positive symptoms, negative symptoms, attentional and preattentional psychophysiological abnormalities, a latent trait predisposing to both schizophrenia and eye movement dysfunctions, and soft neurological signs.

Family studies. Beginning with the pioneering work of Rudin (1916), and others in the Berlin school, over 20 family risk studies have examined the incidence of schizophrenia in relatives of affected individuals. These studies have consistently demon-

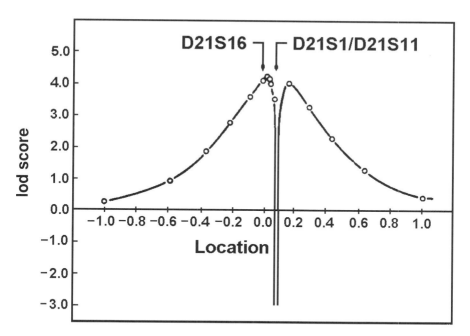

Figure 8–3. Linkage analysis of Alzheimer's disease (AD). Lod scores have been calculated for various locations (in Morgans) of the gene for AD relative to fixed positions for the two chromosome 21 anonymous marker loci, D21S16 and D21S1/D21S11. Composite data are shown for four pedigrees segregating AD. Two maxima are seen, with lod scores of 4.25 and 4.06, respectively; both scores are greater than the critical value of +3 suggesting linkage.
Source. Reprinted from St. George-Hyslop PH, Tanzi RE, Polinsky RJ, et al: "The Genetic Defect Causing Familial Alzheimer's Disease Maps on Chromosome 21." *Science* 235:885–890, 1987. Copyright 1987 by AAAS. Used with permission.

strated an elevated morbid risk for schizophrenia in the first-degree relatives of schizophrenic probands (parents, mean 5.6%; sibs, 10.1%; and children, 12.8%), compared with that for the general population (0.9%), suggesting that schizophrenia is familial (Gottesman and Shields 1982).

Although schizophrenia and other psychotic illnesses, such as bipolar disorder, tend to "breed true" the incidence of both disorders is higher in the families of schizophrenic probands (Rosenthal 1970). Similarly, the incidence of other psychotic disorders (e.g, schizoaffective disorder, paranoid disorder, and atypical psychosis) is increased among the relatives of schizophrenic probands (Kendler et al. 1985), suggesting a genetic predisposition to psychosis itself.

Attentional dysfunction has long been thought to be a central feature of schizophrenia (Kraepelin 1919). Deficits on the Continuous Performance Task (CPT; Kornetsky and Orzack 1978) are estimated to exist in approximately 40% of schizophrenic patients, whereas similar deficits, when found, exist at a lower rate in other psychiatric patients (Nuechterlein and Dawson 1984; Walker 1981). These CPT deficits appear to be trait related, possibly as phenotypic expressions of genetic vulnerability factors to schizophrenia.

A failure to show suppression of the 50 millisecond (msec) preattentional component of the auditory-evoked potential in a conditioning testing paradigm has been implicated as a genetic vulnerability marker (Siegel et al. 1984). Research suggests that this abnormality is trait related in schizophrenia and occurs at a higher rate in schizophrenic patients and their first-degree relatives compared with other psychiatric patients or control subjects (Adler et al. 1985; Baker et al. 1987).

A majority (85%) of patients with chronic schizophrenia and about 50% of those with acute schizophrenia exhibit abnormalities in smooth pursuit eye movements (SPEM) (Holzman et al. 1988; Klein et al. 1976), in contrast to a base rate in the normal population of about 6%–8%. Approximately 50% of the first-degree relatives of schizophrenic patients also exhibit SPEM disruption (Holzman 1987; Iacono 1982), suggesting that it may serve as a genetic marker for schizophrenia or represent the variable expression of an underlying "latent trait" (Matthysse et al. 1986).

Twin studies.   The heritability of schizophrenia is supported by twin study data. MZ and DZ co-twins of probands with schizophrenia differ in their risk for the disorder with weighted mean probandwise concordances of 59.2% and 15.2%, respectively (Kendler 1986). Environmental factors might account for the existence of the discordant MZ twins. Kidd (1978) estimated that up to 25% of cases of schizophrenia may represent phenocopies. Fischer (1971), however, studied the offspring of discordant MZ twins and found equivalent risks for schizophrenia (9.6% and 12.9%), again emphasizing the heritability of schizophrenia.

Adoption studies.   The adoptee study method (Heston 1966; Rosenthal et al. 1968; Tienari et al. 1983) revealed a significant increase in schizophrenia in the offspring of schizophrenic mothers separated at birth compared with the offspring of control mothers. A cross-fostering study found equivalent low rates of severe psychiatric illness among adoptees with healthy biological parents, whether they were reared by adoptive parents with schizophrenia or those without (Wender et al. 1974). The adoptee's family study method, employed by Kety et al. (1975), found that schizophrenia and related disorders were more common among the biological relatives of 34 schizophrenic adoptees than among the biological relatives of matched control adoptees. The rates for these disorders did not differentiate the adoptive relatives of either adoptee group, being low in both. Finally, studies of MZ twins reared apart (Gottesman and Shields 1982) have shown high pairwise concordance for schizophrenia, providing further evidence for a genetic component in the etiology of this disorder.

High-risk studies.   CPT abnormalities have identified individuals at risk for schizophrenia (Erlenmeyer-Kimling and Cornblatt 1987; Nuechterlein 1983). A form of these deficits has also been found in nonpsychotic subjects who have schizotypal features (Golden and Meehl 1979) suggesting that CPT may be a marker of core deficits associated with schizophrenia-related disorders.

Mode of inheritance.   An array of genetic models has been proposed for schizophrenia. Though a dominant gene has been considered (Book 1953; Slater and Cowie 1971; Zerbin-Rudin 1967), the reproductive disadvantage of schizophrenia (Larson and Nyman 1973) would seem to strongly select against this mode of inheritance.

A recessive monogenic model predicts that the incidence of schizophrenia among the offspring of two schizophrenic parents would be comparable to the probandwise concordance for MZ twins, and this is, in fact, what has been observed (Kringlen 1978). Similarly, a recessive model could allow for the maintenance of the abnormal gene in the population despite reduced reproductive fitness of those with the illness. Recessive models have been examined by Rudin (1916), Elston and Campbell (1970), and Stewart et al. (1980). Sex-linked models have been proposed (DeLisi and Crow 1989) based on gender differences in the clinical presentation of the illness (later onset and more benign course in women) and the increased incidence of psychosis in those with sex chromosome aneuploidies.

Oligogenic models were initially proposed by Karlsson (1972), who suggested a two-locus hypothesis for the inheritance of schizophrenia. Matthysse et al. (1979) postulated an intermediate oligogenic model considering a small number of genes with disproportionately large effects on phenotype. More recently, Risch (1990a, 1990b) has suggested that a two- to three-locus epistasis model provides for the pattern of recurrence risk observed among individuals varying in degree of relatedness to schizophrenic probands.

Polygenic models are also compatible with the sharp drop in risk for schizophrenia as one moves from MZ twins, to siblings and offspring, and then to second- and third-degree relatives. They can also account for the observed increase in risk of schizophrenia in relatives with increasing severity in the proband (Gottesman and Shields 1982) and with greater numbers of other affected relatives (Odegaard 1972; but see Essen-Moller 1977).

Formal studies comparing monogenic and polygenic models have included both segregation (Carter and Chung 1980; Tsuang et al. 1982) and pedigree analyses (Elston et al. 1978). On balance these analyses have produced inconclusive results regarding the mode of inheritance of schizophrenia.

Linkage analysis.   Following up on initial suggestions (Turner 1979) of linkage between schizophrenia spectrum disorders and the human leukocyte antigen (HLA) region on chromosome 6p in 6 informative pedigrees, McGuffin et al. (1983) excluded linkage between Present State Examination (PSE; Wing et al. 1974) diagnosed schizophrenia and the HLA region, as well as markers Gc (chromosome 4q) and Gm (chromosome 14q) in 11 informative families segregating the disorder. Chada et al. (1986) and Goldin et al. (1987) excluded linkage to the HLA locus in a total of 18 nuclear families containing at least two members with Research Diagnostic Criteria (RDC; Spitzer et al. 1978) diagnosed schizophrenia. Finally, Andrew et al. (1987), examining 20 phenotypic markers in 20 pedigrees, found no evidence to support linkage between schizophrenia or spectrum disorders and various blood group components and HLA.

Molecular approaches.   A large number of cytogenetic anomalies have been associated with schizophrenia (DeLisi et al. 1988). Aschauer et al. (1989), following up on a translocation 2;18 associated with the disorder, reported linkage between DSM-III (American Psychiatric Association 1980) diagnosed schizophrenia and markers on chromosome 2 in four pedigrees, but results were inconclusive. More recently, W. Byerley and colleagues (personal communication, November 1990) have excluded linkage between schizophrenia and a VNTR marker in the vicinity of the 2;18 breakpoint in 6 pedigrees.

Chromosome 5q has been widely investigated as the location of a potential major susceptibility locus for schizophrenia after a report (Bassett et al. 1988) of an uncle and nephew pair with neuroleptic-responsive DSM-III-R (American Psychiatric Association 1987) schizophrenia and a partial trisomy of chromosome 5. Sherrington et al. (1988) examined five Icelandic and two English pedigrees and found linkage of 5q to schizophrenia, spectrum disorder, and various other psychiatric disorders ("fringe diagnoses"). These fringe diagnoses included alcoholism, major and minor depressive disorders, and anxiety disorders. Others (Aschauer et al. 1990; Kaufmann et al. 1989), however, have failed to replicate this initial linkage finding. Furthermore, they found that the strongest evidence against linkage was achieved with the broadest definition of affection, in direct contrast to the finding by Sherrington et al. (1988). DeLisi and Crow (1989) reported on a study of eight families and excluded linkage to four areas of the X chromosome. They are currently examining markers from the pseudoautosomal regions of the sex chromosomes in suitable families.

Candidates genes have also been examined for linkage to schizophrenia. The regulatory gene, homeobox 2 (chromosome 17p), appears not to be linked to the schizophrenia locus in a Swedish isolate. Similarly, the neurochemical gene tyrosine hydroxylase (TH [11p]) was excluded in these pedigrees (Kennedy et al. 1989), whereas a 13 cM region around the gene for the D_2 receptor (11q) was also excluded (Moises et al. 1991). Recently, the gene for a schizophrenia-associated synaptic antigen, EP10 (chromosome 17), has been excluded in these pedigrees (Kennedy et al. 1991). An earlier study (Feder et al. 1985) had excluded the candidate neurochemical gene, pro-opiomelanocortin (2p23) in other families segregating schizophrenia.

Bipolar Disorder

Bipolar, or manic-depressive, disorder refers to an episodic disturbance in mood alternately characterized by mania (elevated or irritable mood, increased psychomotor activity, distractibility, diminished need for sleep, and often psychosis) and depression (dysphoric mood, diminished psychomotor activity, decreased concentration, sleep and appetite disturbance, and frequently suicidality). Subgroups of bipolar disorder, differing in the severity of disturbance during the manic phase and designated as bipolar I and II, have been identified (Dunner et al. 1976).

Various biological abnormalities have been described in bipolar disorder, ranging from alterations in lateralized brain functions to changes in brain biogenic amines (Goodwin and Jamison 1990). No consistent neuropathological changes have been identified (Jeste et al. 1988).

Epidemiological studies. Estimates of the general population risk (prevalence) of bipolar disorder have ranged from 0.1% to 1.1% with a mean of 0.5%. The population risk for unipolar depression is higher, with values ranging from 3.4% to 18.0%, with a mean of 6.2% (Tsuang and Faraone 1990). It would appear that the risk for mood disorders has increased over time: this seems to be due to a "period effect" (i.e., the effect of some exogenous pathogenic factor over a limited period of time [Lavori et al. 1986]). The risk of bipolar disorder in women is approximately equal to that in men, whereas the risk of unipolar disorder in women is about twice that in men (Weissman et al. 1988). Patients with bipolar illness seem to be overrepresented in the upper social and educational classes: this may reflect certain personality and behavioral patterns (e.g., heightened productivity) associated with a rise in social position in the relatives of bipolar probands (Goodwin and Jamison 1990).

Family studies. Double-blind, controlled family studies (Gershon et al. 1982; Tsuang et al. 1985) have compared the morbid risk of bipolar disorder in the first-degree relatives of bipolar probands with that in the relatives of nonbipolar probands. These studies suggest that the risk to the former group ranges from 3.9% to 8.0%, whereas the risk to the latter group ranges from 0.2% to 0.5%. Morbid risk appears to be especially elevated for the relatives of "early-onset" (i.e., those with onset in childhood) probands (Strober et al. 1988); this cannot be attributed to the period effect mentioned above (Tsuang and Faraone 1990). In addition to bipolar disorder, a number of other psychiatric conditions aggregate in the relatives of bipolar probands including bipolar II disorder (patients with major depression who have had hypomania but not mania); unipolar, cyclothymic, and schizoaffective disorders; and suicide. Some studies have suggested that alcoholism is also part of the bipolar disorder spectrum; others have not (Gershon 1990).

Twin studies. Ten twin studies of mood disorders conducted since 1928 have suggested increased concordance rates in MZ pairs (58%–74%) compared with same-sex DZ pairs (17%–29%) (Tsuang and Faraone 1990). A relative scarcity of unipolar-bipolar pairs argues against these disorders being genotypically identical, although the existence of some of these pairs suggests some relationship between the two disorders. In addition to supporting a major role (51% of the variance) for genetic factors in the development of mood disorders, these twin studies have also suggested an important role (42% of the variance) for shared environmental factors in disease pathogenesis.

Adoption studies. Similarly, two methodologically sound adoption studies (Mendlewicz and Rainer 1977; Wender et al. 1986) of the biological relatives of bipolar probands and control subjects have suggested an important role for genetic factors. Bipolar probands' relatives were at increased risk for bipolar disorder, unipolar disorder, and schizoaffective disorder, further clarifying the boundaries of the bipolar spectrum. The strongest findings among biological relatives appear to be for completed suicide: the rate among relatives of bipolar adoptees may be as much as 15 times the rate among relatives of control adoptees (Wender et al. 1986). Several environmental factors in the adoptive family appear to predict the development of mood disorders: parental alcohol problems for male adoptees and other parental psychiatric problems and parental death before age 19 for female adoptees (Cadoret et al. 1985).

High-risk studies.   High-risk children of bipolar parents appear to have greater degrees of aggressiveness, obsessionality, and affective expression than age-matched control subjects (Goodwin and Jamison 1990). Cognitive deficits, especially on performance subtests of the Wechsler Intelligence Scale for Children-Revised (WISC-R; Wechsler 1974), suggestive of right-hemisphere dysfunction and reminiscent of deficits seen in adult bipolar patients, have also been found in high-risk children (Kestenbaum 1979).

Mode of inheritance.   The absence of male-to-male transmission of bipolar disorder in some families has suggested a dominant X-linked form of the disease (Winokur et al. 1969). Risch et al. (1986) suggested that as many as one-third of bipolar patients may have this X-linked subtype. Segregation analyses have not provided convincing support for either single major locus or polygenetic-multifactorial transmission of bipolar disorder (Tsuang and Faraone 1990). Such analyses have assumed that major depression and bipolar disorder are mild and severe forms of the same disorder. For monogenic transmission these might represent allelic variants at the same locus; for polygenetic transmission these might represent different thresholds on the same continuum of liability to illness. These analyses have been confounded by a secular increase in the rate of affective illness over the past three generations (the aforementioned period effect) and limited by incomplete penetrance and possible nonallelic genetic heterogeneity (Goldin et al. 1984).

Linkage analysis.   Linkage analyses of bipolar disorder have included anonymous marker studies, implicating chromosome 11p15; favored locus studies, implicating chromosome Xq28; and candidate gene studies, arguing against the tyrosine hydroxylase and D_2 receptor genes. Egeland et al. (1987) reported linkage between bipolar I and related disorders (bipolar II disorder; schizoaffective disorder, bipolar type; and unipolar major depression) and the chromosome 11 *HRAS1* oncogene in 19 of 81 members of an extended Old Order Amish pedigree.

Other studies (Detera-Wadleigh et al. 1987; Hodgkinson et al. 1987) have excluded linkage between a major locus for bipolar disorder and these chromosome 11 markers. Kelsoe et al. (1989) reevaluated the original Egeland report with the following changes: new onset of mood disorder in 2 members of the original pedigree, additional genotype data on 10 previously incompletely typed members of the original pedigree, new genotype data on 6 individuals in a newly included sibship (the "left" extension), and new genotype data on 31 additional relatives (the "right" extension). Linkage was excluded to the chromosome 11 markers in these 118 pedigree members.

Turning to X chromosome studies, Baron et al. (1987) reported strong evidence for linkage between bipolar disorder and two Xq phenotypic markers (red-green color vision and G6PD deficiency) in Israeli-Jewish pedigrees. Furthermore, Mendlewicz et al. (1987) provided weaker evidence for linkage between bipolar disorder and a more centromeric X chromosome locus, the hemophilia B (Factor IX) locus. One explanation for disparate locations in the two X chromosome studies is that the confidence intervals associated with these two linkage findings are so wide that they may implicate the same locus (Baron et al. 1990).

Molecular approaches.   Linkage studies have looked at tyrosine hydroxylase (TH) as a candidate gene for bipolar disorder: it is both neurochemically plausible, because it is the rate-limiting enzyme in catecholamine synthesis, and cytologically plausible, because it is in the same chromosomal region of 11p as *HRAS1* and *INS*. Because TH is farther from the bipolar disorder locus than *HRAS1*, it would appear that it is not the bipolar disorder gene. Candidate gene studies have also looked at the D_2 receptor gene: it is both neurochemically plausible, because elevations in D_2 receptor density have been seen antemortem in patients with bipolar disorder on PET scans, and cytologically plausible, because chromosomal rearrangements (balanced translocations) involving the region of the D_2 receptor gene on chromosome 11q have been associated with mood disorders in two separate pedigrees (St. Clair et al. 1990). Preliminary linkage evidence argues against the D_2 receptor gene as the bipolar disorder gene.

Narcolepsy

Narcolepsy probably results from a defect in the rapid-eye-movement (REM)-inhibiting mechanisms of sleep, although it is at times mistakenly considered to be a psychological phenomenon. Onset can be at any age but peaks in young adulthood or late adolescence: 85% of cases begin before age 25. Narcolepsy that includes cataplexy is classic narcolepsy. Hallmark features of narcolepsy are irresistible excessive daytime sleepiness and polysomnographic EEG evidence of abnormal REM sleep. Other phenomena include onset of REM within 10 minutes of sleep initiation that precipitates hypnagogic hallucinations, sleep paralysis, and cataplexy. Much less frequently there are blackouts with automatic behaviors. Abnormalities in brain monoaminergic and cholinergic functioning have been implicated in the pathophysiology of narcolepsy.

Epidemiological studies.   The prevalence of narcolepsy varies from 10/100,000 to 100/100,000 in the United States and Europe to 160/100,000 in Japan and 0.2/100,000 in Israel. The frequency of narcolepsy varies greatly and correlates with the geographical variation of the incidence of HLA-DR2. Twenty percent of unaffected Britons carry this particular HLA (Kramer et al. 1987), and only 11%–12% of Israelis yet 34% of the Japanese population display this HLA type.

Family studies.   There is strong familial clustering of narcolepsy: 30%–50% of affected probands have an affected relative (Baraitser and Parkes 1978; Yoss and Daly 1957). The clinical expression of the disorder can vary markedly, however, even within the same family.

Mode of inheritance.   The inheritance of narcolepsy is probably dominant with variable penetrance. Concordant identical twins are rare in the literature (Douglass et al. 1989; Montplaisir and Poirier 1987), and nongenetic factors likely play a major role in the expression of narcolepsy. Onset follows an illness or psychological factor in about one-half of patients (Passouant and Billiard 1976), although this association may be coincidental.

Linkage analysis.   Nearly 100% of narcoleptic individuals have HLA-DR2, except among blacks, almost all of whom have LA-DQw1 (Langdon et al. 1984; Neely et al. 1987; Parkes et al. 1986). These chromosome 6p antigens are part of the major histo-compatibility complex, essential to cell recognition and the organization of immune responses. The association of these HLA types and narcolepsy is among the highest known for HLA-linked syndromes.

Molecular approaches.   The HLA-DR2, Dw2 gene has been cloned (Uryu et al. 1989); no difference in sequence between narcoleptic and normal individuals has been found. This indicates that narcolepsy is not the result of a mutation at this site; it is possible, however, that the narcolepsy gene lies near the HLA-D region in linkage disequilibrium with it.

CONCLUSIONS

Environmental and hereditary factors that contribute to neuropsychiatric disease often act in concert to produce a given disorder. Nonetheless, the role of environmental factors is large in some illnesses, such as PD, and smaller in others, such as HD. Traditionally, epidemiology has focused on exogenous influences and genetics on endogenous influences. In reality, the fields often overlap and genetic epidemiology is merely a discipline within epidemiology.

In defining environmental effects on disease, epidemiology proceeds in a stepwise manner. First, it establishes an association between exposure to a particular factor and development of the disease. Next, it determines whether this association is valid or the consequence of chance, bias, or confounds through the introduction of suitable control subjects and "blinds." Finally, it judges whether this association represents a cause-effect relationship by means of its magnitude, consistency, and biological plausibility (Hennekens and Buring 1987).

Likewise, genetic studies proceed to uncover heritable effects, first by establishing the association of familial and genetic "exposure" to the disease and then by validating this association, again with appropriate control subjects and "blinds." Subsequently, genetic studies specify the genes mediating these effects by one of two paths, colloquially known as "forward" and "reverse" genetics. With some disorders, the abnormal gene product (e.g., a defective enzyme) may be known, and the disease gene coding for that product thereby may be isolated.

For other disorders, the abnormal gene product is unknown and may be coded for by any of the estimated 50,000 genes that contribute to CNS function. In these disorders, the search for the disease gene begins with establishing its chromosomal location. The gene may then be isolated through the rapidly evolving techniques of molecular genetics. A causal role for the gene in the etiopathogenesis of the disorder requires its specific and consistent association with the disorder, its biological plausibility, and, ideally, its ability to transmit the disorder. The last postulate may be achieved through the creation of an abnormal (cellular) phenotype following the introduction of the disease gene or the reversal of the abnormal phenotype with the introduction of the normal allele.

The "reverse" genetic approach has been particularly successful with so-called simple disorders (i.e., those with a known mode of inheritance, complete penetrance, consistent expression, and etiologic homogeneity). A number of the disorders discussed in this chapter lack one or more of these features, and may be referred to as "complex" disorders. A preliminary categorization of neuropsychiatric diseases into simple and complex disorders is provided in Table 8–2.

Simple disorders appear to be caused by single-gene mutations, inherited in either an autosomal dominant, recessive, or X-linked manner. Complex disorders may result from a few major (oligo)genes (as has been postulated for schizophrenia) or from the combined effects of many (poly)genes. Similarly, complex disorders are characterized by incomplete penetrance, with the concordance rate for MZ twins perhaps representing an upper boundary. The advent of sophisticated structural and functional imaging techniques, however, may extend this boundary upward, as subclinical forms of disease (so-called endophenotypes) are identified.

Both simple and complex disorders may demonstrate variable expression. Thus simple disorders may vary in the presence or absence of neuropsychiatric symptoms, and whether and which neuropsychiatric symptoms are present may depend on the age of the affected individual. This may reflect (nonallelic) etiologic heterogeneity, with different forms of the disorder having both different presentations and different ages at onset, although disorders arising from a single locus may still demonstrate varying phenotypes. Thus variable expression appears to characterize HD families linked to D4S10. This may result from allelic variants at the disease locus or from the effect of distant modifying gene loci. Alternatively, it may reflect the interaction of a fixed molecular lesion with a brain in various states of maturation (Weinberger 1987).

Variable expression may be characterized as one genotype resulting in several phenotypes. Conversely, one phenotype may derive from several genotypes. This is the case with etiologic heterogeneity. The phenotype may be symptomatological or pathophysiological. Thus psychosis may be a heritable clinical feature common to both schizophrenia and bipolar disorder. Likewise, parkinsonism may be a heritable syndrome common to both PD and AD.

Table 8–2.   Simple and complex neuropsychiatric disorders

Simple	Complex
Acute intermittent porphyria,	Alzheimer's disease
Gerstmann-Strassler syndrome	Bipolar disorder
Huntington's disease	Dyslexia
Lesch-Nyhan syndrome	Epilepsy
Metachromatic leukodystrophy	Parkinson's disease
Myotonic dystrophy	Pick's disease
Narcolepsy	Schizophrenia
Wilson's disease	Tourette's syndrome

It is clear that abnormalities in single autosomal or sex genes cannot account for the full presentation of simple and complex disorders. There may be mitochondrial genes at work in some forms of HD and PD, perhaps affecting age at onset or penetrance. Nonetheless, the establishment of linkage between disease and major loci contributing to pathogenesis has become the holy grail of neuropsychiatric genetics. To date, a variety of potential linkages have been discovered: some (e.g, chromosome 4 in HD) have been well replicated; others (e.g., chromosome 11 in bipolar disorder) have not. Only with replication can these preliminary findings be considered valid. Once linkage has been established, the full armamentarium of modern molecular biology may be brought to bear on isolating disease genes. We can expect that this new knowledge will radically alter existing nosologies as genotype-phenotype associations are clarified.

REFERENCES

Adler LE, Waldo MC, Freedman R: Neuropsychologic studies of sensory gating in schizophrenia: comparison of auditory and visual responses. Biol Psychiatry 20:1284–1296, 1985

Amaducci LA, Fratiglioni L, Rocca WA, et al: Risk factors for clinically diagnosed Alzheimer's disease: a case study of an Italian population. Neurology 36:922–931, 1986

American Psychiatric Association: Diagnostic and Statistical Manual of Mental Disorders, 3rd Edition. Washington, DC, American Psychiatric Association, 1980

American Psychiatric Association: Diagnostic and Statistical Manual of Mental Disorders, 3rd Edition, Revised. Washington, DC, American Psychiatric Association, 1987

Anderson VE, Chern MM, Schwanebeck E: Multiplex families and the problem of heterogeneity, in Genetic Research Strategies for Psychobiology and Psychiatry. Edited by Gershon ES, Matthysse S, Breakefield XO, et al. Pacific Grove, CA, Boxwood, 1981, pp 341–351

Andrew B, Watt DC, Gillespie C, et al: A study of genetic linkage in schizophrenia. Psychol Med 17:363–370, 1987

Aschauer H, Aschauer-Treiber G, Cloninger CR, et al: Heterogeneity of schizophrenia: preliminary evidence for multiple genetic loci. Schizophrenia Research 2:39–51, 1989

Aschauer HN, Aschauer-Treiber G, Isenberg KE, et al: No evidence for linkage between chromosome 5 markers and schizophrenia. Hum Hered 40:109–115, 1990

Baker N, Adler LE, Franks RD, et al: Neurophysiological assessment of sensory gating in psychiatric inpatients: comparison between schizophrenia and other diagnoses. Biol Psychiatry 22:603–617, 1987

Baraitser M, Parkes JO: Genetic study of narcoleptic syndrome. J Med Genet 15:254–59, 1978

Baron M, Asnis L, Gruen R: Plasma amine oxidase and genetic vulnerability to schizophrenia. Arch Gen Psychiatry 40:275–279, 1983

Baron M, Risch N, Hamburger R, et al: Genetic linkage between X-chromosome markers and bipolar affective disorder. Nature 326:289–292, 1987

Baron M, Hamburger R, Sandkuyl LA, et al: The impact of phenotypic variation on genetic analysis: application to X-linkage in manic depressive illness. Acta Psychiatr Scand 82:196–203, 1990

Bassett AS, Jones B, McGillivray BC, et al: Partial trisomy chromosome 5 cosegregating with schizophrenia. Lancet 1:799–801, 1988

Bekkelund SI, Selseth B, Mellgren SI: Parkinson's disease in a population group in northern Norway. Tidsskr Nor Laegeforen 109:561–563, 1989

Bleuler E: Dementia Praecox or the Group of Schizophrenias. Leipzig, Deuticke, 1911

Book JA: A genetic and psychiatric investigation of a north Swedish population with special regard to schizophrenia and mental deficiency. Acta Genet 4:1–139, 1953

Botstein D, White RL, Skolnick M, et al: Construction of a genetic linkage map using restriction fragment length polymorphisms. Am J Hum Genet 32:314–331, 1980

Cadoret RJ, O'Gorman TW, Heywood E, et al: Genetic and environmental factors in major depression. J Affect Disord 9:155–164, 1985

Carter CL, Chung CS: Segregation analysis of schizophrenia under a mixed genetic model. Hum Hered 30:350–356, 1980

Cavalli-Sforza LL, Bodmer WF: The Genetics of Human Populations. San Francisco, CA, Freeman, 1971

Chada R, Kulhara P, Singh T, et al: HLA antigens in schizophrenia: a family study. Br J Psychiatry 149:612–615, 1986

Collewijn H, Went LN, Tamminga EP, et al: Oculomotor defects in patients with Huntington's disease and their offspring. J Neurol Sci 86(2–3):307–320, 1988

Coyle JT, Schwarcz R: Lesion of striatal neurons with kainic acid provides a model for Huntington's chorea. Nature (London) 263:244–246, 1976

Coyle JT, Price DL, Delong MR: Alzheimer's disease: a disorder of the cholinergic innervation of cortex. Science 219:1184–1190, 1983

Crutcher KA, Neaderhauser J, Schmidt P, et al: Neurite outgrowth on postmortem human brain chryostat sections: studies of non-Alzheimer's and Alzheimer's tissue. Exp Neurol 114:228–236, 1991

DeLisi LE, Crow TJ: Evidence for a sex chromosome locus for schizophrenia. Schizophr Bull 15:431–440, 1989

DeLisi LE, Reiss AL, White BJ, et al: Cytogenetic studies of males with schizophrenia: screening for the fragile X chromosome and other chromosomal abnormalities. Schizophrenia Research 1:277–281, 1988

Detera-Wadleigh SD, Berrettini WH, Goldin LR, et al: Close linkage of c-Harvey-ras-1 and the insulin gene to affective disorder is ruled out in three North American pedigrees. Nature 325:806–808, 1987

Douglass AB, Harris L, Pazderka F: Monozygotic twins concordant for the narcoleptic syndrome. Neurology 39:149–141, 1989

Dunner DL, Gershon ES, Goodwin FK: Heritable factors in the severity of affective illness. Biol Psychiatry 11:31–42, 1976

Duyk GM, Kim S, Pritchard C, et al: Isolation of Huntington's disease candidate genes by Exon Trapping. Am J Hum Genet 47 (suppl):A249, 1990

Egeland JA, Gerhard DS, Pauls DL, et al: Bipolar affective disorders linked to DNA markers on chromosome 11. Nature 325:783–787, 1987

Elston RC, Campbell MA: Schizophrenia: evidence for the major gene hypothesis. Behav Genet 1:3–10, 1970

Elston RC, Stewart J: A general model for the genetic analysis of pedigree data. Hum Hered 21:523–542, 1971

Elston RC, Namboodiri KK, Spence MA, et al: A genetic study of schizophrenic pedigrees, II: one-locus hypotheses. Neuropsychobiology 4:193–206, 1978

Elston RC, Pericak-Vance MA, Meyers DA, et al: Pedigree analysis of Huntington disease allowing for variable age of onset. Am J Hum Genet 32:142A, 1980

Embry C, Bruyland S: Presumed Alzheimer's disease beginning at different ages in two twins. J Am Geriatr Soc 33:61–62, 1985

Erlenmeyer-Kimling LE, Cornblatt B: The New York High Risk Project: a follow-up report. Schizophr Bull 13:451, 1987

Essen-Moller E: Evidence for polygenic inheritance in schizophrenia. Acta Psychiatr Scand 55:202–207, 1977

Farrer LA, O'Sullivan DM, Cupples A, et al: Assessment of genetic risk for Alzheimer's disease among first-degree relatives. Ann Neurol 25:485–493, 1989

Feder J, Gurling HMD, Darby J: DNA restriction fragment analysis of the proopiomelanocortin gene in schizophrenia. Am J Hum Genet 37:286–294, 1985

Fischer M: Psychoses in the offspring of schizophrenic monozygotic twins and their normal co-twins. Br J Psychiatry 118:43–52, 1971

Gershon E: Genetics, in Manic-Depressive Illness. Edited by Goodwin FK, Jamison KR. New York, Oxford University Press, 1990, pp 373–401

Gershon ES, Hamovit J, Guroff JJ, et al: A family study of schizoaffective, bipolar I, bipolar II, unipolar, and normal control probands. Arch Gen Psychiatry 39:1157–1167, 1982

Gilliam TC, Freimer NB, Kaufmann CA, et al: Deletion mapping of DNA markers to a region of chromosome 5 that co-segregates with schizophrenia. Genomics 5:940–944, 1989

Goate A, Chartier-Harlin MC, Mullan M, et al: Segregation of a missense mutation in the amyloid precursor protein gene with familial Alzheimer's disease. Nature 349:704–706, 1991

Golbe LI, Farrell TM, Davis PH: Follow-up study of early-life protective and risk factors in Parkinson's disease. Mov Disord 5:66–70, 1990a

Golbe LI, Di Iorio G, Bonavita V, et al: A large kindred with autosomal dominant Parkinson's disease. Ann Neurol 27:276–282, 1990b

Golden RR, Meehl PE: Detection of the schizoid taxon with MMPI indicators. J Abnorm Psychol 88:217–233, 1979

Goldin LR, Kidd KK, Matthysse S, et al: The power of pedigree segregation analysis for traits with incomplete penetrance, in Genetic Research Strategies for Psychobiology and Psychiatry. Edited by Gershon ES, Matthysse S, Breakefield XO, et al. Pacific Grove, CA, Boxwood, 1981, pp 305–317

Goldin LR, Cox NJ, Pauls DL, et al: The detection of major loci by segregation and linkage analysis: a simulation study. Genet Epidemiol 1:285–296, 1984

Goldin LR, DeLisi LE, Gershon ES: Relationship of HLA to schizophrenia in 10 nuclear families. Psychiatry Res 20:69–77, 1987

Goldsmith JR, Herishanu Y, Abarbanel JM, et al: Clustering of Parkinson's disease points to environmental etiology. Arch Environ Health 45(2):88–94, 1990

Goodwin FK, Jamison KR: Manic-Depressive Illness. New York, Oxford University Press, 1990

Gottesman II, Shields J: Schizophrenia: The Epigenetic Puzzle. Cambridge, Cambridge University Press, 1982

Gowers WR: A Manual of Diseases of the Nervous System, 2nd Edition. Philadelphia, PA, Blakiston, 1903

Gusella JF, Wexler NS, Conneally PM, et al: A polymorphic DNA marker genetically linked to Huntington's disease. Nature 306:234–238, 1983

Haines J, Tanzi R, Wexler N, et al: No evidence of linkage heterogeneity between Huntington's disease (HD) and G8 (D4S10) (abstract). Am J Hum Genet 39:A156, 1986

Hennekens CH, Buring JE: Epidemiology in Medicine. Boston, MA, Little, Brown, 1987

Heston LL: Psychiatric disorders in foster home reared children of schizophrenic mothers. Br J Psychiatry 112:819–825, 1966

Heston LL: Genetic studies of dementia: with emphasis on Parkinson's disease and Alzheimer's neuropathology, in The Epidemiology of Dementia. Edited by JA Mortimer, LM Schuman. New York, Oxford University Press, 1981, pp 101–114

Heston LL, Mastri AR: The genetics of Alzheimer's disease: associations with hematologic malignancy and Down's syndrome. Arch Gen Psychiatry 34:976–981, 1977

Heyman A, Wilkinson WEE, Hurwitz BJ, et al: Alzheimer's disease: genetic aspects and associated clinical disorder. Ann Neurol 14:507–515, 1983

Hodgkinson S, Sherrington R, Gurling H, et al: Molecular genetic evidence for heterogeneity in manic depression. Nature 325:805–806, 1987

Hofman A, Collette HJ, Bartelds AI: Incidence and risk factors of Parkinson's disease in the Netherlands. Neuroepidemiol 8(6):296–299, 1989a

Hofman A, Schulte W, Tanja TA, et al: History of dementia and Parkinson's disease in 1st-degree relatives of patients with Alzheimer's disease. Neurology 39:1589–1592, 1989b

Holzman PS: Recent studies of psychophysiology and schizophrenia. Schizophr Bull 13:49–75, 1987

Holzman PS, Kringlen E, Matthysse S, et al: A single dominant gene can account for eye tracking dysfunctions and schizophrenia in offspring of discordant twins. Arch Gen Psychiatry 45:641–647, 1988

Huff FJ, Auerbach J, Chakravarti A, et al: Risk of dementia in relatives of patients with Alzheimer's disease. Neurology 38:786–790, 1988

Iacono WG: Bilateral electrodermal habituation/dishabituation and resting EEG in remitted schizophrenics. J Nerv Ment Dis 170:91–101, 1982

Jeffreys AJ, Wilson V, Thien SL: Hypervariable "minisatellite" regions in human DNA. Nature 314:67–73, 1985

Jeste DV, Lohr JB, Goodwin FK: Neuroanatomical studies of affective disorders: a review and suggestions for further research. Br J Psychiatry 153:444–459, 1988

Johnson WG, Hodge SE, Duvoisin R: Twin studies and the genetics of Parkinson's disease—a reappraisal. Mov Disord 5:187–194, 1990

Jorm AF, Korten AE, Henderson AS: The prevalence of dementia: a quantitative integration of the literature. Acta Psychiatr Scand 76:465–479, 1987

Josiassen RC, Shagass C, Roemer RA, et al: A sensory evoked potential comparison of persons "at risk" for Huntington's disease and hospitalized neurotic patients. Int J Psychophysiol 6(4):281–289, 1988

Karlsson JL: A two-locus hypothesis for inheritance of schizophrenia, in Genetic Factors in Schizophrenia. Edited by Kaplan AR. Springfield, IL, Charles C Thomas, 1972, pp 246–255

Kaufmann CA, Malaspina D: Molecular genetics of schizophrenia, in Molecular Approaches to Neuropsychiatric Disease. Edited by Brosius J, Fremeau RT Jr. New York, Academic Press, 1991, pp 307–345

Kaufmann CA, DeLisi LE, Lehner T, et al: Physical mapping and linkage analysis of a putative susceptibility locus for schizophrenia on chromosome 5q. Schizophr Bull 15:441–452, 1989

Kelsoe JR, Ginns EI, Egeland JA, et al: Re-evaluation of the linkage relationship between chromosome 11p and the gene for bipolar affective disorder in the Old Order Amish. Nature 342:238–243, 1989

Kendler KS: Genetics of schizophrenia, in Psychiatry Update: American Psychiatric Association Annual Review, Vol 5. Edited by Frances AJ, Hales RE. Washington, DC, American Psychiatric Press, 1986, pp 25–41

Kendler KS, Gruenberg AM: An independent analysis of the Copenhagen sample of the Danish adoption study, VI: the pattern of psychiatric illness, as defined by DSM-III in adoptees and relatives. Arch Gen Psychiatry 41:555–564, 1984

Kendler KS, Gruenberg AM, Tsuang MT: Psychiatric illness in first-degree relatives of schizophrenic and surgical control patients. Arch Gen Psychiatry 42:770–779, 1985

Kennedy JL, Giuffra LA, Moises HW, et al: Molecular genetic studies of schizophrenia. Schizophr Bull 15:383–391, 1989

Kennedy JL, Honer WG, Gelernter J, et al: Linkage studies of two new genes of neuropsychiatric interest. Biol Psychiatry 29:57S, 1991

Kestenbaum CJ: Children at risk for manic-depressive illness: possible predictors. Am J Psychiatry 136:1206–1208, 1979

Kety SS, Rosenthal D, Wender PH, et al: Mental illness in the biological and adoptive families of adopted individuals who have become schizophrenic: a preliminary report based on psychiatric interviews, in Genetic Research in Psychiatry. Edited by Fieve RR, Rosenthal D, Brill H. Baltimore, MD, Johns Hopkins University Press, 1975, pp 147–166,

Kidd KK: A genetic perspective on schizophrenia, in The Nature of Schizophrenia: New Approaches to Research and Treatment. Edited by Wynne LC, Cromwell RL, Matthysse S. New York, Wiley, 1978, pp 70–75

Kidd KK: Genetic models for psychiatric disorders, in Genetic Research Strategies for Psychobiology and Psychiatry. Edited by Gershon ES, Matthysse S, Breakefield XO, et al. Pacific Grove, CA, Boxwood, 1981, pp 369–382

Kimura M, Sato M, Akatsuka A, et al: Restoration of myelin formation by a single type of myelin basic protein in transgenic shiverer mice. Proc Natl Acad Sci U S A 86:5661–5665, 1989

Klein RH, Salzman LF, Jones F, et al: Eye tracking in psychiatric patients and their offspring. Psychophysiology 13:186, 1976

Kornetsky C, Orzack M: Physiological and behavioral correlates of attentional dysfunction in schizophrenic patients. J Psychiatr Res 14:69–79, 1978

Kraepelin E: Dementia Praecox and paraphrenia (1919). Translated by Barclay RM. Edinburgh, Livingstone, 1971

Kramer ER, Dinner DS, Braun WE, et al: HLA-DR2 and narcolepsy. Arch Neurol 44:853–855, 1987

Kringlen E: Adult offspring of two psychotic parents, with special reference to schizophrenia, in The Nature of Schizophrenia. Edited by Wynne LC, Cromwell RL, Matthysse S. New York, Wiley, 1978, pp 9–24

Kurtzke JF, Goldberg ID: Parkinsonism death rates by race, sex, and geography. Neurology 38:1558–1561, 1988

Langdon N, Welsa KI, van Dam M, et al: Genetic markers in narcolepsy. Lancet 2:1170–1180, 1984

Larson CA, Nyman GE: Differential fertility in schizophrenia. Acta Psychiatr Scand 49:272–280, 1973

Lavori PW, Klerman GL, Keller MB, et al: Age-period-cohort analysis of secular trends in onset of major depression: findings in siblings of patients with major affective disorder. J Psychiatr Res 21:23–35, 1986

Lishman WA: Organic Psychiatry: The Psychological Consequences of Cerebral Disorder, 2nd Edition. Oxford, England, Blackwell Scientific, 1987

Lyons AS, Petrucelli RJ II: Medicine: An Illustrated History. New York, Harry N Abrams, 1987

MacDonald ME, Cheng SV, Zimmer M, et al: Clustering of multiallele DNA markers near the Huntington's disease gene. J Clin Invest 84:1013–1016, 1989

McGuffin P, Festenstein H, Murray R: A family study of HLA antigens and other genetic markers in schizophrenia. Psychol Med 13:31–43, 1983

McKusick V: Mendelian Inheritance in Man, 6th Edition. Baltimore, MD, Johns Hopkins University Press, 1983

Marsden CD, Jenner PG: The significance of 1-methyl-4-phenyl-1,2,3,6-tetrahydropyridine. Ciba Found Symp 126:239–256, 1987

Martin WE, Young WI, Anderson VE: Parkinson's disease—a genetic study. Brain 96:495–506, 1973

Marttila RJ, Rinne UK: Parkinson's disease and essential tremor in families of patients with early-onset Parkinson's disease. J Neurol Neurosurg Psychiatry 51:429–431, 1988

Marttila RJ, Kaprio J, Koskenvuo M, et al: Parkinson's disease in a nationwide twin cohort. Neurology 38:1217–1219, 1988

Matthysse S, Lange K, Wagener DK: Continuous variation caused by genes with graduated effects. Proc Natl Acad Sci U S A 76:2862, 1979

Matthysse S, Holzman PS, Lange K: The genetic transmission of schizophrenia: application of Mendelian latent structure analysis to eye-tracking dysfunctions in schizophrenia and affective disorders. J Psychiatr Res 20:57–65, 1986

Mendlewicz J, Rainer JD: Adoption study supporting genetic transmission in manic-depressive illness. Nature 268:327–329, 1977

Mendlewicz J, Simon P, Sevy S, et al: Polymorphic DNA marker on X chromosome and manic depression. Lancet 1:1230–1232, 1987

Misra VP, Baraitser M, Harding AE: Genetic prediction in Huntington's disease: what are the limitations imposed by pedigree structure? Mov Disord 3:233–236, 1988

Mohs RC, Breitner JCS, Silverman JM, et al: Alzheimer's disease: morbid risk in relatives approximates 50% by age 90. Arch Gen Psychiatry 44:405–408, 1987

Moises HW, Gelernter J, Giuffra LA, et al: No linkage between D_2 dopamine receptor gene region and schizophrenia. Arch Gen Psychiatry 48:643–647, 1991

Montplaisir J, Poirier G: Narcolepsy in monozygotic twins. Neurology 37:1089, 1987

Morton NE, Mi MP: Multiplex families with two or more probands. Am J Hum Genet 20:361–367, 1968

Nakamura Y, Leppert M, O'Connell P, et al: Variable number of tandem repeat (VNTR) markers for human gene mapping. Science 235:1616–1622, 1987

Nee LE, Eldridge R, Sunderland T, et al: Dementia of the Alzheimer type: clinical and family study of 22 twin pairs. Neurology 37:359–363, 1987

Neely S, Rosenberg R, Spire JP, et al: HLA antigens in narcolepsy. Neurology 37:1858–60, 1987

Ngim CH, Devathasan G: Epidemiologic study on the association between body burden mercury level and idiopathic Parkinson's disease. Neuroepidemiol 8:1281–141, 1989

Nuechterlein K: Signal detection in vigilance tasks and behavioral attributes among offspring of schizophrenic mothers and among hyperactive children. J Abnorm Psychol 92:4–28, 1983

Nuechterlein KH, Dawson ME: Information processing and attentional functioning in the developmental course of schizophrenic disorders. Schizophr Bull 10:160–203, 1984

Odegaard O: The multifactorial theory of inheritance in predisposition to schizophrenia, in Genetic Factors in Schizophrenia. Edited by Kaplan AR. Springfield, IL, Charles C Thomas, 1972, pp 256–275

Parkes JD, Langdon N, Lock C: Narcolepsy and immunity. BMJ 292:359–360, 1986

Passouant P, Billiard M: The evolution of narcolepsy with age, in Narcolepsy. Edited by Guilleminault C, Dement WC, Passouant P. New York, Spectrum, 1976, pp 179–196

Pericak-Vance MA, Bebout JL, Haynes CA, et al: Linkage studies in familial Alzheimer's disease: evidence for chromosome 19 linkage. Am J Hum Genet 47 (suppl): A194, 1990

Quinn N, Critchley P, Marsden CD: Young onset Parkinson's disease. Mov Disord 2(2):73–91, 1987

Reich T, Cloninger CR, Guze S: The multifactorial model of disease transmission, I: description of the model and its use in psychiatry. Br J Psychiatry 127:1–10, 1975

Reik W: Genomic imprinting: a possible mechanism for the parental origin effect in Huntington's chorea. J Med Genet 25:805–808, 1988

Rich DP, Anderson MP, Gregory RJ, et al: Expression of cystic fibrosis transmembrane conductance regulator corrects defective chloride channel regulation in cystic fibrosis airway epithelial cells. Nature 347:358–363, 1990

Ridley RM, Frith CD, Crow TJ, et al: Anticipation in Huntington's disease is inherited through the male line but may originate in the female. J Med Genet 25:589–595, 1988

Rieder RO, Kaufmann CA: Genetics, in American Psychiatric Press Textbook of Psychiatry. Edited by Talbott JA, Hales RE, Yudofsky SC. Washington, DC, American Psychiatric Press, 1988, pp 33–65

Risch N: Linkage strategies for genetically complex traits, I: multilocus models. Am J Hum Genet 46:222–228, 1990a

Risch N: Genetic linkage and complex diseases, with special reference to psychiatric disorders. Genet Epidemiol 7:3–16, 1990b

Risch N, Baron M, Mendlewicz J: Assessing the role of X-linked inheritance in bipolar-related major affective disorder. J Psychiatr Res 20:275–288, 1986

Rosenthal D: Genetic Theory and Abnormal Behavior. New York, McGraw-Hill, 1970

Rosenthal D, Wender PH, Kety SS, et al: Schizophrenics' offspring reared in adoptive homes. J Psychiatr Res 6:377–391, 1968

Rudin E: Zur Vererbung und Neuenstehung der Dementia Praecox. Berlin, Springer Verlag, 1916

Schellenberg GD, Deeb SS, Boehnke ML, et al.: Association of apolipoprotein CII allele with familial dementia of the Alzheimer type. Neurogenetics 4:97–108, 1987

Schellenberg GD, Bird TD, Wijisman EM, et al: The genetics of Alzheimer's disease. Biomed Pharmacother 43:463–468, 1989

Schoenberg BS: Descriptive epidemiology of Parkinson's disease: disease distribution and hypothesis formulation. Adv Neurol 45:277–283, 1987

Seltzer B, Sherwin I: A comparison of clinical features in early and late onset primary degenerative dementia: one entity or two? Arch Neurol 40:143–146, 1983

Sherrington R, Brynjolfsson J, Petursson H, et al: Localization of a susceptibility locus for schizophrenia on chromosome 5. Nature 336:164–167, 1988

Siegel C, Waldo M, Minzner G, et al: Deficits in sensory gating in schizophrenic patients and their relatives: evidence obtained with auditory-evoked responses. Arch Gen Psychiatry 41:607–612, 1984

Slater E, Cowie V: The Genetics of Mental Disorders. London, Oxford University Press, 1971

Snell RG, Lazarou LP, Youngman S, et al: Linkage disequilibrium in Huntington's disease: an improved localisation for the gene. J Med Genet 26:673–675, 1989

Spitzer RL, Endicott J, Robins E: Research Diagnostic Criteria: rational and reliability. Arch Gen Psychiatry 35:773–782, 1978

Sroka H, Elizan TS, Yahr MD, et al: Organic mental syndrome and confusional states in Parkinson's disease. Relationship to computerised tomographic signs of cerebral atrophy. Arch Neurol 38:339–342, 1981

St Clair D, Blackwood D, Muir W, et al: A balanced autosomal translocation associated in a single large pedigree with multiple cases of major mental illness including schizophrenia and schizoaffective disorder. Lancet 336:13–16, 1990

St George-Hyslop PH, Tanzi RE, Polinsky RJ, et al: The genetic defect causing familial Alzheimer's disease maps on chromosome 21. Science 235:885–890, 1987

St George-Hyslop PH, Myers R, Haines JL, et al: Familial Alzheimer's disease: progress and problems. Neurobiol Aging 10:417–25, 1989

Stewart J, Debray Q, Caillard V: Schizophrenia: the testing of genetic models. Am J Hum Genet 32:55–63, 1980

Strober M, Morrell W, Burroughs J, et al: A family study of bipolar I disorder in adolescence: early onset of symptoms linked to increased family loading and lithium resistance. J Affective Disord 15:255–268, 1988

Tanner CM: The role of environmental toxins in the etiology of Parkinson's disease. Trends Neurosci 12(2):49–54, 1989

Tanzi RE, St George-Hyslop PH, Haines JL, et al: The genetic defect in familial Alzheimer's disease is not tightly linked to the amyloid beta-protein gene. Nature 329:156–157, 1987

Thompson LM, Plummer S, Altherr M, et al: Isolation and characterization of cDNA clones representing transcripts from the region /f 4p16.3 containing the Huntington's disease gene. Am J Hum Genet 47 (suppl):A118, 1990

Tienari P, Lahti I, Naarald M: Biological mothers in the Finnish adoption study: alternative definitions of schizophrenia. Paper presented at the VIIth World Congress of Psychiatry, Vienna, Austria, June 1983

Tsuang MT, Faraone SV: The Genetics of Mood Disorders. Baltimore, MD, Johns Hopkins University Press, 1990

Tsuang MT, Bucher KD, Fleming JA: Testing the monogenic theory of schizophrenia: an application of segregation analysis to blind family study data. Br J Psychiatry 140:595–599, 1982

Tsuang MT, Faraone SV, Fleming JA: Familial transmission of major affective disorders: is there evidence supporting the distinction between unipolar and bipolar disorders? Br J Psychiatry 146:268–271, 1985

Turner WD: Genetic markers for schizotaxia. Biol Psychiatry 14:177–205, 1979

Uryu N, Maeda M, Nagata Y, et al: No difference in the nucleotide sequence of the DQB B1 domain between narcoleptic and healthy individuals with DR2, DW2. Hum Immunol 24:175–181, 1989

Walker E: Attentional and neuromotor functions of schizophrenics, schizoaffectives, and patients with other affective disorders. Arch Gen Psychiatry 38:1355–1358, 1981

Ward CD, Duvoisin RC, Ince SE, et al: Parkinson's disease in 65 pairs of twins and in a set of quadruplets. Neurology 33:815–824, 1983

Watt NF, Anthony EJ, Wynne LC, et al: Children at Risk for Schizophrenia: A Longitudinal Perspective. Cambridge, Cambridge University Press, 1984

Weber JL, May PE: Abundant class of human DNA polymorphisms which can be typed using the polymerase chain reaction. Am J Hum Genet 44:388–396, 1989

Wechsler D: WISC-R Manual: Wechsler Intelligence Scale for Children-Revised. New York, Psychological Corporation, 1974

Weinberger DR: Implications of normal brain development for the pathogenesis of schizophrenia. Arch Gen Psychiatry 44:660–669, 1987

Weissman MM, Leaf PJ, Tischler GL, et al: Affective disorders in five United States communities. Psychol Med 18:141–153, 1988

Wender PH, Rosenthal D, Kety SS, et al: Cross-fostering: a research strategy for clarifying the role of genetic and experiential factors in the etiology of schizophrenia. Arch Gen Psychiatry 30:121–128, 1974

Wender PH, Kety SS, Rosenthal D, et al: Psychiatric disorders in the biological and adoptive families of adopted individuals with affective disorders. Arch Gen Psychiatry 43:923–929, 1986

Whitehouse PJ, Price DL, Clark JT, et al: Alzheimer's disease: evidence for selective loss of cholinergic neurons in the nucleus basalis. Ann Neurol 10:122–126, 1981

Wing JK, Cooper JE, Sartorius N: The Measurement and Classification of Psychiatric Symptoms. New York, Cambridge University Press, 1974

Winokur G, Clayton PJ, Reich T: Manic Depressive Illness. St. Louis, MO, CV Mosby, 1969

Wolff G, Deuschl G, Wienker TF, et al: New mutation to Huntington's disease. J Med Genet 26:18–27, 1989

Yamamura Y, Sobue I, Ando K, et al: Paralysis agitans of early onset with marked diurnal fluctuation of symptoms. Neurology 23:239–244, 1973

Yokochi M, Narabayashi H, Iizuka R: Juvenile parkinsonism—some clinical, pharmacological and neuropathological aspects. Adv Neurol 40:407–413, 1984

Yoss RE, Daly DD: Criteria for the diagnosis of the narcoleptic syndrome. Proceedings of the Staff Meeting of the Mayo Clinic 32:320–328, 1957

Youngman S, Sarfarazi M, Bucan M, et al: A new DNA marker (D4S90) is located terminally on the short arm of chromosome 4, close to the Huntington's disease gene. Genomics 5:802–809, 1989

Zerbin-Rudin E: Endogene Psychosen, in Humangenetik: Ein Kurzes Handbuch. Edited by Becker PE. Stuttgart, Georg Thieme Verlag KG, 1967, pp 446–513

Section III

Neuropsychiatric Symptomatologies

Chapter 9

Differential Diagnosis in Neuropsychiatry

Richard L. Strub, M.D.
Michael G. Wise, M.D.

When the brain is damaged or rendered dysfunctional by chemical imbalances, behavior is often modified. Such organically based behavioral changes constitute the foundation of neuropsychiatry (Cummings 1985). Recognizing and understanding these characteristic symptoms, symptom clusters, and syndromes are the essence of the diagnostic process in neuropsychiatry (Benson and Blumer 1982; Frederiks et al. 1985; Heilman and Valenstein 1985). Moreover, patients with different neuropsychiatric disorders require very different plans of management. The patient with simple dementia can be evaluated as an outpatient, the patient with a delirium must be admitted to the hospital, and the patient with a restricted behavioral syndrome (e.g., an aphasia or parietal lobe syndrome caused by a focal brain lesion) should be seen by a neurologist or neurosurgeon.

The diagnostic process itself is no different from that in any other medical specialty. Historical information and examination findings are matched with known syndromes in an effort to establish a clinical diagnosis. In neuropsychiatry, the collection of data must be oriented toward organic disease, and the clinical examination must include an expanded mental status examination that encompasses a comprehensive evaluation of various cognitive functions and common organic behavior signs (Folstein et al. 1975; Strub and Black 1993). The diagnostic process involves, first, the recognition of the patient's symptoms as organic in origin, and second, the understanding that the specific symptoms and symptom clusters are characteristic of a particular clinical syndrome or cerebral localization (Kertesz 1983; Strub and Black 1988).

Although a neuropsychiatrist is usually concerned with a recent change in behavior secondary to a new brain disease or disorder, some neuropsychiatric disorders are the remnants of developmental disorders. For example, the patient with mild mental retardation, dyslexia, or mild autism may have compensated adequately for the disorder until challenged by sufficient stress or a specific demand later in life. At such a point, the congenitally weak neurobiological systems may fail to adjust to the new set of demands, and clinically significant symptoms can be produced. The true nature of the patient's new behavioral problem is not fully understood until the developmental

We wish to thank Mary Usner for her secretarial assistance in preparing this manuscript.

189

history is known and the interaction of the congenital problem with the new challenge is untangled.

Differential diagnosis has three levels of specificity in neuropsychiatry (Figure 9–1). The first is the age-old differential between an organic and a nonorganic mental syndrome. The second is the differential among the various organic mental syndromes, and the third and final step is the establishment of a specific diagnosis or identification of a specific organic mental disorder. This final step involves ordering and interpreting appropriate medical, neurodiagnostic, and psychological tests.

Most psychiatrists have greater skill and are more comfortable in analyzing verbal, affective, and interpersonal and interactive data than they are with testing cognitive symptoms. For this reason, we discuss these symptoms at length and include several diagnostic algorithms in this chapter to assist in the organization of the differential diagnostic process.

TYPES AND SPEED OF BEHAVIORAL CHANGE

The rapidity of the onset of behavioral change is a very important element in the differential diagnosis in neuropsychiatry. Behavioral changes can occur acutely as in stroke, subacutely as in delirium, or chronically as in dementia. In each of these clinical situations there is a logical decision-making process that will lead the ex-

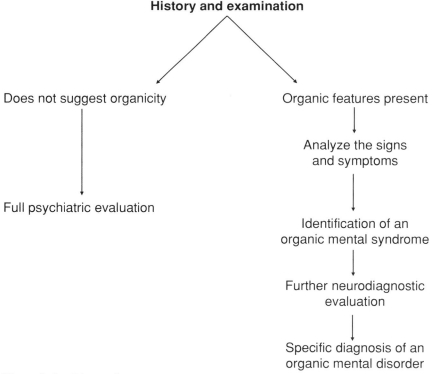

Figure 9–1. Diagnostic process.

aminer to the correct diagnosis. The decision tree in Figure 9–2 has been developed for evaluating a patient with chronic behavioral change.

The types of behavioral changes in neuropsychiatry have been separated into two general categories: cognitive and noncognitive. Evaluating patients who have developed changes in noncognitive spheres is often more difficult than evaluating patients who have changes in cognitive function. Noncognitive change is usually subjective and is often primarily psychiatric and not neuropsychiatric. Certain features help the clinician to identify patients who have noncognitive changes secondary to organic disease (such as brain pathology), medical illness, or medications. The first is knowledge of the epidemiology of common psychiatric disorders. The second is a careful

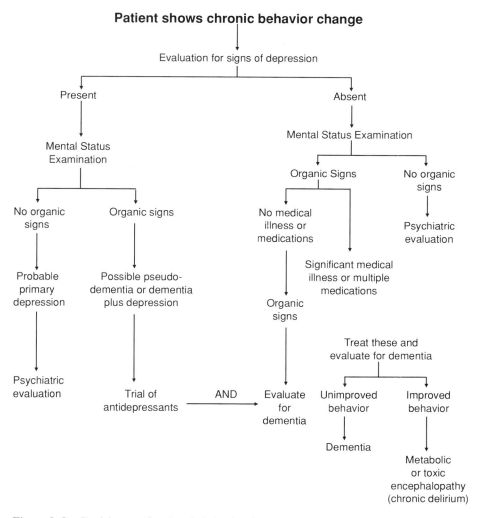

Figure 9–2. Decision tree for chronic behavior change.
Source. Reprinted from Weisberg LA, Strub RL, Garcia CA: *Decision Making in Adult Neurology.* Toronto, Ontario, Decker, 1987, pp. 70–71. Used with permission.

history. The examiner must have a complete medical history and know all medications that the patient is taking. Third, a careful mental status examination and neurological examination are essential.

SPECIFIC SYMPTOMS AND THEIR GENERAL SIGNIFICANCE IN NEUROPSYCHIATRY

Because most individual symptoms can be produced by a variety of causes and can be seen in different neuropsychiatric conditions (Tables 9–1 and 9–2), one can generate an enormous differential diagnosis for each specific symptom. In this section we discuss these major neuropsychiatric symptoms and allude to their most common causes.

Cognitive

Cognitive symptoms include those pertaining to consciousness, attention, speech and language, memory, and orientation in space.

Altered level of consciousness. Psychiatric consultation is often sought by members of the medical and surgical services for patients who have experienced "a recent change in mental status." In most instances this means the patient is either lethargic or agitated and disruptive. In addition to the change in the level of consciousness, such

Table 9–1.   Medications that cause behavioral change

Analgesics	**Anti-inflammatory drugs**	**Sedative-hypnotics**
Meperidine	Adrenocorticotropic	Barbiturates
Opiates	hormone (ACTH)	Benzodiazepines
Pentazocine	Corticosteroids	Glutethimide
Anticholinergic drugs	**Antiparkinsonian drugs**	**Sympathomimetics**
Antihistamines	Amantadine	Aminophylline
Antiparkinsonian drugs	Bromocriptine	Amphetamines
Benztropine	Carbidopa	Cocaine
Biperiden	Levodopa	Ephedrine
Antispasmodics	**Cardiac drugs**	Phenylephrine
Atropine/homatropine	Captopril	Phenylpropanolamine
Belladonna alkaloids	Clonidine	Theophylline
Chlorpheniramine	Digitalis	**Miscellaneous drugs**
Diphenhydramine	Disopyramide	Alcohol
Phenothiazines	Lidocaine	Cimetidine
(especially thioridazine)	Mexiletine	Hallucinogens
Promethazine	Methyldopa	Metoclopramide
Scopolamine	Propranolol	Metrizamide
Tricyclic antidepressants	Reserpine	Yohimbine
(especially amitriptyline)	**Drug withdrawal**	
Trihexyphenidyl	Alcohol	
Anticonvulsant drugs	Barbiturates	
Phenobarbital	Benzodiazepines	

Note. Almost any medication that enters the central nervous system has the potential to induce cognitive or noncognitive change. The medications listed in this table do so more frequently.

patients often exhibit an alteration in thought content or what has been called the *content of consciousness.* This change in both level of alertness and content of consciousness produces the clouded consciousness that typifies the confusional behavior seen in delirium (Lipowski 1990). Presented with such a patient, the clinician must begin the diagnostic processes used in assessing a patient with a delirium or coma (Plum and Posner 1980).

Any patient who is difficult to arouse or will not remain alert without constant stimulation is likely to be physically ill. Other clinical situations, however, can mimic a medically significant decreased level of consciousness. For example, sleepiness, boredom, simple intoxication, or a primary sleep disorder will all produce lethargy at times. In addition, depressed patients with significant psychomotor retardation may be withdrawn and slow to respond; they are, however, rarely confused or lethargic in the sense used here.

Inattention. The capacity to direct and maintain one's attention while screening out extraneous and irrelevant stimuli is a very basic yet highly complex neuropsychological function. Inattention (the breakdown of selective attention) and distractibility are common and clinically very significant neuropsychiatric symptoms. In addition to its clinical importance, inattention can also complicate the entire evaluation process (Mesulam 1985; Pribram and McGuinness 1975). For example, an inattentive patient will frequently fail tests of memory or calculation on the basis of inattention alone.

Inattention is probably the least specific of any symptom in neuropsychiatry. This symptom is seen in conditions as diverse as simple anxiety or fatigue, delirium, dementia, schizophrenia, mania, and focal brain lesions, particularly those localized in the inferior frontal or parietal lobes. In addition to these forms of global inattention, some patients are inattentive to only half of their body and the extrapersonal space on the same side. This syndrome, called *hemiattention* or *hemineglect,* is most frequently

Table 9–2. Clinical conditions that may produce behavior change

Neurological disease	
Infections	Degenerative
Encephalitis	Alzheimer's disease
Meningitis	Pick's disease
Brain abscess	Huntington's disease
Acquired immunodeficiency syndrome (AIDS)	Demyelinating—multiple sclerosis
Syphilis	**Medical illness**
Creutzfeldt-Jakob disease	Infectious—sepsis
Vascular	Toxins
Cerebral vascular accident	Alcohol and illicit drugs
Multi-infarct dementia	Organic compounds
Large arteriovenous malformations	Metallic poisons
Tumors	Metabolic disease
Trauma	Thyroid
Subdural hematoma	Parathyroid
Intracerebral hemorrhage	Pituitary
Frontal and temporal contusions	Adrenal
General closed head injury	Immune disorders
Hydrocephalus	Systemic lupus erythematosus
	AIDS
	Cancer—indirect effects

manifested as a left hemiattention in a patient who has suffered a right-hemisphere brain lesion (Weinstein and Friedland 1977).

Speech and language disorders.   Because verbal language is the primary means of communication between people, any departure from the patient's accustomed manner of verbal interchange is readily recognized. There are many ways in which verbal communication can change, and each has its own clinical significance neuropsychiatrically. For example, certain patients can have a pure speech disorder (such as stuttering, in which basic language function is normal), whereas others demonstrate a primary language disorder (such as aphasia) (Holland 1984). In a third type of patient, basic speech and language are intact but changes in timbre, pitch, and speed of delivery may reflect an underlying affective disorder (Table 9–3).

Changes in the affective tone and speed of speech production have always been important symptoms. Organic lesions, however, can produce similar changes. For example, decreased melodic quality of speech can occur in patients with a right-hemisphere lesion, particularly a lesion that involves the temporal and parietal lobes. A right temporal lesion can cause patients to produce speech with a flat, almost monotonic or aprosodic character (Young 1983). As part of their overall apathy and psychomotor retardation, patients with frontal lobe lesions can also demonstrate a speech delivery that is very flat.

Dysarthria refers to any alteration in speech production caused by a lesion or disease process that interferes with the muscles of articulation. Dysarthria can occur secondarily in disease of the vocal apparatus, in certain neurological disorders, or in a metabolic or toxic condition such as alcohol intoxication. Neurological conditions that can produce dysarthria include parkinsonism, amyotrophic lateral sclerosis, multiple strokes, myasthenia gravis, and oculopharyngeal dystrophy. Articulatory disturbances frequently signal significant neurological or otolaryngological disease.

Stuttering (dysfluency) is usually a developmental disorder of childhood, but it appears de novo in adulthood. When stuttering does present in an adult, it is often due to a new brain lesion, such as a stroke. Mutism can be seen in both classic neurological disease such as stroke (akinetic mutism) (Segarra and Angelo 1970) or basal ganglion disease (parkinsonism), as well as in emotional disorders such as depression or psychosis. Language disorders in general are discussed extensively in Chapter 12. However, it is important to emphasize that the appearance of an aphasia (a disorder of comprehension, word choice, or syntax) (Albert et al. 1981; Goodglass and Kaplan 1983), alexia (acquired reading disorder), or agraphia (acquired writing disorder) usually indicates acquired brain damage or dysfunction involving the patient's language dominant hemisphere. Aphasia, alexia, and agraphia are virtually always organic symptoms that should lead the examiner to search for a specific neurological cause.

Table 9–3   Common speech and language disorders

Change in affective tone	Language disorders
Speech disorders	Aphasia
Dysarthria	Alexia
Stuttering (dysfluency)	Agraphia
Mutism	Schizophrenic language
Aprosodia	Confusional or incoherent language

Memory loss. Memory loss can be difficult to assess because it has many different causes. Because of the complexity of the differential diagnosis of memory loss, its evaluation serves as an excellent example of the diagnostic process used by the skilled neuropsychiatrist. The algorithm in Figure 9–3 demonstrates the most frequently encountered types of memory loss and the line of investigation that should be followed to arrive at a correct diagnosis. It is important to remember that memory loss can be symptomatic of either a psychogenic or an organic condition.

The assessment of memory loss is one of the most important clinical skills that the neuropsychiatrist must acquire. Haphazard testing can lead to erroneous findings. For example, a patient may be given an improper diagnosis of dementia when the memory problem may actually be due to anxiety or depression. This is especially true in the elderly patient. A diagnosis is only as good as the data used to make it (Strub and Black 1993; Squire and Butters 1984; Victor et al. 1989).

Disorientation in space. There are varied neuropsychological mechanisms by which this single cognitive function, spatial orientation, can be impaired. For example, a man who loses his car in a large parking lot may be perfectly "normal" but was merely preoccupied at the time he parked and failed to note the location. In others, the symptom is not so innocent, such as a woman with mild delirium who, from her clouded consciousness and its attendant muddled thinking, may be disoriented in all spheres and lose her car as a symptom of her disorder. In like fashion, patients with dementia or amnesia may not be able to remember because of their recent memory or new learning deficit.

A completely different type of spatial disorientation occurs in patients with parietal lobe damage (DeRenzi 1985). Such patients have a true geographic disorientation and fail to find their car because of visual spatial disorientation. They have visual perception deficits as well as problems integrating visual perception with the location of objects in extrapersonal space. This true spatial disorientation is more common among patients with a lesion in the right parietal lobe but can occur with lesions in other areas of the brain. An additional type of spatial disorientation is seen in patients with hemineglect or hemiattention. These patients usually have right parietal lesions and fail to pay attention to the left side of their environment.

Noncognitive

Affect and mood. Affect is the description of an individual's emotional state at a particular point in time, such as depressed, euphoric, or angry; whereas mood describes an individual's pervasive, sustained emotional state over an extended span of time, such as a week or month. Alteration in mood can occur as a reaction or adjustment to a stressful situation; this is usually classified as an adjustment disorder. Mood alteration can also occur as a result of organic factors. When organic factors such as medications, medical disorders, or neurological disease cause a change in mood, the disorder is classified as an organic mood disorder (according to DSM-III-R criteria [American Psychiatric Association 1987]), or secondary mood disorder. In a study of 755 hospitalized patients seen in psychiatric consultation (Rundell and Wise 1989), 87% of manic patients and 38% of depressed patients warranted a diagnosis of organic mood disorder.

Patient with memory loss

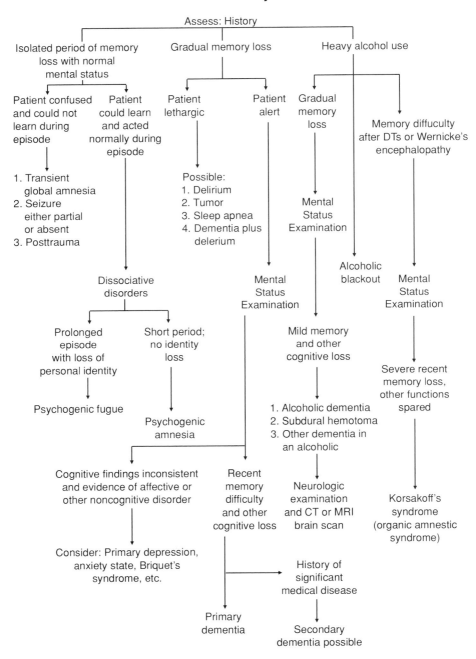

Figure 9–3.   Decision tree for memory loss. DT = delirium tremens; CT = computed tomography; MRI = magnetic resonance imaging.
Source.   Reprinted from Weisberg LA, Strub RL, Garcia CA: *Decision Making in Adult Neurology.* Toronto, Ontario, Decker, 1987, pp. 72–74. Used with permission.

Medical illness, medications, and neurological disease can cause clinical depression and mania (Goodwin and Jamison 1990). For example, patients who have had strokes are at high risk for depression and may also experience mania. Failure to recognize and treat poststroke depression can impact long-term recovery (Parikh et al. 1990). Medical illnesses, such as thyroid disease, can markedly affect mood. A patient with hyperthyroidism may become manic or depressed. Many medications are also implicated as causes for depression, and numerous medications are known to cause mania (Krauthammer and Klerman 1978). The classic examples of medications that cause depression are reserpine and α-methyldopa (Benson et al. 1983). On the other hand, corticosteroids—particularly when given in high doses, such as after organ transplantation—not uncommonly cause mood elevation and may even cause a manic episode (Rundell and Wise 1989).

When a patient presents with a mood disorder, a methodical search for causal factors is important. The clinician must gather a thorough history to include prior mood episodes, medications (both over-the-counter and prescribed), drugs (including illicit drugs, alcohol, and caffeine), associated and past medical disorders, and family history of mood disorders. Complete physical, neurological, and mental status examinations, as well as laboratory investigation for abnormalities, are necessary.

Personality change.   Any central nervous system (CNS) traumatic injury or disease has the potential to cause a change in personality. Diagnostically, this is referred to as an *organic personality syndrome* or *secondary personality syndrome*. Typical injury or lesions associated with personality change are head trauma, partial complex seizures (temporal lobe seizures), CNS tumors, multiple sclerosis, dementia, and strokes. Mild cognitive impairment may or may not be present in secondary personality disorders; global cognitive deficits suggest a diagnosis of dementia (Dian et al. 1990).

Injury to particular regions of the frontal lobes as a result of head trauma or CNS pathology is sometimes associated with characterological change (Blumer and Benson 1975). Lesions in the orbital region of the frontal lobes can cause varying degrees of disinhibition in patients, from mild irritability to outright aggression. Such patients behave inappropriately and exhibit poor impulse control. Because of lack of motivation, such patients often appear depressed, but are not; thus the term *pseudodepression* has been used (Stuss and Benson 1986).

The clinician must rely heavily on past history to decide whether the observed behavior is a change from the patient's previous behavior. If the abnormal characterological behavior is new, then the patient is diagnosed as having an organic personality syndrome. History may reveal, however, that the individual has exhibited sociopathic behavior since age 9, long before the alleged injury, and that the current behavior merely typifies his life-long behavior pattern.

Anxiety.   Anxiety is a ubiquitous phenomenon that occurs in individuals as a normal part of living. When anxiety is excessive and unrealistic, it is often associated with autonomic nervous system and motoric overactivity; cognitive dysfunction, such as difficulties with attention and concentration; and feelings of dread, terror, panic, or apprehension. Such extreme forms of anxiety occur in primary and secondary anxiety disorders and occur concomitantly with other psychiatric disorders. For example, a patient with dementia may become extremely anxious when faced with a difficult task. The patient may abreact and have a "catastrophic reaction." This reaction does not represent an anxiety disorder, but occurs because of the patient's inability to cope with his or her cognitive dysfunction.

Anxiety caused by a specific organic factor is referred to as an *organic anxiety disorder* or *secondary anxiety disorder.* Secondary anxiety syndromes may be caused by medications, substance abuse (both ingestion and withdrawal), and medical or neurological illnesses (Wise and Taylor 1990). Certain medications (e.g, sympatho-mimetic agents, the theophyllines, and thyroid) are potentially anxiogenic. Substance abuse can cause anxiety syndromes in two ways. First, some drugs are anxiogenic when ingested in sufficient quantity. This is particularly true of caffeine and other stimulants, such as amphetamines. Second, anxiety typically accompanies withdrawal syndromes, particularly withdrawal from sedative-hypnotic–type drugs and alcohol (Rickels et al. 1990).

Medical and neurological disorders sometimes cause pathological anxiety. For example, anxiety may be caused by endocrine conditions (such as pheochromo-cytoma and thyroid dysfunction) and neurological disorders (such as subarachnoid hemorrhage, tumors in the vicinity of the third ventricle, and seizures) (Lishman 1987). Medically ill patients with an organic anxiety syndrome can often be differen-tiated from patients with primary psychiatric disorders or adjustment disorders by careful scrutiny of their histories (Geringer and Stern 1988).

Thought disorder.   Disordered thinking is reflected in speech, communications, or content of thought, such as thought derailment, ideas of reference, hallucinations, delusions, poverty of thoughts, loosening of associations, and perseveration (Stone 1988). A thought disorder can be seen in organic disorders such as delirium, dementia, and psychoactive substance use, or in primary thought disorders such as schizophre-nia, mania, and psychotic depression (Black et al. 1988). The division of thought disorders into a functional-versus-organic dichotomy is no longer realistic; therefore, the terms primary thought disorder (manic episode due to bipolar disorder) and sec-ondary thought disorder (manic episode due to steroids) are used.

Certain clinical characteristics in patients suggest a primary thought disorder. Such patients are usually younger, have no related medical illness, no clouding of consciousness, and no disorientation, but they do have a prior psychiatric history, predominantly auditory hallucinations, and ego-syntonic delusions and hallucina-tions. Patients with a secondary thought disorder usually have an older age at onset, associated medical illness(es) and medication(s), no prior psychiatric history, a fluc-tuating level of consciousness, disorientation, ego-dystonic hallucinations and delu-sions, hallucinations that predominantly involve sensory modalities other than hearing, and fleeting, poorly systemized delusional beliefs.

Hallucinations.   A hallucination occurs when the patient perceives a stimulus that does not exist. The hallucinatory perception can be visual, auditory, tactile, olfactory, gustatory, or kinesthetic. Although cultural variation must be taken into account, hal-lucinations that occur in an awake individual are almost always symptomatic of a pathological process. Auditory hallucinations are more typical of so-called functional patients with psychiatric disorders. The one notable exception is alcoholic hallucino-sis—vivid auditory hallucinations that occur in a fully oriented alcoholic patient. Hallucinations that involve other sensory modalities are more typically associated with organic disorders (Cummings 1985).

Auditory hallucinations, unlike visual ones, more typically occur in psychotic psychiatric disorders, such as schizophrenia, mania, or a psychotic depression. For example, auditory hallucinations are reported in 28%–72% of schizophrenic patients (Black et al. 1988). The quality and quantity of such hallucinations may help the clinician diagnostically. If patients report clearly audible voices that comment on their actions, argue, repeat thoughts, or are deprecatory, the disorder is likely psychiatric. If patients report hearing their name called or other brief, repetitive auditory hallucinations, this may represent an organic etiology, such as partial complex seizures, ear disease, or may be symptomatic of a number of psychiatric disorders, such as borderline personality disorder, somatization disorder, or multiple personality disorder.

Visual hallucinations are more typically associated with organic brain disease, although they can also occur in nonpsychiatric patients with severe recent visual loss and patients with primary psychiatric disorders. Visual hallucinations are associated with ingestion of hallucinogens, delirium, narcolepsy, epilepsy, migraine, brain stem lesions, optic nerve disease, postocular surgery, and vitreous detachment.

Visual hallucinations can also occur in healthy individuals during sensory or sleep deprivation, hypnosis, or sleep (dreams). Patients with schizophrenia, particularly chronic schizophrenia, frequently report visual hallucinations. Individuals who have an affective disorder such as a mania or depression episode will sometimes report visual hallucinations. Patients with other psychiatric disorders such as conversion disorder, somatization disorder, or borderline personality disorder occasionally report visual hallucinations.

Tactile hallucinations occur commonly in patients who have a limb amputation or are in drug withdrawal delirium. "Phantom limb" sensation, the feeling that the limb is still present, is reported by most amputees. Given time, the amputee's tactile hallucinations diminish and usually disappear (Frederiks 1969). Tactile hallucinations also occur in psychiatric disorders, such as schizophrenia, or organic disorders, such as delirium and complex partial seizures, or after ingestion of hallucinogens.

Olfactory (smell), gustatory (taste), or kinesthetic (body movement) hallucinations are rare and are most commonly experienced by patients with partial complex seizures (Lishman 1987); however, they are sometimes found in patients with psychiatric or other organic disorders. All three types of hallucinations can be found in patients with somatization disorder and are occasionally reported in patients with psychotic psychiatric disorders.

Aggression.   Anger captures the attention of individuals in the patient's environment faster than any other affective state. Actual aggression or alleged aggressive acts require a very thorough inquiry into past and present history. There is a natural tendency for observers to exaggerate such anxiety-provoking experiences, and a calm examination that elicits exact details is invaluable in the evaluation process. The evaluation of a patient who has committed a violent act usually reveals one of several scenarios:

1. The patient meets the diagnostic criteria for an antisocial personality disorder; that is, there exists a life-long history of sociopathic behavior and this violent act is one episode among many.

2. The patient commits the aggressive act under the influence of a disinhibiting psychoactive substance. When this occurs, psychoactive substance abuse or dependence must be suspected as a primary diagnosis.
3. The patient had normal impulse control until a CNS event such as head trauma, tumor, encephalitis, or dementia occurred, and the patient's personality changed.
4. The patient has significant psychosocial stressors and "reached the breaking point."
5. The patient has a primary or secondary thought disorder and misperceives the environment as threatening.

Aggression does not happen in a vacuum, and a combination of factors is often responsible for the final violent outburst. The clinician must be willing to take the time to sort through the past and recent history, as well as to perform a thorough evaluation. Psychological and neuropsychological testing may aid the clinician in determining the role of personality, cognitive function, and thought patterns in the patient's recent aggressive act.

Psychomotor activity.   Psychomotor activity refers to a patient's verbal and nonverbal behavior and includes reaction time, speed of movement, flow of speech, involuntary movements, and handwriting (Lipowski 1990). Psychomotor agitation refers to generalized overactivity, and psychomotor retardation refers to generalized slowing of physical and mental activity. Psychomotor agitation and retardation can occur in organic mental disorders such as delirium and dementia, after psychoactive substance use, and in other psychiatric disorders such as mood disorders. In catatonia, a profound form of psychomotor retardation, the patient may have a severe psychotic depression or encephalitis. The psychomotor behavior is indistinguishable; often only an electroencephalogram (EEG) can differentiate the patient who has the primary psychiatric disorder (normal EEG) from the patient with encephalitis (abnormal EEG) (Wise 1988).

Certain etiologies tend to give rise to either increased or decreased psychomotor activity. For example, patients who are withdrawing from alcohol or other depressant substances have psychomotor agitation, whereas patients who have a metabolic encephalopathy or an infarction in the territory of the right middle cerebral artery tend to have psychomotor retardation. Some patients with delirium will fluctuate between psychomotor agitation and psychomotor retardation, just as catatonic schizophrenic patients might fluctuate from catatonia to frantic activity (catatonic excitement). Patients with depression can display agitation or can have profound psychomotor retardation. Bipolar, manic patients have increased motor responses, rapid speech, and accelerated mental activity. Finally, complex partial seizures (psychomotor seizures) typically involve impairment in the level of consciousness and may involve automatisms (repetitive motor movements).

SYNDROME ANALYSIS

Once a decision is made that the patient has organic disease the next step in the differential diagnosis process is to determine whether the patient's symptoms and signs fit a pattern of one of the classic organic mental syndromes. Because many of the remaining chapters of this book discuss these syndromes in more detail, only a sketchy introduction to the diagnostic process involved is presented here.

Global Syndromes

The most common and well-recognized global syndrome is dementia: a syndrome of slowly progressive deterioration in cognitive function with associated alterations in mood and behavior (Cummings and Benson 1992). Dementia is a syndrome with many etiologies and many clinical variations. The most common type of dementia is Alzheimer's disease.

Dementia is also seen in patients with multiple strokes (multi-infarct dementia). Such patients typically have a stepwise deterioration in mental status with accompanying neurological signs and symptoms. In its classic form, multi-infarct dementia is relatively easy to diagnose, but there are multi-infarct patients with normal neurological history and examination results consistent with Alzheimer's disease. A large percentage of such patients (15%–20%) probably have a mixed dementia with Alzheimer's disease and strokes.

Some dementia patients present predominantly with frontal lobe signs such as Pick's disease, general paresis, Huntington's disease, and normal-pressure hydrocephalus. Other patients, such as those with progressive supranuclear palsy, Huntington's disease, or acquired immunodeficiency syndrome (AIDS), have symptoms that are primarily subcortical. In all of these cases, the basic history is similar: slowly progressive mental change.

Another common global syndrome frequently encountered in a general hospital setting is delirium. The most characteristic symptom cluster for this condition consists of history of short duration, fluctuating course with the examination demonstrating an altered level of consciousness, inattention, and pervasive defects in cognitive function. Patients with delirium tend to ramble and produce disorganized language without aphasia, to be slow in their thought processes, and, on specific testing, to show cognitive deficits in many areas (Lipowski 1990).

Focal Syndromes

Patients whose behavioral symptoms are secondary to a focal brain lesion are also neuropsychiatrically important. The brain has a certain degree of regional specialization for cognitive functions; these are discussed extensively in Chapter 3. Table 9–4 lists some of the common symptoms of focal lesions.

Whenever a patient's history and examination suggest a localized brain abnormality, a destructive neurological lesion such as tumor or stroke must be considered. The speed of onset of the deficit is critical in the differential diagnosis. A sudden focal deficit is usually due to a vascular event, although tumors can hemorrhage and give a similar clinical picture. Slowly progressive focal deficits suggest an expanding lesion such as a tumor.

CONCLUSIONS

The diagnostic process in neuropsychiatry is an orderly one in which the examiner combines data gained from history and examination and then matches it with

Table 9–4.   Common focal behavioral syndromes and their localization

Left hemisphere (language dominant)
   Language problems in almost all right-handed patients and a high percentage of
      left-handed patients (Holland 1984)
      Anterior (frontal) expressive language difficulty
      Posterior (parietal) comprehension both written and verbal
   Writing problems
   Constructional problems
   Calculation difficulties
   Right-left disorientation

Right hemisphere (nondominant)
   Constructional problems; frontal and parietal
   Geographic disorientation in the environment; frontal and parietal
   Dressing problem; parietal
   Right-left disorientation; parietal
   Loss of musical ability (primarily carrying melody); temporal
   Language problems in rare right-handed patients and many left-handed patients; all lobes

Frontal lobes (bilateral) (Stuss 1986)
   Impulse and character changes
   Mild memory disturbances

known neuropsychiatric syndromes. In order for this process to yield valid diagnoses the examiner must not only be skilled and comfortable with the aspects of mental status testing that identify these organically based behavioral changes, but also thoroughly familiar with the clinical syndromes. This chapter is intended to help the examiner make that difficult transition from data to diagnosis. The other chapters of this volume will acquaint the reader with the clinical syndromes encountered in a neuropsychiatric practice so that the examiner can successfully carry out the differential diagnostic process.

REFERENCES

Albert ML, Goodglass H, Helm NA, et al: Clinical Aspects of Dysphasia. Vienna, Springer-Verlag, 1981

American Psychiatric Association: Diagnostic and Statistical Manual of Mental Disorders, 3rd Edition, Revised. Washington, DC, American Psychiatric Association, 1987

Benson DF, Blumer D (eds): Psychiatric Aspects of Neurologic Disease, Vol 2. New York, Grune & Stratton, 1982

Benson D, Peterson LG, Bartay J: Neuropsychiatric manifestations of antihypertensive medications. Psychiatr Med 1:205–214, 1983

Black DW, Yates WR, Andreasen NC: Schizophrenia, schizophreniform disorder, and delusional (paranoid) disorders, in Textbook of Psychiatry. Edited by Talbott JA, Hales RE, Yudofsky SC. Washington, DC, American Psychiatric Press, 1988, pp 357–402

Blumer D, Benson DF: Personality changes with frontal and temporal lobe lesions, in Psychiatric Aspects of Neurologic Disease. Edited by Benson DF, Blumer D. New York, Grune & Stratton, 1975, pp 151–170

Cummings JL: Clinical Neuropsychiatry. New York, Grune & Stratton, 1985

Cummings JL, Benson DF: Dementia: A Clinical Approach, 2nd Edition. Woburn, MA, Butterworths, 1992

DeRenzi E: Disorders of spatial orientation, in Handbook of Clinical Neurology, Vol 1: Clinical Neuropsychology. Edited by Frederiks JAM. Amsterdam, Elsevier, 1985, pp 405–422

Dian L, Cummings JL, Petry S, et al: Personality alterations in multi-infarct dementia. Psychosomatics 31:415–419, 1990

Folstein MF, Folstein SE, McHugh PR: "Mini-Mental State": a practical method for grading the cognitive state of patients for the clinician. J Psychiatr Res 12:189–198, 1975

Frederiks JAM: Disorders of the body schema, in Handbook of Clinical Neurology, Vol 4. Edited by Vinken PJ, Bruyn GW. Amsterdam, North-Holland Publishing, 1969

Frederiks JAM, Vinken PJ, Bruyn GW, et al: Neurobehavioral disorders, in Handbook of Clinical Neurology, Vol 46. Edited by Vinken PJ, Bruyn GW, Klawans HL. Amsterdam, Elsevier, 1985

Geringer ES, Stern TA: Anxiety and depression in critically ill patients, in Problems in Critical Care. Edited by Wise MG. Philadelphia, PA, JB Lippincott, 1988, pp 35–44

Goodglass H, Kaplan E: The Assessment of Aphasia and Related Disorders, 2nd Edition. Philadelphia, PA, Lea & Febiger, 1983

Goodwin FK, Jamison KR: Manic-Depressive Illness. New York, Oxford University Press, New York, 1990

Heilman KM, Valenstein E (eds): Clinical Neuropsychology, 2nd Edition. New York, Oxford University Press, 1985

Holland A (ed): Language Disorders in Adults. San Diego, CA, College Hill Press, 1984

Kertesz A: Localization in Neuropsychology. New York, Academic Press, 1983

Krauthammer C, Klerman GL: Secondary mania. Arch Gen Psychiatry 35:1333–1339, 1978

Lipowski ZJ: Delirium: Acute Confusional States. New York, Oxford University Press, 1990

Lishman A: Organic Psychiatry, 2nd Edition. Oxford, England, Blackwell Scientific, 1987

Mesulam M-M: Attention, confusional states, and neglect, in Principles of Behavioral Neurology. Edited by Mesulam M-M. Philadelphia, PA, FA Davis, 1985, pp 125–140

Parikh RM, Robinson RG, Lipsey JR, et al: The impact of post-stroke depression on recovery in activities of daily living over a 2-year follow-up. Arch Neurol 47:785–789, 1990

Plum F, Posner G: The Diagnosis of Stupor and Coma, 3rd Edition. Philadelphia, PA, FA Davis, 1980

Pribram KH, McGuinness P: Arousal, activation and effort in the control of attention. Psychol Rev 82:116–149, 1975

Rickels K, Schweizer E, Case G, et al: Long-term therapeutic use of benzodiazepines, I: effects of abrupt discontinuation. Arch Gen Psychiatry 47:899–907, 1990

Rundell JR, Wise MG: Causes of organic mood disorder. Journal of Neuropsychiatry and Clinical Neurosciences 1:398–400, 1989

Segarra JM, Angelo JN: Anatomic Determinants of Behavior Change, in Behavior Change in Cerebrovascular Disease. Edited by Benton AL. New York, Harper & Row, 1970, pp 3–26

Squire LR, Butters N (eds): Neuropsychology of Memory. New York, Guilford, 1984

Stone E (ed): American Psychiatric Glossary, 6th Edition. Washington, DC, American Psychiatric Press, 1988, p 104

Strub RL, Black FW: Neurobehavioral Disorders: A Clinical Approach. Philadelphia, PA, FA Davis, 1988

Strub RL, Black FW: The Mental Status Examination in Neurology, 3rd Edition. Philadelphia, PA, FA Davis, 1993

Stuss DT, Benson DF: The Frontal Lobes. New York, Raven, 1986

Victor M, Adams RD, Collins GH: The Wernicke-Korsakoff Syndrome and Related Neurologic Disorders Due to Alcoholism and Malnutrition, 2nd Edition. Philadelphia, PA, FA Davis, 1989

Weinstein EA, Friedland RP (eds): Hemi-Inattention and Hemispheric Specialization (Advances in Neurology Series, Vol 18). New York, Raven, 1977

Weisberg LA, Strub RL, Garcia CA: Decision Making in Adult Neurology. Toronto, Ontario, Decker, 1987, pp 70–71

Wise MG, Taylor SE: Anxiety and mood disorders in medically ill patients. J Clin Psychiatry 51 (suppl):27–32, 1990

Wise MG, Brannan SK, Shanfield SB, et al: Psychiatry aspects of organ transplantation (letter). JAMA 260:3437, 1988

Young AW (ed): Functions of the Right Cerebral Hemisphere. London, Academic Press, 1983

Chapter 10

Neuropsychiatric Aspects of Pain Management

William G. Brose, M.D.
David Spiegel, M.D.

Approximately one-third of all Americans are estimated to suffer with some form of chronic pain. Back pain, arthritis, headaches, and musculoskeletal disorders, as well as pain due to neurological, cardiac, or oncologic disease combined to affect an estimated 97 million people in 1986 (Bonica 1990). Cancer pain affects approximately one-third of cancer patients with primary disease and two-thirds of those with metastatic disease.

Pain perception is influenced by state of consciousness. For example, chronic pain tends to be greater during evenings and weekends when people are not distracted by routine activities. It is usually, of course, reduced in sleep but may in fact interfere with sleep; more severe kinds of pain can substantially reduce sleep efficiency. Many of the more potent drugs that treat pain reduce alertness and arousal, an often unwanted side effect or one that can lead to abuse of analgesic medications.

Pain is the ultimate psychosomatic phenomenon. It is composed of both a somatic signal that something is wrong with the body and a message or interpretation of that signal involving attentional, cognitive, affective, and social factors. The limbic system and cortex provide means of modulating pain signals (Melzack 1982), either amplifying them through excessive attention or affective dysregulation, or minimizing them through denial, inattention, relaxation, or attention control techniques.

COGNITIVE FACTORS INFLUENCING PAIN

Attention to Pain

Health perception is modulated by the cortex, which enhances or diminishes awareness of incoming signals. Recent neuropsychological and brain imaging research has demonstrated at least three attentional centers that modulate perception: a posterior parieto-occipital orienting system, a focusing system localized to the anterior cingulate gyrus, and an arousal-vigilance system in the right frontal lobe (Posner and Petersen 1990). These systems provide, among other things, for selective attention to incoming stimuli allowing competing stimuli to be relegated to the periphery of awareness.

When Melzack and Wall (1965) postulated the gate control theory of pain, they observed that higher cortical input could inhibit pain signals as well. This theory points to the interaction between central processing and perception of noxious stimuli at the periphery.

Meaning

It has been known for half a century that the meaning structure in which pain is embedded influences the intensity of pain. In his classic study, Beecher (1956) noted that soldiers on the Anzio beachhead, who were quite badly wounded, seemed to require very little in the way of analgesic medication. He found that of surgical patients at Massachusetts General Hospital with equal or less serious surgically induced wounds demanded far higher levels of analgesic medication than did the combat soldiers. Beecher concluded that this difference was based on a difference in the meaning of the pain. Patients who interpret pain signals as a sign of the worsening of their disease are likely to experience a greater intensity of pain. This hypothesis has been confirmed, for example, among cancer patients. Those who believe the pain represents a worsening of their disease show more pain (Spiegel and Bloom 1983).

Mood Disorders

Bond and Pearson (1969) reported a correlation between neuroticism on the Maudsley Personality Inventory (Eysenck and Eysenck 1964) and pain among patients who had cervical carcinoma. Other studies (Ahles et al. 1983; Massie and Holland 1987) have reported that patients with pain score higher on measures of depression, anxiety, and other signs of mood disturbance. In particular, depression and anxiety are noted as frequent concomitants of pain (Blumer and Heilbronn 1982; Bond 1973). This early work implied that patients with psychopathology complained more about pain. Later work suggested that there is an interaction and that perhaps chronic pain amplifies or produces depression (Spiegel and Sands 1988).

Depression is the most frequently reported psychiatric diagnosis among chronic pain patients. Reports of depression among chronic pain populations range from 10% to 87% (Dworkin et al. 1990; Pilowski et al. 1977; Reich et al. 1983). The relative severity of the depression observed in chronic pain patients is illustrated by the finding by Katon et al. (1985) that 32% of a sample of 37 pain patients met criteria for major depression and 43% had a past episode of major depression.

Anxiety is often a concomitant of acute pain. Like depression it may be an appropriate response to serious trauma through injury or illness. Pain may serve a signal function or be part of an anxious preoccupation as in the case of the woman with the sarcoma cited above. Similarly, anxiety and pain may reinforce one another, producing a snowball effect of escalating and mutually reinforcing central and peripheral symptoms.

NEUROLOGICAL MECHANISMS OF PAIN

Very complex interactions of many different peripheral and central nervous system structures, from the skin surface to the cerebral cortex, are now known to be involved in the processing of pain. Blockade of any of these pathways and/or antagonism of involved neurotransmitters may now be rationally considered to treat specific pain problems.

Peripheral Sensory Receptors

Each individual can appreciate that when a potentially damaging stimulus is applied to a sensitive area of the body such as the skin, a chain of signals is initiated that results in the identification of the stimulus as painful. Early descriptions of peripheral nerves indicated that they were modality specific and that each class of nerve fiber was responsible for only one sensory modality (Müller 1844). This concept was not supported by anatomical studies of skin surface, which demonstrated that each class of nerve ending is not present in all skin areas. More recent neurophysiological work has established the existence of specific primary afferent nerves for signaling noxious stimulation. These nerves are termed *nociceptors.*

Nociceptors are activated by some form of energy (mechanical, thermal, or chemical). They transduce that energy into an electrical impulse that is conducted through the nerve axon toward the brain. The reflex response and subjective report of pain associated with a noxious stimulus is the result of spinal cord, brain stem, midbrain, and higher cortical processing of signals from the numerous primary afferent nociceptors that were activated by the stimulus. Nociceptors are characterized by 1) high threshold to all naturally occurring stimuli compared with other receptors in the same tissue and 2) progressively augmenting response to repeated or increasingly noxious stimuli (sensitization).

Particular nociceptors respond only to particular types of stimuli. Although the exact pathways involved in the transduction of noxious information nociceptors has not yet been elucidated, it appears that the peripheral terminal of the Aδ mechanical nociceptor is likely to function as a receptor (Fields 1987). Whether this is true for other nociceptors remains the subject of speculation. The presence of vesicles in primary nociceptive afferent terminals has been determined by electron microscopy. These vesicles likely provide the substrate for various peripherally active agents.

Substance P (sP) is an undecapeptide found in small-diameter primary afferent neurons. This peptide is transmitted to the periphery by these nerves, and stimulation of these primary afferents leads to the release of sP from the distal terminus of the nerve. Other chemicals present in the blood and tissues have been demonstrated to be algesic. Serotonin, histamine, acetylcholine, bradykinin, slow-reacting substance of anaphylaxis (SRS-A), calcitonin-gene–related peptide (CGRP), and potassium all excite primary noxious afferents. At this time the definition of "pain" neuropeptide has not been specified. Prostaglandins alone do not excite pain fibers; however, they do appear to sensitize primary afferents to painful substances.

Direct tissue trauma results in potassium release, synthesis of bradykinin in plasma, and synthesis of prostaglandins in the region of damaged tissue (Figure 10–1; *panel A*). Antidromic impulses in primary nociceptor afferents result in an increase in sP from nerve endings. This is associated with increase in vascular permeability and, in turn, results in marked release of bradykinin. There is also an increase in histamine production from mast cells and an increase in serotonin production from platelets; both of these are capable of powerful activation of nociceptors (Figure 10–1; *panel*

B). Histamine release combines with sP release to increase vascular permeability. Local increases in histamine and serotonin, via activation of nociceptors, results in a further increase in sP so that a self-perpetuating cycle can be seen to develop at each region of the nociceptive afferent nerve fiber in the damaged tissue. In surrounding extracellular fluid, increases in histamine and serotonin result in activation of nearby nociceptors, and this is one reason for secondary hyperalgesia (Figure 10–1; *panel C*). Superimposed on all of these events are the effects of increased release of catecholamines from sympathetic nerve endings, which results in sensitization of nociceptors. Evidence from animal models of arthritis and various human data point to the sympathetic postganglionic neuron as being integral in the changes seen in vascular permeability in response to activation of primary afferent nociceptors (Levine et al. 1988).

Primary Afferent Transmission

After a noxious stimulus has been detected by a nociceptor, the resultant impulse travels away from the point of origin via the primary afferent nerve. The primary afferent nerves that carry pain impulses are almost exclusively unmyelinated C fibers and finely myelinated Aδ fibers. Most C fiber afferents originate from polymodal nociceptors that are activated by mechanical, chemical, and thermal noxious stimuli. The conduction velocity of these C fibers is approximately 1 meter per second (m/s), which likely explains the "slow pain" felt 1–2 seconds after the application of a noxious stimulus (Figure 10–2). The finely myelinated Aδ fibers also transmit pain impulses, but the conduction velocity of these neurons is much faster (12–30 m/s). Aδ fibers are particularly sensitive to stimulation with sharp instruments. In addition, 20%–50% of Aδ fibers respond to heat as well as mechanical stimulation. These fiber types carry the impulses that initially report a noxious stimulus. These primary afferent nociceptors make up the majority of fibers in any peripheral nerve.

Lesion of these peripheral nerves does not necessarily correlate with presence or absence of pain. The proposed pathways for injury of the peripheral nerves to evoke a pain response include

1. Increased activity in sympathetic fibers near the damaged area
2. Neuroma formation due to sprouting from damaged axons

Figure 10–1. *(at right)* Events leading to activation, sensitization, and spread of sensitization of primary afferent nociceptor terminals. *Panel A*: Direct activation by intense pressure and consequent cell damage. Cell damage leads to release of potassium (K^+) and to synthesis of prostaglandins (PG) and bradykinin (BK). PGs increase the sensitivity of the terminal to BK and other pain-producing substances. *Panel B*: Secondary activation. Impulses generated in the stimulated terminal propagate not only to the spinal cord, but into other terminal branches, where they induce the release of peptides, including substance P (sP), which causes vasodilation and neurogenic edema with further accumulation of BK. In addition, sP causes the release of histamine (H) from mast cells and serotonin (5-hydroxytryptamine [5-HT]) from platelets. *Panel C*: Histamine and 5-HT levels rise in the extracellular space, secondarily sensitizing nearby nociceptors. This leads to a gradual spread of hyperalgesia and/or tenderness.
Source. Reprinted from Fields HL: *Pain.* New York, McGraw-Hill, 1987, p. 36. Used with permission.

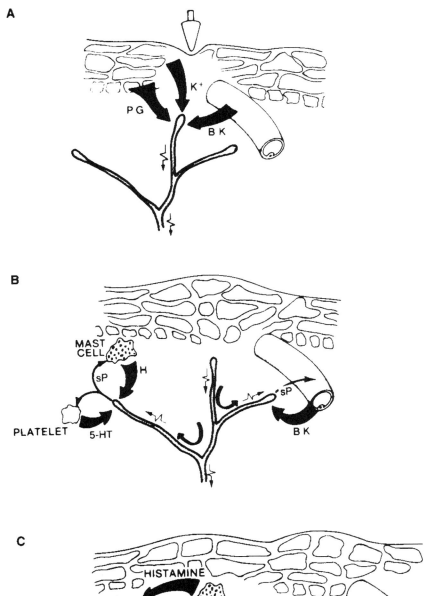

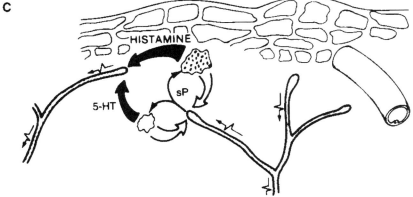

3. Collaterals sprouting from intact neighboring fibers
4. Changes in dorsal root ganglion cells or in central terminals of damaged axons that have lost part of their dorsal input
5. Stimulation of nociceptive nervi nervorum of peripheral nerves

Spinal Cord Terminals of Primary Afferents

Dorsal and ventral roots.   The cell bodies of all somatic primary afferent fibers are in the dorsal root ganglia adjacent to the spinal cord. The only primary afferent cell body outside this position is the trigeminal ganglia, which is the rostral continuation of the dorsal root ganglia. The majority of sensory afferents enter the spinal cord through the dorsal root entry zone. However, nonmyelinated C fiber afferents have also been discovered in the ventral root. The clinical relevance of the fibers that cross or those that enter the ventral root is not known. This heterogeneity in the pathway of the primary afferents associated with pain transmission helps explain the incomplete pain relief that is seen after ablation of a unilateral dorsal root entry zone.

Dorsal horn.   Once the impulses have entered the spinal cord via the dorsal or ventral roots, they terminate in the ipsilateral dorsal horn of the spinal cord. The dorsal

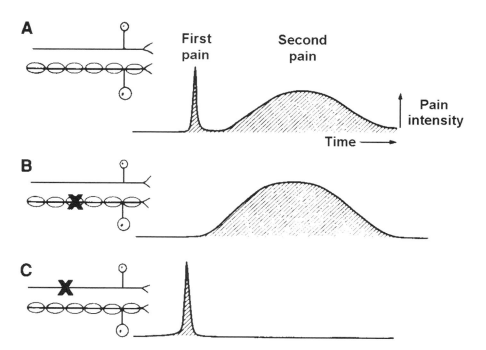

Figure 10–2.   First and second pain are carried by two different primary afferent axons (*panel A*). First pain is abolished by selective blockade of myelinated axons (*panel B*) and second pain by blocking C fibers (*panel C*).
Source.   Reprinted from Fields HL: *Pain.* New York, McGraw-Hill, 1987, p. 26. Used with permission.

horn is organized into distinct laminae, with specific primary afferent terminals in individual laminae. Aδ fibers terminate primarily in lamina I, in ventral portions in lamina II, and through most of lamina III. Unmyelinated C fibers terminate in lamina II.

Lamina I.   Lamina I is a thin superficial layer of neurons that make up the marginal zone. The neurons with cell bodies in lamina I are termed *marginal cells.* These marginal cells receive projections from Aδ and C fiber afferents responsive to noxious mechanical stimuli. In addition, they respond to some polymodal C fiber afferents as well as Aδ temperature impulses. These neurons then project to one of several areas: the thalamus by way of the contralateral spinothalamic tracts, the ipsilateral dorsal white matter, or the ipsilateral dorsal gray matter for an area of several segments.

Lamina II.   Lamina II is also known as the substantia gelatinosa owing to the clear appearance of this section of spinal matter in comparison with surrounding marginal layer and nucleus proprius. This region has undergone extensive evaluation. The neurons of lamina II act as a modulating center for afferent impulses of small and large fibers that terminate in this region. The area is densely packed with cells that make extensive synaptic connections with other cells in the area. The axons of most of these cells are short, and only a few of them project to the thalamus through the contralateral-anterolateral columns. The clinical phenomena of selective spinal cord opiate analgesia are mediated through opioid receptors found in lamina II (Yaksh 1988). Stimulation of these receptors leads to inhibition of marginal cell firing in response to primary afferent signals. Similar inhibition has been postulated with other neurochemicals acting on this lamina, but much more work is needed to delineate the complex interactions involved in processing noxious stimuli here.

Laminae III and IV.   The nucleus proprius is made up of the neurons located in laminae III and IV. One of the predominant populations of cells in the nucleus proprius responds to Aβ, Aδ, and C fiber input; these are termed wide dynamic range neurons (WDRs). Although the receptive fields of the individual afferents may be quite small, the corresponding WDR has a larger receptive field. WDRs project throughout the anterolateral funiculus to the thalamus.

   The convergence of somatic nociceptive afferents and visceral nociceptive afferents on the same neuron in the dorsal horn likely explains the phenomena of referred pain. The presence of viscero-somatic, muscle-somatic, and viscero-viscero convergence seen in the various laminae of the dorsal horn and the development of fairly large receptive fields in some of these second-order neurons also help to explain some of the peculiar characteristics of nonsomatic pain. These are shown schematically in Figure 10–3.

Ascending sensory pathways.   The second-order neurons that arise in the respective laminae of the dorsal horn of the spinal cord subsequently use several specific routes to carry their messages to higher brain centers (Figure 10–4). The specific routes are characterized as tracts and systems that include the neospinothalamic, paleospinothalamic, and spinoreticular systems and dorsal columns.

   Numerous other systems are also involved in the rostral projection of nociceptive information. Important among these other systems would be the dorsal funicular systems and intersegmental systems, which are likely involved in descending inhibitory transmission as well.

Brain stem processing.   The brain stem is involved in transmission of all ascending and descending information. Nociceptive afferent fibers relay to projection neurons in the dorsal horn, which ascend in the anterolateral funiculus to end in the thalamus. During the rostral conduction of these impulses, collaterals activate the nucleus reticularis gigantocellularis, which in turn sends projections to the thalamus, as well as to the periaqueductal gray matter (Figure 10–4).

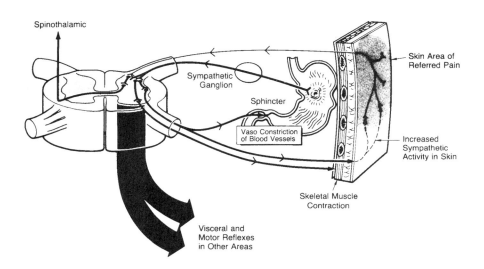

Figure 10–3.   Visceral pain: convergence of visceral and somatic nociceptive afferents. Visceral sympathetic afferents converge on the same dorsal horn neuron as do somatic nociceptive afferents. Visceral noxious stimuli are then conveyed, together with somatic noxious stimuli, via the spinothalamic pathways to the brain.

Note.   1) Referred pain is felt in the cutaneous area corresponding to the dorsal horn neurons on which visceral afferents converge; this is accompanied by allodynia and hyperalgesia in this skin area. 2) Reflex somatic motor activity results in muscle spasm, which may stimulate parietal peritoneum and initiate somatic noxious input to the dorsal horn. 3) Reflex sympathetic efferent activity may result in spasm of sphincters of viscera over a wide area causing pain remote from the original stimulus. 4) Reflex sympathetic efferent activity may result in visceral ischemia and further noxious stimulation; also, visceral nociceptors may be sensitized by norepinephrine release and microcirculatory changes. 5) Increased sympathetic activity may influence cutaneous nociceptors, which may at least be partly responsible for referred pain. 6) Peripheral visceral afferents branch considerably, causing much overlap in the territory of individual dorsal roots; only a small number of visceral afferent fibers converge on dorsal horn neurons compared with somatic nociceptive fibers. Also, visceral afferents converge on the dorsal horn over a large number of segments. This dull, vague visceral pain is very poorly localized and is often called *deep visceral pain.*

Source.   Reprinted from Cousins MJ, Bridenbaugh PO (Eds): *Neural Blockade in Clinical Anesthesia and Management of Pain,* 2nd Edition. Philadelphia, PA, JB Lippincott, 1988, p. 743. Used with permission.

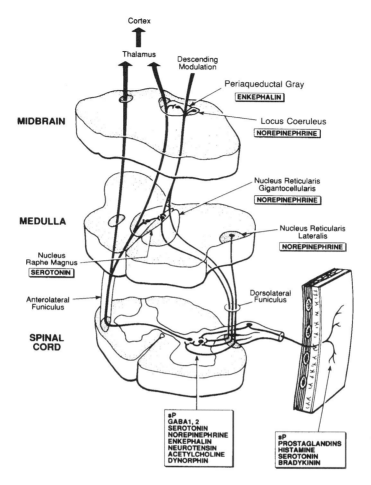

Figure 10–4. Schematic drawing of nociceptive processing, outlining ascending (*left side of diagram*) and descending (*right side of diagram*) pathways. Stimulation of nociceptors in the skin surface leads to impulse generation in the primary afferent. Concomitant with this impulse generation, increased levels of various endogenous algesic agents (substance P [sP], prostaglandins, histamine, serotonin, and bradykinin) are detected near the area of stimulation in the periphery. The noxious impulse is conducted to the dorsal horn or the spinal cord where it is subjected to local factors and descending modulation. The endogenous neurochemical mediators of this interaction at the dorsal horn that have been characterized to date are listed in the figure. Primary nociceptive afferents relay to projection neurons in the dorsal horn that ascend in the anterolateral funiculus to end in the thalamus. En route, collaterals of the projection neurons activate the nucleus reticularis gigantocellularis project to the thalamus and also activate the periaqueductal gray of the midbrain. Enkephalinergic neurons from the periaqueductal gray and noradrenergic neurons from the nucleus reticularis gigantocellularis activate descending serotonergic neurons of the nucleus raphe magnus. These fibers join with noradrenergic fibers from the locus coeruleus reticularis lateralis to project descending modulatory impulses to the dorsal horn via the dorsolateral funiculus. GABA = γ-aminobutyric acid.

Source. Reprinted from Brose WG, Cousins MJ: "Gynecologic Pain," in *Gynecologic Oncology.* Edited by Coppelson M, et al. Edinburgh, Churchill Livingstone, 1992, pp. 1439–1479. Used with permission.

Thalamic relays.   Several nuclear groups of the thalamus are associated with the relay of nociceptive afferent impulses. Included among these are the posterior nuclear complex, the ventrobasilar complex, and the medial intralaminar nuclear complex. In the thalamus, spinothalamic neurons terminate largely on the ventroposteriolateral and the centromedian nuclei. The ventrobasilar complex also receives input from the dorsal columns. The centromedian nucleus is believed to be involved in the qualitative aspects of nociception in that stimulation of this region triggers the unpleasantness associated with tissue damage (Beeson and Chaouch 1987). The projections of the centromedian nucleus are poorly understood at present, but presumably they activate the aversive centers in the limbic system.

Cerebral cortex.   The somatosensory cortex receives processed input from spinothalamic, spinoreticular, and dorsal column systems, as outlined earlier. The majority of attention has been focused on SII as the principal cortical region involved with the reception and perception of noxious information.

Descending modulation.   Up to this point the discussion of pain pathways has been limited to the rostral projection of primary noxious stimuli. The failure of a particular painful stimulus to provoke given behavior in different individuals points out the uncoupling of a simple stimulus-response concept of pain processing. The uncoupling of pain stimulus and response is perhaps best identified by observing the absence of pain in some individuals that are injured in battle or in association with a sporting event. One of the primary focuses of research over the past two decades has been to delineate the physiological explanations for these observed differences in pain response. Through this investigation it has become apparent that the discussion of the afferent limb of the pain pathway mandates consideration of the modulating influences on that pain transmission.

Modulation of pain stimuli can occur at many different levels in the pathway. In their proposal of the gate control theory, Melzack and Wall (1965) predicted modulation of small fiber activity by the presence of large fiber activity in the same region of the dorsal horn. Cutaneous activation of large fiber afferents through transcutaneous nerve stimulation supports this peripheral modulation at the dorsal horn. In addition, the stimulation of dorsal columns that mimics the activation of descending inhibition has also been shown to inhibit the discharge of dorsal horn interneuron nociceptors.

Earlier work by Hagbarth and Kerr (1954) demonstrated the existence of descending long-tract systems to modulate spinal evoked activity. Virtually every pathway carrying nociceptive information, including the spinothalamic and spinoreticular tracts, is under modulatory control from supraspinal systems. Experimental evidence of this supraspinal influence includes inhibition of nociceptive reflexes by electrical stimulation or microinjections of opioid at brain stem sites, both of which are naloxone reversible.

Stimulation of the medullary centers prevents the activation of second-order neurons in the dorsal horn or trigeminal gray matter by primary afferent fibers through this descending inhibition (Beeson and Chaouch 1987). In addition to these different modulating pathways that have been partially characterized, there are undoubtedly additional descending inhibitory influences that have yet to be evaluated. Continued research in this area will help to unravel the complex reaction between pain stimulus and response and perhaps suggest additional therapeutic modalities that may be applied to the treatment of pain.

NEUROPHARMACOLOGY

Pharmacology of Pain

Basic research on the processing of nociceptive information by the central nervous system has led to an improved understanding of pain and pain treatment. Figure 10–4 also summarizes the site of action of several of the chemical substances that have been identified with nociceptive processing. Using this simplified picture of the pain pathway, we can focus on the pharmacological interventions at different points in the pathway and determine a clinical effect on the relief of pain.

Peripheral Desensitization

A rough schematic drawing of the local circuitry involved in the detection of a noxious stimuli from the periphery is shown in Figure 10–5. As discussed previously, following trauma to peripheral site, an inflammatory reaction, including the activation of complement and coagulation-fibrinolytic pathways, will begin. Local release of histamine, serotonin, prostaglandins, and sP occurs. Subsequent

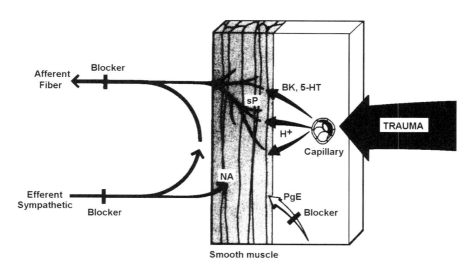

Figure 10–5. Local tissue factors and peripheral pain receptors. The physical stimuli of "trauma," the chemical environment (e.g., H^+), algesic substances (e.g., serotonin [5-hydroxytryptamine (5-HT)], and bradykinin [BK]), and the microcirculatory changes may all modify peripheral receptor activity. Efferent sympathetic activity may increase the sensitivity of receptors by means of noradrenaline (NA; norepinephrine) release. Substance P (sP) may be the peripheral pain transmitter. Points of potential blockade of nociception are shown as "Blocker"; other potential sites involve BK, 5-HT, NA, and sP. PgE = prostaglandin E.
Source.   Reprinted from Cousins MJ, Phillips GD (Eds): *Acute Pain Management.* London, Churchill Livingstone, 1986, p. 742. Used with permission.

changes in the local environment such as decreased tissue pH, changes in the microcirculation, and increase in efferent sympathetic activity all appear to increase the response of peripheral nociceptors.

Numerous drug therapies have been tried to interrupt these peripheral processes. Blockade of pain by aspirin-like drugs is one such peripheral action. Aspirin, indomethacin, ibuprofen, phenylbutazone, diclofenac, and ketorolac are all cyclooxygenase inhibitors. Cyclooxygenase is the enzyme that is responsible for the synthesis of prostaglandins, prostacyclins, and thromboxanes. All these endogenous substances have been proposed as mediators of the local pain response (Juan 1978). Clinical trials with topical capsaicin are also focused on peripheral action. This drug has been shown to deplete sP from cutaneous nerve endings (Gamse et al. 1980). Initially, the effect is a burning pain that is followed by insensitivity to subsequent painful stimuli.

The involvement of the sympathetic nervous system is also suspect. It is known that sympathetic fibers are present in large numbers near cutaneous nociceptors. Blockade of these sympathetic fibers can eliminate the pain of causalgia in some patients. The burning dysesthetic pain and hyperalgesia that are seen with this syndrome, which may be eliminated to sympathetic blockade, can be made to reappear with local application of norepinephrine, the sympathetic neurotransmitter.

Neural Blockade

Neural blockade can occur at any point along the pain pathway. The most common sites of neural block would be peripheral nerves, somatic plexuses, and dorsal roots. These blocks can be performed with relatively short-acting agents such as local anesthetics for acute pain, whereas long-acting (permanent) blockade with alcohol or phenol may be more appropriate for chronic pain. Surgical lesions at any of these points have also been suggested to provide long-lasting interruption of specific pain pathways. The disadvantage of permanent techniques is that they are neither specific for pain fibers nor reliable for protracted pain problems.

Electrical Stimulation

The prediction that large fiber activity could block certain noxious information at the level of the dorsal horn resulted in the introduction of transcutaneous electrical nerve stimulation (TENS). The clinical utility of TENS has yet to be established for individual pain syndromes. Dorsal column stimulation (DCS) excites descending inhibitory pathways with electricity to provide analgesia. The success of DCS has been mixed, but it may have a place in certain deafferentation pain syndromes.

Nonsteroidal Anti-Inflammatory Drugs

The effect of nonsteroidal anti-inflammatory drugs (NSAIDs) to inhibit the synthesis of prostaglandins is currently thought to be the explanation of their pain-relieving properties. The prostaglandins, leukotrienes, and thromboxanes are oxygenated derivatives of arachidonic acid, an essential polyunsaturated fat. The indications for NSAIDs range from the treatment of aches and sprains and dysmenorrhea to long-term therapy for rheumatoid arthritis and osteoarthritis, as well as degenerative joint diseases (e.g., ankylosing spondylitis and gout). Their anti-inflammatory activities have also been shown to relieve pain in cancer patients with bony metastases. In contrast to the opioid drugs, there has not been a clear demonstration of a relationship between blood levels of NSAIDs and pain relief.

The majority of NSAIDs can be classified into one of two groups based on their elimination half-lives (Table 10–1). The NSAIDs in the first group have half-lives between 2 and 4 hours. Acetaminophen is also included in this group, despite its lack of anti-inflammatory properties. The drugs in second group have longer half-lives, ranging from 6 to 60 hours. Patients with renal insufficiency are thought to be at risk for toxicity due to these agents because they are excreted through the kidney.

Dosing of the individual agents has been derived from long-term therapy of rheumatologic disease and represent near maximal anti-inflammatory activity. Although these doses are considered safe for long-term therapy, careful monitoring of side effects is appropriate. Side effects of NSAIDs include gastric irritation, salt and fluid retention, platelet inhibition, and tinnitus.

Antidepressants

Many of the antidepressant drugs act by blocking the uptake of noradrenaline and serotonin in the central nervous system. This effect may also occur in the medulla and increase the concentrations of these neurotransmitters at the synapses involved

Table 10–1. Terminal half-life, recommended dose, influence of food on absorption, and incidence of gastric erosion from nonsteroidal anti-inflammatory drugs (NSAIDS)

Drug	Terminal half-life (hours)	Oral dose and frequency (mg/hour)	Effect of food on absorption[a]	Incidence of gastric erosion (gastritis)
Aspirin	0.2–0.3	600–900/4	1	High
Salicylate	2–3	600/4	1	Intermediate
Diflunisal	8–12	500/12	1	Low
Diclofenac	1.5–2	25–50/8	1	Low
Ibuprofen	2–3	200–400/8	1	Low
Naproxen	12–15	250–375/12	3	Low
Fenoprofen	2–3	400–600/6	2	Low
Indomethacin	6–8	50–75/8	1	Intermediate
Sulindac	6–8	100–200/12	2	Low
Piroxicam	30–60	20–30/24	1	Low
Flufenamic acid	8–10	500/6	1	—
Mefenamic acid	3–4	250/6	1	Intermediate
Ketoprofen	1–4	50/6	1	Low
Ketorolac[b]	5	10–30/6	?	?

[a]1 = decrease in rate of absorption; no change in oral bioavailability;   2 = decrease in rate of absorption and oral bioavailability;   3 = no change in rate of absorption and oral bioavailability.
[b]Not currently available for clinical use; doses based on review of scientific literature.
Source.   Adapted from Gourlay et al. 1987b.

in descending inhibition of dorsal horn cells. Table 10–2 lists the names and properties of some of these antidepressants. Secondary amines are thought to be more effective blockers of norepinephrine, whereas the tertiary amines appear more effective in blocking serotonin reuptake.

Oral tricyclic antidepressants (TCAs) are well absorbed from the gastrointestinal tract. There is conflicting information regarding the existence of therapeutic ranges for antidepressants. All of the currently available pharmacokinetic information refers to the antidepressant activity of these drugs. The time taken for the perception of pain relief after the institution of these drugs is only 2–7 days, compared to the accepted time for antidepressant effect of 3–4 weeks. This observation suggests that different mechanisms may be involved in their analgesic effect and their antidepressant action.

Side effects from TCA use include autonomic, anticholinergic, and adrenergic effects. Dry mouth is the most common side effect and can be relieved by increased fluid intake and salivary stimulants such as sugarless candy. Blurring of vision is also common and usually interferes with reading. Orthostatic hypotension is also common. Patients should be warned to rise slowly and watch for dizziness. Constipation has also been described in association with these agents.

Analgesic Adjuvants

A multitude of agents have been purported to have analgesic qualities. The majority of these agents are thought to potentiate analgesia provided by opioid and nonopioid analgesics. Although the data in support of the use of such compounds may

Table 10–2. Terminal half-life, recommended daily doses, and other properties of antidepressant drugs

Drug	Amine group	Terminal half-life (hours)	Inhibitor concentration[a] NA	Inhibitor concentration[a] 5-HT	Recommended daily dose (mg)[b]
Amitriptyline	Tertiary	20–30	4.6	4.4	50–150
Nortriptyline	Secondary	18–36	0.9	17.0	50–150
Protriptyline	Secondary	50–90	—	—	10–50
Clomipramine	Tertiary	20–30	4.6	0.5	50–75
Imipramine	Tertiary	20–30	4.6	0.5	50–75
Desipramine	Secondary	12–24	0.2	35.0	75–150
Doxepin	Tertiary	10–25	6.5	20.0	75–150
Dothiepin	Tertiary	20–30	—	—	50–100
Mianserin	Tertiary	10–20	20.0	130.0	20–50
Nomifensine	Primary and tertiary	2–4	2.0	120.0	75–150
Zimelidine	Tertiary	5–10	630.0	14.0	200–300

[a]Inhibitor concentration (IC50) represents the antidepressant concentration (x 10^{-8} m) required to inhibit the uptake of either noradrenaline (NA) or serotonin (5-hydroxytryptamine [5-HT]) by 50% using rat midbrain synaptosomes.
[b]It is generally recommended that the antidepressant be administered as a single dose at night, unless significant side effects occur where a night and morning dose (divided dose) may be appropriate.
Source. Adapted from Gourlay et al. 1987b.

be anecdotal, a small number of these drugs do appear to have clinical utility in the management of cancer pain. Table 10–3 summarizes some of the currently available coanalgesics.

Corticosteroids are the first group of drugs to be considered as coanalgesics. These drugs have been used successfully for the management of neuropathic pain from direct neural compression and from pain due to increased intracranial pressure. Systemic steroids are thought to reduce perineural edema and lymphatic edema that may be contributing to pain by compressing individual nerves. This treatment appears to be especially helpful in cases of spinal cord compression. Treatment of such neural compression involves relatively high doses of dexamethasone (near 30 mg/day). Steroids are best employed on a trial basis. A single morning dose or twice daily dose of 2–4 mg/day of dexamethasone can be used over a 10- to 14-day period.

Anticonvulsants are also often advocated as analgesic adjuvants. They suppress neuronal firing and have been successfully employed for treatment of neuropathic

Table 10–3.   Coanalgesic medications

Drugs by classification	Indications	Comments
Antidepressant Amitriptyline Imipramine Mianserin Clomipramine Doxepin	Chronic pain neuropathic pain associated with neuropathy and headache	Improves sleep, may improve appetite
Corticosteroid Dexamethasone Prednisolone Fludrocortisone	Neuropathic pain secondary to direct neural compression, pain secondary in increased intracranial pressure	May stimulate appetite, limit trial to 2 weeks and reassess efficacy
Anticonvulsant Carbamazepine Phenytoin Valproate Clonazepam	Neuropathic pain with paroxysmal character	Start slowly, increase gradually while observing for side effects
Membrane stabilizer Lidocaine 2-Chloroprocaine Tocainide Mexiletine	Neuropathic pain associated with peripheral neuropathy	Efficacy of oral preparations is not established
Phenothiazine Levomepromazine	Insomnia unresponsive to antidepressant or short-acting benzodiazepines	Increase dose slowly to achieve desired effect
Butyrophenone Haloperidol	Acute confusion, nausea, and vomiting	Prolonged use may be complicated by tardive dyskinesia
Antihistamine Hydroxyzine	Nausea, pruritus, and anxiety	Anticholinergic side effects
CNS stimulant Dextroamphetamine Cocaine Caffeine	Opioid-induced sedation, potentiation of NSAID, potentiation of opioid analgesia not proven in cancer	Should only be used as short-term therapeutic trial

Note.   CNS = central nervous system; NSAID = nonsteroidal anti-inflammatory drug.

pain states, including trigeminal neuralgia and peripheral neuropathies. Anticonvulsant drugs probably exert their effects by blocking voltage-dependent sodium channels and thereby interfering with transduction and perhaps spontaneous depolarization seen in damaged neurons. These drugs need to be started slowly and increased gradually, with particular attention being paid to the development of possible side effects. Common side effects can include dizziness, ataxia, drowsiness, blurred vision, and gastrointestinal irritation. In addition, carbamazepine has associated bone marrow toxicity, whereas sodium valproate is known to produce hepatic toxicity.

The use of lidocaine and 2-chloroprocaine in the treatment of certain peripheral neuropathies that have been refractory to other analgesic medications has led to the investigation of another group of drugs, which may be loosely classified as membrane stabilizers. In addition to intermittent intravenous infusion of these two local anesthetics, oral administration of the lidocaine congeners mexiletine and tocainide has been reported as useful in certain patients (Dejard et al. 1988; Lindstrom and Lindblom 1987).

Antipsychotics have long been purported to potentiate the analgesic effect of opioids. Most studies employing these drugs are uncontrolled, however, and the enthusiasm for their continued use is in contrast to available literature. The phenothiazines are the most commonly employed antipsychotics for analgesia. Dundee and colleagues (Dundee et al. 1963; Moore and Dundee 1961) published data regarding the analgesic potency of 14 different phenothiazines in an uncontrolled trial of experimental pain. The results of these studies suggested that the action of a few potentially analgesic phenothiazines was initially antianalgesic and after 2–3 hours only mildly analgesic (Atkison et al. 1985).

Review of phenothiazines in both experimental and clinical pain reveals that only levomepromazine (methotrimeprazine) has established analgesic properties. Levomepromazine appears to have analgesic potency about one-half that of morphine in patients with cancer pain (Beaver et al. 1966).

Benzodiazepines are often discussed as coanalgesics. These drugs do not have any demonstrated analgesic effect. Diazepam has been studied extensively with respect to analgesic activity, and it does not alter sensitivity to pain or potentiate the analgesic activity of opioids. These drugs do decrease affective responses to acute pain, however, and may produce extended relief in chronic pain due to musculoskeletal disorders, perhaps due to their muscle relaxant properties.

Hydroxyzine is an antihistaminic agent. It has proven analgesic properties at high doses. It does not consistently improve analgesia obtained with opioids, but it does potentiate the effect of opioids on the affective components of pain.

The final group of analgesic adjuvants to be considered are the stimulants. This group includes amphetamines, cocaine, and caffeine. Chronic cancer pain has been treated for nearly a century with combinations of opioid and stimulant in Brompton's cocktail. This mixture contains morphine, cocaine, and a phenothiazine. Despite years of clinical experience with such a mixture, no controlled studies have demonstrated superior analgesia with this combination compared with opioid alone. Potentiation of analgesia by sympathomimetics has been well described. Caffeine is known to increase the analgesic effects of aspirin and acetaminophen, and one study suggested that dextroamphetamine doubled the analgesic potency of morphine (Forrest et al. 1977). The long-term use of these stimulants in pain has not been systematically evaluated. The use of these drugs should probably be limited to a therapeutic trial period of several days to determine efficacy for individual patients.

Opioids

In recent years researchers have identified multiple endogenous opioid chemicals with analgesic effects (Yaksh 1988). Among these are the enkephalins and β-endorphin. At least four different types of opioid receptors have also been located in the brain and spinal cord. Although opium has been known for centuries to possess analgesic properties, the location of the active sites for opium was not known. Microinjection techniques used in the 1960s have identified the periaqueductal gray of the midbrain and midline medullary nuclei to be the most sensitive sites.

Table 10–4 summarizes the pharmacodynamic effects obtained when opioid receptors are stimulated. In 1973 Pert and Snyder demonstrated opioid receptors in the brain and brain stem. Afterward Yaksh and Rudy (1976) reported long-lasting analgesia following the introduction of intrathecal opioids. The discovery that spinally administered opioids produced dose-dependent, stereospecific, naloxone-reversible analgesia has led to development of an important clinical tool to combat pain.

Opioids administered systemically will produce inhibition of nociceptive reflexes in spinal transected animals. Also, administration of opioids to the dorsal horn of the spinal cord will inhibit the discharge of nociceptive neurons. Multiple discrete populations of opioid receptors have been identified. Stimulation of μ (mu) and κ (kappa) systems present in the spinal cord depresses the response to noxious stimulation (Yaksh 1981).

Table 10–4. Pharmacodynamic effects obtained when an opioid agonist interacts with the various types of opioid receptors

Effect	Receptor subtype			
	Mu (μ)	Kappa (κ)	Sigma (σ)	Delta (δ)
Pain relief	Yes	Yes, especially at spinal cord level	Yes	Yes
Sedation	Yes	Yes	—	—
Respiratory effects	Depression	Depression, but not as much as for μ (may reach plateau)	Stimulation	Depression
Affect	Euphoria	—	Dysphoria	—
Physical dependence	Marked	Less severe than with μ	—	Yes
Prototype agonist (other drugs with predominantly agonist activity)	Morphine (Meperidine) (Methadone) (Fentanyl) (Heroin) (Codeine) (Propoxyphene) (Buprenorphine)	Ketocyclazocine (Nalbuphine) (Dynorphin) (Butorphanol) (Nalorphine) (Pentazocine)	SKF 10,047	Enkephalins

Note. SKF = SmithKline & French.
Source. Adapted from Gourlay et al. 1987b.

Opiate systems appear to be active in the modulation of noxious impulses presented to the substantia gelatinosa via both direct action and indirect descending inhibition via serotonergic and noradrenergic systems (Yaksh 1988). In addition, other nonopioid systems appear to be functioning at this level to produce analgesic effects. Baclofen and clonidine also rely on both ascending and descending effects for antinociception (Sawynok and Labella 1981). Chemical mediators that have been shown to be associated with analgesia at this level include serotonin, norepinephrine, γ-aminobutyric acid (GABA), neurotensin, and acetylcholine. Some of the proposed endogenous and exogenous ligands for these neurotransmitter systems are shown in Table 10–5.

Many misconceptions surround the use of opioid drugs, which results in a marked tendency for inadequate doses and inappropriately long dosing intervals. Once a decision has been made to use opioid medications, it is both logical and essential to use an effective dosage regimen. In addition to planning effective analgesic therapy with opioids individualized to a particular patient, the use of opioids often involves management of side effects. The major side effects that limit the effectiveness of opioid therapy are nausea, vomiting, sedation, and respiratory depression. The incidence and severity of the side effects seen with the different μ agonists are probably similar at equianalgesic doses. Rather than restrict the dose of opioids to the point at which a patient is free from side effects but experiencing pain, one should consider administering other medications to treat these side effects.

DELIVERY SYSTEMS

The continued reports of inadequate pain relief, despite the vast numbers of newly developed opioids, point to the problems associated with opioid delivery rather than to any defect in the individual drugs, per se. There are many different delivery systems and dosing regimens that can provide good pain relief when used properly. The association between stable blood levels of opioids and continuous analgesia

Table 10–5.   Spinal neurotransmitters, receptors, and ligands

Neurotransmitter systems	Proposed receptor	Endogenous ligand	Exogenous ligand
Opioid	μ	β-Endorphin; Met/Leu-enkephalin	Morphine
	δ	Met/Leu-enkephalin	DADL
	κ	Dynorphin	U50488H
Adrenergic	α_1	Norepinephrine	Methoxamine
	α_2	Norepinephrine	Clonidine
	β	Epinephrine	Isoproterenol
Serotonergic	5-HT	Serotonin	Serotonin
GABAergic	A	GABA	Baclofen
	B	GABA	Muscimol
Neurotensin	—	Neurotensin	Neurotensin
Cholinergic	Muscarinic	Acetylcholine	Oxotremorine

Note.   GABA = γ-aminobutyric acid; 5-HT = 5-hydroxytryptamine.
Source.   Adapted from Yaksh 1988.

must be remembered when planning any systemic opioid therapy. The effective dose of opioid medication is the minimum dose that provides acceptable pain relief with a low incidence of side effects.

Oral Opioids

The rapid clearance of most of opioids, combined with the extensive hepatic metabolism, has important implications for oral dosing. Drugs are absorbed from the gastrointestinal tract directly into the portal circulation, where they travel to the liver. Therefore, allowing oral dosing, a significant percentage of the dose is metabolized to inactive products before the opioids reach the systemic circulation (Mather and Gourlay 1984). This phenomenon is referred to as the hepatic *first-pass effect,* which, with the poor bioavailability seen with certain opioids, lead to perceptions that oral administration of opioids is ineffective. Satisfactory analgesia with oral dosing can be obtained, however, if attention is focused on the pharmacokinetics of the particular opioid to be administered, the oral bioavailability of the drug, and titration of the drug to achieve adequate analgesia in each patient.

Sublingual Administration

Ongoing interest in the improved pain management of patients with terminal malignancy has led to the investigation of sublingual administration. The sublingual route is particularly useful in patients who cannot tolerate oral medication because it causes nausea, vomiting, or dysphagia. This method of administration has theoretical advantages in that the oral cavity is well perfused, providing rapid onset of action; subsequent absorption results in systemic rather than portal drug delivery. The sublingual absorption of lipid-soluble drugs (methadone, fentanyl, and buprenorphine) from alkaline solution was shown to provide analgesic concentrations very quickly (Weinberg et al. 1988). The utility of this technique in comparison with other methods of administration still needs to be assessed.

Rectal Administration

Rectal administration of opioids has been advocated for patients who cannot swallow or for those who have a high incidence of nausea or vomiting with oral administration. Studies of rectal administration of meperidine have indicated a bioavailability similar to that seen following oral dosing: 50% (Ripamonti and Bruera 1991).

Intramuscular Administration

The most commonly used approach for managing postoperative pain is intramuscular administration of morphine or meperidine. The typical prescription would read: "Morphine 10 mg (or meperidine 100 mg) intramuscularly every 3–4 hours as needed for pain."This approach has been shown to provide inadequate analgesia for many reasons. The patient may not request medication despite experiencing severe pain. The nurse may not administer the medication. The dose may not be adequate for the patient's needs. Even controlling all of these potential problems, the variable blood levels seen after intramuscular dosing usually results in periods of pain, alternating with periods of toxicity (Austin et al. 1980).

Subcutaneous Administration

Subcutaneous administration of opioids has been used for decades to provide analgesia. More recent attention has been focused on this technique with the availability of small infusion pumps for delivering continuous opioids to ambulatory patients. Recent applications include subcutaneous infusion for cancer pain and subcutaneous patient-controlled analgesia (PCA). Subcutaneous infusion appears to act clinically like a continuous infusion, but more carefully controlled trials need to be carried out to determine if this similarity is true for all opioids.

Intravenous Administration

The use of intravenous opioids, by intermittent injection as well as continuous infusion, has been known for years to provide more rapid and effective analgesia. The clinical utility of this technique in the management of cancer pain was recently reviewed by the Sloan Kettering Group (Portenoy et al. 1986). The pharmacokinetic support for this clinical observation has been developed over the last several years.

Patient-Controlled Analgesia

The wide interpatient variability of the pharmacokinetic parameters discussed thus far is a primary reason that individual titration of opioid dosing is required to achieve adequate analgesia. Although the physician can do this by evaluating patients at a given time after the therapy has been initiated, the option of patient-controlled analgesia (PCA) is well suited to accommodate the differences between the theory and practice of pain relief. Using PCA, the physician decides the drug to be employed and the dose to be given. The patient can decide when a dose should be administered and the timing between doses.

Spinal Administration

The use of spinal opioids for acute pain management dates back only into the last decade. As compared with all of the delivery systems discussed above, which use indirect delivery of the opioid to the receptor site via the systemic circulation, spinal delivery is a system in which the opioids are delivered directly to the receptors in the spinal cord via local mechanisms. Clinical reports of long-lasting analgesia obtained with spinal opioids indicate frequent side effects, including nausea, vomiting, sedation, pruritus, urinary retention, and respiratory depression. The term *spinal opioid* is used to describe intrathecal, epidural, and intracerebroventricular administration of opioids; the rest of this discussion focuses on epidural opioids.

Much of the concern about the utilization of spinal opioids has focused on the concern for respiratory depression. This can be early (associated with the peak blood levels following epidural administration) or late (perhaps due to the rostral migration of morphine into sensitive respiratory centers). Outcome studies (Rawal et al. 1987) generated from large groups of patients in Sweden who received spinal opioids indicate that the incidence of severe delay respiratory depression after epidural morphine is approximately 1 in 1,000 patients. Although certain demographic characteristics of at-risk populations have been identified, the inability to predict the occurrence of delayed respiratory depression in healthy patients points out the need for increased surveillance of all patients who are receiving opioid analgesia.

The spinal administration of opioids is appropriate for pain in virtually any region of the body. Spinally administered morphine has been shown to migrate over the entire distance of the spinal cord, even when injected in the lumbar epidural space (Gourlay et al. 1985, 1987a). Pain relief from such spinal opioid systems has been shown for pain in cervical dermatomes and even in the trigeminal system.

Continued efforts to refine and evaluate spinal opioids should help to determine the appropriate utilization of this therapy. The high quality of analgesia and the tremendous reports of patient satisfaction seen following epidural morphine analgesia provide ample support for research in this field.

NEURODESTRUCTIVE PROCEDURES

The continued progress in pain management with multidisciplinary therapies has decreased utilization of neurodestructive procedures. Despite the continued success of less invasive and nondestructive techniques, neurolytic blockade still provides valuable adjunctive treatment of nociceptive and neuropathic pain in terminal cancer (Cousins 1988). Often, a properly performed neurodestructive procedure can markedly decrease medication use and control the unwanted side effect associated with high doses of analgesics. Virtually all neurodestructive techniques should be confined to the treatment of nociceptive pain. The central and peripheral changes associated with neuropathic pain are not only never relieved by neurodestructive techniques, they are often aggravated by such procedures. Neurolytic blocks are mainly indicated for localized unilateral pain, except for pituitary ablation, which is suitable for diffuse areas of pain.

HYPNOSIS

Central psychological approaches to pain control can also be effective and are underutilized. It has been known since the middle of the 1800s that hypnosis is effective in controlling even severe surgical pain (Esdaile 1846). Hypnosis and similar techniques work through two primary mechanisms: muscle relaxation and a combination of perceptual alteration and cognitive distraction. Pain is not infrequently accompanied by reactive muscle tension. Patients frequently splint the part of their body that hurts. Yet because muscle tension can by itself cause pain in normal tissue and because traction on a painful part of the body can produce more pain, techniques that induce greater physical relaxation can reduce pain in the periphery. Therefore, having patients enter a state of hypnosis so they can concentrate on an image that connotes physical relaxation such as floating or lightness often produces physical relaxation and reduces pain.

The second major component of hypnotic analgesia is perceptual alteration. Patients can be taught to imagine that the affected body part is numb. This is especially useful for extremely hypnotizable individuals who can, for example, relive an experience of dental anesthesia and reproduce the drug-induced sensations of numbness in their cheek, which they can then transfer to the painful part of their body. Temperature metaphors are often especially useful, which is not surprising given the fact that pain and temperature sensations are part of the same sensory system, as noted above. Thus imagining that an affected body part is cooler or warmer using an image of dipping it in ice water or heating it in the sun can often help patients transform pain signals. Some patients prefer to imagine that the pain is a substance with dimensions that can be moved or can flow out of the body as if it were a viscous liquid. Others like to imagine that they can step outside their body to, for example, visit another room in the house. Less hypnotizable individuals often do better with distraction techniques that help them focus on competing sensations in another part of the body.

Although not all patients are sufficiently hypnotizable to benefit from these techniques, two out of three adults are at least somewhat hypnotizable (Spiegel and Spiegel 1987), and it has been estimated that hypnotic capacity is correlated at a .5 level with effectiveness in medical pain reduction (Hilgard and Hilgard 1975).

SECONDARY GAIN

Secondary gain is a major problem with chronic pain. The term refers to the secondary reinforcements that accompany a primary loss involving physical function, ability to work, ability to engage in sexual activity, or other concomitants of injury and illness. A pain syndrome can set off a downward social spiral in which a patient loses the ordinary reinforcement that comes from contact with colleagues at work and the self-esteem that comes from being productive. Increasing depression can result in a loss of energy and an inability to interact rewardingly with others, leading to social withdrawal. Social contact becomes increasingly organized around pain complaints. Patients who seem to lose the ability to elicit enjoyable and rewarding social interactions increasingly coerce attention from health care providers, family, and friends over their disabilities, which contributes part of the secondary gain. Additional secondary gain may come in the form of being able to avoid unwanted responsibilities such as the pressures of work or unwelcome aspects of social interaction such as sexual activity.

Another major form of secondary gain is financial reinforcement. Disability systems frequently intensify this form of secondary gain by creating an adversarial system in which any evidence of the patient's ability to return to normal function endangers financial support, which in essence requires complete disability. In such an adversarial system, efforts at rehabilitation are used as evidence that there was never any serious disability in the first place. Furthermore, attaining disability status is often a protracted and unpleasant process. During a consolidation phase after an acute injury when patients might be able to return to some level of functioning despite continuing symptoms, they are instead engaged in a battle to prove the extent of their disability. Any improvement results in the reduction or elimination of the case for some disability payment.

Many patients are victims of this system. Others manipulate it, exaggerating their disability to obtain financial benefits, further reinforcing the system's adversarial nature. On the other hand, many more patients are accused of such exaggeration than actually commit it.

Secondary gain factors, both social and financial, substantially complicate treatment, and it is best to do everything possible to minimize them. Useful social strategies include the behavioral therapy principle of requesting health care personnel and family members to provide attention and positive reinforcement for non-pain-related behaviors (Fordyce et al. 1973) while diminishing reinforcement for pain-related interactions.

CONCLUSIONS

As we continue to enrich the knowledge base on which we understand the causes, transmission, and processing of pain signals, we can make pain treatment more comprehensive, humane, and effective. There are multiple levels at which the pain problem can be approached, including removing the cause of the pain at the periphery, reducing muscle tension that exacerbates pain input, blocking pain transmission through competitive electrical stimulation, infusions into the central nervous system, and drugs that block pain transmission or perception. There are also important cognitive interventions that can help reduce patients' focus on pain and ameliorate their reaction to it.

REFERENCES

Ahles TA, Blanchard EB, Ruckdeschel JC: Multidimensional nature of cancer-related pain. Pain 17:277–288, 1983

Atkison JH, Kremer EF, Garfin SR: Current concepts review: psychopharmacologic agents in the treatment of pain. J Bone Joint Surg [Am] 67:337–339, 1985

Austin KL, Stapleton JV, Mather LE: Multiple intramuscular injections: a major source of variability in analgesic response to pethidine. Pain 8:4–19, 1980

Beaver WT, Wallenstein SL, Houde RW, et al: A comparison of the analgesic effects of methotrimeprazine and morphine in patients with cancer. Clin Pharm Therapeut 7:436–446, 1966

Beecher HK: Relationship of significance of wound to pain experienced. JAMA 161:1609–1616, 1956

Beeson JM, Chaouch A: Peripheral and spinal mechanisms of nociception. Physiol Rev 67(1):67, 1987

Blumer D, Heilbronn M: Chronic pains as a variant of depressive disease: the pain prone disorder. J Nerv Ment Dis 170:381–406, 1982

Bond MR: Personality studies in patients with pain secondary to organic disease. J Psychosom Res 17:257–263, 1973

Bond MR, Pearson IB: Psychological aspects of pain in women with advanced cancer of the cervix. J Psychosom Res 13:13–19, 1969

Bonica JJ: Evolution and current status of pain programs. Journal of Pain Symptom Management 5:368–374, 1990

Brose WG, Cousins MJ: Gynecologic pain, in Gynecologic Oncology. Edited by Coppelson M, et al. Edinburgh, Churchill Livingstone, 1992, pp 1439–1479

Cousins MJ: Chronic pain and neurolytic blockade, in Neural Blockade in Clinical Anesthesia and Management of Pain, 2nd Edition. Edited by Cousins MJ, Bridenbaugh PO. Philadelphia, PA, JB Lippincott, 1988, p 1053

Cousins MJ, Bridenbaugh PO (eds): Neural Blockade in Clinical Anesthesia and Management of Pain, 2nd Edition. Philadelphia, PA, JB Lippincott, 1988

Cousins MJ, Phillips GD (eds): Acute Pain Management. London, Churchill Livingstone, 1986

Dejard A, Peterson P, Kestrup J: Mexiletine for the treatment of chronic painful diabetic neuropathy. Lancet 1:9–11, 1988

Dundee JW, Love WJ, Moore J: Alterations in response to somatic pain associated with anesthesia, XV: further studies with phenothiazine derivatives and similar drugs. Br J Anaesth 35:597–610, 1963

Dworkin SF, Von Koroff M, LeResche L: Multiple pains and psychiatric disturbance: an epidemiologic investigation. Arch Gen Psychiatry 47:239–244, 1990

Esdaile J: Hypnosis in Medicine and Surgery (1846), Reprinted. New York, Julian Press, 1957

Eysenck HJ, Eysenck BG: Manual of the Eysenck Personality Inventory. London, University of London Press, 1964

Fields HL: Pain. New York, McGraw-Hill, 1987

Fordyce WE, Fowler RS, Lehmann JR, et al: Operant conditioning in the treatment of chronic pain. Arch Phys Med Rehabil 54:399–408, 1973

Forrest WH, Brown BW, Brown CR, et al: Dextroamphetamine with morphine for the treatment of postoperative pain. N Engl J Med 296:712–715, 1977

Gamse R, Holzer P, Lembeck F: Decrease of substance P in primary afferent neurones and impairment of neurogenic plasma extravasation by capsaicin. Br J Pharmacol 68:207–213, 1980

Gourlay GK, Cherry DA, Cousins MJ: Cephalad migration of morphine in CSF following lumbar epidural administration in patients with cancer pain. Pain 23:317–326, 1985

Gourlay GK, Cherry DA, Plummer JL, et al: The influence of drug polarity on the absorption of opioid drugs into the CSF and subsequent cephalad migration following lumbar epidural administration: application to morphine and pethidine. Pain 31:297–305, 1987a

Gourlay GK, Cousins MJ, Cherry DA: Drug therapy, in Handbook of Chronic Pain Management. Edited by Burrows GD, Elton D, Stanley GV. Amsterdam, Elsevier North-Holland, 1987b

Hagbarth KE, Kerr DIB: Central influences on spinal afferent conduction. J Neurophysiol 17:295, 1954

Hilgard ER, Hilgard JR: Hypnosis in the Relief of Pain. Los Altos, CA, William Kaufmann, 1975

Juan H: Prostaglandins as modulators of pain. Journal of General Pharmacology 9:403, 1978

Katon W, Egan K, Miller D: Chronic pain: lifetime psychiatric diagnosis and family history. Am J Psychiatry 142:1156–1160, 1985

Levine JD, Coderre JJ, Basbaum AI: The peripheral nervous system and the inflammatory process, in Proceedings of the Fifth World Congress on Pain. Edited by Dubner R, Gebhart GF, Bond MR. Amsterdam, Elsevier North-Holland, 1988, p 33

Lindstrom P, Lindblom U: The analgesic effect of tocainide in trigeminal neuralgia. Pain 28:45–50, 1987

Massie MJ, Holland JC: The cancer patient with pain: psychiatric complications and their management. Cancer Pain 71:243–258, 1987

Mather LE, Gourlay GK: The biotransformation of opioids, in Opioid Agonist/Antagonist Drugs in Clinical Practice. Edited by Nimmo WS, Smith G. Amsterdam, Excerpta Medica, 1984

Melzack R: Recent concepts of pain. J Med 13:147–160, 1982

Melzack R, Wall PD: Pain mechanisms: a new theory. Science 150:971–979, 1965

Moore J, Dundee JW: Alterations in response to somatic pain associated with anesthesia, V: the effect of promethazine. Br J Anaesth 33:3–8, 1961

Müller J: Von den Ergentumlichkeiten der ein zelnen Nerve, in Handbuch der Physiologie de Menschen. Edited by Kobling L. Coblenz, Holscher, 1844

Pert CB, Snyder SH: Opiate receptors: demonstration in nervous tissue. Science 179:1011–1014, 1973

Pilowski I, Chapman CR, Bonica JJ: Pain, depression and illness behavior in a pain clinic population. Pain 4:183–192, 1977

Portenoy RK, Moulin DE, Rodgers A, et al: IV infusion of opioids for cancer pain: clinical review and guidelines for use. Cancer Treat Rev 70:575, 1986

Posner MI, Petersen SE: The attention system of the human brain. Annual Review of Neuroscience 13:125–142, 1990

Rawal N, Arner S, Gustaffson LL, et al: Present state of extradural and intrathecal opioid analgesia in Sweden: a nationwide follow-up survey. Br J Anesth 59:791–799, 1987

Reich J, Tupin JP, Abramowitz SI: Psychiatric diagnosis of chronic pain patients. Am J Psychiatry 140:1495–1498, 1983

Ripamonti C, Bruera E: Rectal, buccal and sublingual narcotics for the management of cancer pain. J Palliat Care 7:30–35, 1991

Sawynok J, Labella L: GABA and baclofen potentiate the K^+-evoked release of methionine-enkephalin from rat striatal slices. Eur J Pharmacol 70(2):103–110, 1981

Spiegel D, Bloom JR: Pain in metastatic breast cancer. Cancer 52:341–345, 1983

Spiegel D, Sands S: Pain management in the cancer patient. Journal of Psychosocial Oncology 6:205–216, 1988

Spiegel H, Spiegel D: Trance and Treatment: Clinical Uses of Hypnosis. Washington, DC, American Psychiatric Press, 1987

Weinberg DS, Inturrisi CE, Reidenberg B, et al: Sublingual absorption of selected opioid analgesics. Clin Pharmacol Ther 44:335–342, 1988

Yaksh TL: Spinal opiates analgesia: characteristics and principles of action. Pain 11:293, 1981

Yaksh TL: Neurologic mechanisms of pain, in Neural Blockade in Clinical Anesthesia and Management of Pain, 2nd Edition. Edited by Cousins MJ, Bridenbaugh PO. Philadelphia, PA, JB Lippincott, 1988, p 79

Yaksh TL, Rudy TA: Narcotic analgesia produced by a direct action on the spinal cord. Science 192:1357–1358, 1976

Chapter 11

Delirium

Michael G. Wise, M.D.
George T. Brandt, M.D.

Delirium may well be the most common psychiatric syndrome found in a general medical hospital. Its mortality and morbidity may surpass all other psychiatric diagnoses. Only dementia, when followed for several years, has a higher mortality rate (Roth 1955; Varsamis et al. 1972). Although commonly seen by consultation psychiatrists and other physicians, delirium remains an ignored, underresearched phenomenon.

Figure 11–1 presents a conceptual overview of delirium. Note the wide variety of different physiological insults that can produce the symptom cluster of the delirium syndrome. This multifactorial etiology accounts both for the high incidence of the syndrome and for the evolution of so many "equivalent" diagnostic terms. Delirium can manifest clinically as a hypoactive state (decreased arousal), hyperactive state (increased arousal), or as a mixed state with fluctuations between hypoactive and hyperactive forms. Accurate diagnosis, of course, precedes treatment. The prognosis for delirium, without proper diagnosis and treatment, is bleak.

DEFINITION

Defining *delirium* is not an easy task because many terms have been used to describe this clinical syndrome. The diagnostic criteria for delirium found in DSM-III-R (American Psychiatric Association 1987) are outlined in Table 11–1. Both DSM-III (American Psychiatric Association 1980) and DSM-III-R criteria evolved from a committee effort but underrepresent the wide array of neuropsychiatric abnormalities found in the delirious patient. In the section of this chapter on clinical features we attempt to amplify and expand these criteria. DSM-III-R does unite a broad spectrum of clinical states (i.e., hypoactive, hyperactive, and mixed confusional states) under the diagnostic umbrella of delirium. This approach is not accepted by many of our medical colleagues, particularly neurologists. Adams and Victor (1989), for example, suggested that the diagnosis of delirium should be reserved for a subgroup of confused patients with agitation, autonomic instability, and hallucinations. Delirium tremens (DTs) was the conceptual model they used. Patients who become acutely confused, incoherent, and disoriented, but without autonomic instability and hallucinations, would be said to have "acute confusional states," not delirium.

Pending further research, the unified approach of DSM-III-R, which labels both hyperactive and hypoactive forms as delirium, seems appropriate. Several other aspects of the syndrome must be incorporated into a definition. Delirium usually has a sudden onset, a brief duration, and is reversible. Therefore, delirium is herein defined as *a transient, essentially reversible dysfunction in cerebral metabolism that has an acute or subacute onset and is manifest clinically by a wide array of neuropsychiatric abnormalities.*

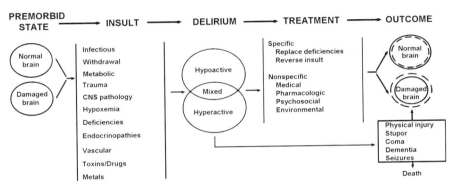

Figure 11–1.   Conceptual overview of delirium.

Table 11–1.   DSM-III-R diagnostic criteria for delirium

A. Reduced ability to maintain attention to external stimuli (e.g., questions must be repeated because attention wanders) and to appropriately shift attention to new external stimuli (e.g., perseverates answer to a previous question).

B. Disorganized thinking, as indicated by rambling, irrelevant, or incoherent speech.

C. At least two of the following:
   (1)   reduced level of consciousness, e.g., difficulty keeping awake during examination
   (2)   perceptual disturbances: misinterpretations, illusions, or hallucinations
   (3)   disturbance of sleep-wake cycle with insomnia or daytime sleepiness
   (4)   increased or decreased psychomotor activity
   (5)   disorientation to time, place, or person
   (6)   memory impairment, e.g., inability to learn new material, such as the names of several unrelated objects after five minutes, or to remember past events, such as history of current episode of illness

D. Clinical features develop over a short period of time (usually hours to days) and tend to fluctuate over the course of a day.

E. Either (1) or (2):
   (1)   evidence from the history, physical examination, or laboratory tests of a specific organic factor (or factors) judged to be etiologically related to the disturbance
   (2)   in the absence of such evidence, an etiologic organic factor can be presumed if the disturbance cannot be accounted for by any nonorganic mental disorder, e.g., manic episode accounting for agitation and sleep disturbance

---

Source.   Reprinted from American Psychiatric Association: *Diagnostic and Statistical Manual of Mental Disorders,* 3rd Edition, Revised. Washington, DC, American Psychiatric Association, 1987, p. 103. Used with permission.

EPIDEMIOLOGY

Incidence and Prevalence

The frequency of delirium varies depending on the type of insult and the predisposition of the individual involved. Engel (1967) estimated that 10%–15% of patients on acute medical and surgical wards were delirious. Lipowski (1990) agreed with this estimate but noted that the increasing age of the population may make the estimate low.

Anthony et al. (1982) used the Mini-Mental State Exam (MMSE; Folstein et al. 1975) and tested consecutively admitted patients to a general medical ward of the Johns Hopkins Hospital. They found a point prevalence for delirium of 24% and also found that 34% of patients had some cognitive impairment on the day of admission. Cameron et al. (1987), using DSM-III diagnostic criteria, found 13.5% of 133 consecutive patients admitted to a medical ward were delirious and that an additional 3.3% became delirious during hospitalization.

Predisposing Factors

Six groups of patients have a high risk of developing a delirium: 1) elderly patients, 2) postcardiotomy patients, 3) burn patients, 4) patients with preexisting brain damage (e.g., dementia and strokes), 5) patients with drug dependency who are experiencing withdrawal, and 6) patients with acquired immunodeficiency syndrome (AIDS). Advancing age increases the risk, with persons aged 60 or over usually cited as the highest risk group (Lipowski 1980a, 1990). If children are excluded, the incidence of delirium increases with the age of the patient population studied.

Postcardiotomy delirium has been the focus of more neuropsychiatric research than any other aspect of delirium (Smith and Dimsdale 1989). In a thorough review of postcardiotomy delirium, Dubin et al. (1979) reported that the frequency across studies varied from 13% to 67%. Several factors, in addition to increased age and preexisting brain damage, may increase the risk of postcardiotomy delirium. These include time on bypass (Heller et al. 1970; Kornfeld et al. 1974), severity of postoperative illness (Kornfeld et al. 1974), serum levels of anticholinergic drugs (Tune et al. 1981), increased levels of central nervous system (CNS) adenylate kinase and subclinical brain injury (Aberg et al. 1982, 1984), decreased cardiac output (Blachly and Kloster 1966), complexity of the surgical procedure (Dubin et al. 1979), complement activation (Chenoweth et al. 1981), embolism (Nussmeier et al. 1986), and nutritional status as measured by albumin levels (M. G. Wise, N. H. Cassem, K. Gray, 1980–1981, unpublished observations). Preoperative psychiatric interviews may reduce postoperative psychosis by 50% (Layne and Yudofsky 1971; Smith and Dimsdale 1989). According to Andreasen (1974), about 30% of adult burn patients have symptoms of delirium and the "frequency increases with both the age of the patient and the severity of the burn" (Andreasen et al. 1972, p. 68). Blank and Perry (1984) described an 18% incidence of delirium in burn patients.

The presence of preexisting brain damage, whether preoperative CNS neurological abnormalities (Branthwaite 1972) or dementia (Purdie et al. 1981), lowers the patient's threshold for developing a delirium. Koponen et al. (1989a) found that 81% of delirious patients in their study had dementia. Rapid drug withdrawal in a patient with drug dependence, particularly rapid withdrawal from alcohol and benzodiazepines, is without question a risk factor for developing delirium. Perry (1990) reported a 90% frequency of organic mental disorders in patients with far-advanced AIDS. In another study (Fernandez et al. 1989), delirium was found to be the most frequent neuropsychiatric complication of AIDS.

Additional factors, such as sleep deprivation and perceptual (sensory) deprivation, are believed to facilitate the development of a delirium. After a thorough review of the literature on the relationship between sleep and delirium Lipowski (1990) stated, "In summary, experimental and clinical studies indicate a relationship between sleep disturbance and delirium but fail to clarify its exact nature" (p. 123). Harrell and Othmer (1987) found that sleep disturbance developed after patients' scores on the MMSE decreased (i.e., after the delirium developed) and not before. Both sensory deprivation and sensory overload are believed to be facilitating factors in delirium (Lipowski 1980a, 1990).

The predisposition associated with personality and psychological variables has been investigated as well. In their review of the postoperative literature, Dubin et al. (1979) indicated that no specific personality profile correlated with delirium. Lipowski (1980a) agreed, reporting that "it may be stated that so far not a single psychological variable has been conclusively shown to predispose one to delirium" (p. 115).

CLINICAL FEATURES OF DELIRIUM

Fluctuating Course

The clinical features of delirium are protean and, to complicate the picture further, vary rapidly over time. This variability and fluctuation is characteristic of delirium and can lead to diagnostic confusion. However, the appearance of lucid intervals in the clinical course of a patient is an important observation and is diagnostic of a delirium.

There is a subgroup of patients who manifest what has been called "reversible dementia" (Cummings et al. 1980; Task Force Sponsored by the National Institute on Aging 1980). These patients lack the dramatic fluctuations that are so typical of delirium and, as a result, are often misdiagnosed as having dementia.

Prodrome

The patient will often manifest symptoms such as restlessness, anxiety, irritability, or sleep disruption before the onset of a delirium.

Attentional Deficits

The patient with a delirium has difficulty sustaining attention. Further, such a patient is easily distracted by incidental activities in the environment. The patient's inability to sustain attention undoubtedly plays a key role in memory and orientation difficulties.

Impaired Memory

The ability of a delirious patient to register events into memory is severely impaired. Whether because of attentional deficits, perceptual disturbances, or malfunction of the hippocampus, the patient will fail tests of immediate and recent memory. After recovery, some patients will be amnestic for the entire episode; others will have islands of memory for events during the episode.

Disorientation

The patient with a delirium, except for lucid intervals, is usually disoriented to time, often disoriented to place, but very rarely, if ever, disoriented to person. It is not unusual for a delirious patient to feel that he or she is in a familiar place (e.g., "a room in the attic of my house") while also nodding agreement that he or she is being monitored in a surgical ICU. The extent of the patient's disorientation will fluctuate with the severity of the delirium.

Arousal Disturbance and Psychomotor Abnormalities

In delirium, the reticular activating system of the brain stem may be hypoactive, in which case the patient would appear apathetic, somnolent, and quietly confused. In other patients, the brain stem's activating system may be hyperactive, in which case the patient is agitated and hypervigilant, exhibiting psychomotor hyperactivity. Some patients have a mixed picture, with swings back and forth between hypoactive and hyperactive states. The patient with a retarded (hypoactive) type of delirium is less apt to be diagnosed as delirious and is often labeled as depressed, uncooperative, or character disordered.

Sleep-Wake Disturbance

Sleep-wake disturbance is not only symptomatic of a delirium, it exacerbates the confusion via sleep deprivation. The sleep-wake cycle of the delirious patient is often reversed. The patient may be somnolent during the day and active during the night. Restoration of the normal diurnal sleep cycle is an important part of delirium treatment.

Disorganized Thinking and Impaired Speech

The delirious patient's thought patterns are disorganized and reasoning is defective. Using DSM-III-R terminology, the patient's consciousness is *clouded.* In addition, as the severity of the delirium increases, spontaneous speech becomes "incoherent, rambling, and shifts from topic to topic" (Cummings 1985, p. 68).

Altered Perceptions

The delirious patient will often experience misperceptions that involve illusions, delusions, and hallucinations. Virtually all patients with a delirium will have misperceptions. The patient will often weave these misperceptions into a loosely knit delusional, often paranoid system. Visual hallucinations are common and can involve simple visual distortions or complex scenes. During a delirium, visual hallucinations occur more frequently than auditory hallucinations. Tactile hallucinations are the least frequent.

Neurological Abnormalities

A number of neurological abnormalities are found in delirium. Testing for these signs at the bedside can be done by drawing a large circle on an unlined blank sheet of paper and asking the patient to draw a clock face with the hands showing 10 minutes before 11 o'clock (Figure 11–2). Or the patient can be asked to name objects (testing for dysnomia) or to write a sentence (testing for dysgraphia). In Chedru's and Geschwind's study (1972), 33 of 34 acutely confused patients had impaired writing. Patten and Lamarre (1989) examined 250 psychiatric patients and noted that dysgraphia is not specific to delirium and can occur with dementia and acute psychiatric disorders. However, dysgraphia in delirious patients tended to be more severe. Delirious patients may not have motor system abnormalities,

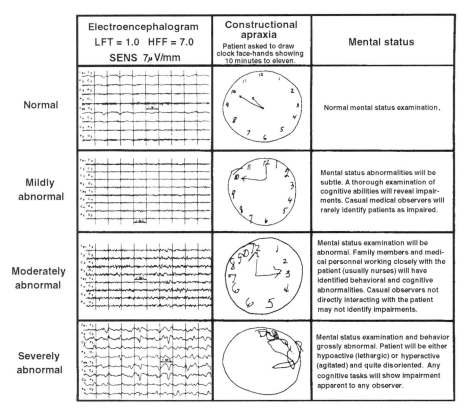

	Electroencephalogram LFT = 1.0　HFF = 7.0 SENS 7μV/mm	Constructional apraxia Patient asked to draw clock face-hands showing 10 minutes to eleven.	Mental status
Normal			Normal mental status examination.
Mildly abnormal			Mental status abnormalities will be subtle. A thorough examination of cognitive abilities will reveal impairments. Casual medical observers will rarely identify patients as impaired.
Moderately abnormal			Mental status examination will be abnormal. Family members and medical personnel working closely with the patient (usually nurses) will have identified behavioral and cognitive abnormalities. Casual observers not directly interacting with the patient may not identify impairments.
Severely abnormal			Mental status examination and behavior grossly abnormal. Patient will be either hypoactive (lethargic) or hyperactive (agitated) and quite disoriented. Any cognitive tasks will show impairment apparent to any observer.

Figure 11–2. Comparison of electroencephalogram, constructional apraxia, and mental status.

although many patients manifest tremor, myoclonus, asterixis, or reflex and muscle tone changes.

Other Features

Emotional disturbances are common among delirious patients. Emotional responses include anxiety, panic, fear, anger, rage, sadness, apathy, and (rarely, except in steroid-induced delirium) euphoria. Medical caregivers may identify the emotional or behavioral disturbance of the critically ill patient without recognizing the underlying confusional state.

PATHOPHYSIOLOGY AND EEG ABNORMALITIES

From 1944 to 1947, Engel, Romano, and others (Engel et al. 1947; Romano and Engel 1944) wrote a series of classic papers that correlated the severity of delirium (i.e., cognitive dysfunction) with electroencephalography (EEG) findings. Their clinical research established that 1) a correlation existed between the electrical abnormality and disturbance of consciousness, which they termed "the primary psychological symptom of delirium"; 2) EEG changes were reversible to the extent that the clinical delirium was reversible; 3) the character of the EEG change appeared to be independent of the specific underlying disease process; 4) the character of the EEG changes was determined by the intensity, duration, and reversibility of the noxious factors as modified by the essential premorbid integrity of the CNS; and 5) clinical interventions (e.g., administration of oxygen in congestive heart failure and pulmonary insufficiency) improved (normalized) the EEG and improved the mental status. Spectral EEG analyses, which measure the quality of alpha, beta, theta, and delta background activity, have further supported Engel's and Romano's proposed correlation between EEG slowing and cognitive deterioration (Koponen et al. 1989b).

Engel's and Romano's classic article (1959)—"Delirium, a Syndrome of Cerebral Insufficiency"—proposed that the basic etiology of all delirium was a derangement in functional metabolism that was manifest at the clinical level by characteristic disturbances in cognitive functions and at the physiological level by characteristic slowing of the EEG. The EEG slowing illustrated in Figure 11–2 is typical for deliriums caused by toxic-metabolic etiologies.

Since Engel's and Romano's 1959 hypothesis that delirium represents a metabolic derangement, little additional research information has been forthcoming. When Lipowski (1980a) reviewed the studies on cerebral metabolism, cerebral blood flow, and delirium, he suggested that studies of regional cerebral blood flow (rCBF) in delirium have only begun. This is still an accurate assessment. Lipowski (1990) stated, "Unfortunately, this superior research technique [positron-emission tomography] has not yet been used to study delirium and to elucidate its pathophysiology" (p 146).

Some neurologists (Adams and Victor 1989; Mesulam 1985; Mori and Yamadori 1987) divide the DSM-III-R concept of delirium into two different types, an acute confusional state (ACS) and an acute agitated delirium (AAD). Mori and Yamadori (1987) studied 41 consecutive patients with infarction in the territory of the right middle artery. They concluded that ACS reflects a disturbance of attention secondary to damage of the frontostriatal region and that AAD is a disturbance of emotion and affect secondary to injury of the middle temporal gyrus. Koponen (1989c) noted that delirium was more common with vascular lesions of the high-order association areas of the prefrontal and posterior parietal regions.

DIFFERENTIAL DIAGNOSIS

The differential diagnosis of delirium is so extensive that there may be a tendency to avoid the search for etiologies. It is also important to realize that confusional states, particularly in the elderly, may have multiple causes. Each potential contributor to the delirium needs to be pursued and reversed independently. Koponen (1989a) found clear organic etiologies in 87% of delirious patients and also found that patients who became confused because of psychological and environmental events were severely demented. The task for the clinician is to organize the wide array of potential causes of delirium into a usable diagnostic system.

Emergent Items (WHHHHIMP)

A two-tiered differential diagnostic system is very helpful when consulting on a delirious patient. The first level of this diagnostic system is represented by the mnemonic *WHHHHIMP*. Diagnoses using this mnemonic must be made early in the course of a delirium because failure to do so may result in irreversible damage to the patient.

W—Wernicke's encephalopathy or Withdrawal. A patient with Wernicke's encephalopathy will have a triad of findings consisting of confusion, ataxia, and ophthalmoplegia (usually lateral gaze paralysis). If Wernicke's encephalopathy is not promptly treated with parenteral thiamine, the patient will be left with a permanent Korsakoff's psychosis. A precise history of alcohol intake is critical for the diagnosis of alcohol withdrawal or DTs. Other findings that increase the suspicion of alcohol withdrawal or DTs are a history of alcohol-related arrests, alcoholic blackouts, medical complications associated with alcohol abuse, liver function abnormalities, and elevated red cell mean corpuscular volume (MCV). Hyperreflexia and increased sympathetic tone (e.g., tachycardia, tremor, sweating, and hyperarousal) at the time of examination should lead the clinician to suspect a hyperadrenergic withdrawal state.

HHHH—Hypoxemia, Hypertensive encephalopathy, Hypoglycemia, or Hypoperfusion. A check of the arterial blood gases, and current and past vital signs, should quickly establish whether hypoxemia or hypertensive encephalopathy is present. The patient with hypoglycemic-induced delirium almost always has a history of insulin-dependent diabetes mellitus. A number of clinical phenomena can singularly, or additively, decrease brain perfusion. These phenomena cause "relative" hypotension (relative to usual perfusion pressures), such as decreased cardiac output from a myocardial infarction, cardiac failure or arrhythmias, and anemia.

I—Intracranial bleeding or Infection. If the patient has had a brief period of unconsciousness, with or without headache, and is now delirious, or if the patient had or now has focal neurological signs, an intracranial bleed or infection must be suspected. Also, the clinician must look for signs of an infectious process, such as fever or an elevated white blood cell count.

M—Meningitis or encephalitis.   These are typically acute febrile illnesses (check vital signs for fever) and usually have either nonspecific localizing neurological signs (e.g., meningismus with stiff neck) or more focal neurological signs.

P—Poisons or medications.   When a delirious patient is encountered in the emergency room, the clinician must consider a toxic organic reaction and order a toxic screen. Other considerations such as pesticide or solvent poisoning are less likely but should be considered. Among hospital and emergency room patients, a very common cause of delirium is prescribed medications. The importance of taking a thorough medication history cannot be overemphasized. For hospitalized patients who become delirious, correlation of behavior with medication administration or discontinuation can be helpful in sorting through a difficult case.

Critical Items (I WATCH DEATH)

Space limitations in this text preclude a complete discussion of each category contained within the *I WATCH DEATH* mnemonic. Table 11–2 lists many of the insults that can cause delirium. Because the list is lengthy, it may be helpful for the clinician to carry a card containing the entire differential diagnosis of delirium.

MAKING THE DIAGNOSIS OF DELIRIUM

Regardless of the suspected diagnosis, the neuropsychiatric evaluation of a patient follows a particular generic process (Table 11–3). In addition to the usual mental status examination, the examiner should, at a minimum, test for construction praxis (Figure 11–2), writing ability, and the ability to name objects. If a delirium is present, every effort should be made to identify the specific etiology (etiologies). Fran-

Table 11–2.   Differential diagnosis for delirium: critical items (I WATCH DEATH)

Infectious	Encephalitis, meningitis, and syphilis
Withdrawal	Alcohol, barbiturates, sedative-hypnotics
Acute metabolic	Acidosis, alkalosis, electrolyte disturbance, hepatic failure, and renal failure
Trauma	Heat stroke, postoperative, and severe burns
CNS pathology	Abscesses, hemorrhage, normal pressure hydrocephalus, seizures, stroke, tumors, and vasculitis
Hypoxia	Anemia, carbon monoxide poisoning, hypotension, and pulmonary or cardiac failure
Deficiencies	Vitamin B_{12}, niacin, and thiamine and hypovitaminosis
Endocrinopathies	Hyper- or hypoadrenocorticism and hyper- or hypoglycemia
Acute vascular	Hypertensive encephalopathy and shock
Toxins or drugs	Medications, pesticides, and solvents
Heavy metals	Lead, manganese, and mercury

cis et al. (1990) noted that 56% of delirious patients had a single definite or probable etiology and the remaining 44% had an average of 2.8 etiologies per patient.

The gold standard for diagnosis is the clinical evaluation, and the most useful diagnostic laboratory measure is the EEG. The Mini-Mental State Exam (MMSE; Folstein et al. 1975) is a screening tool for organicity and is also used to follow the patient's clinical course serially. A score on the MMSE of 24 or less out of 30 indicates cognitive impairment in a patient who has at least an eighth grade education and a good understanding of English. The major problem with the MMSE is its lack of sensitivity (i.e., high rate of false negatives). The Delirium Rating Scale (DRS; Trzepacz et al. 1988) and the Confusion Assessment Method (CAM; Inouye et al. 1990) are two recently developed tests. Both tests translate DSM-III-R diagnostic criteria for delirium into an assessment instrument.

The laboratory evaluation of a delirious patient can be conceptualized as having two levels. The basic laboratory battery will be ordered in virtually every patient with a diagnosis of delirium. When information concerning the patient's mental and physical status is combined with the basic laboratory battery, the specific etiology (etiolo-

---

Table 11–3.   Neuropsychiatric evaluation of the patient

Mental status
   Interview (assess level of consciousness, psychomotor activity, appearance, affect, mood, intellect, and thought processes)
   Performing tests (memory, concentration, reasoning, motor and constructional apraxia, dysgraphia, and dysnomia)

Physical status
   Brief neurological exam (reflexes, limb strength, Babinski reflex, cranial nerves, meningeal signs, and gait)
   Review past and present vital signs (pulse, temperature, blood pressure, and respiration rate)
   Review chart (labs, abnormal behavior noted and if so when it began, medical diagnoses, VDRL, or FTA-ABS+?)
   Review medication records (correlate abnormal behavior with starting or stopping medications)

Laboratory examination—basic
   Blood chemistries (electrolytes, glucose, calcium, albumin, blood urea nitrogen, ammonia [NH_4^+], and liver functions)
   Blood count (hematocrit, white count and differential, mean corpuscular volume, and sedimentation rate)
   Drug levels (need toxic screen? medication blood levels?)
   Arterial blood gases
   Urinalysis
   Electrocardiogram
   Chest X ray

Laboratory examination—based on clinical judgment
   Electroencephalogram (seizures? focal lesion? and confirm delirium)
   Computed tomography (normal pressure hydrocephalus, stroke, and space occupying lesion)
   Additional blood chemistries (heavy metals, thiamine and folate levels, thyroid battery, LE prep, antinuclear antibodies, and urinary porphobilinogen)
   Lumbar puncture (if indication of infection or intracranial bleed)

Note.   FTA-ABS = fluorescent treponemal antibody absorption; VDRL = Venereal Disease Research Laboratory; LE prep = lupus erythematosus prep.

gies) is often apparent. If not, the clinician should review the case and consider ordering further diagnostic studies.

COURSE (PROGNOSIS)

The clinical course of a delirious patient is variable. The possibilities are 1) full recovery, 2) progression to stupor and/or coma, 3) seizures, 4) chronic brain syndromes, 5) death, or 6) *1* through *4* above with associated morbidity (e.g., fracture or subdural hematomas from falls). The majority of patients who experience delirium probably have a full recovery (Lipowski 1990), although the actual probability of this outcome is unknown. Seizures can accompany delirium but are more likely to occur with drug withdrawal, particularly alcohol, and burn encephalopathy (Antoon et al. 1972).

Morbidity

Although there are no direct studies of morbidity in delirium, research does indicate that hospitalization is prolonged (Kay et al. 1956). In one study (Titchener et al. 1956), 38.9% of acute brain syndromes became chronic brain syndromes. Fernandez et al. (1989) found that only 37% of AIDS patients who became delirious had a complete recovery of cognitive function.

Rogers et al. (1989) found that patients who became delirious gained no functional benefit from the surgery (Berggren et al. 1987). Gustafson et al. (1988) found that delirium seemed to be the best predictor of outcome in patients who presented with femoral neck fractures. They reported that delirious patients had longer hospital stays than patients who were not delirious (21.7 days vs. 13.5 days) and were more likely to require walking aids, be bedridden, die, or require rehabilitation. Delirious patients can also pull out intravenous lines, nasogastric tubes, arterial lines, nasopharyngeal tubes, and intra-aortic balloon pumps. Inouye et al. (1989) reported that the risk of complications such as decubiti and aspiration pneumonia was more than six times greater for the delirious elderly patient compared with elderly patients who were not delirious.

Mortality

Most psychiatrists, and physicians in general, underestimate the mortality associated with delirium. Of 77 patients who received a DSM-III diagnosis of delirium from a consultation psychiatrist, 19 (25%) died within 6 months (Trzepacz et al. 1985). A patient diagnosed with delirium during a hospital admission has a 5.5 times greater hospital mortality rate than a patient diagnosed with dementia (Rabins and Folstein 1982). Patients who survive hospitalization have a very high death rate during the months immediately after discharge. Patients with a diagnosis of delirium followed for several months showed a mortality rate equal to that of dementia patients followed for several years (Roth 1955; Varsamis et al. 1972). Cameron et al. (1987) reported that 13 of 20 (65%) delirious patients died during hospitalization.

TREATMENT

Etiologies Known

Because many causes of delirium have specific treatments, the clinician must systematically attempt to establish a diagnosis. For example, without an organized approach to diagnosis, one might attempt to treat the agitation and hallucinations of the patient having DTs with chlorpromazine. This would increase the likelihood of withdrawal seizures.

Etiologies Unknown

Nonspecific treatments can help the patient medically and psychologically through the ordeal of a delirium. These interventions are divided into medical, pharmacological, psychosocial, and environmental categories.

Medical.   In addition to ordering the laboratory tests essential to identify the cause of a delirium, one of the important roles of the neuropsychiatrist is to raise the level of awareness of the medical and nursing staff concerning the morbidity and mortality associated with a delirium. The patient should be placed in a room near the nursing station. Obtaining frequent vital signs is essential. Increased observation of the patient ensures closer monitoring for medical deterioration and for dangerous behaviors, such as trying to crawl over bed rails or pulling out intravenous lines. Fluid input and output must be monitored, and good oxygenation must be ensured. All nonessential medications should be discontinued.

Pharmacological.   There is no consensus in the literature on the pharmacological treatment of delirium when the etiology is unknown. Therefore, we must rely on clinical experience, known properties of drugs (particularly side effects), and anecdotal reports of various treatments. The scenario for pharmacological intervention often involves consultation on an agitated, combative, hallucinating, paranoid, medically ill patient whose behavior is a threat to continuing medical treatment.

Review of the literature and clinical experience indicate that haloperidol is the drug of choice when treating an agitated delirium with an unknown etiology (Lipowski 1980b, 1990). Haloperidol is a potent antipsychotic with virtually no anticholinergic or hypotensive properties, and it can be given parenterally. In fact, intravenous haloperidol has been used in very high doses for many years in seriously ill patients without harmful side effects (Fernandez et al. 1988; Sos and Cassem 1980; Tesar et al. 1985). (Haloperidol is not approved by the Food and Drug Administration for intravenous use.)

Severe refractory agitation has also been controlled with a continuous intravenous infusion of haloperidol (Fernandez et al. 1988). Although extrapyramidal side effects are more likely with the higher-potency antipsychotic drugs, the actual occurrence rate of these side effects in medically ill patients, particularly when using intravenous administration, is strikingly low.

Other antipsychotic medications that have been found useful are thiothixene (Navane) and droperidol (Inapsine). Droperidol, like haloperidol, is a butyrophenone and has comparable antipsychotic potency. Droperidol is approved for intravenous use but is more sedating than haloperidol and has a slight risk of hypotension. In a double-blind study (Resnick and Burton 1984) that compared intramuscular haloperidol to droperidol in actively agitated patients, droperidol appeared to give more rapid relief. Antipsychotic medications that are less potent, such as chlorpromazine and thioridazine, are more likely to cause hypotension and anticholinergic effects.

Benzodiazepines are the drugs of choice in DTs. However, the sedation that accompanies benzodiazepines may further impair the delirious patient's sensorium. Therefore, except in cases of drug-withdrawal states, benzodiazepines are not recommended as a sole agent in the treatment of delirium. Benzodiazepines have been used with success as adjuncts to high-potency neuroleptics like haloperidol (Adams 1984; Garza-Trevino et al. 1989). Intravenous lorazepam, particularly in patients who have not responded to high doses of haloperidol alone, has been found useful.

Psychosocial. The psychological support of a patient both during and after a delirium is important. Having a calm family member remain with the paranoid, agitated patient is reassuring to the patient and can stop mishaps. In lieu of a family member, close supervision by reassuring nursing staff is crucial.

After the delirium has resolved, helping the patient understand the bizarre experience can be therapeutic (MacKenzie and Popkin 1980). An explanation to the family about delirium can reduce anxiety and calm fears. Many patients, if they remember the delirious period, will be reluctant to discuss their experiences. A simple explanation about delirium is usually all that is required to reduce post-traumatic morbidity.

Environmental. Environmental interventions are sometimes helpful but should not be considered as the primary treatment. Both nurses and family members can frequently reorient the patient to date and surroundings. Placing a clock, calendar, and familiar objects in the room may be helpful. Adequate light in the room during the night will usually decrease frightening illusions. A private room for the delirious patient is appropriate only if adequate supervision can be assured. If the patient normally wears eyeglasses or a hearing aid, improving the quality of sensory input by returning these devices may help the patient better understand the surroundings.

A common error occurring on medical and surgical wards is to place delirious patients in the same room. This makes reorientation of these patients impossible and often leads to confirmation, based on conversations with a paranoid roommate, that strange things are indeed happening in the hospital.

CONCLUSIONS

The need for future research into delirium is clear, given its high morbidity, mortality, and cost. Basic questions still need to be answered. Does delirium represent the final common pathway in brain dysfunction? Are hyperactive and hypoactive forms of delirium truly different entities, or is delirium similar to bipolar disorder in its dichotomous clinical presentations? What are the predisposing physiological, personality, emotional, genetic, and environmental factors in the development of a delirium? The resurgence of interest in the neurosciences, neuropsychiatry, and geriatric psychiatry may provide the impetus that is needed to perform this crucial research.

REFERENCES

Aberg T, Ronquist G, Tyden H, et al: Release of adenylate kinase into cerebrospinal fluid during open-heart surgery and its relation to postoperative intellectual function. Lancet 1:1139–1141, 1982

Aberg T, Ronquist G, Tyden H, et al: Adverse effects on the brain in cardiac operations as assessed by biochemical, psychometric, and radiologic methods. J Thorac Cardiovasc Surg 87:99–105, 1984

Adams F: Neuropsychiatric evaluation and treatment of delirium in the critically ill cancer patient. Cancer Bulletin 36:156–160, 1984

Adams RD, Victor M: Principles of Neurology. New York, McGraw-Hill, 1989

American Psychiatric Association: Diagnostic and Statistical Manual of Mental Disorders, 3rd Edition. Washington, DC, American Psychiatric Association, 1980

American Psychiatric Association: Diagnostic and Statistical Manual of Mental Disorders, 3rd Edition, Revised. Washington, DC, American Psychiatric Association, 1987

Andreasen NJC: Neuropsychiatric complications in burn patients. Int J Psychiatry Med 5:161–171, 1974

Andreasen NJC, Noyes R, Hartford C, et al: Management of emotional reactions in seriously burned adults. N Engl J Med 286:65–69, 1972

Anthony JC, LeResche L, Niaz U, et al: Limits of the Mini-Mental State as a screening test for dementia and delirium among hospital patients. Psychol Med 12:397–408, 1982

Antoon AY, Volpe JJ, Crawford JD: Burn encephalopathy in children. Pediatrics 50:609–616, 1972

Berggren D, Gustafson Y, Eriksson B, et al: Postoperative confusion after anesthesia in elderly patients with femoral neck fractures. Anesth Analg 66:497–504, 1987

Blachly PH, Kloster FE: Relation of cardiac output to postcardiotomy delirium. J Thorac Cardiovasc Surg 52:423–427, 1966

Blank K, Perry S: Relationship of psychological processes during delirium to outcome. Am J Psychiatry 141:843–847, 1984

Branthwaite MA: Neurological damage related to open-heart surgery: a clinical survey. Thorax 27:748–753, 1972

Cameron D, Thomas R, Mulvihill M, et al: Delirium: a test of the Diagnostic and Statistical Manual III criteria on medical inpatients. J Am Geriatr Soc 35:1007–1010, 1987

Chedru F, Geschwind N: Writing disturbances in acute confusional states. Neuropsychologia 10:343–353, 1972

Chenoweth DE, Cooper SW, Hugli TE, et al: Complement activation during cardiopulmonary bypass. N Engl J Med 304:497–502, 1981

Cummings J, Benson DF, LoVerme S: Reversible dementia. JAMA 243:2434–2439, 1980

Cummings JL: Acute confusional states, in Clinical Neuropsychiatry. Edited by Cummings JL. New York, Grune & Stratton, 1985, pp 68–74

Dubin WR, Field NL, Gastfriend DR: Postcardiotomy delirium: a critical review. J Thorac Cardiovasc Surg 77:586–594, 1979

Engel GL: Delirium, in Comprehensive Textbook of Psychiatry. Edited by Friedman AM, Kaplan HS. Baltimore, MD, Williams & Wilkins, 1967

Engel GL, Romano J: Delirium, a syndrome of cerebral insufficiency. Journal of Chronic Disease 9:260–277, 1959

Engel GL, Romano J, Ferris EB: Effect of quinacrine (Atabrine) on the central nervous system. Archives of Neurology and Psychiatry 58:337–350, 1947

Fernandez F, Holmes V, Adams F, et al: Treatment of severe, refractory agitation with a haloperidol drip. J Clin Psychiatry 49:239–241, 1988

Fernandez F, Levy J, Mansell P: Management of delirium in terminally ill AIDS patients. Int J Psychiatry Med 19(2):165–172, 1989

Folstein MF, Folstein SE, McHugh PR: Mini-Mental State: a practical method for grading the cognitive state of patients for the clinician. J Psychiatr Res 12:189–198, 1975

Francis J, Martin D, Kapoor W: A prospective study of delirium in hospitalized elderly. JAMA 263:1097–1101, 1990

Garza-Trevino E, Hollister L, Overall J, et al: Efficacy of combinations of intramuscular anti-psychotics and sedative-hypnotics for control of psychotic agitation. Am J Psychiatry 146:1598–1601, 1989

Gustafson Y, Berggren D, Brannstrom B, et al: Acute confusional states in elderly patients treated for femoral neck fracture. J Am Geriatr Soc 36:525–530, 1988

Harrell R, Othmer E: Postcardiotomy confusion and sleep loss. J Clin Psychiatry 48:445–446, 1987

Heller SS, Frank KA, Malm JR, et al: Psychiatric complications of open-heart surgery. N Engl J Med 283:1015–1020, 1970

Inouye S, Horwitz R, Tinetti M, et al: Acute confusional states in the hospitalized elderly: incidence, factors, and complications. Clin Res 37(2):524A, 1989

Inouye S, van Dyck C, Alessi C, et al: Clarifying confusion: the Confusion Assessment Method. Ann Intern Med 113:941–948, 1990

Kay DWK, Norris V, Post F: Prognosis in psychiatric disorders of the elderly. Journal of Mental Science 102:129–140, 1956

Koponen H, Stenback U, Mattila E, et al: Delirium among elderly persons admitted to a psychiatric hospital: clinical course during the acute stage and one-year follow-up. Acta Psychiatr Scand 79:579–585, 1989a

Koponen H, Partanen J, Paakkonen A, et al: EEG spectral analysis in delirium. J Neurol Neurosurg Psychiatry 52:980–985, 1989b

Koponen H, Hurri L, Stenback U, et al: Computed tomography findings in delirium. J Nerv Ment Dis 177:226–231, 1989c

Kornfeld DS, Heller SS, Frank KA, et al: Personality and psychological factors in postcardiotomy delirium. Arch Gen Psychiatry 31:249–253, 1974

Layne OL, Yudofsky SC: Postoperative psychosis in cardiotomy patients: the role of organic and psychiatric factors. N Engl J Med 284:518–520, 1971

Lipowski ZJ: Delirium: Acute Brain Failure in Man. Springfield, IL, Charles C Thomas, 1980a

Lipowski ZJ: Delirium updated. Compr Psychiatry 21:190–196, 1980b

Lipowski ZJ: Delirium: Acute Confusional States. New York, Oxford University Press, 1990

MacKenzie TB, Popkin MK: Stress response syndrome occurring after delirium. Am J Psychiatry 137:1433–1435, 1980

Mesulam M-M: Attention, confusional states, and neglect, in Principles of Behavioral Neurology. Edited by Mesulam M-M. Philadelphia, PA, FA Davis, 1985, pp 125–168

Mori E, Yamadori A: Acute confusional state and acute agitated delirium. Arch Neurol 44:1139–1143, 1987

Nussmeier N, Arlund C, Slogoff S: Neuropsychiatric complications after cardiopulmonary bypass: cerebral protection by a barbiturate. Anesthesiology 64(2):165–170, 1986

Patten S, Lamarre C: Dysgraphia (letter). Can J Psychiatry 34:746, 1989

Perry S: Organic mental disorders caused by HIV: update on early diagnosis and treatment. Am J Psychiatry 147:696–710, 1990

Purdie F, Honigman B, Rosen P: Acute organic brain syndrome: a review of 100 cases. Ann Emerg Med 10:455–461, 1981

Rabins PV, Folstein MF: Delirium and dementia: diagnostic criteria and fatality rates. Br J Psychiatry 140:149–153, 1982

Resnick M, Burton B: Droperidol vs haloperidol in the initial management of acutely agitated patients. J Clin Psychiatry 45:298–299, 1984

Rogers M, Liang M, Daltroy L: Delirium after elective orthopedic surgery: risk factors and natural history. Int J Psychiatry Med 19:109–121, 1989

Romano J, Engel GL: Delirium, I: electroencephalographic data. Archives of Neurology and
    Psychiatry 51:356–377, 1944
Roth M: The natural history of mental disorder in old age. Journal of Mental Science 101:281–
    301, 1955
Smith L, Dimsdale J: Postcardiotomy delirium: conclusions after 25 years? Am J Psychiatry
    146:452–458, 1989
Sos J, Cassem NH: Managing postoperative agitation. Drug Therapy 10(3):103–106, 1980
Task Force Sponsored by the National Institute on Aging: Senility reconsidered. JAMA
    244:259–263, 1980
Tesar GE, Murray GB, Cassem NH: Use of high-dose intravenous haloperidol in the treatment
    of agitated cardiac patients. J Clin Psychopharmacol 5:344–347, 1985
Titchener JL, Swerling I, Gottschalk L, et al: Psychosis in surgical patients. Surg Gynecol
    Obstet 102:59–65, 1956
Trzepacz P, Teague G, Lipowski Z: Delirium and other organic mental disorders in a general
    hospital. Gen Hosp Psychiatry 7:101–106, 1985
Trzepacz P, Baker R, Greenhouse J: A symptom rating scale for delirium. Psychiatry Res 23:89–
    97, 1988
Tune LE, Dainlouh NF, Holland A, et al: Association of postoperative delirium with raised
    serum levels of anticholinergic drugs. Lancet 2:651–653, 1981
Varsamis J, Zuchowski T, Maini KK: Survival rates and causes of death in geriatric psychiatric
    patients: a six-year follow-up study. Canadian Psychiatric Association Journal 17:17–21,
    1972

Chapter 12

Neuropsychiatric Aspects of Aphasia and Related Language Impairments

D. Frank Benson, M.D.

By definition, aphasia is *the loss or impairment of language caused by brain damage. Language,* the key word in the definition, pertains to the ability to handle (decode, encode, and interpret) the symbols used within a cultural group for communication of information, feelings, and thoughts. In most cases, focal structural damage is the source of the impairment.

More than 100,000 Americans acquire aphasia each year, and, because the underlying disorders are often stable, their numbers accumulate over the years. Aphasia represents a numerically prominent and behaviorally significant cause of chronic medical disability. The problems of the aphasic patient encompass the entire spectrum of neuropsychiatry, from the circumscribed effects of focal brain destruction on linguistic processing through emotional and motivational problems based on disordered subcortical networks to the personal predicaments produced by the considerable change in life-style. Unfortunately, little more than sympathy and superficial support have been available for most aphasic patients and their families, and yet the neuropsychiatric complications are often crucial to the well-being and ultimate outcome of the aphasic condition.

HISTORY

With Broca's original description (1861) of a patient who had lost the ability to speak and demonstration that a focal brain injury involved the frontal region, a novel technique—the correlation of clinical behavior with a focal brain defect—became available. Broca's observations were rapidly replicated and a body of clinical and anatomical data developed. Important observations, particularly the dominance of the human left hemisphere for language function (Broca 1865), were established, and after Wernicke (1874) an anterior-posterior dichotomy of language function was solidly demonstrated. Many investigators presented classifications of brain-language correlations. With limited exception, all language functions were localized to the cerebral cortex and were diagrammed in a phrenological, mosaic manner (see Chapter 3).

The early 20th century saw a reaction against the mechanical dictum that a focal brain lesion produces a specific clinical finding. Marie (1906), stating that Broca's original patient was not aphasic, presented a holistic theory of language function. For half a century Marie's thesis of a single aphasia was championed by many investigators. Aphasia was considered the product of a disordered central language area with clinical variation based on damage to surrounding areas carrying out basic functions (e.g., auditory, visual, and motor) (Figure 12–1). Language was considered a single, unitary, nondivisible function.

In the 1960s, with Geschwind's rediscovery and powerful demonstration (1965) that separation (disconnection) of cortical areas could produce distinctive language impairments, the 19th-century localizationist approach was reborn (Figure 12–2). Concomitant with renewed interest in the localizationist approach, the field of neuropsychology expanded, major advances occurred in linguistics (neurolinguistics and psycholinguistics), and cognitive science was born.

Terminology and Classification

The study of aphasia has been plagued by terms invented to describe variations in language disorder. Head (1926) described the situation as "chaos," then compounded the problem with a totally different classification using elementary linguistic terminology. Others solved the classification problem by declaring that all aphasia represented a single, holistic entity, but this approach proved inadequate.

More recently, reintroduction, augmentation, and clarification of the 19th-century classification efforts, primarily through the work of the Boston Aphasia Group, has established a practical classification with consistent terms based on clini-

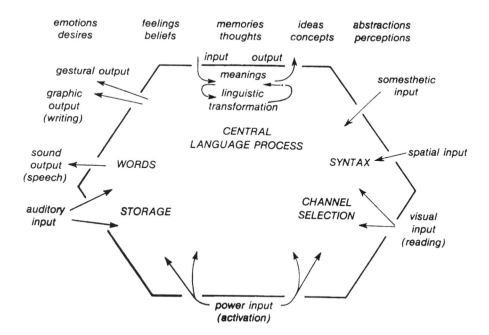

Figure 12–1. Hypothetical model of cerebral mechanisms of speech—attributed to J. R. Brown.
Source. Reprinted from Maruszewski M: *Language, Communication and the Brain.* The Hague, Netherlands, Mouton, 1975. Used with permission.

cal and anatomical correlates that provided a stable structure for later investigations (Benson and Geschwind 1971). Table 12–1 presents an abridged version of this classification with the major language abnormalities, basic neurological dysfunctions, and characteristic anatomical findings associated with each syndrome. Detailed descriptions are available in some neurological textbooks and in a number of texts dedicated to aphasiology and behavioral neurology (Benson 1979; Heilman and Valenstein 1979; Kertesz 1979; Kirshner 1986; Lecours et al. 1983; Mesulam 1985.)

The entities outlined in Table 12–1 are syndromes, not disease entities. A *syndrome* is a collection of clinical findings that, when occurring together, suggest a specific disorder to a physician. A syndrome is not fixed and does not have constant constituents. All aphasic patients vary in symptom presentation, and yet, for most of them, one syndrome better describes the clinical status than do the others. The syndromes of aphasia were invented by 19th-century investigators on the basis of postmortem correlations. Contemporary neurologists have both supported and corrected the early observations linking brain damage locus to specific language syndromes (Alexander and Benson 1991; Kertesz 1979). The original syndrome classification of aphasia was upheld and strengthened by the introduction of new brain-imaging techniques; it remains the gold standard for aphasia deliberations.

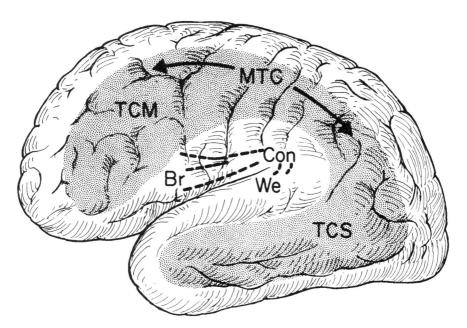

Figure 12–2. Outline of left lateral hemisphere outlining central (*clear,* perisylvian) and outer, border zone language areas (*stippled*). The letters indicate most common situation of structural pathology in the syndromes of aphasia. Br = Broca's area; We = Wernicke's area; Con = supramarginal gyrus-conduction aphasia; TCM, TCS, and MTC demarcate areas most involved in cases of transcortical motor, transcortical sensory, and mixed transcortical aphasias, respectively.
Source. Reprinted from Benson DF, Geschwind N: "The Aphasias and Related Disturbances," in *Clinical Neurology,* Vol 1. Edited by Baker AB, Joynt R. Philadelphia, PA, Harper & Row, 1985, Chapter 10, pp. 1–34. Used with permission.

Table 12–1. Aphasia syndromes

| Syndrome | Major language characteristics | | | | | | Major neurological characteristics | | | Site of pathology (dominant hemisphere) |
	Spontaneous speech	Repetition	Comprehension	Naming	Reading	Writing	Motor	Sensory	Visual field	
Broca	NF	0	+	±	0	0	0	±	++	Posterior inferior frontal lobe
Wernicke	F, P	0	0	0	0	0	++	±	±	Posterior superior temporal lobe
Conduction	F, P	0	++	±	+	±	+	±	+	Deep to supramarginal gyrus
Global	NF	0	0	0	0	0	0	0	0	Combinations of above three
Transcortical motor	NF	+	++	±	+	0	0	+	++	Frontal, anterior, or superior to Broca's area
Transcortical sensory	F	+	0	0	0	0	+	0	0	Parietal-temporal junction
Transcortical mixed	NF	+	0	0	0	0	0	0	0	Combination of above two
Anomic	F	+	+	0	±	±	±	±	±	Multiple sites
Subcortical	F, P, or NF, P	+	±	±	±	±	±	±	±	Putamen and thalamus

Note. NF = nonfluent; F = fluent; P = paraphasic; ++ = normal; + = relatively normal; ± = variable; 0 = abnormal.
Source. Reprinted from Benson DF: "Aphasia Management: The Neurologist's Role," in *Seminars in Speech, Language and Hearing,* Vol 2. Edited by Wertz RT. New York, Thieme-Stratton, 1981, pp. 237–247. Used with permission.

Syndromes of Aphasia

Broca's aphasia. The best known syndrome of language impairment—Broca's aphasia—shows strikingly nonfluent verbal output (sparse, effortful, dysarthric, dysprosodic, short-phrase length, and agrammatic) with relatively preserved comprehension (relational words may be poorly understood), distinct disturbance in repetition and naming, usually a disturbance in reading and writing. Most patients with Broca's aphasia have right-sided weakness and some have mild sensory loss. Pathology involves the dominant hemisphere frontal opercular area. If the lesion is superficial, the prognosis for improvement is good; if the lesion is sufficiently deep to involve the basal ganglia and internal capsule, the language defect tends to be permanent.

Wernicke's aphasia. Wernicke's aphasia features a fluent verbal output with normal word count and phrase length; no effort, articulatory problems, or prosodic difficulties; but difficulty in word finding and frequent paraphasic substitutions. Wernicke's aphasia is a disturbance of comprehension, ranging from total word deafness to partial difficulty in understanding. Often there are no basic neurological defects, but a superior quadrantopia may be present. Pathology involves the dominant posterior superior temporal lobe.

Conduction aphasia. Conduction aphasia features fluent verbal output and good ability to comprehend, but severe disturbance in repetition. Paraphasias are common, particularly substitutions of phonemes. Naming tends to be limited by paraphasic intrusions. Reading aloud is severely disturbed, but reading comprehension may be normal. Writing is often abnormal. Most cases have pathology involving anterior inferior parietal lobe (supramarginal gyrus) (Damasio and Damasio 1980). Paresis and visual field defects are variable, but cortical sensory loss is frequently present.

Global aphasia. In global aphasia, all language modalities—verbal output, comprehension, repetition, naming, reading, and writing—are seriously impaired. Most often this condition is caused by a total middle cerebral artery occlusion.

Transcortical aphasias. The major factor underlying the transcortical aphasias is preservation of the ability to repeat spoken language in the face of distinct language impairment. *Transcortical motor aphasia* resembles Broca's aphasia except for near-normal ability to repeat. Pathology is most frequently seen in the supplementary motor area of the dominant hemisphere or in the frontal tissues between that region and the dominant hemisphere opercular area. *Transcortical sensory aphasia* features significant comprehension disorder, fluent paraphasic verbal output, and good ability to repeat. Pathology is in the dominant parietal region (angular gyrus). *Mixed transcortical aphasia (isolation of the speech area)* combines motor and sensory forms: the patient has a global aphasia except for preservation of the ability to repeat. Pathology in the mixed transcortical syndrome involves the vascular border zone area in both the frontal and parietal lobes.

Anomic aphasia. In this syndrome the primary problem concerns difficulty with word finding causing multiple pauses, a tendency to circumlocution, and stumbling verbal output. Verbal output is fluent with repetition and comprehension relatively intact, but naming to confrontation is disturbed. There is no specific location for pathology.

Subcortical aphasia.   Although computed tomography (CT) scans demonstrate that subcortical lesions (hemorrhage or infarction) can produce aphasia, symptomatology varies considerably depending on the structures involved. Most subcortical aphasias are initiated by mutism followed by abnormal motor speech (hypophonia and articulatory problems), with either fluent or nonfluent output with many paraphasias. Repetition is near normal (without paraphasia); comprehension, naming, reading, and writing may or may not show abnormality. If the lesion is entirely subcortical, recovery is good. If there is concomitant cortical involvement, aphasia may persist.

In addition, several disturbances affecting communication can result from right-hemisphere damage. Two of these produce psychiatrically significant symptomatology: amelodia and verbal dysdecorum.

Amelodia (affective motor aprosodia) is characterized by a flat, monotonous verbal output; inability to produce a melody when singing; decreased facial grimacing; and sparse use of gestures. This emotionless response is easily misinterpreted as depression. Pathology involves the right frontal opercular area or its connections, the right-hemisphere equivalent of Broca's area. The causative lesion may be small and otherwise silent.

Verbal dysdecorum features decreased ability to monitor and control verbal output. Individuals speak too freely, discuss improper topics, and make snide or cruel (but often true) remarks about themselves and others without realizing the social consequences. The presenting complaint is an inability to maintain friendships; even a short exposure to such an individual identifies the problem. Current evidence suggests a right-hemisphere frontal, probably lateral convexity, site of pathology (Alexander et al. 1989).

NEUROPSYCHIATRIC ASPECTS OF APHASIA

Since aphasia is obviously "organic," not psychogenic, aphasic patients have been largely excluded from the "talk therapy" approach of 20th-century psychiatry, and aphasia has been largely ignored by psychiatrists. Psychological considerations, however, often prove crucial to the outcome of aphasia rehabilitation and are almost invariably significant in long-term care. Some problems are general *(psychosocial)*; others are directly related to the type of aphasia (neurobehavioral).

Psychosocial Aspects

Altered life-style.   An important but easily overlooked factor that affects most individuals with acquired aphasia stems from the sudden, unexpected, and truly calamitous alteration of life-style produced by the language disorder. Employment status, social and family position, recreational opportunities, and physical and sexual status are all threatened. The sudden onset of aphasia is catastrophic, and the acute change in life-style caused by the disorder produces massive psychosocial problems.

Threatened economic status.   Aphasia often occurs at an age when a person's earning capacity is near its prime. Although medical and disability insurance, family savings, and other sources of income may be available, the awareness that economic independence is permanently lost can be a crushing blow. Financial problems themselves may become a serious psychological threat.

Social position.   Most aphasic individuals have well-established relationships with co-workers, employees, neighbors, social and recreational associates, and others in their social community. This status changes abruptly with the onset of aphasia. Even if it takes the individual some time to recognize them, changes in social position produced by the disorder represents an important psychosocial vexation.

Family position.   Alteration of family position affects most aphasic individuals and represents a significant behavioral factor. Most individuals who become aphasic have developed a stable role in a family setting. If the language disturbance is severe, the spouse or some other family member must assume much of the leadership and decision making. Aphasia can place an individual in a passive, childlike position within the family. Reaction to this downgrading can be violent, with negative, hostile, paranoid, and downright cruel behavior directed toward family members. The spouse also may feel and express anger because of decreased income, altered social position, and added responsibilities.

Physical status.   Some aphasic individuals suffer significant alterations in physical capability. A previously active, self-caring individual may become hemiparetic, must learn to stand and to walk again, and can never again hope to participate freely in physical activities such as athletics, dancing, hiking, or even just walking. Balance insecurity, visual field defect, unilateral attention disorder, paresthesias, vague or not-so-vague pain, epileptic seizures, and many other physical problems plague the aphasic patient. Physical disability produces a significant psychological distress that affects self-esteem.

Recreational status.   Physical disability, communication problems, concern for underlying disease processes, and similar problems force most aphasic individuals to change their established recreational patterns. Demanding physical activities (e.g., hiking, swimming, tennis, and bowling) may be precluded by physical problems; less demanding activities (e.g., card games, reading, and going to parties) may not be possible or enjoyable because of communication disability. For a normally active adult, the physical limitations of the postaphasic state produce aggravating adjustment problems.

Sexual status.   Aphasia-producing pathology does not, by itself, affect sexual competency in most individuals. Nonetheless, a major degree of paralysis, an inability to communicate accurately, and an underlying uncertainty of residual sexual competency hinder healthy sexual relationships. Although lack of sexuality is usually physiologically unfounded, the spouse may refuse to partake in sexual activities based on fear of causing additional brain damage. Sexual maladjustment may be a significant problem and is routinely overlooked by most physicians and therapists.

Neurobehavioral Aspects

Early neurobehavioral alterations. The patient with aphasia is often lethargic and/or confused in the early post-onset stage. A prolonged period ensues in which the patient fails to fully realize the situation. A combination of decreased mental functioning (clouding of consciousness) and disturbed language decoding capability (comprehension defect) is present.

After a few days or weeks, the clouding of consciousness clears, leaving an alert patient who remains unaware of the full extent of the problem. The patient cannot participate rationally in plans for the future because of decreased reality appreciation. In some patients, particularly those with large posterior dominant-hemisphere lesions, disturbed language comprehension is long lasting, but for most the realization problem disappears, which can lead directly into a reactive depression. Reactive depression never becomes serious for many aphasic patients, but some do develop a characteristic depression featuring intense feelings of personal worthlessness and hopelessness. Feelings of self-deprecation may lead to a severe dysphoria.

As a rule, depression does not develop immediately, but builds over a variable period after onset of aphasia. The reaction typically starts with feelings of futility that lead to an unwillingness to participate in self-care or rehabilitation. Withdrawal and negativism are the key features. In rare instances the negative reaction becomes catastrophic, and the patient may cry and moan for hours, forcefully avoid attention, refuse to eat or take medications, and actively fight off therapists, attendants, and family.

The onset of a reactive depression should immediately be followed by strong, radical support measures. Challenging therapies (e.g., language, occupational, and physical) should be replaced by activities the patient can perform successfully. Critical to treatment are early recognition and prompt response. Hospital personnel and family members should take countermeasures at the first sign of negativism, withdrawal, poor appetite, or other signs of depression. Language therapy should be continued, with an emphasis on positive language competency. Similar approaches are appropriate for physical and occupational therapy. Reactive depression is best controlled by intelligent manipulation since it is self-limited and generally runs its course in a few days. Antidepressant medications are rarely necessary. Despite its morbid appearance, reactive depression is a healthy sign because it indicates sufficient recovery of intellectual competency, allowing for recognition of the severity of the problem and paving the way for more problem-oriented rehabilitation measures.

Long-term neurobehavioral complications. Two distinct and powerful behavioral reactions can be correlated with the anatomical locus of pathology. One accompanies nonfluent (anterior) aphasia, the other fluent (posterior) aphasia (Benson 1973).

The *anterior aphasia behavioral reaction* is definitive with time. With time, most nonfluent aphasic individuals become aware of their new problems. They know what they wish to say, but their output is restricted and barely intelligible. Unable to explain their wishes or thoughts, they experience both frustration and depression. This depression can extend well beyond a time-limited reactive depression and represents a serious problem. Suicide intentions suggested by aphasic patients must be accepted as real possibilities.

Recognition and appropriate alteration of management can combat the depression of anterior aphasia. Careful monitoring is needed, and suicide precautions may become necessary. Institution of appropriate antidepressant medication may be of value. The depression of nonfluent aphasia deserves the comprehensive management given to stroke patients with left frontal pathology (Robinson and Chait 1985).

Depression is far more common in anterior than posterior aphasia (Robinson and Benson 1981). This can be explained by the patient's ability to recognize the disability, the frustration of not being able to express thoughts and desires, and the realization that this frustrating status may continue indefinitely. Robinson and Szetela (1981) demonstrated a correlation between the anatomical locus of brain damage and depression in stroke patients; the more anterior a left cerebral infarct extends, the more likely the patient is to suffer significant depression. Robinson et al. (1975) suggested damage to dopamine and/or norepinephrine channels as the cause of the depression. Whether explained neurochemically or psychodynamically, the increased frequency of depression in left anterior stroke patients must be considered in their care.

Patients with *posterior aphasia* (fluent aphasia), on the other hand, typically have difficulty comprehending spoken language and are frequently unaware of the deficit, producing an unconcern that is pathological. Unaware of their own comprehension disturbance, these individuals tend to blame their communication difficulties on others. Some believe that persons they observe talking together must be using a special code because their conversation cannot be understood. Placing blame outside the self is a paranoid reaction, not unlike the well-recognized paranoia of acquired deafness. Some posterior aphasia patients display impulsive behavior which makes them potentially dangerous, both to themselves and others. Almost all aphasic patients who need custodial management because of dangerous behavior have a posterior, fluent aphasia (Benson and Geschwind 1971).

The cause of behavior typical of posterior aphasia remains conjectural. Impulsive paranoid behavior is particularly common when the left temporal lobe is involved. A psychodynamic interpretation would stress that the unawareness of disability accounts for the tendency to place blame for the problem on others. A neurological interpretation would suggest that damage to the left temporal tissues decreases behavioral control, complicating the language comprehension problem.

Suicide.   A potential complication of aphasia is suicide. The depression, frustration, and catastrophic reaction of the patient with anterior aphasia suggest a strong potential for suicide, but suicide is rarely reported in this group. It occurs more often among patients with posterior aphasia, particularly when they are paranoid and impulsive. Treatment of potential suicide in posterior aphasia patients is extremely difficult because their aphasia precludes traditional psychotherapy measures. Standard precautions should be taken (e.g., removal of self-destructive devices, careful monitoring of activities, transfer to a more secure situation). Efforts should be made to establish and/or maintain interpersonal relationships and minimize frustration.

Legal Aspects

Intelligence in aphasia.   The psychiatrist may be asked to give expert opinion concerning the mental competency of an individual with aphasia. Whether an aphasic

patient retains sufficient intelligence for personal decision making to warrant investment in a long-term rehabilitation program has produced considerable disagreement.
Following Bastian (1898), who stated, "We think in words," many experts emphasize
the symbolic nature of language and declare that defective use of language symbols
produces defective thinking. However, although most aphasic individuals perform
poorly on standard tests of intellectual competency, many retain considerable nonverbal capability. Numerous studies to determine intelligence in aphasia have been attempted but, at best, provide nebulous results (Basso et al. 1981; Lebrun 1974;
Zangwill 1964). Most studies treat aphasia as a single, unitary disturbance, failing to
note that intellectual dysfunction varies considerably with the neuroanatomical locus
of damage. Posterior language area pathology is more likely to interfere with intellectual competency than is anterior damage (Benson 1979).

Most aphasic patients are severely penalized by the verbal nature of intelligence
tests. Standard IQ tests tend to exaggerate any intellectual disorder that may be present. Tests that are used to define the concept of intelligence are more likely to indicate
defective intelligence. However, if the test equates intelligence with thought processing or other performance capabilities, aphasic patients may perform in the normal
range. The examiner must base a decision concerning the intelligence of an aphasic
patient on observations as test results alone are not competent. Important information
such as the retention of social graces; counting; making change; exhibiting appropriate concern about family, business, and personal activities; finding the way about;
socializing; and showing self-concern provide valuable indications of residual intelligence in the individual with aphasia.

Legal competency. Determination of whether an aphasic patient is sufficiently
sound mentally to sign checks or business papers, to dispense money, to manage property or other holdings, to make a will or other testamentary documents, and so on often
hinges on informed medical opinion. Many aphasic patients can manage their own
affairs whereas others are obviously unable to make decisions and deserve the protection of a conservator or a guardian, a status that demands medical opinion. An intermediate group is seriously disabled but can make decisions with appropriate
assistance.

If a legal act—such as signing a will or entering into a contract—is to be performed by an aphasic patient, a physician should evaluate and carefully record the
patient's ability to comprehend both spoken and written language and to express
personal decisions. The document should be reviewed with an attorney present until
both the physician and attorney are satisfied that the patient understands the basic
meaning. The document should be kept short, simple, and as free of legal jargon as
possible.

An even more difficult problem arises when a physician is asked to provide retrospective testimony about an aphasic patient's legal competency. Since the
physician's testimony can relate only to observations of the patient's mental and language capabilities recorded at or near the time of the signing of the document, it may
not be possible to present a firm opinion of mental competency. The final decision
ultimately depends on whether the document reflects the patient's wishes at the time
of signing; this is a legal decision based on testimony from individuals dealing with
the patient at the time.

TREATMENT

In the past several decades neurological rehabilitation has become standardized and disciplined. Many different treatment modalities are available which can influence behavior. Some aphasic patients need considerable physical therapy, gait training, and/or mechanical aids such as crutches and leg braces; most need occupational therapy, particularly instruction and training in daily living activities. Two primary approaches to the treatment of neuropsychiatric complications are in use: pharmacological management and traditional psychotherapy.

Pharmaceutical Approach

The entire panoply of pharmaceuticals currently used by psychiatrists may find use in aphasia. Antidepressant medications are often used, particularly in patients with left anterior lesions. The risk of adrenergic or anticholinergic side effects with antidepressants demands concern.

Tranquilizers also may be helpful. Benzodiazepines may help control anxiety and/or hyperactivity, but their addicting qualities and potential suppression of learning ability (amnesia) demand caution; they are not frequently used in aphasic patients. Psychotropic medications (e.g., phenothiazines and butyrophenones) are useful, particularly with patients with posterior aphasia who have impulsive, paranoid behavior. Patients treated with these medications appear less agitated and are more compliant. Dosage should be kept low to avoid interference with residual mental functions. Stimulants are infrequently used but may be appropriate in selected cases. When brain damage causes apathy, lethargy, and decreased drive, judicious use of a stimulant such as methylphenidate may be beneficial.

Crucial to the pharmaceutical treatment of psychiatric complications of aphasia is the possibility of adverse reactions or cross-reactions. Many patients with aphasia are being treated for conditions such as heart failure, arrhythmia, and hypertension. Some are treated with anticoagulants, and many take aspirin as antiembolus therapy. Some have more esoteric problems such as liver or renal failure, collagen disorder, arteritis, brain tumor, and pulmonary insufficiency; all are likely to be treated with potent medications. The neuropsychiatrist asked to evaluate and treat a patient with aphasia must be aware of the medications and the potential complications of these or additional pharmaceuticals.

In general, drugs should be recognized as adjuncts to more formal rehabilitation measures, not as primary treatment modalities. Judicious use of pharmaceutical products can be rewarding in treatment of psychiatric complications of aphasia.

Psychotherapy Approach

Despite the language disturbance, many forms of psychotherapy can help aphasic patients. Group psychotherapy can be attempted if the group is made up of individuals with similar language disorders and stresses practice of language skills. Inclusion with other individuals with a similar disturbance can provide psychic assurance and decrease feelings of isolation. Seeing the improving status of members of the group offers hope and seeing one's own status becoming better in comparison with others provides encouragement.

Family members can be a valuable asset for psychotherapy in aphasia. An intelligent, well-motivated spouse or child can provide mental support and encouragement. Unfortunately, the opposite (disturbed family members) can pose a problem. Not infrequently the spouse or children are sufficiently upset by the patient's aphasia to represent a serious negative influence. Family counseling, distancing of certain family members from the patient, and/or suggestion for their own psychiatric care may be needed.

Finally, attention should be given to the position of the language therapist in psychotherapy. The aphasic patient gets considerable emotional support by working with a person who understands aphasia and is dedicated to the improvement of the patient's language deficit. A positive transference between the patient with aphasia and the therapist can be used therapeutically. Most language therapists are neither trained nor experienced in psychiatric management; they need coaching and encouragement to maintain treatment of a psychiatrically disturbed patient. Many language therapists attempt to "dump" a disturbed patient into the psychiatrist's lap, correctly claiming that the patient's psychiatric problems obviate good language rehabilitation. It should be recognized, however, that the professional best capable of dealing with the aphasic patient is one trained in language disorders. Whenever possible, the bulk of psychotherapy provided to an aphasic patient should be performed by the language therapist.

CONCLUSIONS

The aphasic patient often suffers significant psychiatric complications, based on both damage to the brain and altered personal status. The complications hamper rehabilitation and may produce significant behavioral problems. Formulation of a rational treatment demands understanding of both the neurological and the psychological aspects, the realm of the neuropsychiatrist.

REFERENCES

Alexander MP, Benson DF: The aphasias and related disturbances, in Clinical Neurology, Vol 1. Edited by Joynt R. Philadelphia, PA, JB Lippincott, 1991, Chapter 10, pp 1–58

Alexander MP, Benson DF, Stuss DT: Frontal lobes and language. Brain Lang 37:643–691, 1989

Basso A, Capitani E, Luzzatti C, et al: Intelligence and left hemisphere disease: role of aphasia, apraxia and size of lesion. Brain 104:721–734, 1981

Bastian HC: Aphasia and Other Speech Defects. London, HK Lewis, 1898

Benson DF: Psychiatric aspects of aphasia. Br J Psychiatry 123:555–566, 1973

Benson DF: Aphasia, Alexia, and Agraphia. New York, Churchill Livingstone, 1979

Benson DF: Aphasia management: the neurologist's role, in Seminars in Speech, Language and Hearing, Vol 2. Edited by Wertz RT. New York, Thieme-Stratton, 1981, pp 237–247

Benson DF, Geschwind N: The aphasias and related disturbances, in Clinical Neurology. Edited by Baker AB, Baker LH. New York, Harper & Row, 1971, Chapter 8, pp 1–33

Benson DF, Geschwind N: The aphasias and related disturbances, in Clinical Neurology, Vol 1. Edited by Baker AB, Joynt R. Philadelphia, PA, Harper & Row, 1985, Chapter 10, pp 1–34

Broca P: Remarques sur le siège de la faculté du langage articulé, suivies d'une observation d'aphemie. Bulletin-Societé Anatomique de Paris 2:330–357, 1861

Broca P: Sur la faculté du langage articulé. Bulletin Societé Anthropologie 6:337–393, 1865

Damasio H, Damasio A: The anatomical basis of conduction aphasia. Brain 103:337–350, 1980

Geschwind N: Disconnexion syndromes in animals and man. Brain 88:237–294, 585–644, 1965

Head H: Aphasia and Kindred Disorders of Speech, Vols I and II (1926). New York, Hafner, 1963

Heilman KM, Valenstein E (eds): Clinical Neuropsychology. New York, Oxford University Press, 1979

Kertesz A: Aphasia and Associated Disorders. New York, Grune & Stratton, 1979

Kirshner HS: Behavioral Neurology: A Practical Approach. New York, Churchill Livingstone, 1986

Lebrun Y: Intelligence and Aphasia. Amsterdam, Swets and Zeitlinger, 1974

Lecours AR, Lhermitte F, Bryans B (eds): Aphasiology. London, Bailliere-Tindall, 1983

Marie P: Revision de la question de l'aphasie. Semaine Médicale 26:241–247, 493–500, 565–571, 1906

Maruszewski M: Language, Communication and the Brain. The Hague, Netherlands, Mouton, 1975

Mesulam M-M: Principles of Behavioral Neurology. Philadelphia, PA, FA Davis, 1985

Robinson RG, Benson DF: Depression in aphasic patients: frequency, severity, and clinical-pathological correlations. Brain Lang 14:282–291, 1981

Robinson RG, Chait RM: Emotional correlates of structural brain injury with particular emphasis on post-stroke mood disorders. CRC Critical Review of Clinical Neurobiology 4:285–318, 1985

Robinson R, Szetela B: Mood change following left hemisphere brain injury. Ann Neurol 9:447–453, 1981

Robinson RG, Shoemaker WJ, Schlumpf M, et al: Effect of experimental cerebral infarction in rat brain: effect on catecholamines and behavior. Nature 255:332–334, 1975

Wernicke C: Das Aphasiche Symptomenkomplex. Breslau, Cohn and Weigart, 1874

Zangwill OL: Intelligence in aphasia, in Disorders of Language. Edited by De Reuck AV, O'Connor M. Boston, Little, Brown, 1964, pp 261–274

Chapter 13

Neuropsychiatric Aspects of Memory and Amnesia

Arthur P. Shimamura, Ph.D.
Felicia B. Gershberg, Sc.B.

Advances in our understanding of brain organization and memory have come from many diverse fields, including neuroanatomy, physiology, behavioral neurology, biological psychiatry, neuropsychology, and cognitive science. In this chapter we review some of these recent advances. In the first section we review neurobehavioral findings concerning the "amnestic syndrome" and describe how these findings contribute to our understanding of normal memory functions. In the second section we highlight advances in neuroanatomical, physiological, and biochemical approaches and describe biological mechanisms that mediate memory functions.

THE AMNESTIC SYNDROME

Memory and the Hippocampus

Across a lifetime, we retain and recollect a plethora of memories, many of which have been held for more than several decades. How does the brain accomplish such extraordinary feats of learning and remembering? An important clue to this process was discovered serendipitously with the investigation of patient H.M., who in 1953 underwent surgery for relief of severe epilepsy (Scoville and Milner 1957). The surgery involved bilateral excision of the medial temporal region, which reportedly included removal of the uncus (including the amygdala), anterior two-thirds of the hippocampus, and hippocampal gyrus (Figure 13–1).

After surgery, H.M. exhibited a profound *anterograde amnesia* (i.e., he was unable to remember events and information encountered since his operation) (Corkin 1984; Milner 1959; Milner et al. 1968). Despite this severe impairment in new learning ability, there was no detectable impairment in intellectual or language abilities. There was some *retrograde amnesia,* which refers to impairment of memory for events that occurred before the onset of amnesia. For example, H.M. could not recognize previously familiar members of the medical staff nor could he remember the

This work was supported by a Biomedical Research Support Grant (No. 89-6-82), a National Institute on Aging Grant (AG-09055), and a National Science Foundation Predoctoral Fellowship (to F. B. Gershberg).

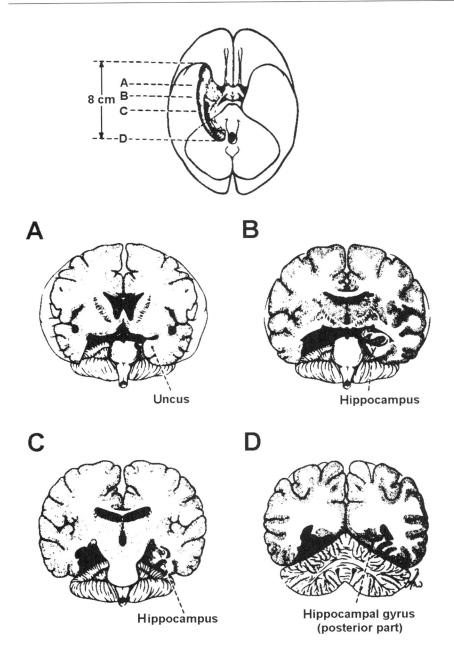

Figure 13–1. Diagram of the extent of tissue removal in the bilateral medial temporal lobe surgery of patient. Surgery included removal of anterior two-thirds of the hippocampus, uncus (including the amygdala), and hippocampal gyrus. Lesioned area is indicated by the darkened region in the area of the left medial temporal lobe of each orbital view, although actual lesion was bilateral.

Source. Reprinted from Milner B: "The Memory Defect in Bilateral Hippocampal Lesions." *Psychiatric Research Reports* 11:43–52, 1959. Used with permission.

layout of the hospital ward, which was also familiar to him before surgery. However, H.M.'s retrograde amnesia was not severe, as indicated by the fact that he performed as well as control subjects on a test of memory for faces of celebrities who became famous before 1950 (Marslen-Wilson and Teuber 1975).

The central feature of H.M.'s memory disorder was new learning impairment, which affects information received from all sensory modalities and includes impairment of both verbal and nonverbal memory. For example, H.M. exhibited severe impairment on tests of word and picture recall, paired-associate learning, and recognition memory. In conjunction with these findings from psychometric tests, clinical observations of H.M. indicated that memory for ongoing events was severely impaired. For example, 30 minutes after eating lunch, H.M. could not recall what he had eaten or whether he had even had lunch. H.M. was aware of his disorder and reflected on his impairment as always "waking from a dream."

Despite the severity of his amnesia, H.M. could think and act normally, as indicated by his preserved IQ. Indeed, even some memory functions were spared, such as *immediate memory,* which is exemplified by intact performance on tests of digit span. Nevertheless, as soon as information is out of conscious experience, it is forgotten. The analysis of H.M.'s amnesia stands as a milestone in our progress to understanding memory in the brain. He provided the crucial evidence for the specific role of the medial temporal region in the process of memory formation and storage. Indeed, the analysis of H.M. by Milner and colleagues provided the impetus for thousands of animal studies on the role of the hippocampus in learning and memory.

Other neurological disorders can produce an amnestic syndrome similar to that seen in patient H.M. The DSM-III-R diagnostic criteria (American Psychiatric Association 1987) for this syndrome are shown in Table 13–1. The diagnostic criteria define anterograde amnesia as impairment of "short-term" memory and retrograde amnesia as impairment of "long-term" memory. (These terms are avoided here so as not to confuse readers familiar with the way in which psychologists and neuroscientists use the terms "short-term memory," which refers to memory that lasts for seconds, and "long-term memory," which refers to memory that lasts beyond the span of short-term or immediate memory.)

Table 13–1. DSM-III-R diagnostic criteria for amnestic syndrome

---

A. Demonstrable evidence of impairment in both short- and long-term memory; with regard to long-term memory, very remote events are remembered better than more recent events. Impairment in short-term memory (inability to learn new information) may be indicated by inability to remember three objects after five minutes. Long-term memory impairment (inability to remember information that was known in the past) may be indicated by inability to remember past personal information (e.g., what happened yesterday, birthplace, occupation) or facts of common knowledge (e.g., past presidents, well-known dates).

B. Not occurring exclusively during the course of delirium, and does not meet the criteria for dementia (i.e., no impairment in abstract thinking or judgment, no other disturbances of higher cortical function, and no personality change).

C. There is evidence from the history, physical examination, or laboratory tests of a specific organic factor (or factors) judged to be etiologically related to the disturbance.

Source. Reprinted from American Psychiatric Association: Diagnostic and Statistical Manual of Mental Disorders, 3rd Edition, Revised. Washington, DC, American Psychiatric Association, 1987, p 109. Used with permission.

Tumors, head injuries, or vascular disorders that impinge on the medial temporal region can produce an amnestic syndrome. Also, a persistent and selective amnesia can occur following viral encephalitis, ischemia, or hypoxia (Shimamura 1989). In such cases, anterograde amnesia is typically the outstanding cognitive impairment, but retrograde amnesia can also occur (Squire and Shimamura 1986). General intellectual abilities and immediate memory (i.e., digit span) are often intact. Although the medial temporal region is typically affected in these disorders, damage to other brain regions can also occur.

Advances in in vivo neuroimaging techniques, such as magnetic resonance imaging (MRI) and positron-emission tomography (PET), have allowed more detailed analysis of the brain areas that are damaged in neurological patients (Damasio and Damasio 1989). For example, a new technique has been developed for high-resolution MRI imaging of the hippocampus (Press et al. 1989). This technique involves positioning the head so the image plane is perpendicular to the long axis of the hippocampal formation. As a result, a clear cross-sectional image of the hippocampal formation can be obtained. This technique has already provided remarkable data concerning the extent of hippocampal damage in patients with amnesia (Press et al. 1989). For example, quantitative analyses of MRI scans using this new technique have revealed that, compared with control subjects, patients with amnesia exhibit an average loss of 49% of tissue in the area of the hippocampal formation. Despite this tissue loss, the average area of the temporal lobe in these patients was nearly identical to that of the control subjects. These data confirm and extend the findings from patient H.M. and offer a new approach to the analysis of amnestic disorders.

Diencephalic Amnesia

Damage to the diencephalic midline can also produce an amnestic disorder that is often indistinguishable from the behavioral consequences of medial temporal damage. Patients with thalamic infarction in the area surrounding the paramedian arteries often exhibit an amnestic syndrome (Graff-Radford et al. 1990). Also, a noted patient with amnesia (patient N.A.), who sustained left-thalamic damage after a penetrating head injury with a miniature fencing foil, exhibited a severe amnesia for verbal information (Kaushall et al. 1981). The two structures within the diencephalon that have been implicated as critical for memory processes are the mediodorsal nucleus of the thalamus and the mammillary bodies of the hypothalamus.

The best-studied cases of amnesia due to diencephalic damage are those of patients with Korsakoff's syndrome. Korsakoff's syndrome can develop after nutritional deficiency resulting from many years of chronic alcohol abuse (Butters and Cermak 1980; Victor et al. 1989). Neuropathological studies have indicated bilateral lesions along the walls of the third and fourth ventricles, typically involving the dorsomedial thalamic nuclei and mammillary bodies (Mair et al. 1979; Mayes et al. 1988; Victor et al. 1989). In addition, cortical atrophy and cerebellar damage are often observed. A study (Shimamura et al. 1988) using quantitative analyses of computed tomography (CT) data from patients with Korsakoff's syndrome corroborated these neuropathological findings by identifying increased fluid volume and low density values in the medial thalamic region and the frontal and temporal lobes.

Patients with Korsakoff's syndrome exhibit severe anterograde amnesia in the presence of relatively preserved intellectual abilities. Extensive retrograde amnesia can occur and encompass memory loss that can span several decades (Albert et al. 1979). One factor that complicates the characterization of the memory impairment in Korsakoff's syndrome is generalized cortical atrophy, which is presumed to be a consequence of chronic alcohol abuse. Indeed, some memory functions, such as memory for temporal order, immediate memory, and stimulus encoding, are impaired in patients with Korsakoff's syndrome but not in other patients with amnesia (Shimamura 1989). Moreover, patients with Korsakoff's syndrome are often emotionally flat, apathetic, and lacking insight about their deficit (Talland 1965).

Transient Amnesias

Not all amnestic syndromes are permanent. Traumatic head injury, for example, can cause a transient and selective memory impairment. After the initial stages of unconsciousness or confusion, both anterograde and retrograde amnesias occur, and the severity of anterograde amnesia is often correlated with the temporal extent of retrograde amnesia (Russell and Nathan 1946). Retrograde amnesia tends to follow *Ribot's Law* (Ribot 1881), which states that memory for the recent past is affected more severely than memory for the distant past. Amnesia following head trauma can last for minutes, days, or even weeks. In mild trauma cases, new learning ability recovers to premorbid levels. In more severe cases, both amnesia and other cognitive impairment can be long lasting and sometimes permanent.

Another form of memory impairment is *transient global amnesia* (TGA), which closely resembles the permanent amnestic syndrome seen in patients with medial temporal or diencephalic amnesia. The onset of anterograde and retrograde amnesias is sudden, and the amnesia typically lasts for several hours. Patients can appear neurologically intact when examined on the day after a TGA attack (Kritchevsky et al. 1988). Both epileptic seizures and transient cerebrovascular disorder have been considered as causes of TGA, but vascular etiology is widely favored (Whitty et al. 1977).

Amnesia can also occur after electroconvulsive therapy (ECT). After a postictal confusional period of 3–60 minutes, amnesia is present as a relatively circumscribed disorder (Squire 1977). ECT causes both anterograde and retrograde amnesias. Anterograde amnesia can be quite severe, particularly in patients who receive bilateral ECT. Retrograde amnesia is often temporally graded, affecting memory for recent events more than memory for very remote events. By several months after ECT treatment, there is extensive recovery of new learning capacity. In fact, performance on memory tests given 6–9 months after ECT is similar to pre-ECT performance. Retrograde amnesia also resolves considerably when testing occurs 6–9 months after ECT.

Despite good recovery of memory functions, however, patients prescribed ECT often complain that their memory is not as good as it used to be (Squire and Chace 1975). These complaints may be mediated by 1) the permanent absence of memory for events during the amnesic lacuna, 2) misattributions of instances of normal forgetting to the ECT treatment, or 3) subtle, persisting memory problems that are too mild to detect on psychometric tests. Although the biological factors that cause the transient amnesic disorder after ECT are not well understood, it is known that the hippocampus has one of the lowest seizure thresholds of all brain structures (Inglis 1970). Thus hippocampal functioning may be disproportionately compromised after ECT.

Preserved Memory Functions in Amnesia

One of the most striking findings of the past decade is evidence of preserved memory functions in patients with amnesia (Schacter 1987; Shimamura 1986; Squire 1987). Specifically, amnesic patients can perform in an entirely normal fashion on certain "implicit" or "nondeclarative" memory tests, such as tests of skill learning, classical conditioning, and priming. For example, H.M. showed considerable retention of perceptual-motor skill on a mirror-drawing task in which he was required to trace the outline of a star while viewing the star in a mirror (Milner 1962).

Preserved skill learning has been observed in other cases of amnesia as well (Parkin 1982). Cohen and Squire (1980) observed preserved skill learning by amnesic patients who were asked to read mirror-reversed words. Patients with Korsakoff's syndrome, patients prescribed ECT, and patient N.A. improved their reading speed of mirror-reversed words across training sessions to the same extent as control subjects (Figure 13–2). Moreover, amnesic patients exhibited normal retention of the mirror-reading skill even when they were tested 1 month after learning. Despite preserved skill learning, recognition memory for the words used in the task was severely impaired in amnesic patients. Moreover, the patients often did not recognize the testing apparatus nor did they have conscious recollection of having engaged in the task before. These findings indicate that skill learning can be preserved even when the patient has little or no recollection of having acquired the skill.

There are several other forms of preserved memory function in amnesia. One form is illustrated by an early anecdote of "unconscious" memory that was reported by Claparede (1911). During an interview with an amnesic patient, Claparede hid a pin between his fingers and surreptitiously pricked the patient on the hand. At a later time during the interview, he once again reached for the patient's hand, but the patient quickly withdrew her hand. The patient did not acknowledge the previous incident, and, when asked why she withdrew her hand, she simply stated, " . . . sometimes pins are hidden in people's hands." This anecdote is an example of stimulus-response learning without awareness.

Another form of such learning was demonstrated by Weiskrantz and Warrington (1979), who assessed classical conditioning of the blink response in two amnesic patients. These patients retained the conditioned response for as long as 24 hours, even though they did not recognize the test apparatus. A memory phenomenon known as *priming* is also preserved in amnesia (Schacter 1987; Shimamura 1986). Priming is a facilitation or bias in performance as a result of recently encountered information. The seminal evidence for preservation of priming in amnesia came from Warrington and Weiskrantz (1968, 1970). Amnesic patients were asked to identify words or pictures that were presented in a degraded form. If the subjects could not identify a stimulus,

Figure 13–2. *(at right)* Acquisition of a mirror-reading skill during three daily sessions and retention of the skill 3 months later. The skill in reading nonrepeated mirror-reversed words was acquired at a normal rate by patient N.A., patients with Korsakoff's syndrome, and patients prescribed electroconvulsive therapy (ECT).
Source. Reprinted from Cohen NJ, Squire LR: "Preserved Learning and Retention of Pattern Analyzing Skill in Amnesia: Association of Knowing How and Knowing That." *Science* 210:207–209,1980. Copyright 1980 by the AAAS. Used with permission.

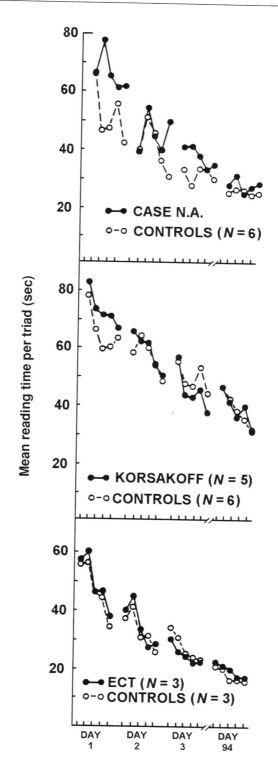

a succession of less degraded versions of the stimulus were shown until identification was successful. When amnesic patients were asked to identify the same degraded words or pictures at a later time, their performance was facilitated by the previous experience; that is, they were able to identify the stimuli more quickly. This priming effect occurred despite failure to discriminate previously presented stimuli from new ones in a recognition memory test.

A variety of priming paradigms have since been used to demonstrate preserved priming in amnesia. For example, Shimamura and Squire (1984) presented words (e.g., *baby*) and later asked subjects to "free associate" to related words (e.g., *child*). Amnesic patients exhibited a normal bias to use recently presented words, suggesting that semantic associations can also be used to prime information in memory. This priming effect, as well as others, are short lasting, and decline to baseline levels after a 2-hour delay. Although patients with circumscribed diencephalic or medial temporal lesions exhibit normal priming effects, patients with the clinical diagnosis of Alzheimer's disease do not. For example, impaired word association priming has been observed in patients with probable Alzheimer's disease (Salmon et al. 1988; Shimamura et al. 1987). These findings suggest that priming effects may depend critically on neocortical areas that are damaged in Alzheimer's disease.

Demonstrations of preserved memory functions in amnesic patients suggest that some memory processes can be dissociated from the brain regions that are damaged in amnesia. Various taxonomies have been used to distinguish the memory forms that are impaired in amnesia from those that are preserved (Squire 1987). For example, many distinguish *conscious* recollection from *unconscious* or *automatic memory*. Squire and colleagues (Cohen and Squire 1980; Squire 1987) suggested that amnesia impairs declarative memory and spares procedural or nondeclarative memory. Others have used related terms such as *explicit* and *implicit memory* (Schacter 1987) or *memory* and *habit* (Mishkin et al. 1984). Such descriptions provide a framework for theoretical views about the organization of memory in the brain.

NEURAL MECHANISMS OF MEMORY

Memory at the Neural Systems Level

One important feature of memory is the ability to report explicitly knowledge about facts and events of previous experiences (e.g., "I ate a chocolate doughnut for breakfast this morning at the cafeteria"). Such memories involve the formation, association, and organization of various pieces of information, including information about what occurred, when it occurred, and where it occurred. Thus to establish, maintain, and ultimately recollect such (declarative) memories, it is critical to have an efficient neural mechanism by which new pieces of information can be associated with each other and with previously stored information.

One particular area that has received extensive analysis is the hippocampal formation, which includes the entorhinal cortex, dentate gyrus, subicular complex, and hippocampus proper (Figure 13–3). These structures form the *trisynaptic circuit* (Squire et al. 1989; Swanson et al. 1982). In this circuit, the axons of entorhinal neurons form a fiber bundle known as the *perforant path,* which projects to the dentate gyrus granule cells where it forms its first set of synapses. The granule cells give rise to the mossy fibers, which synapse onto neurons in the CA_3 field of the hippocampus. The CA_3 neurons give rise to the Schaffer collaterals, which project to pyramidal cells of the CA_1 field. The CA_1 cells complete the circuit with projections to the subiculum and entorhinal cortex. The subiculum gives rise to the projections that exit through the fornix to diencephalic structures such as the mammillary bodies and the anterior thalamic nuclei. The complete neural circuitry of the hippocampal formation is exceedingly complex; however, this basic neural architecture (i.e., the trisynaptic circuit) is typical of hippocampal circuitry along its rostral-caudal extent.

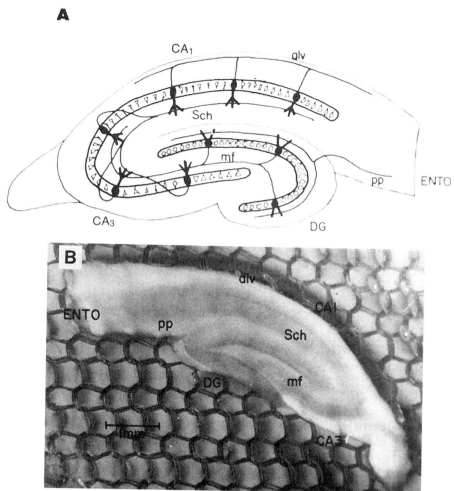

Figure 13–3. *Panel A*: Schematic diagram of the trisynaptic circuit in the hippocampus (ENTO = entorhinal cortex; pp = perforant path; DG = dentate gyrus; mf = mossy fibers; Sch = Schaffer collaterals; alv = alveus). *Panel B*: Photograph of a hippocampal tissue slice preparation.

Source. Reprinted from Teyler TJ: "Memory Electrophysiological Analogs," in *Learning and Memory: A Biological View.* Edited by Martinez JL Jr, Kesner RP. New York, Academic Press, 1984, pp. 237–265. Used with permission.

What is the functional role of hippocampal circuitry? As illustrated in Figure 13–4, many areas of neocortex, such as the cingulate cortex, superior temporal gyrus, orbitofrontal cortex, and insula, project directly to the entorhinal cortex. In addition, the entorhinal cortex receives projections from adjacent cortical areas, such as the perirhinal cortex (areas 35 and 36) and the parahippocampal gyrus (areas TF/TH), which are located rostral and caudal to the entorhinal cortex, respectively. These adjacent areas themselves receive projections from many neocortical regions (as shown in the upper half of Figure 13–4). All of these projections to the entorhinal cortex have reciprocal projections back to neocortical regions. The neocortical regions that project to the entorhinal cortex have been classified as "polysensory associational cortices," which indicates that the entorhinal cortex receives highly processed, multimodal information (Squire et al. 1989).

A functional model of the neural system within the medial temporal region has been developed from these anatomical findings. The entorhinal cortex receives a vast amount of information from various polysensory areas in neocortex, either directly or by way of the perirhinal cortex and parahippocampal gyrus. Neural activity courses through the trisynaptic circuit, enabling a process that acts to conjoin or index the information from various inputs. The product of this process influences or modulates activity in polysensory neocortical regions. In other words, the medial temporal region—particularly the hippocampus—is privy to extensive cortical activity from a variety of areas, and one possibility is that the hippocampus acts to associate or index cortical activity that otherwise would not occur because of the geographical disparity of the cortical sites (Squire et al. 1989). In the following sections we further delineate findings concerning the functional role of hippocampal circuitry.

MEMORY AT THE SYNAPTIC LEVEL

Knowledge about memory at the synaptic level has benefited from physiological analyses of hippocampal tissue slice preparations. Hippocampal slice preparations are made by cutting thin slices (350–500 μm) perpendicular to the long axis of the hippocampus (Figure 13–3). With this slice preparation, electrophysiological stimulations and recordings can be performed selectively on each component of the trisynaptic circuit. For example, excitatory postsynaptic potentials (EPSPs) can be reliably recorded after electrical stimulation of the perforant path in hippocampal slice preparations. Such recordings can be made for as long as the tissue survives, which can be for several hours or even days.

Studies of hippocampal physiology have demonstrated that neural transmission along the trisynaptic circuit is excitatory (Swanson et al. 1982). Many of the pyramidal cell connections are mediated by excitatory amino acids, such as glutamic acid and aspartic acid. In addition, inhibitory interneurons in the hippocampus synapse on hippocampal pyramidal cells and thus may act to modulate excitatory activity in the trisynaptic circuit. Many of these interneurons, such as basket cells, modulate excitatory transmission with the neurotransmitter γ-aminobutyric acid (GABA).

An important discovery regarding the nature of hippocampal function has been the finding of *long-term potentiation* (LTP), a phenomenon in which long-lasting changes in synaptic efficacy are induced by brief, high-frequency stimulation (Lynch 1986; Teyler 1984). LTP is characterized by lowered firing thresholds and can be

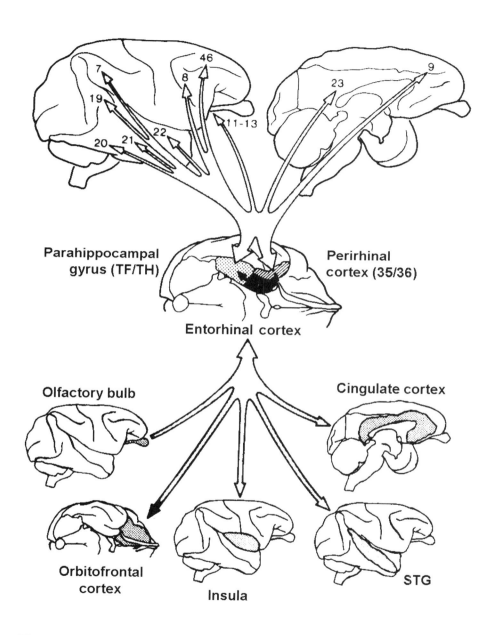

Figure 13–4. Diagram of the cortical areas that project to the entorhinal cortex either directly as shown by the projections below (e.g., orbitofrontal cortex and cingulate cortex or indirectly by way of the parahippocampal gyrus or perirhinal cortex (e.g., Brodmann areas shown above). The entorhinal cortex projects to the hippocampus and also sends reciprocal projections back to cortical areas. STG = superior temporal gyrus.

Source. Reprinted from Squire LR, Shimamura AP, Amaral DG: "Memory and the Hippocampus," in *Neural Models of Plasticity: Experimental and Theoretical Approaches.* Edited by Byrne JH, Berry WO. New York, Academic Press, 1989, pp. 208–239. Used with permission.

induced at every component of the trisynaptic circuit. Because LTP involves long-lasting synaptic changes, it has been useful as a model of memory formation at the synaptic level. Studies of the nature of LTP have demonstrated several important properties of hippocampal physiology—and perhaps of the process by which declarative memory is formed (Lynch 1986). First, LTP can be induced quickly and can last for as long as the cell survives. Second, LTP is cumulative such that successive episodes of high-frequency stimulation increase the degree of synaptic efficacy.

A third property of LTP is cooperativity; that is, more effective potentiation occurs when stimulation is delivered to a group of axons that terminate at overlapping synaptic fields than when stimulation is restricted to a small number of axons (Lynch 1986; McNaughton and Morris 1987). This property suggests that excitation from different axons that terminate on the same synaptic area can cooperate to facilitate LTP. Finally, LTP is selective (i.e., it does not induce a general increase in the efficacy of all synapses on the postsynaptic membrane). Thus there is regional localization of LTP induction.

In summary, LTP provides a useful model for the physiology of hippocampal function and thus may be associated with the kinds of plastic changes that occur naturally in the formation of long-lasting memories. The properties of LTP—namely the fact that it is long-lasting, forms quickly, acts cooperatively, and has regional selectivity—are all features that would be advantageous for the formation of memory.

Memory at the Biochemical Level

At the biochemical level, many neural and intracellular processes must contribute to the formation, maintenance, and retrieval of memory. Indeed, it is most likely that many biochemical processes influence memory either directly or indirectly, via modulation of general activational or metabolic processes that occur throughout the brain (Dunn 1986). These direct and indirect effects include modulation of neurotransmitters, such as acetylcholine, norepinephrine, and serotonin, and modulation of intracellular processes, such as protein synthesis, enzymatic reactions, and cell metabolism (Kandel and Schwartz 1982; Lynch 1986). Even peripheral effects, such as hormonal influences, can affect memory functions rather dramatically (McGaugh 1990).

One important issue of memory at the biochemical level concerns mechanisms by which physiological activity leads to structural changes. One prominent candidate for an intracellular mechanism of long-term plasticity is protein phosphorylation (Dunn 1986; Kandel and Schwartz 1982). Protein phosphorylation involves a cascade of processes that begins with the binding of neurotransmitters onto receptors. The binding of neurotransmitters onto receptors activates adenylate cyclase, which produces cyclic adenosine monophosphate (cAMP). The cAMP activates a protein kinase that phosphorylates proteins. The mechanism of protein phosphorylation is quite specific, depending on the cAMP-dependent protein kinase that is activated. For example, Kandel and Schwartz (1982) suggested that synaptic efficacy in the invertebrate *Aplysia californica* is induced by a specific form of protein phosphorylation that restricts potassium ion channels and thereby lowers the firing threshold of the neuron. This and other related mechanisms could lead to cellular or structural modifications that are long lasting (Dunn 1986).

Another biochemical mechanism of cellular plasticity was proposed by Lynch (1986), who offered an elegant model of the way in which LTP increases synaptic efficacy. It was proposed that LTP involves a calcium-mediated process that produces structural changes in the cell membrane of the postsynaptic neuron. The model is supported by the finding that LTP increases the number of postsynaptic synapses and also produces changes in the shape of dendritic spines. The importance of calcium was suggested because injection of a calcium chelator was effective in greatly reducing the likelihood of LTP. It is presumed that calcium ions activate a proteolytic enzyme (calpain) within the postsynaptic neuron, which acts to break down the postsynaptic membrane, expose previously concealed or inactive glutamate receptors, and thus increase synaptic efficacy. The model is also supported by the finding that leupeptin, an inhibitor of calpain, prevents the morphological changes that occur in the postsynaptic membrane. Interestingly, when leupeptin was injected by intraventricular cannulas into living rats, memory on a maze learning task was significantly impaired (Lynch 1986).

The model proposed by Lynch (1986) has recently received further support from research on the biochemistry of glutamate receptors. One type of receptor channel is called the N-methyl-D-aspartate (NMDA) receptor, because of its affinity for binding with NMDA. Other related glutamate receptors are the so-called quisqualate and kainate receptors. All of these receptor types can be found in the hippocampus, but the NMDA receptors have unique properties that may contribute to the formation of long-term memory. NMDA receptors are most highly concentrated in the hippocampus—especially in the CA_1 field—although they are also found in moderate proportions throughout the brain, including the neocortex, corpus striatum, thalamus, hypothalamus, and cerebellum (Olverman et al. 1984).

Several findings have suggested a relationship between NMDA receptors and memory. First, the formation of LTP is blocked by an antagonist of NMDA, 2-amino-5-phosphonovalerate (APV), though APV does not interfere with normal synaptic transmission (Harris et al. 1984). Second, rats that were given infusions of APV in sufficient doses to block LTP performed poorly on a spatial memory task (Morris et al. 1986). Third, the action of glutamate on NMDA receptors may be responsible for its excitotoxic effects on hippocampal cells during episodes of anoxia or ischemia (Meldrum 1985). Experimental prophylactic methods have been proposed that involve the injection of glutamate antagonists to protect against neuronal death following an anoxic or ischemic event. These methods may prove extremely useful in the prevention of amnesia following anoxia or ischemia.

CONCLUSIONS

The study of memory and amnesia is one of the most productive areas in neuropsychiatric research. Progress has occurred as a result of extensive interdisciplinary research—drawing on neuroanatomy, neurophysiology, psychiatry, neurology, psychology, and cognitive science. Based on this progress, investigations concerning memory assessment and rehabilitation have been conducted, but further studies in these clinical areas are needed (Glisky et al. 1986; Wilson 1987). In addition to providing clinical benefits, the research reviewed in this chapter has been of paramount importance in the elucidation of the neural organization of normal memory functions. Further developments in clinical and basic research are certainly forthcoming with the advent of better neuroanatomical and physiological techniques as well as more precise analyses of behavior.

REFERENCES

Albert MS, Butters N, Levin J: Temporal gradients in the retrograde amnesia of patients with alcoholic Korsakoff's disease. Arch Neurol 36:211–216, 1979

American Psychiatric Association: Diagnostic and Statistical Manual of Mental Disorders, 3rd Edition, Revised. Washington, DC, American Psychiatric Association, 1987

Butters N, Cermak LS: Alcoholic Korsakoff's Syndrome: An Information Processing Approach. New York, Academic, 1980

Claparede E: Reconnaissance et moiite. Archives de Psychologie 11:79–90, 1911 (Recognitive and "me-ness," translation in Organization and Pathology of Thought. Edited by Rapaport D. New York, Columbia University Press, 1951)

Cohen NJ, Squire LR: Preserved learning and retention of pattern analyzing skill in amnesia: association of knowing how and knowing that. Science 210:207–209, 1980

Corkin S: Lasting consequences of bilateral medial temporal lobectomy: clinical course and experimental findings in H.M. Semin Neurol 4:249–259, 1984

Damasio H, Damasio AR: Lesion Analysis in Neuropsychology. New York, Oxford University Press, 1989

Dunn AJ: Biochemical correlates of learning and memory, in Learning and Memory. Edited by Martinez JL, Kesner RP. San Diego, CA, Academic, 1986, pp 165–201

Glisky EL, Schacter DL, Tulving E: Learning and retention of computer-related vocabulary in memory-impaired patients: method of vanishing cues. J Clin Exp Neuropsychol 8:292–312, 1986

Graff-Radford NR, Tranel D, VanHoesen GW, et al: Diencephalic amnesia. Brain 113:1–25, 1990

Harris EW, Ganong AH, Cotman CW: Long-term potentiation in the hippocampus involves activation of N-methyl-D-aspartate receptors. Brain Res 323:132–137, 1984

Inglis J: Shock, surgery, and cerebral symmetry. Br J Psychiatry 117:143–148, 1970

Kandel ER, Schwartz JH: Molecular biology of learning: modification of transmitter release. Science 218:433–442, 1982

Kaushall PI, Zetin M, Squire LR: A psychosocial study of chronic circumscribed amnesia. J Nerv Ment Dis 169: 383–389, 1981

Kritchevsky M, Squire LR, Zouzounis JA : Transient global amnesia: characterization of anterograde and retrograde amnesia. Neurology 38:213–219, 1988

Lynch G: Synapses, Circuits, and the Beginnings of Memory. Cambridge, MA, MIT Press, 1986

McGaugh JL: Significance and remembrance: the role of neuromodulatory systems. Psychological Science 1:15–25, 1990

McNaughton B, Morris RGM: Hippocampal synaptic enhancement and information storage within a distributed memory system. Trends Neurosci 10:408–415, 1987

Mair WGP, Warrington EK, Weiskrantz L: Memory disorder in Korsakoff's psychosis: a neuropathological and neuropsychological investigation of two cases. Brain 102:749–783, 1979

Marslen-Wilson WD, Teuber H: Memory for remote events in anterograde amnesia: recognition of public figures from news photographs. Neuropsychologia 13: 353–364, 1975

Mayes AR, Meudell PR, Mann D, et al: Location of lesions in Korsakoff's syndrome: neuropsychological and neuropathological data on two patients. Cortex 24:367–388, 1988

Meldrum B: Excitatory amino acids and anoxic/ischaemic brain damage. Trends Neurosci 8:47–48, 1985

Milner B: The memory defect in bilateral hippocampal lesions. Psychiatric Research Reports 11:43–52, 1959

Milner B: Les troubles de la memoire accompagnant des lesions hippocampiques bilaterales (Memory impairment accompanying bilateral hippocampal lesions), in Physiologie de l'Hippocampe. Paris, Centre Nationale de la Recherche Scientifique, 1962, pp 257–272

Milner B, Corkin S, Teuber H: Further analysis of the hippocampal amnesic syndrome: 14-year follow-up study of H.M. Neuropsychologia 6:215–234, 1968

Mishkin M, Malamut B, Bachevalier J: Memories and habits: two neural systems, in The Neurobiology of Learning and Memory. Edited by McGaugh JL, Lynch G, Weinberger N. New York, Guilford, 1984, pp 65–77

Morris RGM, Anderson E, Lynch GS, et al: Selective impairment of learning and blockade of long-term potentiation by an N-methyl-D-aspartate receptor antagonist, AP5. Nature 319:774–776, 1986

Olverman HJ, Jones AW, Watkins JC: L-Glutamate has higher affinity than other amino acids for [3H]-D-AP5 binding sites in rat brain membranes. Nature 307:460–462, 1984

Parkin AJ: Residual learning capability in organic amnesia. Cortex 18:417–440, 1982

Press, GA, Amaral DG, Squire LR: Hippocampal abnormalities in amnesic patients revealed by high-resolution magnetic resonance imaging. Nature 341:54–57, 1989

Ribot T: Les Maladies de la Memoire. Paris, Germer Baillere, 1881 (translation: Diseases of Memory. New York, Appleton-Century-Crofts, 1882)

Russell WR, Nathan PW: Traumatic amnesia. Brain 69: 280–300, 1946

Salmon DP, Shimamura AP, Butters N, et al: Lexical and semantic priming deficits in patients with Alzheimer's disease. J Clin Exp Neuropsychol 10:477–494, 1988

Schacter DL: Implicit memory: history and current status. J Exp Psychol [Learn Mem Cogn] 13:501–518, 1987

Scoville WB, Milner B: Loss of recent memory after bilateral hippocampal lesions. J Neurol Neurosurg Psychiatry 20:11–21, 1957

Shimamura AP: Priming in amnesia: evidence for a dissociable memory function. Q J Exp Psychol 38 (A):619–644, 1986

Shimamura AP: Disorders of memory: the cognitive science perspective, in Handbook of Neuropsychology. Edited by Boller F, Grafman J. Amsterdam, Elsevier Sciences, 1989, pp 35–73

Shimamura AP, Squire LR: Paired-associate learning and priming effects in amnesia: a neuropsychological study. J Exp Psychol [Gen] 113:556–570, 1984

Shimamura AP, Salmon DP, Squire LR, et al: Memory dysfunction and word priming in dementia and amnesia. Behav Neurosci 101:347–351, 1987

Shimamura AP, Jernigan TL, Squire LR: Korsakoff's Syndrome: radiological, CT findings and neuropsychological correlates. J Neurosci 8:4400–4410, 1988

Squire LR: ECT and memory loss. Am J Psychiatry 134: 997–1001, 1977

Squire LR: Memory and Brain. New York, Oxford University Press, 1987

Squire LR, Chace P: Memory functions six to nine months after electroconvulsive therapy. Arch Gen Psychiatry 32:1557–1564, 1975

Squire LR, Shimamura AP: Characterizing amnesic patients for neurobehavioral study. Behav Neurosci 100:866–877, 1986

Squire LR, Shimamura AP, Amaral DG: Memory and the hippocampus, in Neural Models of Plasticity: Experimental and Theoretical Approaches. Edited by Byrne JH, Berry WO. New York, Academic, 1989, pp 208–239

Swanson LW, Teyler TJ, Thompson RF: Hippocampal long-term potentiation: mechanisms and implications for memory. Neuroscience Research and Progress Bulletin 20:613–765, 1982

Talland GA: Deranged Memory. New York, Academic, 1965

Teyler TJ: Memory: electrophysiological analogs, in Learning and Memory: A Biological View. Edited by Martinez JL Jr, Kesner RP. New York, Academic, 1984, pp 237–265

Victor M, Adams RD, Collins GH: The Wernicke-Korsakoff Syndrome, 2nd Edition. Philadelphia, PA, FA Davis, 1989

Warrington EK, Weiskrantz L: New method of testing long-term retention with special reference to amnesic patients. Nature 217:972–974, 1968

Warrington EK, Weiskrantz L: The amnesic syndrome: consolidation or retrieval? Nature 228:628–630, 1970

Weiskrantz L, Warrington EK: Conditioning in amnesic patients. Neuropsychologia 17:187–194, 1979

Whitty CWM, Zangwill OL (eds): Amnesia. London, Butterworths, 1977

Wilson BA: Rehabilitation of Memory. New York, Guilford, 1987

Section IV

Neuropsychiatric Disorders

Chapter 14

Neuropsychiatric Aspects of Traumatic Brain Injury

Jonathan M. Silver, M.D.
Robert E. Hales, M.D.
Stuart C. Yudofsky, M.D.

More than 2 million people sustain traumatic brain injuries in the United States each year; 500,000 of these persons require hospitalization, and 70,000–90,000 of the survivors are afflicted with the chronic sequelae of such injuries (Department of Health and Human Services 1989). In this population, psychosocial and psychological deficits are commonly the major source of disability to the victims and of stress to their families. The psychiatrist, neurologist, and neuropsychologist are often called on to treat these patients. In this chapter, we review the role these professionals play in the prevention, diagnosis, and treatment of the cognitive, behavioral, and emotional aspects of traumatic brain injury.

EPIDEMIOLOGY

Disorders arising from traumatic injuries to the brain are more common than any other neurological disease, with the exception of headaches. Traumatic brain injury (including brain trauma and transient and persistent postconcussion syndromes) has an annual incidence of 370 per 100,000 (Kurtzke 1984), a rate that is at least three times greater than that of schizophrenia and a prevalence that is greater than that for the individual prevalences for schizophrenia, mania, and panic disorder (Regier et al. 1988; Silver et al. 1990a).

Motor vehicle accidents account for approximately one-half of traumatic injuries; other common causes are falls (21%), assaults and violence (12%), and accidents associated with sports and recreation (10%) (Department of Health and Human Services 1989). Children are highly vulnerable in accidents as passengers and, as pedestrians, to falls, to impact from moving objects (e.g., rocks or baseballs), and to sports injuries (Hendrick et al. 1965). Tragically, among infants, most head injuries are the result of child abuse (64%) (Department of Health and Human Services 1989).

The total economic cost of brain injury is staggeringly high: an estimated $25 billion a year (Department of Health and Human Services 1989). Because the victims of traumatic brain injury most commonly are young adults, they may require prolonged rehabilitation. The costs of 5–10 years of these services can exceed $4 million for each survivor (Department of Health and Human Services 1989).

NEUROANATOMY AND NEUROCHEMISTRY
OF TRAUMATIC BRAIN INJURY

Patients who sustain brain injury from trauma may incur damage through several mechanisms including penetrating injuries, contusions, diffuse axonal injuries, hematomas, and hypoxia. Contusions affect specific areas of the brain and usually occur as the result of low-velocity injuries, such as falls. Courville (1945) examined the neuroanatomical sites of contusions and found that most injuries were in the temporal and frontal lobes. Most of these lesions were the result of the location of bony prominences that surround the orbital, frontal, and temporal areas along the base of the skull. Contrecoup injuries are contusions that occur when the opposite side of the head is struck. A typical example is the patient who falls on the back of his head and injures the frontal and temporal lobes as the result of brain tissue abrading on the bony prominences.

Diffuse axonal injury refers to damage to the axons in cerebral white matter that commonly occurs during acceleration or deceleration injuries. The axon is vulnerable to injury during high-velocity accidents when there is twisting and turning of the brain around the brain stem (as can occur in "whiplash" car accidents). Diffuse axonal injury often results in sudden loss of consciousness and can occur in minor brain injury or "concussion" (Jane et al. 1985). Among cases of traumatic brain injury without diffuse axonal injury, there is a lower incidence of skull fractures, contusions, and intracranial hematomas (Adams et al. 1982).

Subdural hematomas (acute, subacute, and chronic) and intracerebral hematomas have effects that are specific to their locations and degree of neuronal damage. In general, subdural hematomas affect arousal and cognition. During hypoxia, free radicals and excitotoxic neurotransmitters, such as glutamate, are released and result in further damage to neurons (Faden et al. 1989).

Studies of neurochemical changes after traumatic brain injury indicate that such injuries can affect the neurotransmitter systems that mediate mood and affect, including norepinephrine, serotonin, dopamine, and acetylcholine (Silver et al. 1991). Specific lesions may deplete norepinephrine and serotonin by interrupting the nerve tracts of these pathways (Morrison et al. 1979). The norepinephrine nerve tracts course from the brain stem anteriorly to curve around the hypothalamus, the basal ganglia, and the frontal cortex. Similarly, the serotonin system has projections to the frontal cortex. Diffuse axonal injury or contusions can affect both of these systems. Secondary neurotoxicity that is caused by excitotoxins and lipid peroxidation may further damage the neuronal systems that mediate norepinephrine and serotonin.

NEUROPSYCHIATRIC ASSESSMENT OF TRAUMATIC BRAIN INJURY

History Taking

Although brain injuries subsequent to serious automobile, occupational, or sports accidents may not result in diagnostic enigmas for the psychiatrist, less severe trauma may first present as relatively subtle behavioral or affective change. Confusion, intellectual changes, affective lability, or psychosis may occur directly after the trauma or many years afterward. Patients may fail to associate the traumatic event with subsequent symptoms. For all psychiatric patients, the clinician must specifically inquire whether the patient has been involved in situations that are associated with head trauma. The practitioner should ask about automobile, bicycle, or motorcycle accidents; falls; assaults; playground accidents; and participation in sports that are associated frequently with brain injury (e.g., football, rugby, and boxing). Patients must be asked whether there was any loss of consciousness after these injuries, whether they were hospitalized, and whether they had posttraumatic symptoms, such as headache, dizziness, irritability, problems with concentration, and sensitivity to noise or light.

Because many patients are either unaware of, minimize, or deny the severity of behavioral changes that occur after traumatic brain injury, family members also must be asked about the effects of injury on the behavior of their relative. For example, in evaluating the social adjustment of patients years after severe brain injury, Oddy et al. (1985) found that patients reported different symptoms than did their relatives. Forty percent of relatives of 28 patients with traumatic brain injury reported that their relative behaved childishly. However, this symptom was not reported by patients themselves. Although 28% of the patients complained of problems with their vision after the injury, this difficulty was not reported by relatives.

Family members also are more aware of emotional changes than are the victims of brain injury. Whereas individuals with traumatic brain injury tend to view the cognitive difficulties as more severe than the emotional changes (Hendryx 1989), mood disorders and frustration tolerance are viewed as more disabling than cognitive disabilities by families (Rappaport et al. 1989).

Documentation and Rating of Symptomatology

Symptom rating scales, electrophysiological imaging, and neuropsychiatric assessments should be used to define symptoms and signs that result from traumatic brain injury. Severity of injury may be measured by several parameters, including duration of unconsciousness, initial score on the Glasgow Coma Scale (GCS; Teasdale and Jennett 1974), and degree of posttraumatic amnesia.

The GCS is a 15-point scale that documents eye opening, verbal responsiveness, and motor response to stimuli and can be used to measure the depth of coma, both initially and longitudinally. Mild head injury is usually defined as loss of consciousness for less than 15–20 minutes, brief or no hospitalization, no prominent residual neurobehavioral deficits, and a GCS score of 13–15. With severe traumatic brain injury, posttraumatic amnesia or loss of consciousness may persist for at least 1 week or longer or, in extreme cases, may last weeks to months; GCS scores for severe traumatic brain injury are less than 10.

Laboratory Evaluation

Imaging techniques.   Brain imaging techniques are frequently used to demonstrate the location and extent of brain lesions. Computed tomography (CT) is now widely available and may document contusions and hematomas. The timing of such imaging is important, because lesions may be visualized months after the injury that cannot be seen during the acute phase. Thus for a significant number of patients with severe brain injury, initial CT evaluations may not detect lesions that are observable on CT scans performed 1 and 3 months after the injury (Cope et al. 1988).

Magnetic resonance imaging (MRI) has been shown to detect clinically meaningful lesions in patients with severe brain injury when CT scans have not demonstrated anatomical bases for the degree of coma (Wilberger et al. 1987). MRI is especially sensitive in detecting lesions in the frontal and temporal lobes, loci that are frequently related to neuropsychiatric consequences (Levin et al. 1987).

New techniques in brain imaging, such as regional cerebral blood flow (rCBF) and positron-emission tomography (PET), can detect areas of abnormal function when even CT and MRI scans fail to show abnormalities (Ruff et al. 1989). Single photon emission computed tomography (SPECT) also shows promise in documenting brain damage after traumatic brain injury.

Electrophysiological techniques. Electrophysiological assessment of the patient after traumatic brain injury may also assist in the evaluation. Electroencephalography (EEG) can detect the presence of seizures or abnormal areas of functioning. To enhance the sensitivity of this technique, the EEG should be performed after sleep deprivation, with photic stimulation and hyperventilation and with anterotemporal and/or nasopharyngeal leads (Goodin et al. 1990). Computed interpretation of the EEG (CEEG) and brain electrical activity mapping (BEAM) may be useful in detecting areas of dysfunction not shown in the routine EEG.

Neuropsychological testing. Neuropsychological assessment of the patient with traumatic brain injury is essential to document cognitive and intellectual deficits and strengths. Tests are administered to assess the patient's attention, concentration, memory, verbal capacity, and executive functioning. This latter capacity is the most difficult to assess and includes problem-solving skills, abstract thinking, planning, and reasoning abilities. A valid interpretation of these tests includes assessment of the patient's premorbid intelligence and other higher levels of functioning.

Patients' complaints may not be easily or accurately categorized as either *functional* (i.e., primarily due to a psychiatric disorder), or *neurological* (i.e., primarily caused by the brain injury). In reality, most symptoms result from the interaction of many factors including neurological, social, emotional, educational, and vocational. Because important insurance and other reimbursement decisions may hinge on whether or not disabilities stem from brain injury, the clinician should take care that his or her impressions are based on data and not misapplied to deprive the patient of deserved benefits. For example, mood disorders and cognitive sequelae of brain injury are often miscategorized as "mental illnesses" that are not covered by some insurance policies.

CLINICAL FEATURES

The neuropsychiatric sequelae of traumatic brain injury include problems with attention, concentration, executive functioning, intellectual changes, cognitive dysfunctions, personality changes, affective disorders, anxiety disorders, psychosis, posttraumatic epilepsy, aggression, and irritability. The severity of the neuropsychiatric sequelae of the brain injury has multiple determinants, including extent, severity and anatomical location of brain lesion, preinjury behavior, anosmia, and psychosocial conditions. The duration of posttraumatic amnesia correlates with subsequent cognitive recovery (Levin et al. 1982). The presence of total anosmia in a group of patients with closed head injury predicted major vocational problems at least 2 years after these patients had been given medical clearance to return to work (Varney 1988). Posttraumatic anosmia may occur as a result of damage to the olfactory nerve that is located adjacent to the orbitofrontal cortex.

The interaction between the brain injury and the psychosocial factors cannot be underestimated. Preexisting emotional and behavioral problems are exacerbated after injury. Although many victims of traumatic brain injury may not have a previous history of psychiatric problems, a significant percentage of patients have had histories of learning disabilities, attentional deficits, behavioral problems, and drug or alcohol abuse. Ruff et al. (1990) found that victims of traumatic brain injury who had a history of alcohol abuse had a poorer outcome, including increased mortality, and a higher prevalence of mass lesions. Factors such as levels of education, levels of income, and an individual's socioeconomic status are positive factors in the ability to return to work after minor head injury (Rimel et al. 1981).

Personality Changes

Unlike many primary psychiatric illnesses that have gradual onset, traumatic brain injury often occurs suddenly and devastatingly. Although some patients recognize that they no longer have the same abilities and thus potentials that they had before the injury, many others with significant disabilities deny that there have been any changes. Prominent behavioral traits such as disorderliness, suspiciousness, argumentativeness, isolativeness, disruptiveness, and anxiousness often become more pronounced after brain injury.

In a survey of the relatives of victims of severe traumatic brain injury, McKinlay et al. (1981) found that 49% of 55 patients developed personality changes 3 months after the injury. After 5 years, 74% of these patients were reported to have changes in their personality (Brooks et al. 1986). More than one-third of these patients had problems of "childishness" and "talking too much" (Brooks et al. 1986; McKinlay et al. 1981).

Thomsen (1984) found that 80% of 40 patients with severe traumatic brain injury had personality changes that persisted 2–5 years, and 65% had changes lasting 10–15 years after the injury. These changes included childishness (60% and 25%, respectively), emotional lability (40% and 35%, respectively), and restlessness (25% and 38%, respectively). Approximately two-thirds of patients had less social contact, and one-half had loss of spontaneity and poverty of interests after 10–15 years.

Because of the vulnerability of the prefrontal and frontal regions of the cortex to contusions, injury to these regions is common and gives rise to changes in personality known as the *frontal lobe syndrome* (Table 14–1). For the prototypic patient with the frontal lobe syndrome, the cognitive functions are preserved while personality changes abound.

Certain behavioral syndromes have been related to damage to specific areas of the frontal lobe (Auerbach 1986). The orbitofrontal syndrome is associated with behavioral excesses, such as impulsivity, disinhibition, hyperactivity, distractibility, and mood lability. Injury to the dorsolateral frontal cortex may result in slowness, apathy, and perseveration. Outbursts of rage and violent behavior occur after damage to the inferior orbital surface of the frontal lobe and anterior temporal lobes. Patients also develop changes in sexual behavior after brain injury. Kreutzer and Zasler (1989) assessed 21 male patients for the psychosexual consequences of traumatic brain injury. A majority of subjects had decreased sex drive, erectile function, and frequency of intercourse.

Intellectual Changes

Problems with intellectual functioning are perhaps the most subtle manifestations of brain injury. Changes can occur in the capacity to concentrate, use language, abstract, calculate, reason, remember, plan, and process information (Levin et al. 1985). Mental sluggishness, poor concentration, and memory problems are common complaints of both patients and relatives (Brooks et al. 1986; Thomsen 1984).

Children who survive head trauma often return to school with behavioral and learning problems (Mahoney et al. 1983). Even children who have sustained mild head injuries show neuropsychological sequelae when carefully tested (Gulbrandsen 1984). In those who survive moderate to severe brain injury, the degree of memory impairment often exceeds the level of intellectual dysfunction (Levin et al. 1988).

Affective Changes

The diagnostic issues that must be considered in the evaluation of the patient who appears depressed after traumatic brain injury are reviewed in greater detail elsewhere (Silver et al. 1991). Sadness is a common reaction after traumatic brain in-

Table 14–1.   Personality and cognitive changes in patients with frontal lobe syndrome

Social and behavioral changes
  Exacerbation of preexisting behavioral traits such as disorderliness, suspiciousness, argumentativeness, disruptiveness, and anxiousness
  Apathy, loss of interest in social interactions, and global lack of concern for consequences of behavior
  Uncharacteristic lewdness with loss of social graces and inattention to personal appearance and hygiene
  Intrusiveness, boisterousness, increased volume of speech, and pervasive, uncharacteristic profanity
  Increased risk taking, unrestrained drinking of alcoholic beverages, and indiscriminate selection of foods and gluttony
  Impulsivity and distractibility
Affective changes
  Apathy, indifference, and shallowness
  Lability of affect, irritability, and manic states
  Dyscontrol of rage and violent behavior
  Intellectual changes
  Reduced capacity to utilize language, symbols, and logic
  Reduced ability to use mathematics, to calculate, to process abstract information, and to reason
  Diminished ability to focus, to concentrate, and to be oriented in time or place

Source.   Adapted from MacKinnon and Yudofsky 1991. Used with permission.

jury, as patients describe "mourning" the loss of their "former selves," often a reflection of deficits in intellectual functioning and motoric abilities.

The clinician must distinguish mood lability that occurs commonly after brain injury from major depression. Lability of mood and affect may be caused by temporal limbic and basal forebrain lesions (Ross and Stewart 1987) and have been shown to be responsive to standard pharmacological interventions of depression (discussed below). In addition, apathy secondary to brain injury (which includes decreased motivation and pursuit of pleasurable activities or schizoid behavior) and complaints of slowness in thought and cognitive processing may resemble depression.

The clinician should determine whether or not a patient may have been having an episode of major depression before an accident. Traumatic injury may occur as a result of the depression and suicidal ideation. Alcohol use, which frequently occurs with and complicates depressive illness, is also a risk factor for motor vehicle accidents. One common scenario is depression leading to poor concentration, to substance abuse, and to risk taking (or even overt suicidal behavior), which together contribute to the motor vehicle accident and brain injury.

For mild traumatic brain injury, estimates of depressive complaints range from 6% to 39% (Rutherford et al. 1977; Schoenhuber et al. 1988). For depression after severe traumatic brain injury, in which patients often have concomitant cognitive impairments, reported rates of depression vary from 10% to 77% (Brooks et al. 1986; Kinsella et al. 1988; Oddy et al. 1985; van Zomeren and van den Burg 1985; Varney et al. 1987; Weddell et al. 1980). Varney et al. (1987) found that duration of loss of consciousness after closed head injury ranged from a few minutes to 8 days; 77% of patients with these injuries fulfilled the DSM-III (American Psychiatric Association 1980) diagnostic criteria for major depressive disorder. Of those patients with depression, 46% believed their the depression did not begin until more than 6 months after the injury.

Studies consistently report increased risk of suicide subsequent to traumatic brain injury. Data from a follow-up study (Brooks 1990) of 42 patients with severe traumatic brain injury showed that 1 year after injury, 10% of those surveyed had spoken about suicide, and 2% had made suicide attempts. Five years after the traumatic event, 15% of the patients had made suicide attempts. In addition, many other patients expressed hopelessness about their condition and that life was not worth living. The medical team, family, and other caregivers must work closely together to gauge suicide risk on a regular and ongoing basis.

Manic episodes and bipolar disorders have also been reported to occur after traumatic brain injury, although the occurrence is less frequent than that of depression after brain injury (Bamrah and Johnson 1991; Clark and Davison 1987). Predisposing factors for the development of mania after brain injury include damage to the basal region of the right temporal lobe (Starkstein et al. 1990) and right orbitofrontal cortex (Starkstein et al. 1988) in patients who have family histories of bipolar disorder.

Delirium and Psychotic Changes

Psychosis can occur either immediately after brain injury or after a latency of many months of normal functioning. When the psychiatrist is consulted during the time period in which the patient with a brain injury is emerging from coma, the usual clinical picture is one of delirium, with restlessness, agitation, confusion, disorientation, delusions, and/or hallucinations. Although delirium in patients with traumatic brain injury is most often the result of the effects of the injury on brain tissue chemistry, the psychiatrist should be aware that there may be other causes for the delirium (e.g., side effects of medication, withdrawal, or intoxication from drugs ingested before the traumatic event) and environmental factors (e.g., sensory monotony). Table 14–2 lists common factors that can result in posttraumatic delirium.

Psychosis that occurs after a span of time subsequent to the trauma is more difficult to diagnose and treat. Lishman (1987) reported schizophrenic-like symptoms of patients after traumatic brain injury that were "indistinguishable" from symptoms of the "naturally occurring" disorder. Psychotic symptoms may persist despite improvement in the cognitive deficits caused by trauma (Nasrallah et al. 1981).

Review of the literature (Davison and Bagley 1969) revealed that 1%–15% of schizophrenic inpatients have histories of brain injury. Wilcox and Nasrallah (1987) found that a group of patients diagnosed with schizophrenia had a significantly greater history of brain injury with loss of consciousness before the age of 10 than did patients who were diagnosed with mania or depression or patients who were hospitalized for surgery. Homeless mentally ill individuals are also at increased risk for brain injury. We believe that the cognitive deficits subsequent to traumatic brain injury in conjunction with psychosis increase the risk for becoming homeless; in addition, being homeless and living in a shelter carries a definite risk for trauma (Kass and Silver 1990).

Posttraumatic Epilepsy

A varying percentage of patients—depending on the location and severity of injury—will have seizures during the acute period after trauma. Posttraumatic epilepsy, with repeated seizures and the requirement for anticonvulsant medication, occurs in approximately 12%, 2%, and 1% of patients with severe, moderate, and mild head injuries, respectively, within 5 years of the injury (Annegers et al. 1980). Risk factors for posttraumatic epilepsy include skull fractures and wounds that penetrate the brain.

Salazar et al. (1985) studied 421 Vietnam veterans who had sustained brain-penetrating injuries and found that 53% had posttraumatic epilepsy. In 18% of these patients, the first seizure occurred after 5 years; in 7%, the first seizure occurred after 10 years. In addition, 26% of those patients with epilepsy had an organic mental syndrome as defined in DSM-III. Patients who develop posttraumatic epilepsy have also been shown to have more difficulties with physical and social functioning and to require more intensive rehabilitation efforts (Armstrong et al. 1990).

Posttraumatic epilepsy is associated with psychosis, especially when seizures arise from the temporal lobes. Brief episodic psychoses may occur with epilepsy;

Table 14–2. Etiologies for posttraumatic delirium

Fluid and electrolyte imbalance	Decreased oxygenation
Infections	Side effects of medications
Blood disorders (e.g., anemias and coagulopathies)	Drug intoxication or withdrawal
	Sensory monotony

about 7% of patients with epilepsy have persistent psychoses (McKenna et al. 1985). These psychoses exhibit a number of atypical features, including confusion and rapid fluctuations in mood.

Anticonvulsant drugs can result in cognitive and emotional symptoms (Reynolds and Trimble 1985; Smith and Bleck 1991). Phenytoin has more profound effects on cognition than does carbamazepine (Gallassi et al. 1988), and negative effects on cognition have been found in patients who received phenytoin after traumatic injury (Dikmen et al. 1991). Treatment with more than one anticonvulsant (polytherapy) has been associated with increased adverse neuropsychiatric reactions (Reynolds and Trimble 1985).

Patients who have a seizure immediately after brain injury often are placed on an anticonvulsant drug for seizure prophylaxis. Temkin et al. (1990) showed that the administration of phenytoin acutely after traumatic injury had no prophylactic effect on seizures that occurred subsequent to the first week after injury. Therefore, any patient with traumatic brain injury who is treated with anticonvulsant medication requires regular reevaluations to substantiate continued clinical necessity.

Anxiety Disorders

Several anxiety disorders may develop after traumatic brain injury. Approximately 60% of the relatives of 55 patients with severe traumatic brain injury reported that the patients were tense or anxious within the first year after injury (McKinlay et al. 1981). There was no change in this percentage 5 years after the trauma (Brooks et al. 1986). However, only 18% of 57 patients in another study complained of anxiety 2 years after severe traumatic brain injury (van Zomeren and van den Burg 1985). Patients with mild traumatic brain injury do not appear to be at an increased risk for complaints of anxiety (Dikmen et al. 1986; Schoenhuber and Gentili 1988).

Because of the potential life-threatening nature of many of the causes of traumatic brain injury, including motor vehicle accidents and assaults, patients are at increased risk of developing posttraumatic stress disorder (PTSD). Typical symptoms of PTSD, according to DSM-III-R (American Psychiatric Association 1987), include reexperiencing the traumatic event, social withdrawal, and autonomic hyperactivity. Patients may also develop anxiety or phobias related to the situation that caused the injury, such as severe anxiety when driving for a person who was injured in a motor vehicle accident.

Minor Brain Injury (Postconcussion Syndrome)

Patients with "minor" brain injury may present with somatic, perceptual, cognitive, and emotional symptoms that have been characterized as the *postconcussion syndrome* (Table 14–3). By definition, minor brain injury is associated with a brief duration of loss of consciousness (less than 20 minutes) or no loss of consciousness, and the patient usually does not require hospitalization after the injury. The psychiatrist is often called to assess the patient years after the injury, and brain-related symptoms such as depression and cognitive dysfunction may not be associated with the injury. The results of laboratory tests, such as brain imaging studies, often do not reveal significant abnormalities.

Nonetheless, patients with a history of "mild" injury or "brief" loss of consciousness can experience severe cognitive sequelae, possibly from diffuse axonal injury. In the evaluation of neuropsychological deficits in 53 patients who were experiencing postconcussive problems from 1 to 22 months after injury, Leininger et al. (1990) detected significantly poorer performance on tests of reasoning, information processing, and verbal learning than that found in a control population.

Although there is often substantial resolution of postconcussion symptoms within 3 months after injury, Schoenhuber et al. (1988) found that of 103 patients with minor head injury, 54% complained of irritability, 47% complained of memory loss, and 39% complained of depression after 1 year. However, many patients return to work despite the continuation of psychiatric symptoms (Hugenholtz et al. 1988).

Patients with minor traumatic brain injury usually vividly recall the traumatic event, and this may contribute to the development of PTSD in addition to postconcussive symptoms. There is overlap between these two syndromes, and determining the predominate diagnosis may be difficult. In general, postconcussion symptoms should decrease within 3 months, whereas symptoms of PTSD may not diminish until 3–6 months after the trauma.

Aggression

Irritability and aggressiveness are major sources of disability to patients with traumatic head injuries and of stress to their families. McKinlay et al. (1981) found that irritability and aggressiveness occur in as many as 70% of the people who experience brain damage from blunt trauma in the first year after injury. After 5 years, 64% of relatives complained that irritability was still problematic (Brooks et al. 1986). Thomsen (1984) found that 48% of patients had irritability 10–15 years after severe injury. For patients with minor brain injury, 54% complained of irritability after 1 year (Schoenhuber et al. 1988).

Explosive and violent behaviors have long been associated with focal brain lesions as well as with diffuse damage to the central nervous system (Elliott 1976). The current DSM-III-R classification of this disorder is *organic personality syndrome, explosive type*. However, most of the criteria in this DSM-III-R category refer to changes that are related to injury to the prefrontal and frontal regions of the brain.

Table 14–3.   Symptoms of postconcussion syndrome[a]

Somatic symptoms	Perceptual symptoms
Headache	Tinnitus
Dizziness	Sensitivity to noise
Fatigue	Sensitivity to light
Insomnia	**Emotional symptoms**
Cognitive symptoms	Depression
Memory difficulties	Anxiety
Impaired concentration	Irritability

[a]Adapted from Lishman (1988).
Source.   Reprinted from Silver JM, Hales RE, Yudofsky SC: "Psychiatric Consultation to Neurology," in *American Psychiatric Press Review of Psychiatry,* Vol 9. Edited by Tasman A, Goldfinger SM, Kaufmann CA. Washington, DC, American Psychiatric Press, 1990, pp. 433–465. Used with permission.

Dyscontrol of aggression may occur with damage to many other cortical and subcortical structures, without the associated personality disturbances specified in DSM-III-R (Weiger and Bear 1988).

Because of the prominence of this syndrome, we have proposed a specific diagnostic category of *organic aggressive syndrome*, which describes the specific condition of dyscontrol of rage and violence secondary to brain lesions and avoids reference to the variety of emotional and behavioral changes described in DSM-III-R (Table 14–4). The characteristic features of this syndrome differ from aggression related to diagnoses not associated with brain injury (Yudofsky et al. 1990). Characteristics of organic aggressive syndrome include reaction to modest or trivial stimuli that is without premeditation and does not serve any obvious purpose, brief and explosive outbursts punctuated by periods of relative calm, and feelings of remorse or embarrassment after the outburst (Yudofsky and Silver 1985; Yudofsky et al. 1989).

TREATMENT

Many useful therapeutic approaches are available for people with brain injuries. Brain-injured patients may develop neuropsychiatric symptoms based on the location of their injury, the emotional reaction to their injury, their preexisting strengths and difficulties, and social expectations and supports. Comprehensive rehabilitation centers address many of these issues with therapeutic strategies that are developed specifically for this population.

Although these programs meet many of the needs of patients with traumatic brain injury, comprehensive neuropsychiatric evaluation (including the daily evaluation and treatment of the patient by a psychiatrist) is rarely available. Although we propose a multifactorial, multidisciplinary, collaborative approach to treatment, for purposes of exposition we have divided treatment into psychopharmacological, behavioral, and psychological and social interventions.

Psychopharmacological Treatment

Psychopharmacological agents are commonly prescribed and may be highly effective in the treatment of specific psychiatric syndromes and symptomatologies. A key principle is that patients with brain injury of any type are far more likely to be

Table 14–4.   Diagnostic criteria for proposed organic aggressive syndrome

Persistent or recurrent aggressive outbursts, whether of a verbal or physical nature.

The outbursts are out of proportion to the precipitating stress or provocation.

Evidence from history, physical examination, or laboratory tests of a specific organic factor that is judged to be etiologically related to the disturbance.

The outbursts are not primarily related to the following disorders: paranoia, mania, schizophrenia, narcissistic personality disorder, borderline disorder, conduct disorder, or antisocial personality disorder.

Source.   Reprinted from Yudofsky SC, Silver JM, Yudofsky B: "Organic Personality Disorder, Explosive Type," in *Treatments of Psychiatric Disorders: A Task Force Report of the American Psychiatric Association.* Washington, DC, American Psychiatric Association, 1989, pp. 839–852. Used with permission.

sensitive to the side effects (and, occasionally, the therapeutic effects) of medications than are patients without brain injury. For example, the sedative and anticholinergic side effects (especially memory impairment) of thioridazine (Mellaril and others) or amitriptyline (Elavil and others) occur at much lower doses for patients with brain injury than for those without brain injury. Therefore, doses of psychotropic medications must be raised and lowered in small increments over protracted periods of time, although patients ultimately may require the same doses and serum levels that are used for patients without brain injury to achieve therapeutic response (Silver et al. 1990a, 1990b, 1991).

Many psychotropic medications affect seizure threshold (Silver and Yudofsky 1988). This can be of concern because of the frequent problem of posttraumatic seizures after traumatic brain injury. Of all the antipsychotic drugs, molindone and fluphenazine have consistently demonstrated the lowest potential for lowering the seizure threshold (Oliver et al. 1982; Silver and Yudofsky 1988). Clozapine treatment is associated with a significant dose-related incidence of seizures (ranging from 1% to 2% of patients who receive doses below 300 mg/day, and 5% of patients who receive 600–900 mg/day). Patients treated with the antidepressants maprotiline and bupropion also possibly have a higher incidence of seizures.

Wroblewski et al. (1990) reviewed the records of 68 patients with traumatic brain injury who received tricyclic antidepressant (TCA) treatment for at least 3 months. The frequency of seizures were compared for the 3 months before, during, and after treatment. Seizures occurred among 6 patients during the baseline period, 16 during TCA treatment, and 4 after treatment. Fourteen patients (19%) had seizures shortly after the initiation of TCA treatment. For 12 of these patients, no seizures occurred after TCA treatment was discontinued. Importantly, 7 of these patients were receiving anticonvulsant medication before and during TCA treatment. The occurrence of seizures was related to greater severity of brain injury. The authors concluded and we concur that TCAs should be used with caution in patients with severe traumatic brain injury. Nonetheless, other investigators found that seizure control did not appear to worsen if psychotropic medications were introduced cautiously and if the patient was on an effective anticonvulsant regimen (Ojemann et al. 1987).

Affective illness (depression, mania, mood lability). The literature regarding the effects of antidepressant agents in the treatment of patients with brain damage and, specifically, traumatic brain injury is sparse (Silver et al. 1991). Somatic therapies can be effective in the treatment of depression in patients with other neurological diseases. These treatments include antidepressants, stimulants, and electroconvulsive therapy (ECT) (Silver et al. 1990b).

Varney et al. (1987) found that 82% of 51 patients with major depressive disorder and traumatic brain injury who received treatment with either TCAs or carbamazepine reported at least moderate relief of depressive symptoms. Cassidy (1989) reported on an open trial using fluoxetine with 9 patients with severe traumatic brain injury and associated depression. He found that 2 had marked improvement and 3 had moderate improvement. Interestingly, half the patients experienced sedative side effects, and 3 out of 8 patients reported an increase in the levels of anxiety.

Antidepressants should be carefully monitored to ensure that the patient receives an adequate dose of medication. The choice of medication depends on the desired side effect profile. For this reason, antidepressants with the fewest sedative, hypotensive, and anticholinergic side effects are preferred. We suggest nortriptyline (initial doses of 10 mg/day), or desipramine (initial doses of 10 mg tid), and a careful plasma monitoring to achieve plasma levels in the therapeutic range for the parent compound and its major metabolites (e.g., nortriptyline levels 50–100 ng/ml; desipramine levels greater than 125 ng/ml) (American Psychiatric Association 1985). If the patient becomes sedated, confused, or severely hypotensive, the dosage of these drugs should be reduced. Fluoxetine (Prozac) or sertraline (Zoloft), with no anticholinergic effects, is also recommended. ECT remains a highly effective and underutilized modality for the treatment of depression overall, and can be used effectively after acute traumatic brain injury (Ruedrich et al. 1983).

Manic episodes that occur after traumatic brain injury have been successfully treated with lithium carbonate, carbamazepine (Stewart and Nemsath 1988), valproic acid (Pope et al. 1988), and ECT (Clark and Davison 1987). Many of these drugs have neurological side effects. Lithium has been reported to aggravate confusion in patients with brain damage (Schiff et al. 1982), as well as to induce nausea, tremor, ataxia, and lethargy.

Brain damage increases the susceptibility to neurotoxicity induced by combination therapy with carbamazepine and lithium (Parmelee and O'Shannick 1988). These symptoms frequently include lethargy, confusion, drowsiness, weakness, ataxia, nystagmus, and increased seizures. For patients with affective disorders following brain injury, we limit the use of lithium to those with mania or with recurrent depressive illness that preceded brain damage. To avoid lithium-related side effects, we begin with low doses (300 mg/day) and assess the response to low therapeutic blood levels (e.g., 0.2–0.5 mEq/L). For patients who have a seizure disorder in addition to mania, carbamazepine or valproic acid should be considered.

Antidepressants can be used to treat the labile mood that often occurs with neurological disease. Schiffer et al. (1985) conducted a double-blind crossover study with amitriptyline and placebo in 12 patients with pathological laughing and crying secondary to multiple sclerosis. Eight patients had a dramatic response to amitriptyline, at a maximum dose of 75 mg/day. Hornstein et al. (1990) reported that patients with "emotional incontinence" secondary to several neurological disorders responded to treatment with fluoxetine. In our experience, antidepressants such as nortriptyline, desipramine, and sertraline can also be effective for this condition. It may be necessary to administer these medications at standard antidepressant dosages to obtain full therapeutic effects.

Cognitive function and arousal. Stimulants, such as dextroamphetamine and methylphenidate, and dopamine agonists, such as amantadine and bromocriptine, may be beneficial in treating the patient with apathy and impaired concentration (Evans et al. 1987; Weinstein and Wells 1981). Gualtieri (1988) recommended stimulant medication for brain-injured patients with attention-deficit disorder with hyperactivity, anergia or apathy, and/or frontal lobe syndrome. These medications are not without side effects: patients may develop agitation and irritability or may become depressed on discontinuation. Therefore, stimulants should never precipitously be discontinued and should always be tapered slowly. When prescribed in usual dosages, stimulants do not appear to lower seizure threshold.

Psychosis.   The psychotic ideation resulting from traumatic brain injury is generally responsive to treatment with antipsychotic medications. However, side effects such as hypotension, sedation, and confusion are common. Also, patients with brain injury are particularly subject to dystonias, akathisias, and other parkinsonian side effects— even at relatively low doses of antipsychotic medications. Antipsychotic medications may also impede the neuronal recovery that follows brain injury (Feeney et al. 1982). Therefore, we advise that antipsychotics be used sparingly during the acute phases of recovery after the injury. Haloperidol (Haldol) 0.5 mg bid, or fluphenazine (Prolixin) 0.5 mg bid, may be used as initial treatment. In general, we recommend a low-dose neuroleptic strategy for all patients (Silver and Yudofsky 1988).

Anxiety disorders and PTSD.   We prefer to treat complaints of anxiety in patients with brain injury with supportive psychotherapy and social interventions. When the symptoms are so severe that they require pharmacological intervention, treatment with benzodiazepines or buspirone may be considered. Side effects of benzodiazepines include sedation and memory impairment, which often affect the cognitive performance of patients with brain injury. Benzodiazepines with briefer half-lives may be used, if those agents are indicated. Buspirone has less effect on cognitive functioning than do benzodiazepines, but its therapeutic effects occur after a latency of several weeks.

   Patients with brain injury may also develop other anxiety disorders, such as panic disorder, obsessive-compulsive disorder, PTSD, and phobias. Medications, particularly antidepressants, are often indicated for these disorders, with the caveat that these patients are more susceptible to side effects. The most important step in the treatment of the patient with PTSD is the careful assessment and diagnosis of comorbid DSM-III-R Axis I or II conditions. When there is no pervasive comorbid condition, antidepressant medications should be the initial pharmacological treatment. The positive symptoms of PTSD, including reexperiencing of the event and increased arousal, often improve with medication. The negative symptoms of avoidance and withdrawal usually respond poorly to pharmacotherapy.

Sleep.   Sleep patterns of patients with brain damage are often disordered, with impaired rapid-eye-movement (REM) recovery and multiple nocturnal awakenings (Prigatano et al. 1982). Hypersomnia that occurs after severe penetrating head injury most often resolves within the first year after injury, whereas insomnia that occurs in patients with long periods of coma and diffuse injury has a more chronic course (Askenasy et al. 1989). Barbiturates, alcohol, and long-acting benzodiazepines should be prescribed with great caution. These drugs interfere with REM and stage 4 sleep patterns, and may contribute to persistent insomnia (Buysse and Reynolds 1990). Clinicians should advise patients against using over-the-counter preparations for sleeping and for colds because of the prominent anticholinergic side effects of these remedies.

Aggression.   Although the Food and Drug Administration (FDA) has not approved any medication specifically for the treatment of aggression, medications are widely used (and commonly misused) in the management of acute aggressive episodes as well as for chronically aggressive patients. Before any therapeutic intervention is planned for the treatment of violent behavior, the clinician must carefully document these behaviors, including spontaneous day-to-day and week-to-week fluctuations. The Overt Aggression Scale (OAS) (Figure 14–1) can help the clinician monitor the efficacy of interventions and designate specific time frames for the initiation and discontinuation of pharmacotherapy of acute episodes and the initiation of pharmacotherapy for chronic aggressive behavior (Yudofsky et al. 1986). Sedation-producing medication must be time limited to avoid seriously disabling side effects, ranging from oversedation to tardive dyskinesia.

Table 14–5 summarizes our recommendations for the use of various classes of medication in the treatment of aggressive disorders. In treating aggression, the clinician, where possible, should diagnose and treat underlying disorders and use, where possible, antiaggressive agents specific for those disorders.

Antipsychotics are the most commonly used medications in the treatment of aggression. Although these agents are appropriate and effective when aggression is related to active psychosis, the use of neuroleptic agents to treat chronic aggression, especially due to organic brain injury, is often ineffective and entails significant risks for the patient to develop serious complications. In these cases, the sedative side effects, rather than the antipsychotic properties of the drugs, are used to "treat" (i.e., mask) the aggression.

Often, patients develop tolerance to the sedative effects of the neuroleptics and, therefore, require increasing doses. As a result, extrapyramidal and anticholinergic-related side effects occur. Paradoxically (and frequently), because of the development of akathisia, the patient may become more agitated and restless as the dose of neuroleptic is increased, especially when a high-potency antipsychotic is administered. The akathisia is often mistaken for increased irritability and agitation, and a vicious cycle of increasing neuroleptics and worsening akathisias occurs.

Although other investigators have recommended antipsychotic drugs such as haloperidol for the treatment of agitation with closed head injury (Rao et al. 1985), we recommend the use of antipsychotic agents only for the management of aggression stemming from psychotic ideation or for the intermittent management of brief aggressive events related to organic dyscontrol (through the sedative effects of neuroleptics). Table 14–6 summarizes the most disabling side effects that occur when neuroleptics are used to treat chronic aggression in patients with traumatic brain injury.

The literature concerning the effects of the benzodiazepines in the treatment of aggression is inconsistent. Reports of increased hostility and paradoxical induction of rage are balanced by reports that this phenomenon is rare and that benzodiazepines may be effective in controlling aggression (Dietch and Jennings 1988; Silver and Yudofsky 1988; Yudofsky et al. 1987). If sedation is necessary in the management of acute aggression, medications such as paraldehyde, chloral hydrate, or diphenhydramine may be preferable to sedative antipsychotic agents.

The sedative properties of benzodiazepines are especially helpful in the acute management of agitation and aggression. Intramuscular lorazepam has been suggested as an effective medication in the emergency treatment of the violent patient (Bick and Hannah 1986). Lorazepam in 1 or 2 mg doses may be administered, if necessary, in combination with a neuroleptic medication (haloperidol, 2–5 mg). Table 14–6 summarizes the problems associated with the use of benzodiazepines. Clonazepam may be effective in the long-term management of aggression, although controlled, double-blind studies have not been conducted (Freinhar and Alvarez

OVERT AGGRESSION SCALE (OAS)

Stuart Yudofsky, M.D., Jonathan Silver, M.D., Wynn Jackson, M.D., and Jean Endicott, Ph.D.

IDENTIFYING DATA

Name of patient	Name of rater
Sex of patient: 1 Male 2 Female	Date / / (mo/da/yr) Shift: 1 Night 2 Day 3 Evening

❐ No aggressive incident(s) (verbal or physical against self, others, or objects during the shift. (Check here)

AGGRESSIVE BEHAVIOR (check all that apply)

VERBAL AGGRESSION	PHYSICAL AGGRESSION AGAINST SELF
❐ Makes loud noises, shouts angrily	❐ Picks or scratches skin, hits self, pulls hair (with no or minor injury only)
❐ Yells mild personal insults, e.g., "You're stupid!"	❐ Bangs head, hits fist into objects, throws self onto floor or into objects (hurts self without serious injury)
❐ Curses viciously, uses foul language in anger, makes moderate threats to others or self	❐ Small cuts or bruises, minor burns
❐ Makes clear threats of violence toward others or self (I'm going to kill you.), or requests to help to control self	❐ Mutilates self, makes deep cuts, bites that bleed, internal injury, fracture, loss of consciousness, loss of teeth

PHYSICAL AGGRESSION AGAINST OBJECTS	PHYSICAL AGGRESSION AGAINST OTHER PEOPLE
❐ Slams door, scatters clothing, makes a mess	❐ Makes threatening gesture, swings at people, grabs at clothes
❐ Throws objects down, kicks furniture without breaking it, marks the wall	❐ Strikes, kicks, pushes, pulls hair (without injury to them)
❐ Breaks objects, smashes windows	❐ Attacks others causing mild-moderate physical injury (bruises, sprains, welts)
❐ Sets fires, throws objects dangerously	❐ Attacks others causing severe physical injury (broken bones, deep lacerations, internal injury)

Time incident began: _____:_____ AM/PM	Duration of incident: _____:_____ (hours/minutes)

INTERVENTION (check all that apply)

❐ None ❐ Talking to patient ❐ Closer observation ❐ Holding patient	❐ Immediate medication given by mouth ❐ Immediate medication given by injection ❐ Isolation without seclusion (time out) ❐ Seclusion	❐ Use of restraints ❐ Injury requires immediate medical treatment for patient ❐ Injury requires immediate treatment for other person

COMMENTS

Figure 14–1.   The Overt Aggression Scale.
Source.   Reprinted from Yudofsky SC, Silver JM, Jackson W, et al: "The Overt Aggression Scale for the Objective Rating of Verbal and Physical Aggression." *American Journal of Psychiatry* 143:35–39, 1986. Used with permission.

1986). We use this medication when aggression and anxiety occur together as pronounced symptoms in patients with brain injury.

In preliminary reports, buspiron—a serotonin subtype (5-HT$_{1A}$)—agonist has been reported to be effective in the management of aggression and agitation in patients with head injury (Levine 1988), dementia (Colenda 1988), and developmental disabilities (Ratey et al. 1989). We have also noted that some patients become more aggressive when treated with buspirone. Therefore, buspirone should be initiated at low dosages (i.e., 5 mg bid) and increased by 5 mg every 3–5 days. Dosages of 45–60 mg/day may be required before there is improvement in aggressive behavior.

Several reports discuss the use of antidepressants to control aggressive behavior. In open studies, Mysiw et al. (1988) and Jackson et al. (1985) reported that amitrip-

Table 14–5. Psychopharmacological treatment of aggression

Agent	Indications	Special clinical considerations
Acute aggression		
Antipsychotics	Psychotic symptoms Acute management of violence using sedative side effects	Oversedation and multiple side effects
Benzodiazepines	Acute management of violence using sedative side effects	Paradoxical rage
Chronic aggression		
Anticonvulsants		
Carbamazepine (CBZ); valproic acid (VPA)	Seizure disorder	Bone marrow suppression (CBZ) and hepatotoxicity (CBZ and VPA)
Lithium	Manic excitement or bipolar disorder	Neurotoxicity and confusion
Buspirone	Persistent, underlying anxiety and/or depression	Delayed onset of action
Antidepressants	Depression or mood lability with irritability	May need usual clinical doses
Propranolol (and other β-blockers)	Chronic or recurrent aggression	Latency of 4–6 weeks

Source. Adapted from Yudofsky et al. 1990. Used with permission.

Table 14–6. Side effects of drugs used in the management of aggression

Neuroleptics	Benzodiazepines
Oversedation	Oversedation
Hypotension (falls)	Motor disturbances (poor coordination)
Confusion	Mood disturbances
Neuroleptic malignant syndrome	Memory impairment and confusion
Parkinsonian side effects	Dependency, overdoses, and withdrawal syndromes
Akathisia	Paradoxical violence
Dystonia	
Tardive dyskinesia	

Source. Reprinted from Yudofsky SC, Silver JM, Hales RE: "Pharmacologic Management of Aggression in the Elderly." *Journal of Clinical Psychiatry* 51 (10, Suppl.):22–28, 1990. Copyright 1990 by Physicians Postgraduate Press. Used with permission.

tyline (maximum dose 150 mg/day) was effective in the treatment of patients with recent severe brain injury whose agitation had not responded to behavioral techniques. Trazodone is another antidepressant that has been reported effective in treating aggression that occurs with organic mental disorders (Pinner and Rich 1988). Preliminary reports have been published on the use of fluoxetine (a potent serotonergic antidepressant) in the treatment of aggressive behavior in a patient with brain injury (Sobin et al. 1989), as well as patients with personality disorders (Coccaro et al. 1990). Fluoxetine is started with low doses (5 mg/day) by diluting the contents of a 20 mg capsule in water, and raising the dose as tolerated every week to doses as large as 80 mg/day.

Although lithium is known to be effective in controlling aggression related to manic excitement, many studies have suggested that it may also have a role in the treatment of aggression in selected, nonbipolar patient populations. These include patients with head injury (Haas and Cope 1985), mental retardation and self-injurious behavior (Luchins and Dojka 1989), and other organic brain syndromes (Silver and Yudofsky 1988; Yudofsky et al. 1987). Because of the potential for neurotoxicity and its relative lack of efficacy in many patients with aggression secondary to brain injury, we recommend the use of lithium in those patients whose aggression is related to manic effects or recurrent irritability related to cyclic mood disorders.

Carbamazepine, an anticonvulsant effective for the treatment of bipolar disorders and generalized and complex partial seizures, has been advocated for the control of aggression in both epileptic and nonepileptic populations (Gleason and Schneider 1990; Silver and Yudofsky 1988). This is a highly effective medication to treat aggression in patients with brain injury, particularly for those patients who have aggressive episodes and seizures or epileptic foci.

Although a specific antiaggressive response to carbamazepine has not yet been demonstrated according to the most strict scientific criteria, a vast amount of clinical experience strongly suggests its efficacy in this area. However, the clinician should be aware of the potential risks associated with carbamazepine treatment, particularly bone marrow suppression (including aplastic anemia) and hepatotoxicity. Complete blood counts and liver function tests should be appropriately monitored (Silver and Yudofsky 1988). In our experience and that of others (Giakas et al. 1990), the anticonvulsant valproic acid may also be helpful to some patients with organically induced aggression.

Since the first report of the use of β-adrenergic receptor blockers in the treatment of aggression in 1977, over 25 papers have appeared in the neurological and psychiatric literature reporting experience with over 200 patients (Silver and Yudofsky 1988; Yudofsky et al. 1987). Most of these patients had been unsuccessfully treated with antipsychotics, minor tranquilizers, lithium, and/or anticonvulsants before treatment with β-blockers. The β-blockers that have been investigated include propranolol (a lipid-soluble, nonselective receptor antagonist), nadolol (a water soluble, nonselective receptor antagonist), pindolol (a lipid-soluble, nonselective β-adrenergic receptor antagonist with partial sympathomimetic activity), and metoprolol (a lipid soluble, selective β-adrenergic receptor antagonist). A list of β-blockers and their pharmacological properties is shown in Table 14–7.

A growing body of evidence suggests that β-adrenergic receptor blockers are effective agents for the treatment of aggressive and violent behaviors, particularly those related to organic brain syndrome. When a patient requires the use of a once-a-day medication because of compliance difficulties, long-acting propranolol (i.e., Inderal LA) or nadolol (Corgard) can be used in once-a-day regimens. When patients develop bradycardia that prevents prescribing therapeutic dosages of propranolol, pindolol (Visken) can be substituted, using one-tenth the dosage. The intrinsic sympathomimetic activity of pindolol stimulates the β-receptor and restricts the development of bradycardia.

Brain Injury. Historically, pharmacological treatment has been directed towards controlling the resultant symptomatologies (e.g., depression, aggression, and psychosis) that occur after brain injury. Over the past several years, there have been significant developments in the pharmacotherapy of brain injury; we anticipate that, in the near future, initial treatment of victims of brain trauma will be directed toward minimizing damage rather than treating the neuropsychiatric sequelae of the injury.

As discussed above, many intracellular events occur during injury, including hypoxia and release of excitotoxic substances, such as glutamate (Albers et al. 1989). Glutamate binds to the N-methyl-D-aspartate (NMDA) receptor, and causes neuronal swelling and intracellular calcium entry, leading to further toxicity and cell destruction. In addition, glutamate may lead to the production of free radicals, which also are neurotoxic. NMDA receptor antagonists, such as MK-801 and dextrorphan can block this toxicity. Interestingly, phencyclidine, a potent psychotomimetic agent, is an NMDA antagonist. Lazaroides, such as U74006F, inhibit lipid peroxidation that occurs after injury.

Table 14–7. Pharmacological characteristics of β-adrenergic receptor antagonists

Drug (generic/trade)	Potency[a]	Local anesthetic activity	ISA[b]	Lipid solubility	Plasma half-life (hours)
Nonselective (β₁- and β₂-adrenergic receptor) antagonists					
Alprenolol/Aptine	0.3–1	+	++	++	2–3
Carteolol/Cartrol	50	0	+	?	6
Nadolol/Corgard	0.5	0	0	0	14–18
Penbutolol/Levatal	4	0	+/–	?	26
Pindolol/Visken	5–10	+/–	++	+	3–4
Propranolol/Inderal	1.0	++	0	++	3–5
Sotalol/Sotalex	0.3	0	0	0	5–12
Timolol/Blocadren	5–10	0	+/–	+	4
Selective (β₁-adrenergic receptor) antagonists					
Acebutalol/Sectral	0.3	+	+	+	3
Atenolol/Tenormin	1.0	0	0	0	6–8
Betaxolol/Kerlone	4	+/–	–	?	14–22
Metoprolol/Lopressor	0.5–2	+/–	0	+	3–7

[a]Propanolol = 1.
[b]ISA = Intrinsic symptomometric activity.
Source. Data from Hoffman and Lefkowitz 1990 and American Medical Association, Department of Drugs, Division of Drugs and Toxicology 1991.

Behavioral and Cognitive Treatments

Behavioral treatments are important in the care of patients with traumatic brain injury. These programs require careful design and execution by a staff well versed in behavioral techniques. Behavioral methods can be used in response to aggressive outbursts and other maladaptive social behaviors (Burke and Lewis 1986). One study (Eames and Wood 1985) found that behavior modification was 75% effective in dealing with disturbed behaviors after severe brain injury.

After brain injury, patients may need specific cognitive strategies to assist with impairments in memory and concentration. As opposed to earlier thoughts that cognitive therapy should "exercise" the brain to develop skills that have been damaged, current therapies involve teaching the patient strategies to compensate for lost or impaired functions. (For more information on cognitive treatments, see Chapter 28.) We emphasize that, for most patients, treatment strategies are synergistic. For example, the use of β-adrenergic receptor antagonists to treat agitation and aggression can enhance a patient's ability to benefit from behavioral and cognitive treatments.

Psychological and Social Interventions

Psychological issues involving patients with brain injury revolve around four major themes: psychopathology that preceded the injury; psychological response to the traumatic event; psychological reactions to deficits brought about by brain injury; and psychological issues related to potential recurrence of brain injury.

Preexisting psychiatric illnesses are frequently intensified with brain injury. The angry, obsessive patient or the patient with chronic depression will exhibit a worsening of these symptoms after brain injury. Specific coping mechanisms used before the injury may no longer be possible because of cognitive deficits caused by the neurological disease. Therefore, patients need to learn new methods of adaptation to stress. In addition, as mentioned above, the social, economic, educational, and vocational status of the patient—and how these are affected by brain lesions—influence the patient's response to the injury.

The events surrounding brain injury often have far-reaching experiential and symbolic significance for the patient. Such issues as guilt, punishment, magical wishes, and fears crystallize about the nidus of a traumatic event. For example, a patient who sustains brain injury during a car accident may view the injury as punishment for long-standing violent impulses toward an aggressive father. In such cases, reassurance and homilies about his or her lack of responsibility for the accident are usually less productive than psychological exploration.

The patient's reactions to being disabled by brain damage have "realistic" as well as symbolic significance. When intense effort is required for a patient to form a word or move a limb, frustration may be expressed as anger, depression, anxiety, or fear. Particularly in cases in which brain injury results in permanent impairment, a psychiatrist may experience countertransferential discomfort that results in failure to discuss directly with the patient and his or her family the implications of resultant disabilities and limitations. Gratuitous optimism, collaboration with denial of the patient, and facile solutions to complex problems can erode the therapeutic alliance and ongoing treatment.

By gently and persistently directing the patient's attention to the reality of the disabilities, the psychiatrist can help the patient begin the process of acceptance and adjustment to the impairment. Clinical judgment will help the psychiatrist in deciding whether and when explorations of the symbolic significance of the patient's brain injury should be pursued. The persistence of anxiety, guilt, and fear beyond the normative stages of adjustment and rehabilitation may indicate that psychodynamic approaches are required.

Families of patients with neurological disorders are under severe stress. The relative with a brain injury may be unable to fulfill his or her previous role or function as parent or spouse, thus significantly affecting the other family members. By treating the psychological responses of relatives to the brain injury, the clinician can foster a supportive and therapeutic atmosphere for the patient as well as significantly help the relative.

For both patients and their families, severe traumatic brain injury results in multifaceted losses. The psychiatrist can be of enormous benefit in treating the family and patient by providing support, insight, and other points of view. Educational and supportive treatment of families can be therapeutic when used together with appropriate social skills training. Patient advocacy groups, such as the National Head Injury Foundation, can provide important peer support for families. Many patients require clear, almost concrete statements describing their behaviors because insight and judgment may be impaired.

Brain injury can and often does recur. With repeated injury, there is an increase in the incidence of neuropsychiatric and emotional symptoms (Carlsson et al. 1987). In fact, trauma from accidents occurs more commonly in patients who have already experienced such events than in those who have not. Therapeutic emphasis should be placed on those actions and activities that will aid in preventing recurrence, including compliance with appropriate medications and abstinence from alcohol and other substances of abuse.

PREVENTION

Motor Vehicle Accidents

The proper use of seat belts with upper torso restraints is 45% effective in preventing fatalities, 50% effective in preventing moderate to critical injuries, and 10% effective in preventing minor injuries when used by drivers and passengers (U.S. Department of Transportation 1984). This would translate to 12,000–15,000 lives saved a year (National Safety Council 1986). It is calculated that the installation of air bag safety devices in automobiles for drivers and passengers would save from 3,000 to 7,000 lives per year (National Safety Council 1986).

Alcohol abuse is a common concomitant of affective and characterological disorders. Alcohol intoxication is frequently found in the patient with brain injury, whether from violence, falls, or motor vehicle accidents (Brismar et al. 1983). In the United States, it is estimated by the National Safety Council that alcohol ingestion is implicated in more than 50% of all automobile-related fatalities (Haddon and Baker 1981). Alcohol-related deaths among people age 19 and 20 can be decreased by over one-third by changing the minimum drinking age from 18 to 21 (Decker et al. 1988).

Drivers in fatal accidents often have a history of alcohol use, previous accidents, moving traffic violations, psychopathology, stress, paranoid thinking, and depression. They often have poor control of hostility and anger, with low tolerance for tension, and a history of high risk taking (Tsuang et al. 1985). Psychiatric patients are at greater risk for motor vehicle accidents because they often have several of these characteristics (Noyes 1985). We strongly advocate that in all psychiatric and other medical histories a detailed inquiry about alcohol use, seat belt use, and driving patterns be present. The use of illicit substances and medications that may induce sedation, such as antihistamines, antihypertensive agents, anticonvulsants, minor tranquilizers, and antidepressants, should also be assessed and documented.

Motorcycle riding—with or without helmets—and using bicycles for commuting purposes are associated with head injuries, even when safety precautions are taken and driving regulations are observed. Nonuse of motorcycle helmets is associated with increased accident rates and fatalities (McSwain and Petrucelli 1984). The use of bicycle helmets can significantly decrease the morbidity and mortality from bicycle-related head injuries (Thompson et al. 1989).

Significant preventive measures to reduce head trauma include counseling a patient about risk taking; the treatment of alcoholism and depression; the judicious prescription of medications and full explanations of sedation, cognitive impairment, and other potentially dangerous side effects; and public information activities on topics such as the proper use of seat belts, the dangers of drinking and driving, and automobile safety measures.

Prevention of Brain Injury in Children

Each year in the United States over 1,400 children under age 13 die as motor vehicle passengers; more than 90% of these children were not using car seat restraints (Insurance Institute for Highway Safety 1983). Child safety seats have been found to be 80%–90% effective in the prevention of injuries to children (National Safety Council 1985).

Children younger than 4 years old who are not restrained in safety seats are 11 times more likely to be killed in motor vehicle accidents (National Safety Council 1985). It is not safe for the child to sit on the lap of the parent, with or without restraints, because the adult's weight can crush the child during an accident. Young children traveling with drivers who, themselves, are not wearing seat belts are four times as likely to be left unrestrained (National Safety Council 1985). Children who ride on bicycle-mounted child seats are highly subject to injuries to the head and face and must wear bicycle helmets (Sargent et al. 1988).

Children are often involved in sports that carry the risk of brain injury. Minor brain injury is not uncommon in football and can result in persistent symptoms and disabilities (Gerberich et al. 1983). Soccer may involve the use of the head with sudden twists to strike the ball that may also result in neuropsychiatric abnormalities (Tysvaer et al. 1989).

The clinician must always be alert to the possibility that patients may be neglectful, use poor judgment, and even be directly violent in their treatment of children. Unfortunately, it is not uncommon for head trauma to result from overt child abuse on the part of parents, other adults, and peers. We must always be alert to such possibilities in our patients and, when discovered, take direct actions to address these problems. We encourage direct counseling of patients who do not consistently use infant and child car seats for their children.

CONCLUSIONS

Invariably, brain injury leads to emotional damage in the patient and in the family. In this chapter, we have reviewed the most frequently occurring psychiatric symptomatologies that are associated with traumatic brain injury. We have emphasized how the informed psychiatrist is not only effective but essential both in the prevention of brain injury and, when it occurs, the treatment of its sequelae. We advocate, in addition to increased efforts devoted to the prevention of brain injury, a multidisciplinary and multidimensional approach to the assessment and treatment of neuropsychiatric aspects of brain injury.

REFERENCES

Adams JH, Graham DI, Murray LS, et al: Diffuse axonal injury due to nonmissile head injury in humans: an analysis of 45 cases. Ann Neurol 12:557–563, 1982

Albers GW, Goldberg MP, Choi DW: N-methyl-D-aspartate antagonists: ready for clinical trial in brain ischemia? Ann Neurol 25:398–403, 1989

American Psychiatric Association: Task Force on the Use of Laboratory Tests in Psychiatry: tricyclic antidepressants: blood level measurements and clinical outcome: an APA Task Force Report. Am J Psychiatry 142:155–162, 1985

American Psychiatric Association: Diagnostic and Statistical Manual of Mental Disorders, 3rd Edition. Washington, DC, American Psychiatric Association, 1980

American Psychiatric Association: Diagnostic and Statistical Manual of Mental Disorders, 3rd Edition, Revised. Washington, DC, American Psychiatric Association, 1987

Annegers JF, Grabow JD, Groover RV, et al: Seizures after head trauma: a population study. Neurology 30:683–689, 1980

Armstrong KK, Sahgal V, Bloch R, et al: Rehabilitation outcomes in patients with posttraumatic epilepsy. Arch Phys Med Rehabil 71:156–160, 1990

Askenasy JJM, Winkler I, Grushkiewicz J, et al: The natural history of sleep disturbances in severe missile head injury. Journal of Neurological Rehabilitation 3:93–96, 1989

Auerbach SH: Neuroanatomical correlates of attention and memory disorders in traumatic brain injury: an application of neurobehavioral subtypes. Journal of Head Trauma Rehabilitation 1:1–12, 1986

Bamrah JS, Johnson J: Bipolar affective disorder following head injury. Br J Psychiatry 158:117–119, 1991

Bick PA, Hannah AL: Intramuscular lorazepam to restrain violent patients (letter). Lancet 1:206, 1986

Brismar B, Engstrom A, Rydberg U: Head injury and intoxication: a diagnostic and therapeutic dilemma. Acta Chir Scand 149:11–14, 1983

Brooks N: Personal communication, reported in Eames P, Haffey WJ, Cope DN: Treatment of behavioral disorders, in Rehabilitation of the Adult and Child with Traumatic Brain Injury, 2nd Edition. Edited by Rosenthal M, Griffith ER, Bond MR, et al. Philadelphia, PA, FA Davis, 1990, pp 410–432

Brooks N, Campsie L, Symington C, et al: The five year outcome of severe blunt head injury: a relative's view. J Neurol Neurosurg Psychiatry 49:764–770, 1986

Burke WH, Lewis FD: Management of maladaptive social behavior of a brain injured adult. Int J Rehabil Res 9:335–342, 1986

Buysse DJ, Reynolds III CF: Insomnia, in Handbook of Sleep Disorders. Edited by Thorpy MJ. New York, Marcel Dekker, 1990, pp 373–434

Carlsson GS, Svardsudd K, Welin L: Long-term effects of head injuries sustained during life in three male populations. J Neurosurg 67:197–205, 1987

Cassidy JW: Fluoxetine: a new serotonergically active antidepressant. Journal of Head Trauma Rehabilitation 4:67–69, 1989

Clark AF, Davison K: Mania following head injury: a report of two cases and a review of the literature. Br J Psychiatry 150:841–844, 1987

Coccaro EF, Astill JL, Herbert JL, et al: Fluoxetine treatment of impulsive aggression in DSM-III-R personality disorder patients. J Clin Psychopharmacol 10:373–375, 1990

Colenda CC: Buspirone in treatment of agitated demented patients. Lancet 1:1169, 1988

Cope DN, Date ES, Mar EY: Serial computerized tomographic evaluations in traumatic head injury. Arch Phys Med Rehabil 69:483–486, 1988

Courville CB: Pathology of the Nervous System, 2nd Edition. Mountain View, CA, Pacific Press, 1945

Davison K, Bagley CR: Schizophrenic-like psychoses associated with organic disorders of the central nervous system: a review of the literature, in Current Problems in Neuropsychiatry: Schizophrenia, Epilepsy, the Temporal Lobe. Edited by Herrington RN. Br J Psychiatry (special publication no 4), 1969

Decker MD, Graitcer PL, Schaffner W: Reduction in motor vehicle fatalities associated with an increase in the minimum drinking age. JAMA 260:3604–3610, 1988

Department of Health and Human Services: Interagency Head Injury Task Force Report. Washington, DC, U.S. Government Printing Office, 1989

Dietch JT, Jennings RK: Aggressive dyscontrol in patients treated with benzodiazepines. J Clin Psychiatry 49:184–189, 1988

Dikmen S, McLean A, Temkin N: Neuropsychological and psychosocial consequences of minor head injury. J Neurol Neurosurg Psychiatry 49:1227–1232, 1986

Dikmen SS, Temkin NR, Miller B, et al: Neurobehavioral effects of phenytoin prophylaxis of posttraumatic seizures. JAMA 265:1271–1277, 1991

Eames P, Wood R: Rehabilitation after severe brain injury: a follow-up study of a behavior modification approach. J Neurol Neurosurg Psychiatry 48:613–619, 1985

Elliott FA: The neurology of explosive rage. Practitioner 217:51–59, 1976

Evans RW, Gualtieri CT, Patterson D: Treatment of chronic closed head injury with psychostimulant drugs: a controlled case study and an appropriate evaluation procedure. J Nerv Ment Dis 175:106–110, 1987

Faden AI, Demediuk P, Panter S, et al: The role of excitatory amino acids and NMDA receptors in traumatic brain injury. Science 244:798–800, 1989

Feeney DM, Gonzalez A, Law WA: Amphetamine, haloperidol, and experience interact to affect rate of recovery after motor cortex injury. Science 217:855–857, 1982

Freinhar JP, Alvarez WA: Clonazepam treatment of organic brain syndromes in three elderly patients. J Clin Psychiatry 47:525–526, 1986

Gallassi R, Morreale A, Lorusso S, et al: Carbamazepine and phenytoin: comparison of cognitive effects in epileptic patients during monotherapy and withdrawal. Arch Neurol 45:892–894, 1988

Gerberich SG, Priest JD, Boen JR, et al: Concussion incidences and severity in secondary school varsity football players. Am J Public Health 73:1370–1375, 1983

Giakas WJ, Seibyl JP, Mazure CM: Valproate in the treatment of temper outbursts (letter). J Clin Psychiatry 51:525, 1990

Gleason RP, Schneider LS: Carbamazepine treatment of agitation in Alzheimer's outpatients refractory to neuroleptics. J Clin Psychiatry 51:115–118, 1990

Goodin DS, Aminoff MJ, Laxer KD: Detection of epileptiform activity by different noninvasive EEG methods in complex partial epilepsy. Ann Neurol 27:330–334, 1990

Gualtieri CT: Pharmacotherapy and the neurobehavioural sequelae of traumatic brain injury. Brain Injury 2:101–129, 1988

Gulbrandsen GB: Neuropsychological sequelae of light head injuries in older children 6 months after trauma. J Clin Neuropsychol 6:257–268, 1984

Haas JF, Cope N: Neuropharmacologic management of behavior sequelae in head injury: a case report. Arch Phys Med Rehabil 66:472–474, 1985

Haddon JW, Baker SP: Injury control, in Preventive and Community Medicine. Edited by Clark D, McMahon B. Boston, MA, Little, Brown, 1981, pp 109–140

Hendrick EB, Harwood-Hash DCF, Hudson AR: Head injuries in children: a survey of 4465 consecutive cases at the Hospital for Sick Children, Toronto, Canada. Clin Neurosurg 11:46–65, 1965

Hendryx PM: Psychosocial changes perceived by closed-head-injured adults and their families. Arch Phys Med Rehabil 70:526–530, 1989

Hoffman BB, Lefkowitz RJ: Adrenergic Receptor Antagonists, in Goodwin and Gilman's The Pharmacological Basis of Therapeutics, 8th Edition. Edited by Gilman AG, Rall TW, Neiw AS, et al. New York, Pergamon, 1990

Hornstein A, Flax J, Seliger G, et al: Treatment of emotional incontinence with fluoxetine. Paper presented at the New Research Program at the annual meeting of the American Psychiatric Association, New York, May 1990

Hugenholtz H, Stuss DT, Stethem LL, et al: How long does it take to recover from a mild concussion? Neurosurgery 22:853–858, 1988

Insurance Institute for Highway Safety: Children in Crashes. Washington, DC, Insurance Institute for Highway Safety, 1983

Jackson RD, Corrigan JD, Arnett JA: Amitriptyline for agitation in head injury. Arch Phys Med Rehabil 66:180–181, 1985

Jane JA, Steward O, Gennarelli T: Axonal degeneration induced by experimental noninvasive minor injury. J Neurosurg 62:96–100, 1985

Kass F, Silver JM: Neuropsychiatry and the homeless. Journal of Neuropsychiatry and Clinical Neurosciences 2:15–19, 1990

Kinsella G, Moran C, Ford B, et al: Emotional disorder and its assessment within the severe head injured population. Psychol Med 18:57–63, 1988

Kreutzer JS, Zasler ND: Psychosexual consequences of traumatic brain injury: methodology and preliminary findings. Brain Injury 3:177–186, 1989

Kurtzke JF: Neuroepidemiology. Ann Neurol 16:265–277, 1984

Leininger BE, Gramling SE, Farrell AD, et al: Neuropsychological deficits in symptomatic minor head injury patients after concussion and mild concussion. J Neurol Neurosurg Psychiatry 53:293–296, 1990

Levin HS, Benton AL, Grossman RG: Neurobehavioral Consequences of Closed Head Injury. New York, Oxford University Press, 1982

Levin HS, High VM, Meyers CA, et al: Impairment of remote memory after closed head injury. J Neurol Neurosurg Psychiatry 48:556–563, 1985

Levin HS, Amparo E, Eisenberg HM, et al: Magnetic resonance imaging and computerized tomography in relation to the neurobehavioral sequelae of mild and moderate head injuries. J Neurosurg 66:706–713, 1987

Levin HS, Goldstein FC, High Jr WM, et al: Disproportionately severe memory deficit in relation to normal intellectual functioning after closed head injury. J Neurol Neurosurg Psychiatry 51:1294–1301, 1988

Levine AM: Buspirone and agitation in head injury. Brain Injury 2:165–167, 1988

Lishman WA: Organic Psychiatry: The Psychological Consequences of Cerebral Disorder, 2nd Edition. Boston, MA, Blackwell Scientific, 1987

Lishman WA: Physiogenesis and psychogenesis in the "post-concussional syndrome." Br J Psychiatry 153:460–469, 1988

Luchins DJ, Dojka D: Lithium and propranolol in aggression and self-injurious behavior in the mentally retarded. Psychopharmacol Bull 25:372–375, 1989

MacKinnon RA, Yudofsky SC: The Psychiatric Evaluation in Clinical Practice, 2nd Edition. Philadelphia, PA, JB Lippincott, 1991

McKenna PJ, Kane JM, Parrish K: Psychotic syndromes in epilepsy. Am J Psychiatry 142:895–904, 1985

McKinlay WW, Brooks DN, Bond MR, et al: The short-term outcome of severe blunt head injury as reported by the relatives of the injured person. J Neurol Neurosurg Psychiatry 44:527–533, 1981

McSwain NE, Petrucelli E: Medical consequences of motorcycle helmet nonusage. J Trauma 24:233–236, 1984

Mahoney WJ, D'Souza BJ, Haller JA, et al: Long-term outcome of children with severe head trauma and prolonged coma. Pediatrics 71:754–762, 1983

Morrison JH, Molliver ME, Grzanna R: Noradrenergic innervation of cerebral cortex: widespread effects of local cortical lesions. Science 205:313–316, 1979

Mysiw WJ, Jackson RD, Corrigan JD: Amitriptyline for post-traumatic agitation. Am J Phys Med Rehabil 67:29–33, 1988

Nasrallah HA, Fowler RC, Judd LL: Schizophrenia-like illness following head injury. Psychosomatics 22:359–361, 1981

National Safety Council: Accident Facts. Chicago, IL, National Safety Council, 1985

National Safety Council: Accident Facts. Chicago, IL, National Safety Council, 1986

Noyes Jr R: Motor vehicle accidents related to psychiatric impairment. Psychosomatics 26:569–580, 1985

Oddy M, Coughlan T, Tyerman A, et al: Social adjustment after closed head injury: a further follow-up seven years after injury. J Neurol Neurosurg Psychiatry 48:564–568, 1985

Ojemann LM, Baugh-Bookman C, Dudley DL: Effect of psychotropic medications on seizure control in patients with epilepsy. Neurology 37:1525–1527, 1987

Oliver AP, Luchins DJ, Wyatt RJ: Neuroleptic-induced seizures: an in vitro technique for assessing relative risk. Arch Gen Psychiatry 39:206–209, 1982

Parmelee DX, O'Shannick GJ: Carbamazepine-lithium toxicity in brain-damaged adolescents. Brain Injury 2:305–308, 1988

Pinner E, Rich CL: Effects of trazodone on aggressive behavior in seven patients with organic mental disorders. Am J Psychiatry 145:1295–1296, 1988

Pope Jr HG, McElroy SL, Satlin A, et al: Head injury, bipolar disorder, and response to valproate. Compr Psychiatry 29:34–38, 1988

Prigatano GP, Stahl ML, Orr WC, et al: Sleep and dreaming disturbances in closed head injury patients. J Neurol Neurosurg Psychiatry 45:78–80, 1982

Rao N, Jellinek HM, Woolston DC: Agitation in closed head injury: haloperidol effects on rehabilitation outcome. Arch Phys Med Rehabil 66:30–34, 1985

Rappaport M, Herrero-Backe C, Rappaport ML, et al: Head injury outcome up to ten years later. Arch Phys Med Rehabil 70:885–892, 1989

Ratey JJ, Sovner R, Mikkelsen E, et al: Buspirone therapy for maladaptive behavior and anxiety in developmentally disabled persons. J Clin Psychiatry 50:382–384, 1989

Regier DA, Boyd JH, Burke Jr JD, et al: One-month prevalence of mental disorders in the United States. Arch Gen Psychiatry 45:977–986, 1988

Reynolds EH, Trimble MR: Adverse neuropsychiatric effects of anticonvulsant drugs. Drugs 29:570–581, 1985

Rimel RW, Giordani B, Barth JT, et al: Disability caused by minor head injury. Neurosurgery 9:221–228, 1981

Ross ED, Stewart RS: Pathological display of affect in patients with depression and right frontal brain damage: an alternative mechanism. J Nerv Ment Dis 176:165–172, 1987

Ruedrich I, Chu CC, Moore SI: ECT for major depression in a patient with acute brain trauma. Am J Psychiatry 140:928–929, 1983

Ruff RM, Buchsbaum MS, Troster AI, et al: Computerized tomography, neuropsychology, and positron emission tomography in the evaluation of head injury. Neuropsychiatry, Neuropsychology, and Behavioral Neurology 2:103–123, 1989

Ruff RM, Marshall LF, Klauber MR, et al: Alcohol abuse and neurological outcome of the severely head injured. Journal of Head Trauma Rehabilitation 5:21–31, 1990

Rutherford WH, Merrett JD, McDonald JR: Sequelae of concussion caused by minor head injuries. Lancet 1:1–4, 1977

Salazar AM, Jabbari B, Vance SC, et al: Epilepsy after penetrating head injury, I: clinical correlates: a report of the Vietnam head injury study. Neurology 35:1406–1414, 1985

Sargent JD, Peck MG, Weitzman M: Bicycle-mounted child seats: injury risk and prevention. Am J Dis Child 142:765–767, 1988

Schiff HB, Sabin TD, Geller A, et al: Lithium in aggressive behavior. Am J Psychiatry 139:1346–1348, 1982

Schiffer RB, Herndon RM, Rudick RA: Treatment of pathologic laughing and weeping with amitriptyline. N Engl J Med 312:1480–1482, 1985

Schoenhuber R, Gentili M: Anxiety and depression after mild head injury: a case control study. J Neurol Neurosurg Psychiatry 51:722–724, 1988

Schoenhuber R, Gentili M, Orlando A: Prognostic value of auditory brain-stem responses for late postconcussion symptoms following minor head injury. J Neurosurg 68:742–744, 1988

Silver JM, Yudofsky SC: Psychopharmacology and electroconvulsive therapy, in The American Psychiatric Press Textbook of Psychiatry. Edited by Talbott JA, Hales RE, Yudofsky SC. Washington, DC, American Psychiatric Press, 1988, pp 767–853

Silver JM, Yudofsky SC: The Overt Aggression Scale: overview and clinical guidelines. Journal of Neuropsychiatry and Clinical Neurosciences 3:S22–S29, 1991

Silver JM, Hales RE, Yudofsky SC: Psychiatric consultation to neurology, in American Psychiatric Press Review of Psychiatry, Vol 9. Edited by Tasman A, Goldfinger SM, Kaufmann CA. Washington, DC, American Psychiatric Press, 1990a, pp 433–465

Silver JM, Hales RE, Yudofsky SC: Psychopharmacology of depression in neurologic disorders. J Clin Psychiatry 51 (1, suppl):33–39, 1990b

Silver JM, Yudofsky SC, Hales RE: Depression in traumatic brain injury. Neuropsychiatry, Neuropsychology, and Behavioral Neurology 4:12–23, 1991

Smith MC, Bleck TP: Convulsive disorders: toxicity of anticonvulsants. Clin Neuropharmacol 14:97–115, 1991

Sobin P, Schneider L, McDermott H: Fluoxetine in the treatment of agitated dementia. Am J Psychiatry 146:1636, 1989

Starkstein SE, Boston JD, Robinson RG: Mechanisms of mania after brain injury: 12 case reports and review of the literature. J Nerv Ment Dis 176:87–100, 1988

Starkstein SE, Mayberg HS, Berthier ML, et al: Mania after brain injury: neuroradiological and metabolic findings. Ann Neurol 27:652–659, 1990

Stewart JT, Nemsath RH: Bipolar illness following traumatic brain injury: treatment with lithium and carbamazepine. J Clin Psychiatry 49:74–75, 1988

Teasdale G, Jennett B: Assessment of coma and impaired consciousness: a practical scale. Lancet 2:81–84, 1974

Temkin NR, Dikmen SS, Wilensky AJ, et al: A randomized, double-blind study of phenytoin for the prevention of post-traumatic seizures. N Engl J Med 323:497–502, 1990

Thompson RS, Rivara FP, Thompson DC: A case-control study of the effectiveness of bicycle safety helmets. N Engl J Med 320:1361–1367, 1989

Thomsen IV: Late outcome of very severe blunt head trauma: a 10–15 year second follow-up. J Neurol Neurosurg Psychiatry 47:260–268, 1984

Tsuang MT, Boor M, Fleming JA: Psychiatric aspects of traffic accidents. Am J Psychiatry 142:538–546, 1985

Tysvaer AT, Storli OV, Bachen NI: Soccer injuries to the brain: a neurologic and electroencephalographic study of former players. Acta Neurol Scand 80:151–156, 1989

U.S. Department of Transportation: Final Regulatory Impact Assessment on Amendments to Federal Motor Vehicle Safety Standard 208, Front Seat Occupant Protection (Publ DOT HS 806 572). Washington, DC, U.S. Government Printing Office, 1984

van Zomeren A, van den Burg W: Residual complaints of patients two years after severe head injury. J Neurol Neurosurg Psychiatry 48:21–28, 1985

Varney NR: Prognostic significance of anosmia in patients with closed-head trauma. J Clin Exp Neuropsychol 10:250–254, 1988

Varney NR, Martzke JS, Roberts RJ: Major depression in patients with closed head injury. Neuropsychology 1:7–9, 1987

Weddell R, Oddy M, Jenkins D: Social adjustment after rehabilitation: a two year follow-up of patients with severe head injury. Psychosom Med 10:257–263, 1980

Weiger WA, Bear DM: An approach to the neurology of aggression. J Psychiatr Res 22:85–98, 1988

Weinstein GS, Wells CE: Case studies in neuropsychiatry: post-traumatic psychiatric dysfunction: diagnosis and treatment. J Clin Psychiatry 42:120–122, 1981

Wilberger JE, Deeb A, Rothfus W: Magnetic resonance imaging in cases of severe head injury. Neurosurgery 20:571–576, 1987

Wilcox JA, Nasrallah HA: Childhood head trauma and psychosis. Psychiatry Res 21:303–306, 1987

Wroblewski BA, McColgan K, Smith K, et al: The incidence of seizures during tricyclic antidepressant drug treatment in a brain-injured population. J Clin Psychopharmacol 10:124–128, 1990

Yudofsky SC, Silver JM: Psychiatric aspects of brain injury: trauma, stroke, and tumor, in Psychiatry Update: American Psychiatric Press Annual Review, Vol 4. Edited by Hales RE, Frances AJ. Washington, DC, American Psychiatric Press, 1985, pp 142–158

Yudofsky SC, Silver JM, Jackson W, et al: The Overt Aggression Scale for the objective rating of verbal and physical aggression. Am J Psychiatry 143:35–39, 1986

Yudofsky SC, Silver JM, Schneider SE: Pharmacologic treatment of aggression. Psychiatric Annals 17:397–407, 1987

Yudofsky SC, Silver JM, Yudofsky B: Organic personality disorder, explosive type, in Treatments of Psychiatric Disorders: A Task Force Report of the American Psychiatric Association. Washington, DC, American Psychiatric Association, 1989, pp 839–852

Yudofsky SC, Silver JM, Hales RE: Pharmacologic management of aggression in the elderly. J Clin Psychiatry 51 (10, suppl):22–28, 1990

Chapter 15

Neuropsychiatric Aspects of Epilepsy and Atypical Spells

Vernon M. Neppe, M.D., Ph.D.
Gary J. Tucker, M.D.

As psychiatrists have become more aware of the multiple physical conditions that can cause behavior change and particularly psychosis, they have become increasingly aware of the behavior changes associated with seizure disorders. The study of seizure disorders for psychiatrists is not only important for diagnostic and treatment purposes, it also has many theoretical implications for the understanding of behavioral disorders in general (Neppe and Tucker 1988b).

Two major historical relationships between epilepsy and psychopathology exist, namely personality and psychosis. There are also several controversies in the psychiatric perception of epilepsy, such as the place of temporal lobe epilepsy and the difficulties of evaluating epilepsy in the modern psychiatric context and the relationship of epilepsy to psychopathology. In this chapter we address all these areas.

EPILEPSY IN MODERN PSYCHIATRY

Seizure disorders have been largely ignored in current psychiatric nosology, and in DSM-III-R (American Psychiatric Association 1987) there is no diagnosis of epilepsy and related conditions and the entity of *epileptic psychosis* does not exist except as a part of the more general concept of organic delusional disorder. Epilepsy with psychosis generally is classified as *atypical psychosis* or organic hallucinosis or organic delusional state. Even a diagnosis of atypical psychosis will only be disputably correct because DSM-III-R refers to "other nonorganic psychotic disorders," and it is unclear whether or not organic disorders can be included under atypical psychosis.

In general, the person with epilepsy is healthy and does not have any psychiatric stigmata. However, one apparently conservative estimation suggested that about one-fifth of epileptic outpatients have major psychopathology, for which about one-half will require hospitalization (Blumer 1975). There is a substantial increase in psychoses in seizure disorders. The incidence in epileptic populations has been variably cited

We gratefully acknowledge the permission given by the American Psychiatric Association and *Hospital and Community Psychiatry* to reproduce here significant, updated sections from our two-part series on epilepsy and psychiatry (Neppe and Tucker 1988a, 1988b).

at frequencies from 2.8% to 27% (with an average of 7%), and the prevalence of epilepsy in psychiatric hospitals is 2%–3%, which is much higher than the general population prevalence rate for seizure disorders of about 1.5% (Pincus and Tucker 1985). These figures would make the lifetime expectancy of psychosis in epilepsy about 10% over a 30-year period, whereas the lifetime risk for schizophrenia in the general population is about 0.8% (McKenna et al. 1985).

Although they constitute a small proportion of the total epilepsy population, patients with underlying coarse organic neurobehavioral syndromes superimposed on or coexisting with the epilepsy, or with behavioral disturbances or psychoses as a consequence of the epilepsy, are the ones most often written about. Epileptic patients without additional psychopathology who work well within the community comprise what we call the "epilepsy standard group" as opposed to the "epilepsy plus group" who have additional organic concomitants or psychotic predispositions. The differentiation is more than academic because associated psychopathology or coarse neurobehavioral syndromes in and of themselves may produce symptoms that may distort interpretations of the psychiatric population with epilepsy when in fact the epilepsy was not causal but only coexisting.

SEIZURE DISORDERS

A person is only epileptic when he or she has seizures recurrently. An epileptic seizure involves paroxysmal cerebral neuronal firing, which may or may not produce disturbed consciousness and/or other perceptual or motor alterations (Neppe 1985a). The diagnosis of epilepsy is made when these seizures are recurrent and in quality. The most classical and most common epileptic seizures are of the *grand mal* or generalized tonic-clonic kind. When preceded by perceptual, autonomic, affective, or cognitive alterations, such seizures are secondarily generalized, as opposed to no original locus of firing, producing focal features before the tonic-clonic movements (generalized from the start) (International League Against Epilepsy Commission 1985).

Although one epileptic seizure does not make a person epileptic, a single seizure does require evaluation to ensure that underlying treatable, discernible etiologies are not present. These causes are best perceived as either nonprogressive or progressive. Important nonprogressive causes include head injury, encephalitis, birth trauma, hyperpyrexic convulsions, genetic predisposition, medication (e.g., neuroleptics and tricyclic antidepressants [TCAs]), and withdrawal states (e.g., from alcohol). Relevant potentially progressive conditions include tumor, metabolic disease (e.g., hypoglycemia and uremia), endocrine disease, Alzheimer's disease and other dementias, multiple sclerosis, cerebral arteriopathy, and other degenerative or infiltrative conditions. The physician should attempt to establish the underlying causes of seizures, particularly those presenting in adulthood (over age 30) (Pincus and Tucker 1985).

The classification of seizures and epilepsy has been controversial. It has shifted away from terms such as *grand mal* to an attempt to correlate clinical seizure type with electroencephalogram (EEG) ictal (i.e., during the seizure) and interictal (i.e., between seizures) changes. The latest classification of epileptic seizures, as recognized by the International League Against Epilepsy (ILAE) in 1981, ignores anatomical aspects; for example, the term *temporal lobe epilepsy* technically no longer exists

(International League Against Epilepsy Commission 1981). It makes a descriptive attempt at classifying epilepsy as generalized or partial seizures and describes the progression of firing; for example, seizures may begin as simple partial, progress on to complex partial, and then secondarily generalize (Table 15–1).

Generalized seizures manifest immediately and spread bilaterally through the cerebral cortex. They are generalized in that subcortical fibers may have been involved and there is simultaneous spread throughout the cerebral cortex.

In partial (focal) seizures (or partial focal attacks), epileptic firing starts in a specific area (focus or locus) of the brain. This evokes the physiological experience that stimulating that focus would produce. When such seizures involve no alteration in consciousness they are *simple partial seizures* (previously called *elementary partial seizures*). When there is a defect in consciousness they are *complex partial seizures* (*CPSs*).

Tonic-clonic seizures (or *grand mal seizures*) are the most common form of generalized seizure. They manifest as total consciousness loss with a tetanic muscular phase (i.e., tonic) followed by a phase of repetitive jerking (i.e., clonic). These seizures may be generalized from the start or begin as partial seizures and secondarily generalize.

Petit mal seizures (or *typical absence seizure*) are a common seizure type (occurring particularly in children) generalized from the start, with loss of consciousness for a few seconds without any motor phase and typical EEG findings (i.e., bilateral, synchronous, 3–4 per second spike wave, and discharge).

Temporal Lobe Epilepsy

The term *temporal lobe epilepsy* is still commonly used in the absence of an adequate alternative. Temporal lobe epilepsy phenomena are not synonymous with its

---

Table 15–1. International League Against Epilepsy revised classification of epileptic seizures

---

1. Partial (focal, local) seizures
   - A.   Simple: motor, somatosensory, autonomic, or psychic
   - B.   Complex
     - a) Impaired consciousness at outset
     - b) Simple partial followed by impaired consciousness
   - C.   Partial seizures evolving to generalized tonic-clonic (GTC)
     - a) Simple to GTC
     - b) Complex to GTC
2. Generalized seizures (convulsive or nonconvulsive)
   - A.   a) Absence seizures
     - b) Atypical absences
   - B.   Myoclonic
   - C.   Clonic
   - D.   Tonic
   - E.   Tonic-clonic
   - F.   Atonic
   - G.   Combinations
3. Unclassified epileptic seizures

Source.   International League Against Epilepsy Commission 1981.

attempted, nonanatomical replacement, *complex partial seizures,* because complex partial seizures are restricted to patients who have focal firing with defects of consciousness (Neppe 1982).

Many patients with temporal lobe epilepsy have no defect of consciousness and have simple partial seizures (e.g., olfactory hallucinations), which may derive from the temporal lobes. In addition, they may have simple partial seizures with psychic symptomatology (e.g., cognitive alterations, such as flashbacks). Temporal lobe epilepsy may also manifest with the *temporal lobe absence* or behavioral arrest that is associated with a brief loss of consciousness of 10–30 seconds (Neppe 1981a). These episodes may be associated with minor automatisms (e.g., chewing movements) and at times with "drop attacks"—the falling associated with loss of muscle tone. Patients with temporal lobe epilepsy often appear to be staring and after the episode may be aware that there was a loss of consciousness. They may experience postictal features such as headache and sleepiness, but certainly they have a perplexity and disorientation (Neppe 1985a).

Temporal lobe epilepsy may also manifest with psychomotor automatisms alone, which may involve a so-called psychic (or cognitive-affective sensory perceptual) phase followed by a motor phase. The psychic phase may be very brief and not recognized by the patient. It may be associated with many perceptual alterations, such as an auditory buzz or hum, more complex verbalizations, or aphasias. Visual abnormalities include diplopia, perceived movement, and changes in perceived object size or shape. These are followed by automatisms of various degrees of complexity. There may be simple buttoning or unbuttoning or masticatory movements, more complex "wandering" fugue states, furor type anger (which is very rare), or speech automatisms (which are far more common than recognized) (Neppe 1981a).

The features of temporal lobe epilepsy are so varied and so protean that it is necessary to classify them. The term *possible temporal lobe symptoms* (PTLSs) has been suggested (Neppe 1983b). These are symptoms that can be induced by stimulating areas of the temporal lobe during neurosurgery (implying a link with the temporal lobe), but without direct EEG confirmation during the episode, they cannot of themselves be demonstrated to derive from the temporal lobe; hence the word *possible.* PTLSs are further subdivided into controversial (dubious), benign (symptoms not of themselves requiring treatment), and disintegrative (symptoms severe enough to require treatment) (Table 15–2). They should be distinguished from nonspecific symptoms such as depersonalization or decreased concentration, which do not of themselves have any localizing value.

A major question about temporal lobe epilepsy is whether behavior disturbances occur more commonly in patients with temporal lobe epilepsy specifically or whether behavior disturbance is related to seizure disorders in general (Neppe and Tucker 1988b). The incidence of psychoses associated with temporal lobe epilepsy is usually noted as four to seven times greater, rarely only at twice as much (McKenna et al. 1985; Sengoku et al. 1983). The confounding variables include increased seizures, increased amount of anticonvulsants, and increased numbers of different types of seizures. Additionally, the temporal lobe constitutes 40% of the cerebral cortex, and the age at onset for temporal lobe seizures somewhat resembles that for psychoses (Neppe 1986; Stevens 1988). These factors could variably be perceived as important causal, predisposing, or incidental features. However, patients with temporal lobe epilepsy

Table 15–2.   Possible temporal lobe symptoms (PTLSs)

Controversial (dubious) PTLSs (CPTLSs)

Hypergraphia

Hyperreligiosity

Polymodal hallucinatory experience

Paroxysmal episodes of

Profound mood changes within hours

Frequent subjective paranormal experiences (e.g., telepathy, mediumistic trance, writing automatisms, visualization of presences or of lights or colors round people, dream extrasensory power, out-of-body experiences, alleged healing abilities, precognition, near-death experiences, and sense of floating)

Intense libidinal change

Uncontrolled, limited precipitated, directed, nonamnesic aggressive episodes

Recurrent nightmares of stereotyped kind

Episodes of blurred vision or diplopia

Intense ecstasy or religious experience

Hyposexuality

Unexplained episodes of dizziness

Flowery or perfumy smells

Benign PTLSs (BPTLSs) *symptoms not necessarily requiring treatment*

Paroxysmal episodes of

Complex visual hallucinations linked to other qualities of perception such as voices, emotions, or time

Olfactory hallucinations with burning, rotting, episodic components or linked to other PTLSs

Any form of

Simple auditory perceptual abnormality

Gustatory hallucinations

Rotation or disequilibrium feelings linked to other perceptual qualities

Unexplained "sinking," "rising," or "gripping" epigastric sensations

Flashbacks

Illusions of distance, size, loudness, tempo, strangeness, unreality, fear, or sorrow

Hallucinations of indescribable modality

Temporal lobe epileptic déjà vu (has associated ictal or postictal features [e.g., headache, sleepiness, and confusion] linked to the experience in clear or altered consciousness)

Any CPTLSs that appear to improve after administration of an anticonvulsant agent such as carbamazepine

Depersonalization or derealization linked with other PTLS features

Any CPTLSs associated with postevent headache (consistent quality), sleepiness, or confusion or with other PTLSs

Disintegrative PTLSs (DPTLSs) *symptoms requiring treatment*

Paroxysmal episodes of

Epileptic amnesia

Lapses in consciousness

Conscious "confusion" (apparent clear consciousness but abnormalities of orientation, attention, and behavior)

Epileptic automatisms

Masticatory-salivary episodes

Speech automatisms

"Fear which comes of itself" linked to other disorders (hallucinatory or unusual autonomic)

Uncontrolled, unprecipitated, undirected, amnesic aggressive episodes

Superior quadrantic homonymous hemianopia

(continued)

Table 15–2. Possible temporal lobe symptoms (PTLSs) *(continued)*

Receptive (Wernicke's) aphasia

Any CPTLSs or BPTLSs with ictal EEG correlates

Seizure-related features

Any typical absence, tonic or clonic, tonic-clonic, or bilateral myoclonic seizures in the absence of metabolic, intoxication, or withdrawal-related phenomena

Note. Patients may have more symptoms than those noted above.

Source. Adapted from Neppe 1991.

have increased difficulties with seizure control and medication, and this may be related to the more primitive embryological structure of the archipallium.

Pseudoseizures

The term *seizure* at times is also applied to other nonepileptic episodic phenomena that do not involve paroxysms of firing of cerebral neurons. The most common nonepileptic seizure is the so-called pseudoseizure or hysterical seizure. The pseudoseizure involves episodic behavioral aberrations that may closely mimic epileptic seizures. The differentiation of these from true seizures is at times difficult; Table 15–3 clarifies the features suggesting nonepileptic seizures (Neppe and Tucker 1988b).

Differentiation of Epileptic Seizures

The ultimate differentiation of epileptic from nonepileptic seizures and of aberrant behavior that may be interpreted as truly epileptic from behavior that is not epileptic is via EEG confirmation. Developments in this regard have been rapid over the past few years with the increasing usage of EEG telemetry. Telemetry involves prolonged monitoring over periods of time varying from 12 hours to 2 weeks while the patient is generally confined to a particular room. Cable telemetry is most com-

Table 15–3. General features of nonepileptic seizures

Setting	Examination
Unconsciously motivated	Restraint accentuates the seizure
Environmental gain (audience usually present)	Inattention decreases over time
Seldom sleep-related	Plantar flexor reflexes
Often triggered (e.g., by stress)	Reflexes intact (corneal, pupillary, and blink)
Suggestive profile on Minnesota Multiphasic Personality Inventory (MMPI; Hathaway and McKinley 1989)	Consciousness preserved
	Autonomic system uninvolved
	Autonomically intact
Attack	**After attack**
Atypical movements, often bizarre or purposeful	No postictal features
Seldom results in injury	Prolactin normal (after 20–30 minutes)
Ends gradually	No or little amnesia
Out-of-phase movements of extremities	Memory exists (hypnosis or Amytal Sodium)
Pelvic thrusting or side-to-side movements	

monly used. This involves, for example, a 25-foot cable connected to the EEG montage on the patient's head.

Often no seizure manifestations are picked up for prolonged periods of time because seizures only occur paroxysmally. Moreover, those patients evaluated in a specialized center with EEG telemetry are invariably so atypical that the hypothesized seizure originates deep within the brain. Frequently, patients go off their anticonvulsants during inpatient monitoring; consequently, the risk of destabilizing seizures exists.

A cheaper, safer alternative or adjunct to inpatient video-EEG monitoring is home ambulatory EEG monitoring. Patients are connected to a small battery and electrically operated EEG recording device over a 2- or 3-day period. Previously, such techniques were limited to 4 or 8 channels resulting in poor sensitivity. However, 16-channel computerized systems with artifact filtered and automatic spike detection now allow seizures and atypical spells to be better diagnosed and evaluated. Moreover, evaluation of the patient in a natural state, either at home or at work, awake or asleep, is an enormous advantage. These patients remain on their anticonvulsant medication although, as with EEGs, they should preferably be off benzodiazepines.

Another recent advance involves measuring blood prolactin levels to differentiate true epileptic seizures from nonepileptic seizures. If the serum prolactin is substantially elevated after a seizure, it is reasonable evidence that, in fact, the person has had an epileptic seizure, although normal prolactin level may occasionally occur in the face of true epileptic seizures, particularly when the seizures were of the simple partial kind. A useful rule in interpreting test results is that the prolactin elevation should be above the upper limit of normal and should be at least double the level at the same time the following day. Also the prolactin should have fallen an hour after the apparent seizure phenomenon.

SEIZURES AND PSYCHIATRIC DISORDERS

Eight major interconnected elements may be responsible for aberrant behavior in the epileptic patient (Neppe 1985a):

1. *Ictal or subictal firing.* In this instance the behavior reflects an actual epileptic effect. The most common example is psychomotor automatism, in which the person is motorically producing deviant behavior as part of the seizure manifestation. In psychiatry this is relatively rare, but it achieves a preeminence in forensic neuropsychiatry.
2. *Kindling-like phenomena.* Kindling is the pathophysiological process whereby repetitive subthreshold electrical or chemical stimuli to certain brain areas will eventually induce threshold responses (Neppe 1985a). These responses are classically in the form of seizures; however, it appears that they may manifest as abnormal behavior before the onset of the seizures (Stevens and Livermore 1978).
3. *The site of the focus.* The area at which the firing of the partial seizure originates or through which it passes may or may not play a substantial role in psychopathology. The temporal lobe is believed by some to be the source of behavioral disturbances (Neppe 1981b; Trimble 1983).

4. *Medication effects.* Overmedication or incorrect medication may lead to side effects. Anticonvulsants produce a variety of cognitive, perceptual, and behavioral side effects that may substantially modify the person's behavior, predisposing the person to a psychiatric presentation.

5. *Other cerebral abnormalities.* The epilepsy may be an epiphenomenon of a psycho-organic syndrome of some kind. The most common example would be mild mental retardation, which may be associated with diffuse organic brain pathology (possibly submicroscopic) and also with a lowered seizure threshold (i.e., a predisposition to epilepsy). An alternative mechanism for other cerebral abnormalities is the induction of cerebral anoxia secondary to status epilepticus, which may cause organic brain damage.

6. *Psychosocial aspects.* Environmental stressors commonly trigger disorganization, personality disintegration, or decompensation in the person with epilepsy. Moreover, even small amounts of alcohol or substance abuse of any kind may precipitate loss of control of the epileptic condition or aggravate psychopathology. Alternatively, persons with epilepsy may feel inadequate or paranoid that people may find out about their seizures and may withdraw into themselves, not having the confidence to interact in a socially appropriate manner.

7. *Predisposition.* Genetic, in utero, or other constitutional or later environmental experiences (e.g., encephalitis, hyperpyrexic convulsions, minor head injury, or drug abuse) may induce, precipitate, or predispose to psychiatric illness in the epileptic patient.

8. *As a complication.* Epilepsy may be associated with psychopathology because numerous psychiatric conditions may secondarily be associated with epilepsy (e.g., the Alzheimer's groups of dementias and the cerebral arteriopathies).

The Ictus and Psychopathology

Peri-ictal phenomena. Classically, the aberrant behavior in epilepsy is measured with regard to whether or not it is associated with the seizure phenomenon. When it appears to be directly linked to a particular seizure phenomenon the behavior is described as peri-ictal; when the phenomenon seems to be occurring between seizures, the behavior is considered interictal (Neppe 1985a). This terminology is rather simplistic because many patients are unaware of whether or not they have had a seizure, and therefore peri-ictal phenomena may be mistaken as interictal. Peri-ictal manifestations can be subdivided into events occurring preictally, ictally, or postictally.

Preictal events. Preictal events immediately precede the seizure manifestation. The epileptic prodrome is a phase before the onset of the actual seizure that may last several days and occasionally more than a week. It is characterized by changes in personality, behavior, or emotionality. Emotions such as mild irritability or poor concentration may be the most common but nonspecific manifestations. In contrast, the aura to the seizure is short. Patients may describe these as lasting up to half an hour, but usually they occur for periods of seconds before the seizure manifestation.

Ictal events. The ictal manifestation that most commonly presents psychiatrically is the psychomotor automatism. This may involve behavioral aberrations, and in the psychiatric presentation these may be complicated and have marked cognitive manifestations. Episodes of altered consciousness involving marked misinterpretations of reality, profound derealization, and depersonalization, as well as significant paranoid symptomatology, may occur.

Postictal events. Clouding of consciousness commonly occurs during this phase and patients may manifest a great deal of aggression, which is generally nonspecific and undirected and will occur only if the person is physically handled or their behavior is put under some kind of restraint (Rodin 1973). Occasionally psychotic manifestations occur during this phase with marked delusional and hallucinatory features. Postictal features are particularly relevant in differentiating true epileptic seizure phenomena from pseudoseizures.

Kindling

Kindling—the pathophysiological process whereby repetitive subthreshold electrical or chemical stimuli to certain brain areas will eventually induce threshold responses (Neppe 1985a)—and related hypotheses have become fashionable and possibly useful ways to explain certain episodic behavioral disturbances. Evidence from animal studies (McNamara et al. 1980) has shown that repetitive intermittent subthreshold stimuli administered to parts of the brain (e.g., the amygdala, piriform, and hippocampal areas) will induce a permanent threshold change allowing a progression of seizure phenomena. Such changes occur throughout the animal kingdom but are more difficult to induce with higher degrees of encephalization. Behavioral manifestations begin to precede seizure manifestations in cats, as contrasted with rats (Stevens and Livermore 1978).

Although kindling has never been demonstrated definitively in man, there is indirect support for the occurrence of kindling phenomena in man (Adamec et al. 1981) in the development of mirror foci, in epilepsy in the generalization of partial seizure phenomena, and in certain models such as alcohol withdrawal and posttraumatic stress reaction (Neppe 1985b). The major evidence against such a phenomenon is the prolonged duration of time it should take (i.e., years) and the fact that certain behavior disturbances appear to occur almost immediately after seizures and do not take such a long period of time.

Drugs that act against kindling act on a variety of processes. The most potent limbic antikindling agent available is carbamazepine, which has psychotropic effects, possibly as a consequence of kindling reduction (Albertson et al. 1980; Albright and Burnham 1980). Carbamazepine has a potent action on the endpoint of the kindled animal preparation; however, it has very little effect in preventing the kindling phenomenon. Certain anticonvulsants may be better at different stages in behavioral disorders in a single person's illness. For patients with histories of hallucinogen abuse, for example, we find phenytoin preferable at times to carbamazepine, and the patient may be resistant to carbamazepine. On the other hand, relatively early in the process, carbamazepine may be the appropriate drug (Scher and Neppe 1989). The role of valproate in these phenomena is not as clear. Its mechanism is different from those of phenytoin, phenobarbital, and carbamazepine (Neppe 1990).

Psychosocial Facets of Epilepsy

The epileptic patient encounters major psychosocial stressors. First is the stress of having a chronic illness. Studies comparing the epileptic patient with groups of patients with other chronic illnesses such as rheumatic heart disease, diabetes mellitus, and cancer have concluded that each of these conditions has its own special stressors (Dodrill and Batzel 1986). However, when comparing any of these populations to patients with organic brain disease, there are also specific difficulties in that organicity in and of itself has its own problems (Szatmari 1985).

The special difficulty of the epileptic patient is the paroxysmal (or episodic) element of the illness. In between episodes the person with epilepsy may be functioning normally. There is a substantial covert stress leading the person with epilepsy to being afraid of performing normal social activities, like dating with a favored friend of the opposite sex during adolescence. The threat is greater than the occurrence (Neppe 1985a). In addition, the actual tonic-clonic seizure is such a frightening experience for many members of the general population, and there is so much folklore associated with the grand mal seizure, that the visualization of such an episode is said to be far more traumatic for the spectator than for the epileptic patient. The consequence of this is that interpretations of the epilepsy may be distorted thereafter, and even an isolated seizure may have grave consequences at an interpersonal level.

Therefore, the psychosocial stressors encountered by the person with epilepsy are very substantial, but they are additionally based on limitation of particular activities. To indicate that epileptic individuals should not operate dangerous machinery, work in jobs that expose them to great heights, swim alone, or, in some instances, even bathe autonomously is obvious. The trauma of not driving is a very substantial one for the average person with epilepsy.

The functional limitations of epilepsy are substantial, and when they are not adhered to the epileptic individual must conquer his or her guilt. Criminal behavior (e.g., driving) puts the person with epilepsy at a high stress-risk level; he or she needs to deceive to survive, and this is not healthy. Also, the phenomenon of dependency on others is often hard to break in the neuropsychological rehabilitation of the epileptic patient. It is sometimes easier to remain ill than to become seizure free and healthy. The patient has to learn to deal with health (Neppe 1985d).

Methodological Issues

Epidemiological studies of seizures, the temporal lobe, and psychopathology have been plagued by methodological flaws. A major difficulty is fundamental definitions. Although epilepsy has been defined as a recurrent paroxysmal condition with biochemical and electrical discharges in the brain and association with alterations in consciousness, behavior, cognition, affect, and motoric functions, its clinical operational definition is more difficult. Psychiatric patients are sometimes dubiously labeled as *epileptic* on the basis of previous psychiatric history: they may have histories of a single seizure; their seizures may have been associated with alcohol or other withdrawal; or they may be on anticonvulsant medication for "blackouts." Such cases are difficult to interpret. Operationally, the term *epileptic psychotic patients* should be limited to individuals with psychoses in clear or altered consciousness plus a confirmed history of epilepsy associated with at least two documented seizures not linked to withdrawal phenomena (Neppe and Tucker 1989).

Clinical evaluation.   The patient should be interviewed carefully for the exact nature of the subjective alterations. Usually in seizures these are repetitive and consistent in quality (Neppe and Tucker 1988b). There may be multiple perceptual and cognitive modalities that are involved, but these are usually simple and consistent in each specific patient. Often a history of amnesia is a clue, although dissociative disorders also produce amnesia. Some memory of the events may occur in patients with seizure disorders, particularly the auras of the experiences (i.e., psychic kinds of experiences). At times the patient will experience some postictal depression or lethargy, wanting to sleep, developing a headache, and feeling perplexed (Tucker et al. 1986).

Seizures and Psychopathology: Classification

Epilepsy and psychiatry have distanced themselves partly as a consequence of the inadequacy of attempts to classify psychopathology in epileptic patients. Slater, Beard, and Glithero (1963) demonstrated that the basic symptoms associated with classical schizophrenic disorders are present in patients with seizure disorders. More recently, Perez and Trimble (1980), in a prospective study, and Toone et al. (1982), in a retrospective study, using the standardized Present State Examination (PSE; Wing et al. 1974) demonstrated that psychoses associated with temporal lobe seizure disorders are indistinguishable from schizophrenia. However, such studies analyze specifically positive and particularly Schneiderian symptoms of schizophrenia; the negative symptoms appear different (Neppe 1986).

We have applied psychopathology in the epileptic patient along a multiaxial framework with the Neppe Multiaxial Epilepsy Schema (Neppe and Tucker 1988b). This bears some similarity to the DSM-III (American Psychiatric Association 1980) multiaxis approach and has, in fact, been modeled on such approaches. Table 15–4 reflects new updated ideas on this classification, which we now call the Tiered Axes for Psychopathology and Epilepsy (TAPE) (Neppe 1981b, 1986; Neppe and Tucker 1989).

Axes I through V of the psychopathology tier are amplifications of current DSM-III-R terminology. Axis VI is the pharmacological response, and Axis VII is the age at onset. These two new axes exist not only on the psychopathology tier, which on Axes I–V closely reflects the DSM-III-R framework, but also on the corresponding epilepsy tier. Axis VI—pharmacological response—can and probably should be applied to any psychopathology. Factors such as compliance, response, blood and other levels, and duration and frequency of all psychotropics, anticonvulsants, and other nonneuropsychiatric medications should be recorded so that pharmacokinetic and dynamic factors are considered. Age at onset of both seizures and the major psychiatric conditions (such as psychotic features) is an important epidemiological consideration for these conditions.

The TAPE classification should be applied to all patients with seizures and psychopathology. It would unify diagnostic and research frameworks in this area and allow an added appreciation of the similarities and differences between the many conditions that manifest with seizures and psychopathology. The classification can also easily be modified for use in any organic condition or pseudoseizures.

Special Conditions

Psychoses. Many empirical similarities exist between seizure disorders and schizophrenia. Schizophrenia and seizure disorders are both hard to define simply; the genetic frequencies are similar for both conditions, with somewhere between 10% and 13% of the offspring of the parents with these conditions having the condition (Metrakos and Metrakos 1961). They are also both basically clinical diagnoses presenting primarily as behavioral disturbances, and there are generally no pathological changes evident in either of these conditions. Furthermore, the peak age at onset is similar with both being disorders of early to late adolescence, although epilepsy often presents in childhood and may present at any age (Neppe and Tucker 1988a). The

---

Table 15–4.   Tiered Axes for Psychopathology and Epilepsy (TAPE)

Psychopathology tier
Axis
I   Psychiatric diagnosis (DSM-III-R; American Psychiatric Association 1987)
       Descriptive psychopathology diagnosis
       Severity of episode (mild, moderate, or severe)
II   Personality or developmental disorder (DSM-III-R)
       Personality description
III   Physical disorders (DSM-III-R) (related or unrelated)
       Symptomatic etiology of psychopathology
IV   Psychosocial stressors (DSM-III-R)
V   Global assessment of functioning (current, past year, during illness, and expected on
       recovery)
VI   Pharmacological response of psychopathology
       Pharmacological compliance
       Neuroleptic dose, levels and response, duration of treatment, and frequency of dosing
       Other treatments or medications responsiveness
       Duration of treatment for each drug
       Combinations and frequency of dosing
VII   Age at onset of current psychopathology (e.g., psychosis)

Epilepsy tier
Axis
I   Seizure classification
       Epilepsy syndrome
       Extent of seizure control (complete, occasional, moderate, or poor)
II   Intelligence (normal or borderline, mild, or moderate mental retardation)
III   Time link of psychopathology and seizures (peri-ictal, interictal, nonictal, or unclear)
IV   Electroencephalographic (EEG) localization
       EEG seizure features
       Neuroradiological or nuclear medicine or other brain tests
V   Course (deteriorating or nondeteriorating)
       Chronicity (single episode, episodic, or chronic)
VI   Pharmacological response of seizures
       Pharmacological compliance with antiseizure medication
       Anticonvulsant doses and frequency of dosing and levels
       Duration of treatment for each drug
VII   Age at onset of seizures

neurotransmitter dopamine is somehow related in both conditions as dopamine antagonists are antipsychotic and mildly epileptogenic, and dopamine agonists are psychotogenic and mildly antiepileptic (Trimble 1977). Perhaps most significantly, both conditions need a team to rehabilitate patients.

Despite more than 100 publications in the scientific literature dealing with core issues of epilepsy in relation to psychosis, the area remains particularly poorly explored and ill defined (McKenna et al. 1985). Several different kinds of psychoses appear to be associated with epilepsy (Table 15–5) (Neppe 1986; Neppe and Tucker 1989). Possibly the most common is the chronic, paranoid hallucinatory psychosis. These patients have paranoid persecutory and sometimes a grandiose delusional schema that are relatively systematized, and they require high doses of neuroleptic medication in addition to the anticonvulsant. It is possible that the anatomic site of the lesion, for example, dominant temporal hemisphere or bilateral damage, may be important. This group may, in fact, turn out to be dichotomous: one group having organic disorders, the other nonorganic disorders. Generally, the psychoses are perceived as interictal, but only because they most commonly occur between seizures, not because they may have a special reciprocal relationship to the peri-ictal phenomena.

It is extremely difficult to place these 10 kinds (and there may be more) of epileptic psychosis in the context of those psychoses that are antagonistic to seizures and those that more commonly occur with seizures. The TAPE classification takes into account not only a multiaxial framework but also responses to appropriate pharmacological and other interventions (Neppe 1986; Neppe and Tucker 1989).

Depression and seizures. The incidence of depression appears higher among persons with epilepsy than in the general population. However, there is little research support for the claim that patients with complex partial seizures are particularly predisposed to depression, especially if this involves nondominant hemisphere lesions (Stevens 1988). Robertson (1987) found that depression generally was moderate and was endogenous-melancholic in approximately two-fifths of 66 epileptic patients studied. Attendant features were high state and trait anxiety and hostility. The EEGs of the patients and a control group were not significantly different. Patients receiving phenobarbital were more depressed compared with those on carbamazepine. The phe-

---

Table 15–5. Examples of "epileptic psychoses"

Interictal, clear consciousness psychoses
1. Mild mental retardation, secondary generalized epilepsy, and unfixed unsystematized delusions
2. Temporal lobe epilepsy with paranoid-hallucinatory psychosis
3. Manic-like episodic interictal psychosis
4. Postsurgical (temporal lobe) psychosis
5. Nonorganic "epileptic psychosis"

Peri-ictal psychoses
6. Complex partial seizure and status epilepticus
7. Preictal psychosis
8. Peri-ictal psychosis without clouding but with delusional syndrome
9. Postictal delirium (not in our definition)
10. Psychotic episode (with clear consciousness) after a seizure (? postictal or ? early interictal)

nomenology of the depression was not clearly influenced by epilepsy variables. Depression in patients with epilepsy represents the outcome of multiple factors in genetically predisposed individuals.

Blumer and Montouris (1992) recently found that depression and related features are the most common psychiatric concomitants in an epilepsy population receiving inpatient EEG monitoring. The term *interictal dysphoric disorder* has been developed, and has been integrated into a comprehensive Axis I classification outlined in Table 15–6 (Neppe and Blumer 1992).

Personality profiles. The consistency of behavioral symptoms is particularly relevant in the light of modern attempts at developing personality profiles in patients with temporal lobe disorders. For example, Waxman and Geschwind (1975) reported a specific interictal syndrome associated with temporal lobe disorders that consists of hypergraphia, hyposexual activity, and a preoccupation with philosophical and moral concerns. This work was continued in a well-known study by Bear and Fedio (see Bear 1986; Bear et al. 1982), who analyzed the above symptoms and 14 other behavior traits. Their 18-point personality inventory measures overall psychopathology rather than a specific syndrome (Rodin and Schmaltz 1984).

Hermann and Riel (1981) found that four traits (sense of personal destiny, dependence, paranoia, and philosophical interest) were significantly elevated in a temporal lobe epilepsy group. Some studies have argued against syndrome specificity, showing that traits were also present in the other populations (Stark-Adamec et al. 1985) or that there may be hemisphere differences in control groups (e.g., left-hemisphericity types

---

Table 15–6.   Summative classification of epilepsy and Axis I disorders

I.   Nonpsychotic disorders of the interictal phase
   1. Interictal dysphoric disorder (IDD) (syndrome)
   2. IDD with predominance in one or two symptoms
   3. IDD with episodic psychotic features
   4. IDD with persistent psychotic features
   5. Simple interictal disorder: isolated (single or dual) symptomology

II. Nonpsychotic disorders of the alternating type
   1. Alternating dysphoric disorder (ADD) (syndrome)
   2. ADD with predominance in one or two symptoms
   3. ADD with episodic psychotic features
   4. ADD with persistent psychotic features
   5. Simple interictal disorder: isolated (single or dual) symptomology

III. Nonpsychotic disorders clearly related to seizures
   1. Preictal disorders
   2. Postictal disorders

IV. Psychotic disorders related to seizures
   1. Peri-ictal psychoses
   2. Postictal psychoses
   3. Parictal psychoses
   4. Alternating psychoses

V.   Psychotic disorders not related to seizures
   1. Interictal psychoses
   2. Postsurgical psychoses
   3. Nonictal psychoses

had greater control over their impulses, were more trusting and imaginative, and viewed themselves in a positive light, whereas right-hemisphericity types were more tense, suspicious, shy, and pragmatic) (Vingiano 1989). Many symptoms may occur in any one specific kind of patient, distorting population studies. For example, in a Caucasian African population, hypergraphia was not commonly found among persons with temporal lobe epilepsy, suggesting that it may be culturally and not organically related (Neppe and Tucker 1988b).

The most common sexual abnormality in temporal lobe epilepsy appears to be hyposexuality; moreover, the relationship of altered sexuality in temporal lobe epilepsy is particularly controversial (Blumer 1975). Alternatively, Roberts and Guberman (1989) reported a remarkable proportion (involving about half the patients they identified) of religious conversions in their epileptic study population. Many psychiatrists who have seen a large number of such patients argue that a specific personality profile has yet to be identified and point out how many of the apparent traits are actually opposites (Stevens 1983, 1988). However, this does not imply that such traits may not occur with increased prevalence or may not reflect nonspecific personality changes in certain subpopulations of patients with temporal lobe epilepsy (Neppe and Tucker 1988b). Certain other subpopulations (e.g., suicidal epileptic patients) may have a higher prevalence of personality disorders (Mendez et al. 1989).

PSYCHOPATHOLOGY IN THE NONEPILEPTIC PATIENT

Clinicians have often noted that the distinctions made by classification systems often are more distinct in theory than in practice. One area of speculation involves the concept of so-called atypical psychosis. Monroe (1982) delineated a group he called "episodic psychotics," and related this to a limbic ictal disorder that was unresponsive to TCAs and neuroleptics. He noted that these patients also had a psychosis of precipitous onset, intense affects, and intermittent course with symptom-free intervals. Tucker et al. (1986) described a series of patients who had documented temporal lobe dysfunction on EEG and symptomatology very similar to episodic psychosis described by Monroe (1982). All of the patients described spell-type episodes. They also experienced marked mood lability, often with suicidal ideation and suicide attempts, as well as psychotic phenomena and cognitive changes. All patients returned to normal baseline with symptom-free intervals. It is extremely important that many of these conditions occur in a state of clear consciousness and do not necessarily present themselves with either a clouding of consciousness or symptoms of disorientation (Neppe and Tucker 1988a).

Such studies of patients with possible temporolimbic dysfunction have been continued from other sources (Wells and Duneau 1980), including chronic nonepileptic psychiatric patients with EEG temporal lobe foci (Neppe 1983a), violent refractory schizophrenic patients (Hakola and Laulumaa 1982), patients with borderline personality disorder (Gardner and Cowdry 1986), and patients who become dysphoric on neuroleptics and have abnormal EEGs (Brodsky et al. 1983). These findings suggest the extended use of anticonvulsant medication, particularly carbamazepine (Neppe 1984).

In psychiatry particularly, patients at times have episodes that are extremely difficult to interpret. These episodes may be very short-lived, lasting seconds or minutes, but on occasion can last for days. Such patients behave out of character and usually exhibit a lability of affect that is profound, with disturbances ranging from depression through mania. They may appear markedly thought disordered, deluded, or hallucinated, and very often these episodes are repetitive and of the same quality each time. These patients may exhibit behavioral alterations perceived as characterological disorders. We have called such episodes *spells* to obviate debate as to whether they are truly ictal (Neppe and Kaplan 1988; Tucker et al. 1986).

These patients may respond to anticonvulsant medication, and trials of anticonvulsants are needed. In our experience many of these patients respond well to carbamazepine, phenytoin, or valproate. This may or may not imply that these patients have seizurelike episodes. It is possible that these patients may occasionally respond to short courses of anticonvulsant therapy and not require permanent treatment (Neppe and Kaplan 1988).

TREATMENT

The heterogeneity of behavior disturbances in epileptic patients implies a heterogeneity of management that is patient based and individually tailored (Neppe and Tucker 1988a). The single most important principle is anticonvulsant monotherapy (Table 15–7) (Neppe 1985a, 1985c).

Anticonvulsants may induce change in the psychiatric patient by both pharmacokinetic and pharmacodynamic interactions with other medications. Pharmacokinetically, enzyme induction tends to affect predominantly the P_{450} cytochrome enzyme system in the liver. This implies that both anticonvulsant metabolism—particularly carbamazepine—and the metabolism of other lipid-soluble compounds are accelerated (Neppe et al. 1988). Three major anticonvulsants, namely phenobarbital, phenytoin, and carbamazepine (in that order), are potent enzyme-inducing agents in the liver. We see little role for barbiturates such as phenobarbital in the management

Table 15–7. Choice of anticonvulsant

Type of seizure	First choice	Alternatives
	Oral	
Typical absences (petit mal [PM])	Ethosuximide	Valproate
		Clonazepam
Generalized tonic-clonic (GTC) seizures	Carbamazepine	Phenytoin
		Valproate
Partial seizures	Carbamazepine	Phenytoin
		Primidone
PM and GTC seizures	Valproate	Carbamazepine plus ethosuximide
	Carbamazepine	
Atypical absences	Carbamazepine	Phenytoin
		Phenytoin
		Primidone
Myoclonus (MC)	Valproate	Clonazepam
Psychiatric overlay (not PM or MC)	Carbamazepine	Clonazepam
	Intravenous	
Status epilepticus	Diazepam	Phenytoin
	Clonazepam	

of seizure disorders today; their only place may be for patients who are already taking them and do not have any side effects.

Pharmacodynamic interactions are even more complex and difficult. Interactions at receptors in the brain may produce modulatory effects at, for example, dopaminergic, serotonergic, and γ-aminobutyric acid (GABA)-ergic levels.

Phenytoin. Diphenylhydantoin sodium (or phenytoin) is now less popular than it was and has limited use in the neuropsychiatric patient despite being an outstanding anticonvulsant to control generalized tonic-clonic and some partial seizures. Its problem, like phenobarbital, is its side-effect profile (Neppe 1985a, 1985c; Neppe et al. 1991). Mild cognitive impairment occurs, particularly in higher doses. Because phenytoin has a small therapeutic range, patients can easily become drug toxic, and (ironically) one of the side effects of significant toxicity is seizures. Additionally, it can make petit mal seizures worse. Gum hyperplasia is a particular problem with chronic use of phenytoin, producing an appearance that can at times be unsightly (Trimble 1979, 1988).

Carbamazepine. The trend in psychiatry has been increasing use of carbamazepine rather than phenytoin, because it is safer, has apparent psychotropic properties, and has proven value in several conditions. Carbamazepine is particularly relevant in the psychiatric context because it appears to include less cognitive, motoric, and affective dysfunction than some of the older anticonvulsants such as phenytoin, phenobarbital, and primidone (Trimble 1979). It is as effective as phenytoin in both generalized tonic-clonic seizures and partial seizures and thus is the drug of choice for such conditions. It is ineffective in petit mal absences where sodium valproate or ethosuximide is generally used. Carbamazepine, however, also appears to have a substantial psychotropic effect (Neppe 1985c; Trimble 1979). This psychotropic effect may or may not relate to its anticonvulsant structure because it is also structurally similar to both TCAs and phenothiazines (Gagneux 1975).

Therapeutic ranges have not been established for anticonvulsants in nonepileptic patients. Only one double-blind study (Neppe 1990) used fixed-dosed carbamazepine in patients with chronic psychoses who were on adjunct neuroleptics; a therapeutic range in the low anticonvulsant range for seizures, namely 6–9 μg/mole, was suggested. Ranges could also vary with different psychiatric conditions.

Carbamazepine and the other anticonvulsants involved in enzyme induction produce important metabolic and endocrine effects. Patients on oral contraceptives may have their steroid level lowered, with the consequence that they may become pregnant. In addition, by virtue of the lipid solubility of cholecalciferol and consequently increased rate of metabolism, patients may become vitamin D deficient, particularly in cold winter climates. Consequently, alterations in calcium metabolism with mild hypocalcemia might result. Furthermore, by virtue of the enzyme induction, folic acid (as a coenzyme vitamin in hepatic enzyme pathways) may be depleted, with the consequence that patients may require small folic acid supplementation, rather like that occurring in pregnancy (Neppe et al. 1988). Finally, both an induction of hepatic enzymes, as well as a deinduction of hepatic enzyme systems, occurs in the context of carbamazepine (Neppe 1990). It is probable that patients going off anticonvulsant medication will experience a reverse process, whereby the liver enzymes will be slowed down, with the consequence that there may be accumulation of higher amounts of psychotropic agent.

Initial concerns about irreversible hemopoietic complications with carbamazepine have lessened. Such complications occur with the same order of frequency as with some TCAs. Extremely common, unrelated to these irreversible effects, and of no practical immunological significance is a small drop in the white cell count (Neppe et al. 1988).

Valproate. Sodium valproate is a good broad spectrum drug that apparently also has a low incidence of cognitive side effects. The drug is an outstanding anticonvulsant and is particularly useful in combined tonic-clonic and petit mal seizures. It also appears effective against partial epilepsy. The role of valproate is far less proven in the nonepileptic psychiatric context than that of carbamazepine. It has become fashionable to use it as a third-line drug in manic-depressive illness, at times with remarkable success. Still, such success is relatively rare, and in our experience the real role of valproate in affective illness is unproven. An added difficulty is the limited value of valproate serum levels even in the patient with seizure disorders. Because of this, dosing is a "guesstimate" at best.

Valproate does not induce enzymes but metabolically competes; thus theoretically it raises psychotropic levels and has its own level raised. It is safe, relatively nontoxic, and generally well tolerated. The major concern with its use is potentially fatal, rare hepatotoxicity in young children, particularly when they are on other anticonvulsants. This may or may not be linked with a deficiency of carnitine.

Use of Other Psychotropics in Seizure Disorders

Neuroleptics. Often a neuroleptic agent is required in epileptic patients with psychosis. All neuroleptics are epileptogenic. Findings suggest that neuroleptics should not be combined in patients with epilepsy (Neppe 1989). Haloperidol has traditionally been used commonly in epileptic patients with good effects. Thiothixene appears to be a good alternative as is thioridazine (Neppe 1989). Prochlorperazine and chlorpromazine have also been used. A drug that may have potential application but is as yet unproven is pimozide (Larkin 1983).

Antidepressants. When used in patients with epilepsy, antidepressants are problematic because they lower the seizure threshold. Monoamine oxidase inhibitors (MAOIs) appear far less epileptogenic than TCAs. In practice, the TCAs are probably far more epileptogenic than the neuroleptics.

β-Adrenergic blockers and the azaperones. On many occasions, patients with epilepsy are not fully controlled on anticonvulsants, despite apparent adequate medication trials. These patients may give a history of seizures occurring more frequently during or after stress. The use of β-blockers (e.g., propranolol) or azaperones (e.g., buspirone) in seizure patients has not formally been researched, but preliminary evidence based on a few cases suggests that they have promise, apparently diminishing seizure frequency. Clearly, formal controlled studies are necessary.

Benzodiazepines. We do not recommend the routine use of benzodiazepines. Despite their initial extremely potent anticonvulsant effects, suggesting they may be ideal in these populations, their use for chronic stress is often protracted. It is at times extremely difficult to remove epileptic patients from benzodiazepines without them having seizures, and the long-term efficacy of maintenance benzodiazepine for stress in epileptic patients is unproven. Moreover, the cognitive, psychomotor, and mnestic impairments induced by anticonvulsants could be accentuated. Nevertheless, a significant proportion of truly intractable epileptic patients with behavior disturbances require benzodiazepines. Many of these patients have been taking them for years and are anticipated to be on them for a lifetime.

Nonpharmacological Perspectives

While management of patients with seizure disorders involves primarily appropriate use of anticonvulsants, counseling and the various aspects of psychosocial support—allowing the patient to live as normal a life as possible and to be supported within the framework of the environment—are also very important. Occasionally techniques such as biofeedback may help.

CONCLUSIONS

Psychopathology occurs only in a minority of persons with epilepsy. Attempted etiological explanations like kindling, lateralization, localization, and biochemical changes are all, therefore, explanations for a small proportion of the epileptic population. Medications used to treat seizure disorders often do not alleviate behavior changes, and at times agents such as neuroleptics help behavior change but not seizure disturbances. The exact etiology of these conditions remains to be determined. Perhaps the use of more sophisticated dynamic imaging techniques such as single photon emission computed tomography (SPECT), positron-emission tomography (PET), magnetic resonance imaging (MRI), and computed tomography (CT) will give better ideas of the source of the behavioral changes (Neppe and Tucker 1988a).

REFERENCES

Adamec RE, Stark-Adamec C, Perrin R, et al: What is the relevance of kindling for human temporal lobe epilepsy? in Kindling 2. Edited by Wada JA. New York, Raven, 1981, pp 303–311

Albertson TE, Peterson SL, Stark LG: Anticonvulsant drugs and their antagonism on amygdalized kindled seizures in rats. Neuropharmacology 19:643–652, 1980

Albright PS, Burnham WM: Development of a new pharmacological seizure model: effects of anticonvulsants on cortical—and amygdala—kindled seizures in the rat. Epilepsia 21:681–689, 1980

American Psychiatric Association: Diagnostic and Statistical Manual of Mental Disorders, 3rd Edition. Washington, DC, American Psychiatric Association, 1980

American Psychiatric Association: Diagnostic and Statistical Manual of Mental Disorders, 3rd Edition, Revised. Washington, DC, American Psychiatric Association, 1987

Bear DM: Behavioural changes in temporal lobe epilepsy: conflict, confusion, challenge, in Aspects of Epilepsy and Psychiatry. Edited by Trimble MR, Bolwig TG. London, John Wiley, 1986, pp 19–29

Bear D, Levin K, Blumer D, et al: Interictal behaviour in hospitalised temporal lobe epileptics: relationship to idiopathic psychiatric syndromes. J Neurol Neurosurg Psychiatry 45:481–488, 1982

Blumer D: Temporal lobe epilepsy and its psychiatric significance, in Psychiatric Aspects of Neurological Disease. Edited by Benson FD, Blumer D. New York, Grune & Stratton, 1975, pp 171–198

Blumer D, Montouris G: Psychiatric morbidity in patients admitted for intensive EEG–video-monitoring for seizures: the interictal dysphoric disorder. Epilepsia 33 (suppl 3):S126–127, 1992

Brodsky L, Zuniga JG, Casenas ER, et al: Refractory anxiety: a masked epileptiform disorder. Psychiatr J Univ Ottawa 8(1):42–45, 1983

Dodrill CB, Batzel LW: Interictal behavioral features of patients with epilepsy. Epilepsia 27 (suppl 2):S64–S76, 1986

Gagneux AR: The chemistry of carbamazepine, in Epileptic Seizures—Behaviour—Pain. Edited by Birkmayer W. Berne, Hans Huber, 1975, pp 120–126

Gardner DL, Cowdry RW: Positive effects of carbamazepine on behavioral dyscontrol in borderline personality disorder. Am J Psychiatry 143:519–522, 1986

Hakola HP, Laulumaa VA: Carbamazepine in treatment of violent schizophrenics. Lancet 1:1356, 1982

Hathaway SR, McKinley JC: Minnesota Multiphasic Personality Inventory–2. Minneapolis, MN, University of Minnesota Press, 1989

Hermann BP, Riel P: Interictal personality and behavioral traits in temporal lobe and generalized epilepsy. Cortex 17:125–128, 1981

International League Against Epilepsy Commission: Proposal for revised clinical and electroencephalographic classification of epileptic seizures. Epilepsia 22:489–501, 1981

International League Against Epilepsy Commission: Proposal for classification of epilepsies and epileptic syndromes. Epilepsia 26:268–278, 1985

Larkin C: Epileptogenic effect of pimozide. Am J Psychiatry 140:372–373, 1983

McKenna PJ, Kane JM, Parrish K: Psychotic syndromes in epilepsy. Am J Psychiatry 142:895–904, 1985

McNamara JO, Byrne MC, Dasheiff RM, et al: The kindling model of epilepsy: a review, in Progress in Neurobiology. Edited by Phillis JW, Kerkut G. London, Pergamon, 1980, pp 139–159

Mendez MF, Lanska DJ, Manon ER, et al: Causative factors for suicide attempts by overdose in epileptics. Arch Neurol 46:1065–1068, 1989

Metrakos K, Metrakos JD: Genetics of convulsive disorders, II: genetics and encephalographic studies in centrencephalic epilepsy. Neurology 11:474–483, 1961

Monroe RR: Limbic ictus and atypical psychoses. J Nerv Ment Dis 170:711–716, 1982

Neppe VM: Review article: symptomatology of temporal lobe epilepsy. S Afr Med J 60(23):902–907, 1981a

Neppe VM: Review article: non-epileptic symptoms of temporal lobe dysfunction. S Afr Med J 60(26):989–991, 1981b

Neppe VM: Differing perspectives to the concept of temporal lobe epilepsy. The Leech 52:6–10, 1982

Neppe VM: Carbamazepine as adjunctive treatment in nonepileptic chronic inpatients with EEG temporal lobe abnormalities. J Clin Psychiatry 44(9):326–331, 1983a

Neppe VM: Temporal lobe symptomatology in subjective paranormal experients. Journal of the American Society for Psychiatric Research 77:1–30, 1983b

Neppe VM: The use of carbamazepine in psychiatry, in Update on Psychiatric Management. Edited by Carlile JB. Durban, South Africa, Medical Association of South Africa, 1984, pp 50–54

Neppe VM: Epilepsy and psychiatry: essential links. Psychiatric Insight 2(2):18–22, 1985a

Neppe VM: The kindling phenomenon implications for animal and human behaviour, in Neuropsychology 2—Proceedings, Second South African Congress of Brain and Behaviour. Edited by Griesel D. Pretoria, South Africa, South African Brain and Behaviour Society, 1985b, pp 47–51

Neppe VM: The management of epilepsy in the psychiatric patient. Psychiatric Insight 2(2):23–26, 1985c

Neppe VM: Non-responsive psychosis: neuropsychological rehabilitation by antikindling agents. in Neuropsychology 2—Proceedings, Second South African Congress of Brain and Behaviour. Edited by Griesel D. Pretoria, South Africa, South African Brain and Behaviour Society, 1985d, pp 52–56

Neppe VM: Epileptic psychosis: a heterogeneous condition. Epilepsia 27:634, 1986

Neppe VM: Carbamazepine, limbic kindling and non-responsive psychosis, in Innovative Psychopharmacotherapy. Edited by Neppe VM. New York, Raven, 1989, pp 123–151

Neppe VM: Carbamazepine in the non affective psychotic and non psychotic dyscontrol, in Carbamazepine and Ox-carbamazepine in Psychiatry: International Clinical Psychopharmacology. Edited by Emrich H, Schiwy W, Silverstone T. London, Clinical Neuroscience Publishers, 1990, pp 43–54

Neppe VM: The Inventory of Neppe of Symptoms of Epilepsy and Temporal Lobe–Manual. Seattle, WA, University of Washington, 1991

Neppe VM, Blumer D: Nomenclature of psychiatric disorders of epilepsy—Axis I: psychopathology. Epilepsia 33 (suppl 3):S17–18, 1992

Neppe VM, Kaplan C: Short-term treatment of atypical spells with carbamazepine. Clin Neuropharmacol 11:287–289, 1988

Neppe VM, Tucker GJ: Modern perspectives on epilepsy in relation to psychiatry: behavioral disturbances of epilepsy. Hosp Community Psychiatry 39:389–396, 1988a

Neppe VM, Tucker GJ: Modern perspectives on epilepsy in relation to psychiatry: classification and evaluation. Hosp Community Psychiatry 39:263–271, 1988b

Neppe VM, Tucker GJ: Atypical, unusual and cultural psychoses, in Comprehensive Textbook of Psychiatry, 5th Edition. Edited by Kaplan HI, Sadock BJ. Baltimore, MD, Williams & Wilkins, 1989, pp 842–852

Neppe VM, Tucker GJ, Wilensky AJ: Fundamentals of carbamazepine use in neuropsychiatry. J Clin Psychiatry 49 (suppl 4):4–6, 1988

Neppe VM, Bowman B, Sawchuk KSLJ: Carbamazepine for atypical psychosis with episodic hostility: a preliminary study. J Nerv Ment Dis 179:339–340, 1991

Perez MM, Trimble MR: Epileptic psychosis: psychopathological comparison with process schizophrenia. Br J Psychiatry 137:245–249, 1980

Pincus JH, Tucker GJ: Behavioral Neurology, 3rd Edition. New York, Oxford University Press, 1985

Roberts JK, Guberman A: Religion and epilepsy. Psychiatr J Univ Ottawa 14(1):282–286, 1989

Robertson MM, Trimble MR, Townsend HR: Phenomenology of depression in epilepsy. Epilepsia 28:364–372, 1987

Rodin EA: Psychomotor epilepsy and aggressive behavior. Arch Gen Psychiatry 28:210–213, 1973

Rodin EA, Schmaltz S: The Bear-Fedio personality inventory and temporal lobe epilepsy. Neurology 34:591–596, 1984

Scher M, Neppe V: Carbamazepine adjunct for nonresponsive psychosis with prior hallucinogenic abuse. J Nerv Ment Dis 177:755–757, 1989

Sengoku A, Yagi K, Seino M, et al: Risks of occurrence of psychoses in relation to the types of epilepsies and epileptic seizures. Folia Psychiatry and Neurology of Japan 37:221–225, 1983

Slater E, Beard AW, Glithero E: The schizophrenia-like psychoses of epilepsy. Br J Psychiatry 109:95–150, 1963

Stark-Adamec C, Adamec R, Graham J, et al: Complexities in the complex partial seizures personality controversy. Psychiatr J Univ Ottawa 10:232–236, 1985

Stevens JR: Epilepsy, personality, behavior and psychopathology—the state of the evidence and directions for future research and treatment. Folia Psychiatr Neurol Jpn 37:203–216, 1983

Stevens JR: Psychiatric aspects of epilepsy. J Clin Psychiatry 49 (suppl 4):49–57, 1988

Stevens JR, Livermore AJ: Kindling of the mesolimbic dopamine system: animal model of psychosis. Neurology 28:36–46, 1978

Szatmari P: Some methodologic criteria for studies in developmental neuropsychiatry. Psychiatr Dev 3:153–170, 1985

Toone BK, Garralda ME, Ron MA: The psychoses of epilepsy and the functional psychoses: a clinical and phenomenological comparison. Br J Psychiatry 141:256–261, 1982

Trimble MR: The relationship between epilepsy and schizophrenia: a biochemical hypothesis. Biol Psychiatry 12:299–304, 1977

Trimble MR: The effects of anticonvulsant drugs on cognitive abilities. Pharmacol Ther 4:677–685, 1979

Trimble MR: Limbic system disorders in man, in Psychopharmacology of the Limbic System. Edited by Trimble MR, Zarifian E. Oxford, England, Oxford University Press, 1983, pp 110–124

Trimble MR: Cognitive hazards of seizure disorders. Epilepsia 29 (suppl 1):S19–S24, 1988

Tucker GJ, Price TP, Johnson VB, et al: Phenomenology of temporal lobe dysfunction: a link to atypical psychosis—a series of cases. J Nerv Ment Dis 174:348–356, 1986

Vingiano W: Hemisphericity and personality. Int J Neurosci 44(3–4):263–274, 1989

Waxman SG, Geschwind N: The interictal behavior syndrome of temporal lobe epilepsy. Arch Gen Psychiatry 32:1580–1586, 1975

Wells C, Duneau GW: Neurology for Psychiatrists. Philadelphia, PA, FA Davis, 1980

Wing JK, Cooper JE, Sartorius N: The Measurement and Classification of Psychiatric Symptoms. New York, Cambridge University Press, 1974

Chapter 16

Neuropsychiatric Aspects of Sleep

Thomas C. Neylan, M.D.
Charles F. Reynolds III, M.D.
David J. Kupfer, M.D.

The relevance of sleep to neuropsychiatry needs little elaboration in that the importance of sleep to mood, cognition, and general health is intuitively obvious. Although the interest in disorders of sleep dates back to the earliest writings of descriptive medicine, the rapid growth in the scientific study of sleep and sleep-related clinical disorders did not begin until the discovery of rapid-eye-movement (REM) sleep by Aserinsky and Kleitman in 1953. Sleep became understood not as just a passive phenomenon arising from a reduction in wakefulness (Sterman and Shouse 1985), but rather as a dynamic process comprised of two major brain states: REM and non-REM (NREM) sleep. Over the past three decades, the field of sleep medicine has grown rapidly and there are now more than 140 sleep disorder centers in the United States.

CLINICAL MANIFESTATIONS OF SLEEP-WAKE DISORDERS

Approximately 50 million Americans complain of some form of sleep disturbance (Bixler et al. 1979), and each year 10 million seek treatment from physicians for a sleep-related disturbance (Institute of Medicine 1979). A thorough medical and psychiatric history is essential for diagnosing conditions that impact on sleep-wake function. Patients' chief complaints are usually related to disrupted or too little sleep, excessive sleepiness, or adverse events associated with the sleep period (Table 16–1).

In obtaining a clinical history from patients, the entire 24-hour time period should be explored. Patients should be asked about symptoms of morning headaches, cataplexy, hypnagogic-hypnopompic hallucinations, sleep paralysis, automatic behavior, or sleep drunkenness. A 2-week sleep-wake log is invaluable for obtaining history of irregular sleep-wake patterns; napping; use of stimulants, hypnotics, or alcohol; diet; activity during the day; number of arousals; and perceived length of sleep time and its relationship to daytime mood and alertness. Additional history should be obtained from bed partners for events usually not perceived by the patient, such as respiratory pauses or unusual body movements.

Supported in part by Grants MH 00295 (to CFR:RSA), MH37869 (to CFR), MH30915 (to DJK), and AG06836 (to CFR).

NORMAL HUMAN SLEEP

Normal sleep consists of recurring 70- to 120-minute cycles of NREM and REM sleep. NREM sleep consists of four stages characterized polysomnographically by the electroencephalogram (EEG), the electrooculogram (EOG), and the electromyogram (EMG) (Rechtschaffen and Kales 1968). During wakefulness, the EEG is characterized by low-voltage fast activity consisting of a mix of alpha (8–13 Hz) and beta ($\geq$13 Hz) frequencies.

Stage 1 of NREM sleep is characterized by the slower theta (4–7 Hz) frequencies. Stage 2 is characterized by a background theta rhythm and the episodic appearance of sleep spindles (brief bursts of 12–14 Hz activity), and K complexes (a K complex is a single high-amplitude, slow-frequency electronegative wave followed by a single electropositive wave). Stages 3 and 4, also called slow-wave or delta sleep, are defined as epochs of sleep consisting of more than 20% and 50%, respectively, of high-amplitude activity in the delta band (0.5–3.0 Hz). Typically, sleep progresses from wakefulness through the four stages of NREM sleep until the onset of the first REM period.

REM sleep is a dramatic physiological state in that the brain becomes electrically and metabolically activated. A generalized muscle atonia can be detected by the disappearance of EMG activity. There are bursts of rapid eye movements, fluctuations in respiratory and cardiac rate, penile and clitoral engorgement, and a suspension of normal temperature regulation such that humans become transiently poikilothermic (Parmeggiani 1980). Finally, REM sleep is the stage in which there are the most vivid and often times bizarre dreams.

Infants at birth spend up to 20 hours a day asleep. REM and NREM stages are not fully differentiated until 3–6 months of age, owing to the relative immaturity of

---

Table 16–1.   Sleep definitions

---

apnea   cessation of airflow for at least 10 seconds.

cataplexy   sudden loss in muscle tone usually precipitated by a sudden emotional response such as fear or laughter.

circadian rhythm   a regular pattern of fluctuation in physiology or behavior that is usually linked to the 24-hour light-dark cycle.

diurnal   a behavior or physiological variable that is tied to daytime.

hypersomnia   excessive sleepiness. Pertains to the propensity to fall asleep.

hypnagogic-hypnopompic hallucinations   hallucinations occurring at the beginning or end of sleep that are usually a manifestation of REM sleep.

hypopnea   reduction in airflow by at least 50% for at least 10 seconds.

insomnia   difficulty with initiating or maintaining sleep.

parasomnia   adverse physiological or behavioral event occurring during sleep.

phase advance or delay   shift of the sleep or wake cycle to an earlier or later position in the 24-hour day.

polysomnogram   the electrophysiological recording of multiple biological parameters during sleep.

Zeitgeber   an environmental factor such as the light-dark cycle that helps entrain biological rhythms to a 24-hour time period.

Source.   American Sleep Disorders Association Diagnostic Classification Steering Committee 1990.

neural structures governing sleep. During the first 3 years, the sleep-wake rhythm develops from an ultradian to a circadian pattern with the principal sleep phase occurring at night. During adolescence there is a precipitous drop in slow-wave sleep (Feinberg 1974). In the third through sixth decades there is a gradual and slight decline in sleep efficiency and total sleep time. With advancing age, sleep becomes more fragmented and lighter in depth with more transient arousals, sleep stage shifts, and a gradual disappearance of slow-wave sleep.

INTERNATIONAL CLASSIFICATION OF SLEEP DISORDERS

In 1979, the Association of Sleep Disorders Centers (ASDC) published its first nosology dividing sleep disorders into four major categories: disorders of initiating and maintaining sleep (insomnias); disorders of excessive somnolence; sleep-wake schedule disorders; and parasomnias (Association of Sleep Disorders Centers and the Association for the Psychophysiological Study of Sleep 1979). In 1990, the International Classification of Sleep Disorders (ICSD; American Sleep Disorders Association Diagnostic Classification Steering Committee 1990) was published which substantially modified the original ASDC nosology with the introduction of a triaxial diagnostic system. Axis A lists the primary sleep diagnosis, Axis B specifies the procedures used to establish the diagnosis, and Axis C lists relevant non-sleep medical and/or psychiatric diagnoses. The proposed DSM-IV classification (Table 16–2) adapts some aspects of the ICSD nosology in that disorders are classified on the basis of presumed pathophysiology as opposed to a predominant symptom such as insomnia. In this chapter we present the major sleep-wake disorders organized around the ICSD nosology.

DIFFERENTIAL DIAGNOSIS OF DYSSOMNIAS

The following section provides a brief review of the dyssomnias that cause insomnia and excessive sleepiness (Table 16–3). The ICSD nosology divides the dys-

---

Table 16–2.   Proposed DSM-IV classification of sleep disorders[a]

I. Primary sleep disorders 　A. Dyssomnias 　　1. Primary insomnia 　　2. Primary hypersomnia 　　3. Narcolepsy 　　4. Breathing-related sleep disorder 　　5. Circadian rhythm sleep disorder 　　6. Dyssomnia not otherwise 　　　specified (NOS) 　B. Parasomnias 　　1. Nightmare disorder 　　2. Sleep terror disorder 　　3. Sleepwalking disorder 　　4. Parasomnia NOS	II. Sleep disorders related to another mental 　disorder (nonsubstance and/or primary) 　A. Insomnia related to [Axis I or Axis II 　　disorder] 　B. Hypersomnia related to [Axis I or 　　Axis II disorder] III. Secondary sleep disorder due to an Axis 　III condition IV. Substance-induced sleep disorder

---

[a]Obtained from personal communication with D. J. Kupfer, Chairman of the DSM-IV Workgroup on Sleep Disorders.

somnias into those caused by so-called intrinsic factors (i.e., originating within the body) and those caused by extrinsic factors (e.g., stimulants or environmental noise that can disrupt sleep), as well as circadian rhythm disruptions.

Intrinsic Sleep Disorders

The intrinsic sleep disorders include the majority of disorders treated by sleep specialists: the major insomnias, sleep apnea, myoclonus, and narcolepsy. Two common forms of insomnia not caused by a primary psychiatric disorder are psychophysiological insomnia and idiopathic (childhood-onset) insomnia referred to as *primary insomnia* in DSM-III-R (American Psychiatric Association 1987).

Table 16–3.   International classification of sleep disorders—dyssomnias

A. Intrinsic sleep disorders
    1. Psychophysiological insomnia
    2. Sleep state misperception
    3. Idiopathic insomnia
    4. Narcolepsy
    5. Recurrent hypersomnia
    6. Idiopathic insomnia
    7. Posttraumatic hypersomnia
    8. Obstructive sleep apnea syndrome
    9. Central sleep apnea syndrome
    10. Central alveolar hypoventilation syndrome
    11. Periodic limb movement disorder
    12. Restless legs syndrome
    13. Intrinsic sleep disorder, not otherwise specified (NOS)

B. Extrinsic sleep disorders
    1. Inadequate sleep hygiene
    2. Environmental sleep disorder
    3. Altitude insomnia
    4. Adjustment sleep disorder
    5. Insufficient sleep syndrome
    6. Limit-setting sleep disorder
    7. Sleep-onset association disorder
    8. Food allergy insomnia
    9. Nocturnal eating (drinking) syndrome
    10. Hypnotic-dependent sleep disorder
    11. Stimulant-dependent sleep disorder
    12. Alcohol-dependent sleep disorder
    13. Toxin-induced sleep disorder
    14. Extrinsic sleep disorder NOS

C. Circadian rhythm sleep disorders
    1. Time zone change (jet lag) syndrome
    2. Shift work sleep disorder
    3. Irregular sleep-wake pattern
    4. Delayed sleep phase syndrome
    5. Advanced sleep phase syndrome
    6. Non-24-hour sleep-wake disorder
    7. Circadian rhythm sleep disorder NOS

Source.   American Sleep Disorders Association Diagnostic Classification Steering Committee 1990.

Psychophysiological insomnia is sometimes referred to as *learned* or *conditioned* insomnia. Typically, it begins during a period of increased stress that manifests in an acute sleep disruption. Patients become preoccupied with sleep and develop anticipatory anxiety about daytime fatigue and diminished performance. The disorder can become chronic, persisting over many years, and cause chronic fatigue, muscle aches, and mood disturbance (Hauri and Fisher 1986).

Idiopathic insomnia does not have any psychosocial antecedents and appears to be a trait phenomenon in which the patient has a constitutional predisposition for fragmented sleep. Often the disorder is lifelong, originating in early childhood (Hauri and Olmstead 1980) and presumed to be secondary to a neurochemical or structural disorder involving neural networks governing sleep-wake states. It is difficult to treat and often requires unconventional or innovative pharmacological intervention (Regestein 1987).

Sleep apnea.   Sleep-disordered breathing is typically an occult disorder that causes daytime somnolence, impaired concentration and intellectual functioning, and morning headaches. It is associated with obesity, loud snoring, systemic and pulmonary hypertension, cardiac arrhythmias, and excessive mortality. It can be caused by an impairment in central respiratory drive (central apnea), intermittent upper-airway obstruction (obstructive apnea), or a combination of the two (mixed apnea). Patients with this disorder experience frequent respiratory pauses during sleep associated with oxygen desaturation.

Sleep apnea is studied polysomnographically by measuring oral and nasal airflow, respiratory effort, oxygen saturation, and architecture with a standard sleep montage (EEG, EOG, and EMG) (Figure 16–1). Daytime sleepiness can be measured objectively with the Multiple Sleep Latency Test (MSLT; Carskadon et al. 1986) (also

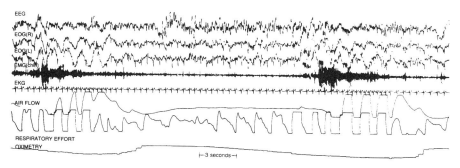

Figure 16–1.   Sleep recording from a 25-year-old man with obstructive sleep apnea syndrome. Despite sustained respiratory effector, upper-airway collapse during sleep prevents airflow, resulting in oxyhemoglobin desaturation, electrocardiogram (EKG) bradytachycardia, and electroencephalogram (EEG) microarousals. This pattern recurs hundreds of times nightly. The resulting sleep fragmentation and loss (through repeated arousals necessary for the resumption of breathing) cause excessive daytime sleepiness. EOG(R) = right electrooculogram; EOG(L) = left electrooculogram; EMG(chin) = electromyogram.
Source.   Reprinted from Reynolds CF, Kupfer DJ: "Sleep Disorders," in *American Psychiatric Press Textbook of Psychiatry.* Edited by Talbott JA, Hales RE, Yudofsky SC. Washington, DC, American Psychiatric Press, 1988, pp. 737–752. Used with permission.

see Chapter 6). Patients typically have evidence of pathological sleepiness as measured by latencies to sleep onset of less than 5 minutes on the MSLT.

There are various behavioral, medical, pharmacological, and surgical treatments for sleep apnea. Behavioral approaches include weight loss, abstinence from sedative-hypnotics, and training to avoid the supine position during sleep. Mechanical approaches include a variety of tongue-retaining devices and continuous positive airway pressure (CPAP). Medical approaches consist of the use of tricyclic antidepressants, particularly protriptyline, and supplemental oxygen. Surgical techniques are currently being refined.

Nocturnal myoclonus and restless legs syndrome.   Sleep can be fragmented by the occurrence of periodic leg movements leading to complaints of either insomnia or daytime sleepiness. Nocturnal myoclonus is repetitive, brief leg jerks that occur in regular 20- to 40-second intervals that are associated with transient arousals leading to sleep fragmentation. It is a common disorder that is seen in association with sleep apnea, narcolepsy, uremia, diabetes, and a variety of disorders affecting the cortex, brain stem, and spinal cord (Coleman et al. 1980). It is typically idiopathic with no evidence of gross central nervous system (CNS) pathology. It is a normal phenomenon at birth, disappears in childhood, and frequently reemerges in old age. The most common treatments for this disorder are benzodiazepines and levodopa (L-dopa).

Restless legs syndrome is characterized by the presence of deep paresthesias in the calf muscles that causes sleep-onset insomnia. It is associated with uremia, anemia, and pregnancy, as well as with nocturnal myoclonus. Treatments under investigation include opioids, carbamazepine, clonidine, benzodiazepines, baclofen, and L-dopa.

Narcolepsy.   Narcolepsy is a common cause of daytime hypersomnolence in which REM sleep repeatedly and suddenly intrudes into wakefulness. The clinical phenomenology of narcolepsy is best understood by a consideration of normal REM physiology (e.g., activated EEG, generalized atonia, and dream cognition). Both cataplexy and sleep paralysis involve muscle atonia occurring at a time when the patient feels awake. Hypnagogic hallucinations are thought to be related to the dreamlike perceptual phenomenon of REM sleep.

Treatment approaches include the use of REM-suppressing agents such as tricyclic antidepressants to control cataplexy. Stimulants such as methylphenidate, amphetamine, and pemoline are useful for controlling daytime somnolence. An important nonpharmacological approach is the use of scheduled naps throughout the wake period.

Extrinsic Sleep Disorders

Extrinsic sleep disorders are caused by external factors, including behavioral patterns, without which there would be no sleep disturbance. The purest forms of these disorders are altitude insomnia and environmental sleep disorder in which there is a clear, easily identifiable external cause for the sleep disturbance. Several of these sleep disorders are related to ingestion of substances that have direct toxic effects on sleep. Both alcohol- and hypnotic-dependent sleep disorders involve the development of tolerance to the sleep-inducing effects of the agent, as well as increased arousals during withdrawal periods. Stimulants cause sleep-onset insomnia during usage and rebound hypersomnia during withdrawal.

Several of these disorders are related to dysfunctional behavior patterns that perturb sleep. Adjustment sleep disorder, experienced by most people at some point in their lives, is typically an insomnia related to acute stress such as a school examination. Inadequate sleep hygiene, one of the most common disorders, is related to habits such as napping or late-evening exercise that adversely affect sleep. Treatment includes implementation of habits promoting good sleep hygiene (Table 16–4).

Circadian Rhythm Sleep Disorders

The sleep-wake cycle, under the circadian control of endogenous regulators or oscillators, can be disrupted by a misalignment between biological rhythms and external demands on waking behavior. Circadian rhythm disorders present with either insomnia or hypersomnolence depending on the juxtaposition of performance demands and the underlying circadian cycle.

Rapid shifts in the sleep-wake schedule cause an acute circadian dysrhythmia. Jet lag is one of the most common of these disorders. Travelers flying across multiple time zones are met with a radical change in the cues called *Zeitgebers*, which help entrain circadian rhythms with respect to both the social schedule and the light-dark

---

Table 16–4. Rules of sleep hygiene

1. Sleep as much as needed to feel refreshed during the following day. Restricting the time in bed seems to solidify sleep, but excessively long times in bed seem related to fragmented and shallow sleep.
2. Get up at the same time each day, 7 days a week. (A regular awake time in the morning leads to regular times of sleep onset.)
3. A steady daily amount of exercise probably deepens sleep.
4. Insulate your bedroom against sounds (carpeting, insulated curtains, and closing the door).
5. Excessively warm rooms may disturb sleep; keep the room temperature moderate.
6. Hunger may disturb sleep. A light snack at bedtime may help sleep.
7. Try to avoid excessive liquids in the evening, in order to minimize the need for nighttime trips to the bathroom.
8. Avoid caffeine-containing beverages in the evening.
9. Avoid alcohol in the evening. Although alcohol helps tense people fall asleep more easily, the ensuing sleep is then broken up.
10. People who feel angry and frustrated because they cannot sleep should not try harder and harder to fall asleep but should turn on the light, leave the bedroom, and do something different like reading a boring book. Don't engage in stimulating activity. Return to bed only when sleepy. Get up at your regular time the next day, no matter how little you slept.
11. The chronic use of tobacco disturbs sleep.
12. If you find yourself waking up and looking at the clock, put the clock under the bed or cover it up.

Note. Adapted from Hauri and Orr 1982.
Source. Reprinted from Reynolds CF, Kupfer DJ: "Sleep Disorders," in *American Psychiatric Press Textbook of Psychiatry.* Edited by Talbott JA, Hales RE, Yudofsky SC. Washington, DC, American Psychiatric Press, 1988, pp. 737–752. Used with permission.

cycle. Similarly, workers who rotate on to different shifts experience an acute mis-alignment in their underlying biological rhythms. These disorders give rise to sleep-wake complaints, mood disturbance, decreased work performance, and general physical malaise. The general treatment approach is to promote good sleep hygiene with the goal of properly aligning patients' circadian system with their sleep-wake schedule.

Some circadian sleep-wake disorders are related to a diminished capacity to re-spond to external Zeitgebers. In the delayed sleep phase syndrome, patients have an innate preference to begin sleeping in the late hours of night and to sleep until the late morning or early afternoon. They experience sleep-onset insomnia and morning hypersomnolence when forced to comply with a conventional sleep-wake schedule. Conversely, patients with advanced sleep phase syndrome experience hypersomno-lence in the early evening hours and mid-night arousal. Treatment involves the re-alignment of the sleep-wake schedule with manipulation or augmentation of external Zeitgebers such as the use of bright light therapy.

DIFFERENTIAL DIAGNOSIS OF PARASOMNIAS

Parasomnias are adverse events that occur during sleep. Many of these disorders are found normally in young children and are labeled as pathological only if they persist into adulthood. Two common parasomnias occurring as a partial arousal from deep sleep are sleepwalking and sleep terrors. In sleepwalking, subjects be-come partially aroused and ambulatory. They are typically difficult to awaken and have amnesia for the events. Sleep terrors involve intense fear, autonomic arousal, and poor dream recall. This is in contradistinction to nightmares, which arise from REM sleep and are characterized by vivid, detailed imagery, associated with good recall. Treatment is directed toward reducing stress, anxiety, and sleep deprivation. In extreme cases low-dose benzodiazepines are effective.

Several prominent parasomnias are characterized by abnormal motor behavior during sleep. Nocturnal paroxysmal dystonia is characterized by stereotypic and vio-lent movements that can resemble seizure activity (Lugaresi et al. 1986). REM-sleep behavior disorder occurs when there is incomplete or absent muscle atonia during REM. The disorder is characterized by violent and dramatic motor activity, which represents the motor expression of dreaming. Benzodiazepines, particularly clonazepam, are useful in reducing these events (Mahowald and Schenck 1989).

MEDICAL AND/OR PSYCHIATRIC SLEEP DISORDERS

Sleep can be adversely affected by a variety of psychiatric, neurological, and med-ical disorders. In each case, the treatment is directed to the underlying disorder.

Affective Disorders

Sleep disturbance is verifiable in 90% of patients with major depression and is characterized by sleep fragmentation, decreased quantity and altered distribution of delta sleep, reduced duration of the first NREM period (e.g., REM latency), redistribution of REM sleep into the first half of the night, and increased density of rapid eye movements (Kupfer and Reynolds 1992; Reynolds and Kupfer 1987). Bipolar patients, in contrast, typically become hypersomnolent during depressive episodes and have comparatively increased sleep efficiency and total sleep time (Detre et al. 1972).

Multiple studies have shown that REM latency is related to state-dependent factors in major depression. Giles et al. (1986) found that REM latency was related to appetite loss, terminal insomnia, anhedonia, and unreactive mood. Kupfer et al. (1988) have shown that REM latency is shorter during the earlier phases of relapse in recurrent major depression. Delusional depression is distinguishable from the nondelusional subtype because of the higher frequency of sleep-onset REM periods and decreased total REM time (Thase et al. 1986).

In addition, there are intriguing data that suggest that short REM latency may be a vulnerability or trait marker for major depression. Several groups (e.g., Hauri et al. 1974; Rush et al. 1986) have found reduced REM latency in patients after clinical remission of their depressive episodes. First-degree relatives of depressed probands with short REM latency have been found to be at increased risk of developing major depression (Giles et al. 1988). Similarly, first-degree relatives concordant for depression have been found to be concordant for REM latency as well (Giles et al. 1987a).

REM latency and other REM measures have been found useful in predicting response to treatment and risk of relapse. Kupfer et al. (1976) showed that the degree of REM latency prolongation and total REM suppression seen during initiation of treatment with amitriptyline predicted clinical response. Similarly, REM suppression by clomipramine has been found to predict response to treatment (Hochli et al. 1986). Short REM latency during an index episode of depression confers a higher risk of relapse after clinical remission (Giles et al. 1987b; Reynolds et al. 1989).

Schizophrenia

Schizophrenic patients have been found to have prolonged sleep latencies, sleep fragmentation with multiple arousals, decreased slow-wave sleep, variability in REM latency, and decreased REM rebound after REM-sleep deprivation (Zarcone 1988).

Several investigators have attempted to find correlations between clinical features of schizophrenia and specific sleep variables. For example, the variability in REM latency has been linked to family history of affective disorder (Keshavan et al. 1990), presence of negative symptoms (Tandon et al. 1988), tardive dyskinesia (Thaker et al. 1989), and neuroleptic withdrawal (Neylan et al., 1992). Diminished slow-wave sleep, one of the most replicated findings in schizophrenia, has been found to be associated with poor performance on neuropsychological tests of attention (Orzack et al. 1977); van Kammen et al. (1988) found an inverse relationship between presence of negative symptoms and slow-wave sleep.

Anxiety Disorders

Sleep in patients with anxiety disorders differs from that seen in patients with major depression in the presence of normal REM latencies and decreased REM percent (Reynolds et al. 1983). Mellman and Uhde (1989) confirmed that panic attacks can arise during sleep, particularly during transitions from stage 2 to delta sleep. Ross et al. (1989) reviewed what is known about sleep in posttraumatic stress disorder (PTSD) and argued that sleep disturbance, particularly disturbing repetitive dreams, may be the essential feature of the disorder. Moreover, they suggested that dysfunctional REM-sleep physiology may contribute to the pathogenesis of the disorder.

Dementia

Sleep in patients with primary degenerative dementia of the Alzheimer's type (PDDAT) represents an exaggeration of the deterioration of sleep seen in normal aging. Compared to age-matched control subjects, patients with PDDAT have more sleep fragmentation and less delta and REM sleep (Reynolds 1989). Patients with PDDAT have more sleep-related phenomena, such as sundowning and nocturnal wanderings, which is often the precipitating factor that provokes families to institutionalize their elderly relatives (Sanford 1975).

There is evidence that the prevalence of sleep apnea is higher in patients with probable Alzheimer's dementia compared with age- and sex-matched control subjects. Furthermore, the severity of dementia is correlated with the severity of apnea (Reynolds et al. 1985). Hoch et al. (1989) showed that sleep EEG predicted mortality in a sample of patients with mixed symptoms of depression and dementia. Patients who had died during a 2-year follow-up period had significantly longer REM latencies, less REM-sleep rebound after sleep deprivation, and higher indices of sleep-disordered breathing.

Other Neuropsychiatric Conditions

Sleep and seizures.   NREM sleep has a well-known activating effect on seizure activity, whereas epileptic discharges usually are suppressed during REM sleep. Many epileptic patients have their seizures predominantly during sleep or on arousal from sleep (Janz 1962). Unusual nocturnal motor behavior, sleep-related incontinence, or nocturnal tongue biting warrants an evaluation for sleep seizures.

Sleep in parkinsonism.   Sleep disturbance is reported in approximately 75% of patients with parkinsonism. Sleep is characterized by increased number of awakenings, decreased delta and REM sleep, and a scarcity of sleep spindles. The resting tremor usually subsides with the onset of stage 1 sleep but, depending on the severity of the disorder, can persist into stage 2 or reemerge during sleep stage changes (April 1966). Nigrostriatal degeneration may have a direct or indirect impact on the neural substrate regulating sleep.

Kleine-Levin syndrome.   A rare form of periodic hypersomnolence is the Kleine-Levin syndrome, which is characterized by intermittent attacks of hypersomnolence and hyperphagia often associated with indiscreet hypersexuality, poor social judgment, mood disturbance, and hallucinations. It occurs most frequently in males in their late adolescence and early 20s and is followed by a gradual decline in the frequency and duration of the episodes (Critchley 1962). The pathophysiology is postulated to involve an underlying disturbance of limbic and hypothalamic function.

NEUROPSYCHIATRIC ASPECTS OF SLEEP DISORDERS

Sleep Deprivation

Short-term effects of 1–2 nights of sleep deprivation include fatigue, irritability, impaired attention with poor performance on dull monotonous tasks, and impairments in short-term memory. Sleep deprivation has well-described mood-elevating effects in more than 50% of endogenous depressive patients (Wu and Bunney 1990) and is increasingly being used by clinicians in the treatment of depression. Long-term sleep deprivation can lead to reversible perceptual abnormalities, irritability, transient paranoia, disorientation, and severe fatigue.

Sleep Apnea

The clinical impact of sleep apnea is related to two important phenomena: hypoxia and sleep fragmentation. Cerebral hypoxia can lead to the intellectual deterioration, impaired attention and memory, and personality changes seen in apnea patients. From a psychosocial perspective, the symptom of hypersomnolence is the most debilitating of symptoms seen in apnea patients. Several investigators have attempted to discern if hypersomnolence is related to sleep hypoxia or to sleep fragmentation. In a study of patients with obstructive sleep apnea, Roehrs et al. (1989) reported that, although the number of arousals and hypoxic events covaried significantly, it was the arousal index that best predicted short latencies on the MSLT. This finding supports the hypothesis that daytime somnolence is secondary to the disruption in quantity and quality of sleep.

Narcolepsy

Narcolepsy has been found to affect psychological state as well as cognition. Patients have been found to have more job-related injuries, problems with occupational or academic performance, and a higher prevalence of anxiety and affective disorders (Richardson et al. 1990). Several studies have shown impaired performance in tasks requiring sustained attention as a result of intrusive microsleeps. However, not all performance decrements can be attributed to impaired arousal because attentional deficits have been found in narcoleptic patients during EEG verified wakefulness (Mendelson 1987).

Sleep-Wake Schedule Disorders and Effects of Shift Work

Sleep-wake schedule disorders can give rise to various neuropsychiatric and medical symptoms. Rotating-shift workers have been found to have 2–3 times the injury rate compared with co-workers who work stable day, evening, or night shifts (Smith and Colligan 1982). Shift workers have high rates of gastrointestinal, cardiac, and reproductive disorders (Czeisler and Allan 1988). Monk (1989) pointed out that the ability to cope with shift work is related to tolerance for circadian desynchronosis, decreased sleep, and domestic pressures often experienced by those who work unconventional hours.

MANAGEMENT OF SLEEP DISORDERS

Given the broad spectrum of pathophysiological processes that affect sleep-wake function, the management of sleep disorders rests on the foundation of the specific diagnosis. The clinical history, exam, and sleep diary remain the cornerstone of the initial assessment. Polysomnography is indicated in any patient with complaints of irresistible daytime sleepiness given the high prevalence of sleep apnea and narcolepsy in this population. The use of polysomnography in patients with insomnia is indicated when initial attempts to improve sleep hygiene, modify sleep-related habits that elicit arousal, or treat clinical affective disorders are unsuccessful.

A detailed discussion of the treatment of sleep disorders secondary to apnea, narcolepsy, nocturnal myoclonus, major depression, parasomnias, and sleep-wake schedule disorders is beyond the scope of this chapter. A broad overview is presented in Table 16–5. (For excellent reviews, see American Psychiatric Association 1989.) In this section we focus on the use of nonpharmacological and pharmacological interventions in patients with insomnia.

Education about healthy sleep habits is potentially a sufficient intervention. However, since patients are usually entrenched in their habits, a more realistic and longer-term approach is needed to help patients gradually make these adjustments. Various relaxation therapies such as hypnosis, meditation, deep breathing, and progressive muscle relaxation can be helpful. Success depends on a high degree of motivation from patients who must devote considerable time to practicing these techniques. Biofeedback can be helpful in those patients who are not sensitive to their internal state of arousal (Hauri and Esther 1990). Patients are provided an external measure of a biological variable such as EMG or EEG, allowing them a means to influence their own level of arousal.

Stimulus control behavior modification is focused on eliminating environmental cues associated with arousal (Bootzin 1972). Patients are instructed to restrict the use of their bed for sleep and intimacy, to go to bed only when sleepy, to remove clocks from sight, and to adhere to a stable sleep-wake schedule. The goal is to limit the amount of wake time spent in bed, thereby reestablishing the association between bed and sleep.

Sleep restriction therapy is similarly aimed at reducing the amount of wake time spent in bed (Spielman et al. 1987). Patients are instructed to restrict their time in bed commensurate to their estimate of their total sleep time. Patients often have their usual difficulties with sleep fragmentation during the first few nights and become sleep deprived. Sleep deprivation helps consolidate sleep on subsequent nights, thereby improving sleep efficiency. Increases in length of time in bed can subsequently be titrated to the presence of daytime fatigue.

The brief use of short–half-life benzodiazepines is an effective and benign treatment for the occasional difficult night in young or middle-aged adults. Benzodiazepines are less well tolerated in geriatric patients because of cognitive side effects, daytime somnolence, and potentiation of sleep-disordered breathing. In this group, the use of 25–50 mg of trazodone or 20–75 mg of nortriptyline can be quite effective (Reynolds et al. 1987). In younger adults, low-dose amitriptyline is effective and less liable for the development of tolerance compared with benzodiazepines.

Finally, in some nonapneic, nongeriatric patients with chronic insomnia, who

Table 16–5. Selected sleep-wake disorders: classification, polysomnographic findings, and treatment

DSM-III-R classification	ICSD classification	Polysomnographic findings	Primary treatment
Primary insomnia	Psychophysiological insomnia and idiopathic insomnia	Varies from normal to moderate sleep continuity disturbance	Biofeedback, stimulus control, temporal control, and short-term benzodiazepines
Myclonic sleep disorder	Periodic limb movement disorder	Periodic leg twitches, electroencephalogram (EEG) microarousals	Benzodiazepines
Hypersomnia disorders related to a physical condition	Obstructive sleep apnea syndrome	Mixed or obstructive apneas, EEG microarousals, and electrocardiogram arrhythmias	Weight loss, continuous positive airway pressure, and surgery
	Narcolepsy	Repeated sleep-onset REM periods (multiple sleep latency test)	Stimulants (e.g., methylphenidate) and tricyclic antidepressants for cataplexy
Insomnia related to a physical condition, (e.g., sleep apnea)	Central sleep apnea syndrome	Central sleep apneas and microarousals	Continuous positive airway pressure and low-flow oxygen
Sleep-wake schedule disorder, delayed type	Delayed sleep phase syndrome	Normal sleep 4–6 hours later than conventional	Chronotherapy
Parasomnias	Parasomnias	Partial arousal out of slow-wave sleep	Various: behavioral or pharmacological
Dyssomnias related to a mental condition (e.g., major depression)	Sleep disorders associated with mood disorders	Short REM latency, prolonged first REM period, and increased rapid eye movements	Pharmacotherapy and/or psychotherapy for depression (with or without adjunctive benzodiazepines)

Note. DSM-III-R = Diagnostic and Statistical Manual of Mental Disorders, 3rd Edition, Revised (American Psychiatric Association 1987); ICSD = International Classification of Sleep Disorders (American Sleep Disorders Association Diagnostic Classification Steering Committee 1990); REM = rapid eye movement.
Source. Adapted from Reynolds and Kupfer 1988.

have not responded to the interventions mentioned above, the long-term use of benzodiazepines is indicated. As has recently been suggested by the American Psychiatric Association's Task Force on benzodiazepines, the abuse potential for these drugs, albeit real, has probably been overstated in the past decade (American Psychiatric Association 1990).

REFERENCES

American Psychiatric Association: Diagnostic and Statistical Manual of Mental Disorders, 3rd Edition, Revised. Washington, DC, American Psychiatric Association, 1987

American Psychiatric Association: Treatment of Psychiatric Disorders: A Task Force Report of the American Psychiatric Association, Vol 3. Washington, DC, American Psychiatric Association, 1989, pp 2419–2453

American Psychiatric Association: Benzodiazepine Dependence, Toxicity, and Abuse: Task Force Report. Washington, DC, American Psychiatric Association, 1990

American Sleep Disorders Association Diagnostic Classification Steering Committee: International Classification of Sleep Disorders: Diagnostic and Coding Manual. Rochester, MN, American Sleep Disorders Association, 1990

April RS: Observations on parkinsonian tremor in all-night sleep. Neurology (NY) 16:720–724, 1966

Aserinsky E, Kleitman N: Regularly occurring periods of eye motility and concomitant phenomena during sleep. Science 118:273–274, 1953

Association of Sleep Disorders Centers and the Association for the Psychophysiological Study of Sleep: Diagnostic classification of sleep and arousal disorders. Sleep 2:1–137, 1979

Bixler EO, Kales A, Soldatos CR, et al: Prevalence of sleep disorders in the Los Angeles metropolitan area. Am J Psychiatry 136:1257–1262, 1979

Bootzin RR: A stimulus control treatment for insomnia, in American Psychological Association Proceedings. Washington, DC, American Psychological Association, 1972, pp 395–396

Carskadon MA, Dement WC, Mitler MM, et al: Guidelines for the Multiple Sleep Latency Test (MSLT): a standard measure of sleepiness. Sleep 9:519–524, 1986

Coleman RM, Pollack CP, Weitzman ED: Periodic movements in sleep (nocturnal myoclonus): relationship to sleep disorders. Ann Neurol 8:416–421, 1980

Critchley M: Periodic hypersomnia and megaphagia in adolescent males. Brain 59:494–515, 1962

Czeisler CA, Allan JS: Pathologies of the sleep-wake schedule, in Sleep Disorders: Diagnosis and Treatment, 2nd Edition. Edited by Williams RL, Karacan I, Moore CA. New York, Wiley, 1988, pp 109–129

Detre TP, Himmelhoch J, Swartzburg M, et al: Hypersomnia and manic-depressive disease. Am J Psychiatry 128:1303–1305, 1972

Feinberg I: Changes in sleep cycle patterns with age. J Psychiatr Res 10:283–306, 1974

Giles DE, Roffwarg HP, Schlesser MA, et al: Which endogenous depressive symptoms relate to REM latency reductions? Biol Psychiatry 21:473–482, 1986

Giles DE, Roffwarg HP, Rush AJ: REM latency concordance in depressed family members. Biol Psychiatry 22:910–924, 1987a

Giles DE, Jarrett RB, Roffwarg HP, et al: Reduced rapid eye movement latency: a predictor of recurrence in depression. Neuropsychopharmacology 1:33–39, 1987b

Giles DE, Biggs MM, Rush AJ, et al: Risk factors in families of unipolar depression, I: psychiatric illness and reduced REM latency. J Affective Disord 14:51–59, 1988

Hauri PJ, Esther MS: Insomnia. Mayo Clin Proc 65:869–882, 1990

Hauri P, Fisher J: Persistent psychophysiologic (learned) insomnia. Sleep 9:38–53, 1986

Hauri P, Olmstead P: Childhood-onset insomnia. Sleep 3:59–65, 1980

Hauri P, Orr WC: The Sleep Disorders: A Current Concepts Monograph. Kalamazoo, MI, Up-john, 1982

Hauri P, Chernik D, Hawkins D, et al: Sleep of depressed patients in remission. Arch Gen Psychiatry 31:386–391, 1974

Hoch CC, Reynolds CF, Houck PR, et al: Predicting mortality in mixed depression and dementia using sleep EEG variables. Journal of Neuropsychiatry and Clinical Neurosciences 1:366–371, 1989

Hochli D, Riemann D, Zulley J, et al: Initial REM sleep suppression by clomipramine: a prognostic tool for treatment response in patients with a major depressive disorder. Biol Psychiatry 21:1217–1220, 1986

Institute of Medicine: Report of a Study: Sleeping Pills, Insomnia and Medical Practice. Washington, DC, U.S. National Academy of Medical Sciences, 1979

Janz D: The grand mal epilepsies and the sleeping-waking cycle. Epilepsia 3:69–109, 1962

Keshavan MS, Reynolds CF, Kupfer KJ: Electroencephalographic sleep in schizophrenia: a critical review. Compr Psychiatry 30:34–47, 1990

Kupfer DJ, Reynolds CF: Sleep and affective disorders, in Handbook of Affective Disorders, 2nd Edition. Edited by Paykel ES. London, Churchill-Livingstone, 1992, pp 311–323

Kupfer DJ, Foster FG, Reich L, et al: EEG sleep changes as predictors in depression. Am J Psychiatry 133:622–626, 1976

Kupfer DJ, Frank E, Grochocinski VJ, et al: Electroencephalographic sleep profiles in recurrent depression: a longitudinal investigation. Arch Gen Psychiatry 45:678–681, 1988

Lugaresi E, Ciriguotta F, Montagna P: Nocturnal paroxysmal dystonia. J Neurol Neurosurg Psychiatry 49:375–380, 1986

Mahowald MW, Schenck CH: REM sleep behavior disorder, in Principles and Practices of Sleep Medicine. Edited by Kryger MH, Roth T, Dement WC. Philadelphia, PA, WB Saunders, 1989, pp 389–409

Mellman TA, Uhde TW: Electroencephalographic sleep in panic disorder. Arch Gen Psychiatry 46:178–184, 1989

Mendelson WB: Human Sleep: Research and Clinical Care. New York, Plenum Medical, 1987

Monk TH: Shift work, in Principles and Practices of Sleep Medicine. Edited by Kryger MH, Roth T, Dement WC. Philadelphia, PA, WB Saunders, 1989, pp 332–337

Neylan TC, van Kammen DP, Kelley ME, et al: Sleep in schizophrenic patients on and off haloperidol: clinically stable versus relapse patients. Arch Gen Psychiatry 4:643–649, 1992

Orzack MN, Hartmann EL, Kornetsky C: The relationship between attention and slow wave sleep in chronic schizophrenia. Psychopharm Bull 13:59–61, 1977

Parmeggiani PL: Temperature regulation during sleep: a study in homeostasis, in Physiology in Sleep. Edited by Orem J, Barnes CD. New York, Academic, 1980, pp 98–143

Rechtschaffen A, Kales A (eds): A Manual of Standardized Terminology, Techniques, and Scoring System for Sleep Stages of Human Subjects. Bethesda, MD, U.S. Department of Health, Education, and Welfare, Public Health Service, 1968

Regestein QR: Specific effects of sedative/hypnotic drugs in the treatment of incapacitating chronic insomnia. Am J Med 83:909–916, 1987

Reynolds CF: Sleep in dementia, in Principles and Practices of Sleep Medicine. Edited by Kryger MH, Roth T, Dement WC. Philadelphia, PA, WB Saunders, 1989, pp 415–416

Reynolds CF, Kupfer DJ: Sleep research in affective illness: State of the art circa 1987. Sleep 10:199–215, 1987

Reynolds CF, Kupfer DJ: Sleep disorders, in American Psychiatric Press Textbook of Psychiatry. Edited by Talbott JA, Hales RE, Yudofsky SC. Washington, DC, American Psychiatric Press, 1988, pp 737–752

Reynolds CF, Shaw DH, Newton TF, et al: EEG sleep in generalized anxiety disorder: a preliminary comparison with primary depression. Psychiatry Res 8:81–89, 1983

Reynolds CF, Kupfer DJ, Taska LS, et al: Sleep apnea in Alzheimer's dementia: correlation with
mental deterioration. J Clin Psychiatry 46:257–261, 1985

Reynolds CF, Perel JM, Kupfer DJ, et al: Open-trial response to antidepressant treatment in
elderly patients with mixed depression and cognitive impairment. Psychiatry Res 21:95–
109, 1987

Reynolds CF, Perel JM, Frank E, et al: Open-trial maintenance nortriptyline in late-life depression: survival analysis and preliminary data on the use of REM latency as a predictor of
recurrence. Psychopharmacol Bull 25:129–132, 1989

Richardson JW: Mayo sleep disorders update. Mayo Clin Proc 65:857–860, 1990

Richardson JW, Fredrickson PA, Siong-Chi L: Narcolepsy update. Mayo Clin Proc 65:991–
998, 1990

Roehrs T, Zorick F, Wittig R, et al: Predictors of objective level of daytime sleepiness in patients
with sleep-related breathing disorders. Chest 95:1202–1206, 1989

Ross RI, Ball WA, Sullivan KA, et al: Sleep disturbance as the hallmark of posttraumatic stress
disorder. Am J Psychiatry 146:697–707, 1989

Rush AJ, Erman MK, Giles DE, et al: Polysomnographic findings in recently drug free and
clinically remitted depressed patients. Arch Gen Psychiatry 43:878–884, 1986

Sanford JRA: Tolerance of debility in elderly dependents by supports at home: significance for
hospital practice. BMJ 3:471–473, 1975

Smith M, Colligan M: Health and safety consequences of shift work in the food processing
industry. Ergonomics 25:133–144, 1982

Spielman AJ, Saskin P, Thorpy MJ: Treatment of chronic insomnia by restriction of time in bed.
Sleep 10:45–56, 1987

Sterman MB, Shouse MN: Sleep centers in the brain: the preoptic basal forebrain area revisited,
in Brain Mechanisms of Sleep. Edited by McGinty DJ, Drucker-Colin R, Morrison A, et al.
New York, Raven, 1985, pp 277–299

Tandon R, Shipley JE, Eiser AS, et al: Association between abnormal REM sleep and negative
symptoms in schizophrenia. Psychiatry Res 27:359–361, 1988

Thaker GK, Wagman AM, Kirkpatrick B, et al: Alterations in sleep polygraphy after neuroleptic
withdrawal: a putative supersensitive dopaminergic mechanism. Biol Psychiatry 25:75–86,
1989

Thase ME, Kupfer KJ, Ulrich RF: EEG sleep in psychotic depression: a valid subtype? Arch
Gen Psychiatry 43:886–893, 1986

van Kammen DP, van Kammen WB, Peters J, et al: Decreased slow-wave sleep and enlarged
lateral ventricles in schizophrenia. Neuropsychopharmacology 1:265–271, 1988

Wu JC, Bunney WE: The biological basis of an antidepressant response to sleep deprivation
and relapse: review and hypothesis. Am J Psychiatry 147:14–21, 1990

Zarcone VP: Sleep and schizophrenia, in Sleep Disorders: Diagnosis and Treatment, 2nd Edition. Edited by Williams RL, Karacan I, Moore CA. New York, Wiley, 1988, pp 165–188

Chapter 17

Neuropsychiatric Aspects of Cerebral Vascular Disorders

Sergio E. Starkstein, M.D., Ph.D.
Robert G. Robinson, M.D.

Cerebrovascular disease represents one of the major health problems in the United States, with an estimated annual incidence for thromboembolic stroke between 300,000 and 400,000 (Wolf et al. 1977). During the past 10 years, however, there has been a steady decline in the incidence of stroke, which is presumed to be related to the improved control of hypertension. Nevertheless, stroke remains the third leading cause of mortality and morbidity in the United States.

There are four major categories of cerebrovascular disease: atherosclerotic thrombosis, cerebral embolism, lacunae, and intracranial hemorrhage. Atherosclerotic thrombosis is often the result of a dynamic interaction between hypertension and atherosclerotic deposition of hyaline-lipid material in the walls of peripheral, coronary, and cerebral arteries. These plaques may lead to stenosis of one or more of these cerebral arteries or to complete occlusion.

Cerebral embolism, which accounts for approximately one-third of all strokes, is usually caused by a fragment breaking away from a thrombus within the heart and traveling up the carotid artery. Lacunae, accounting for nearly one-fifth of strokes, are the result of occlusion of small penetrating cerebral arteries. They are infarcts that may be so small as to produce no recognizable deficits, or, depending on their location, they may be associated with pure motor or sensory deficits. Intracranial hemorrhage is the fourth most frequent cause of stroke. The main causes of intracranial hemorrhage that present as acute strokes include intracranial hemorrhage, usually associated with hypertension; rupture of saccular aneurysms or arteriovenous malformations (AVMs); a variety of hemorrhagic disorders of assorted etiology; and trauma producing hemorrhage.

Finally, there are several less common types of cerebrovascular disease. These may lead to intraparenchymal damage, but frequently bleeds on the surface of the

This work was supported in part by the National Institute of Mental Health Grants Research Scientist Award MH00163 (to RGR), MH40355, and NS15080; a grant from the National Alliance for the Research on Schizophrenia and Depression Young Investigator Award (to SES), and a grant from the Institute of Neurological Investigation "Dr. Raul Carrea," Buenos Aires, Argentina (to SES). The authors thank Thomas R. Price, John R. Lipsey, Rajesh Parikh, Kenneth L. Kubos, Krishna Rao, Godfrey D. Pearlson, Lynn Book Starr, and Paula Andrezewski who participated in many of the studies described.

brain (e.g., subdural hematoma) do not produce permanent parenchymal damage.

We have organized this chapter into two sections: the description and classification of clinical psychiatric disorders associated with cerebrovascular disease, and a more in-depth discussion of the syndromes of depression, mania, and anxiety for which the most empirical data are available.

CLINICAL PSYCHIATRIC DISORDERS
ASSOCIATED WITH CEREBROVASCULAR DISEASE

Various emotional disorders have been associated with cerebrovascular disease (Table 17–1). There have been two primary lines of thought in the study of emotional disorders associated with cerebrovascular disease. One attributes emotional disorders to an understandable psychological reaction to the associated impairment; the other, based on a lack of association between severity of impairment and severity of emotional disorder, suggests a direct causal connection between cerebrovascular disease and neuropsychiatric disorder.

Catastrophic Reaction

The catastrophic reaction, as defined by Goldstein (1939) and Gainotti (1972), consists of behavioral observations and verbal expressions of the patient. The symptoms and signs include restlessness, hyperemotionality, sudden burst of tears, irritation or expressions of anger toward the examiner, cursing or other strong utterances, displacement of anxiety or extraneous events, sharp refusal to continue with the examination, objection to the evaluation, and a tendency to perform the test with bragging or anxious expectancy. Catastrophic reactions were reported more frequently among patients with left-hemisphere lesions and aphasia, particularly those with Broca's type (Gainotti 1972).

Indifference Reaction

The indifference reaction consists of apparent indifference toward failures, lack of interest in events, a tendency to joke in an unconcerned way, explicit denial of illness or lack of awareness of physical or mental impairments, and tendency to attribute physical or mental impairments to insignificant causes such as weariness or a lack of concentration. Robinson et al. (1983a) found that this syndrome also included patient self-reports of anxiety, slowness, and worrying. Indifference reactions were more often associated with neglect for the left half of the body in space and right-hemisphere lesions. In a study of 93 patients with single lesions of the right hemisphere (Starkstein et al. 1989), this syndrome was found in 19 patients.

Aprosodias

The aprosodias have been described by Ross and Mesulam (1979) to be abnormalities in the affective components of language, encompassing prosody and emotional gesturing. Prosody can be defined as the "variation of pitch, rhythm, and stress of pronunciation that bestows certain semantic and emotional meaning to speech" (Ross and Mesulam 1979, p. 144).

Prosody can further be divided into four separate categories. Motor aprosody consists of marked difficulty in spontaneous use of emotional inflection in language (e.g., an absence of normal prosodic variations in speech) or emotional gesturing, while comprehension of emotional inflection or gesturing remains intact. This is associated with posterior inferior lesions of the right frontal lobe. Sensory aprosody, on the other hand, is manifested by intact spontaneous emotional inflection in language

Table 17–1. Clinical syndromes associated with cerebrovascular disease

Syndrome	Clinical symptoms	Associated lesion location
Catastrophic reaction	Anxiety reaction, tears, aggressive behavior, swearing, displacement, refusal, renouncement, and compensatory boasting	Left hemisphere
Indifference reaction	Undue cheerfulness or jokes, anosognosia, minimization, loss of interest, and apathy	Right hemisphere
Major depression	Depressed mood, diurnal mood variation, loss of energy, anxiety, restlessness, worry, weight loss, decreased appetite, early morning awakening, delayed sleep onset, social withdrawal, and irritability	Left frontal lobe Left basal ganglia
Minor depression	Depressed mood, anxiety, restlessness, worry, diurnal mood variation, hopelessness, loss of energy, delayed sleep onset, early morning awakening, social withdrawal, weight loss, and decreased appetite	Right or left posterior parietal and occipital regions
Aprosodias		
Motor	Poor expression of emotional prosody and gesturing, good prosodic comprehension and gesturing, and denial of feelings of depression	Right-hemisphere posterior inferior frontal lobe
Sensory	Good expression of emotional prosody and gesturing, poor prosodic comprehension and gesturing, and difficulty empathizing with others	Right-hemisphere posterior inferior parietal lobe and posterior superior temporal lobe
Pathological laughing and crying	Frequent, usually brief laughing and/or crying; crying not caused by sadness or out of proportion to it; and social withdrawal secondary to emotional outbursts	Frequently bilateral hemispheric lesions Can occur with almost any lesion location
Anxiety disorder	Symptoms of major depression, intense worry and anxious foreboding in addition to depression, associated light-headedness or palpitations and muscle tension or restlessness, and difficulty concentrating or falling asleep	Left cortical lesion, usually dorsal lateral frontal lobe
Mania	Elevated mood, increased energy, increased appetite, decreased sleep, feeling of well-being, pressured speech, flight of ideas, grandiose thoughts	Right basotemporal or right orbitofrontal lesions
Bipolar mood disorder	Symptoms of major depression alternating with mania	Right basal ganglia or right thalamic lesions

and gesturing, while the comprehension of emotional inflection or gesturing is markedly impaired. It is associated with lesions of the right temporal parietal lobe (angular gyrus). In a manner analogous to the organization of propositional language in the left hemisphere, both expression and comprehension of emotional inflection and gesturing are impaired in global aprosody. Repetition is impaired in conduction aprosody. Expression is impaired in transcortical motor aprosody, and comprehension is impaired in transcortical sensory aprosody; repetition remains intact in each of these conditions.

Other Emotional or Cognitive Disorders

Less common mental disorders that occur after cerebrovascular disease include generalized anxiety disorder (Starkstein et al. 1990a), organic hallucinosis (Rabins et al. 1991), and paranoid delusional states (Benson 1976). There are also large numbers of cognitive and language (aphasic) disorders associated with cerebral infarcts. Among patients who have suffered several cerebral infarcts over time, at least two syndromes of dementia have been identified: multi-infarct dementia (associated with cortical infarcts) and Binswanger's subcortical encephalopathy (associated with infarcts of the subcortical white matter). (For a more in-depth discussion, see Cummings and Benson 1992.)

SYNDROMES OF DEPRESSION, MANIA, AND ANXIETY

Poststroke Depression

By far, the most common emotional disorder associated with cerebrovascular disease is poststroke depression (PSD), which occurs in between 30% and 50% of patients after acute stroke, generally within the first few months. Approximately half of them show the symptom cluster of major depression; the other half show the symptom cluster of minor depression (Robinson et al. 1983b).

Robinson and colleagues found that more than 50% of patients who met diagnostic criteria for major PSD reported sadness, anxiety, tension, loss of interest and concentration, sleep disturbances with early morning awakening, loss of appetite with weight loss, difficulty concentrating and thinking, and thoughts of death (Lipsey et al. 1986). The researchers concluded that the phenomenology of depressive disorder in stroke patients is virtually identical to that found in patients with functional mood disorders. In addition, Fedoroff et al. (1991) found that the presence of an acute cerebral infarction did not lead to a significant number of incorrectly diagnosed cases of depression.

Robinson and Price (1982) found that almost one-third of 103 patients were depressed at the time of the initial interview. At an 8–9 month follow-up evaluation, 67% of the patients remained depressed; one year later, however, none of the patients seen for follow-up remained depressed. In a second longitudinal study (Robinson et al. 1987), 26% of acute stroke patients had the symptom cluster of major depression and 20% had the symptom cluster of minor depression. In addition, about 30% of patients who were not depressed in-hospital became depressed after discharge. This study found that the natural course of major depression was approximately 1 year, while the duration of minor depression was more prolonged and in many cases fulfilled the 2-year duration requirement for dysthymic disorder.

Two factors have been identified that can influence the natural course of PSD. One is treatment of depression with antidepressant drugs (discussed below); the second is lesion location. Starkstein et al. (1988e) compared depressed patients who had recovered from depression by the 6th month poststroke with another group that remained depressed. The recovered group had a higher frequency of subcortical and cerebellar/brain stem lesions; the nonrecovered group had a significantly higher frequency of cortical lesions. The nonrecovered group had significantly more severe impairments in activities of daily living (ADLs) in-hospital than did the recovered group.

Biological markers.   The dexamethasone suppression test (DST; Carroll et al. 1981) has been investigated as a possible biological marker for functional melancholic depression. Several studies have demonstrated that although there is a statistical association between major PSD and failure to suppress serum cortisol in response to administration of dexamethasone, the specificity of the test is insufficient to allow it to be diagnostically useful (Lipsey et al. 1985; Olsson et al. 1989).

Barry and Dinan (1990) examined growth-hormone response to desipramine as a biological marker of PSD. They found that growth-hormone responses were significantly blunted in patients with PSD, suggesting that diminished α_2-adrenergic receptor function may be an important marker for PSD. Future studies may further examine the validity of the growth-hormone response to desipramine as a marker of PSD.

Relationship to lesion variables.   The location of the lesion along the anterior-posterior dimension is an important variable in the severity of depression following stroke. Robinson et al. (1984) found that major or minor depression occurred in 14 of 22 stroke patients with a left-hemisphere injury, but in only 2 of 14 patients with a right-hemisphere lesion. The intrahemispheric location of the lesion was also an important determinant: depression was more frequent in patients with left anterior (frontal) lesions than with left posterior lesions. Moreover, there was a significant correlation between the distance of the anterior border of the lesion from the frontal pole and severity of depression. Several other studies (Eastwood et al. 1989; Morris et al. 1992; Sinyor et al. 1986b) support the hypothesis that depressive disorders after stroke are more severe the closer the lesion is to the frontal pole and that left frontal lesions are usually the most likely lesions to show this relationship.

Cortical and subcortical lesions.   Evidence suggests that the frequency of depression is higher among patients with left anterior hemisphere lesions than among patients with right-hemisphere lesions. Starkstein et al. (1987b) found that 44% of patients with left cortical lesions were depressed, whereas 39% of patients with left subcortical lesions, 11% of patients with right cortical lesions, and 14% of patients with right subcortical lesions were depressed. Although the frequencies of depression between patients with left cortical versus left subcortical lesions or right cortical versus right subcortical lesions were not significantly different, patients who had lesions in the left hemisphere had significantly higher rates of depression than patients with right-hemisphere lesions, regardless of the cortical or subcortical location of the lesion. Finally, correlations between depression scores and the distance of the lesion from the frontal pole were significant for both patients with left cortical lesions and patients with left subcortical lesions. These relationships were not significant for patients with right-hemisphere lesions. When other confounding factors are removed (e.g., prior lesions and family or personal history of mood disorder) left dorsal lateral frontal cortical and left basal ganglia lesions produce a similar high frequency of major depression that is greater than that for any other lesion location (Starkstein et al. 1988a).

Middle cerebral circulation versus posterior circulation lesions. Starkstein et al. (1988c) compared 37 patients with posterior circulation lesions—including both those with hemispheric lesions (temporo-occipital) and those with cerebellar/brain stem lesions—to 42 patients with middle cerebral artery lesions. Major or minor depression occurred in 48% of the patients in the middle cerebral artery lesion group and in 35% of patients with cerebellar/brain stem lesions. At 6-months follow-up, frequencies of depression among the patients with in-hospital depression were 82% and 20%, respectively. At follow-up 1 to 2 years poststroke, frequencies of depression were 68% and zero, respectively. Thus patients with lesions in the cerebellar/brain stem region had a significantly shorter course of depression. These findings suggest that the mechanism of depression after middle cerebral artery lesions may differ from the mechanism of depression after cerebellar/brain stem lesions. Starkstein et al. (1988c) speculated that the shorter duration of depression after cerebellar/brain stem lesions may be related to their smaller size and to the possibility that the cerebellar/brain stem lesions produce less injury to the biogenic amine pathways that have been proposed to play an important role in the modulation of emotions.

Right-hemisphere lesions. Starkstein et al. (1989) reported that, of 54 patients with positive computed tomography (CT) scans, 6 of 9 patients (66%) with major depression and 5 of 8 patients (63%) with minor depression had lesions that involved the parietal lobe, compared to 9 of 25 patients (36%) without mood changes and 1 of 12 patients (8%) with undue cheerfulness. Finset (1988) found that patients with lesions in the parietal white matter had a higher frequency of depression than patients with lesions in any other location in the right hemisphere.

Premorbid risk factors and depression. Although a significant proportion of patients with left anterior or right posterior lesions develop PSD, not every patient with a lesion in these locations develops a depressive mood. That raises the questions of why clinical variability occurs and why some but not all patients with lesions in these locations develop depression.

Starkstein et al. (1988d) examined these questions by comparing 13 patients with major PSD to 13 stroke patients without depression, who had lesions of the same size and location. Eleven pairs had left-hemisphere lesions, and 2 pairs had right-hemisphere lesions. Damage was cortical in 10 pairs and subcortical in 3 pairs. The groups did not differ on important demographic variables, such as age, sex, socioeconomic status, or education. They also did not differ on family or personal history of psychiatric disorders or neurological deficits. Patients with major PSD, however, had significantly more subcortical atrophy. Because most patients' CT scans were obtained immediately after the stroke, it is likely that the subcortical atrophy preceded the stroke. Thus a mild degree of subcortical atrophy may be a premorbid risk factor that increases the risk of developing major depression following a stroke.

In the previously described study of patients with right-hemisphere lesions, Starkstein et al. (1989) found that patients who developed major depression after a right-hemisphere lesion had a significantly higher frequency of family history of psychiatric disorders than did either nondepressed patients with a right-hemisphere lesion or patients with major depression after left-hemisphere lesions. This suggests that a genetic predisposition for depression may play an important role in the development of major depression after right-hemisphere lesions.

Relationship to physical impairment.   Both Robinson et al. (1983b) and Eastwood et al. (1989) have reported a low but significant correlation between depression and functional physical impairment. There is little evidence to support the idea that physical impairment is a major cause of PSD. However, if depression develops, the patient's physical recovery tends to be retarded. Sinyor et al. (1986a) reported that although nondepressed stroke patients showed a slight increase or no change in functional status over time, depressed patients had significant decreases in function during the first month after the stroke.

Parikh et al. (1990) compared stroke patients with major or minor depression to nondepressed stroke patients during a 2-year period after the stroke. Although both groups had similar impairments in ADLs during the time they were in-hospital, the depressed patients had significantly less improvement by 2-year follow-up. This finding held true after controlling for important variables such as the type and extent of in-hospital and rehabilitation treatment, the size and location of the lesion, the patients' demographic characteristics, the nature of the stroke, the occurrence of another stroke during the follow-up period, and medical history.

PSD and cognitive impairments.   Numerous investigators have reported that elderly patients with functional major depression have intellectual deficits that improve with treatment of depression (Wells 1979). Bolla-Wilson et al. (1989) administered a comprehensive neuropsychological battery and found that patients with major depression and left-hemisphere lesions had significantly greater cognitive impairments than nondepressed patients with comparable left-hemisphere lesions. These cognitive deficits primarily involved tasks of temporal orientation, language, executive motor, and frontal lobe functions. On the other hand, among those with right-hemisphere lesions, patients with major depression did not differ from nondepressed patients on any of the measures of cognitive impairment.

PSD and aphasia.   Patients with left-hemisphere lesions that produce aphasia have a frequency of depression similar to that of patients with left-hemisphere lesions that do not produce aphasia (Robinson and Benson 1981). Although nonfluent aphasia and PSD do not appear to be causally related, they are both produced by lesions of similar anatomical location (anterior areas of the left hemisphere). Thus patients with nonfluent aphasia are at higher risk of developing PSD than patients with other types of aphasia. Although it may be suggested that the higher frequency of depression among nonfluent aphasic patients is related to their greater awareness of their impairment,

Starkstein and Robinson (1988) concluded that lesion location was the important variable in the association between PSD and nonfluent aphasia. In other words, the association between nonfluent aphasia and PSD is explained by the fact that the lesion that is producing nonfluent language may also produce depression.

Mechanism of PSD.   Although the cause of PSD remains unknown, one of the mechanisms that has been hypothesized to play an etiological role is dysfunction of the biogenic amine system. The noradrenergic and serotonergic cell bodies are located in the brain stem and send ascending projections through the median forebrain bundle to the frontal cortex. The ascending axons then arc posteriorly and run longitudinally through the deep layers of the cortex, arborizing and sending terminal projections into the superficial cortical layers (Morrison et al. 1979). Lesions that disrupt these pathways in the frontal cortex or the basal ganglia may affect many downstream fibers. Based on these neuroanatomical facts and the clinical findings that the severity of depression correlates with the proximity of the lesion to the frontal pole, Robinson et al. (1984) suggested that PSD may be the consequence of severe depletions of norepinephrine and/or serotonin produced by frontal or basal ganglia lesions.

In support of this hypothesis, laboratory investigations in rats have demonstrated that the biochemical response to ischemic lesions is lateralized. Right-hemisphere lesions produce depletions of norepinephrine and spontaneous hyperactivity, whereas comparable lesions of the left hemisphere do not (Robinson 1979). A similar lateralized biochemical response to ischemia in human subjects was reported by Mayberg et al. (1988). Patients with stroke lesions in the right hemisphere had significantly higher ratios of ipsilateral-to-contralateral spiperone binding in noninjured temporal and parietal cortex than patients with comparable left-hemisphere strokes. Patients with left-hemisphere lesions, on the other hand, showed a significant inverse correlation between the amount of spiperone binding in the left temporal cortex and depression scores (i.e., higher depression scores were associated with lower serotonin receptor binding).

Thus a greater depletion of biogenic amines in patients with right-hemisphere lesions as compared with those with left-hemisphere lesions could lead to a compensatory upregulation of receptors that might protect against depression. On the other hand, patients with left-hemisphere lesions may have moderate depletions of biogenic amines but without a compensatory upregulation of 5-HT receptors and, therefore, a dysfunction of biogenic amine systems in the left hemisphere. This dysfunction ultimately may lead to the clinical manifestations of depression.

Treatment of PSD.   In a study of the efficacy of antidepressant treatment of PSD, Lipsey et al. (1984) found that patients treated with nortriptyline showed significantly greater improvement in their scores on the Hamilton Rating Scale for Depression (Hamilton 1960) than did placebo-treated patients. Successfully treated patients had serum nortriptyline levels between 50 and 150 ng/ml. Three patients experienced side effects (including delirium, confusion, drowsiness, and agitation) that were severe enough to require the discontinuation of nortriptyline.

Electroconvulsive therapy (ECT) has also been reported to be effective for treating PSD (Murray et al. 1987). It causes few side effects and no neurological deterioration. Finally, psychological treatment, including group and family therapy, has also been reported to be useful (Oradei and Waite 1974; Watziawick and Coyne 1980). However, controlled studies for these treatment modalities have not been conducted.

Rehabilitation in PSD. Psychosocial adjustment after stroke is an important issue to consider. Thompson et al. (1989) examined 40 stroke patients as well as their caregivers an average of 9 months poststroke. They found that a lack of meaningfulness in life and overprotection by the caregiver were independent predictors of depression. They also found that psychosocial factors could predict depression and motivation in stroke patients and suggested that both cognitive adaptation and social support theories may be useful approaches to understand people's ability to cope after a stroke.

Poststroke Anxiety

Studies of patients with functional (i.e., no known neuropathology) depression have demonstrated that it is important to distinguish depression associated with significant anxiety symptoms (i.e., agitated depressions) from depression without these symptoms (i.e., retarded depressions) because their cause and course may be different (Stravakaki and Vargo 1986).

Starkstein et al. (1990a) found that, of 98 patients with first episode acute stroke lesions, only 6 met the criteria for generalized anxiety disorder in the absence of any other mood disorder. On the other hand, 23 out of 47 patients with major depression also met the criteria for generalized anxiety disorder. Patients were then divided into those with anxiety only, anxiety and depression, depression only, and no mood disorder. No significant between-group differences were found in neurological examination. Examination of patients with positive CT scans revealed that anxious-depressed patients had a significantly higher frequency of cortical lesions (16 of 19) than did either the depression only group (7 of 15) or the control group (13 of 27). On the other hand, the depression only group showed a significantly higher frequency of subcortical lesions compared with the anxious-depressed group.

Subcortical lesions have frequently been associated with abulia, apathy, and indifference (Graff-Radford et al. 1984). On the other hand, lesions of the left frontal cortex have been reported to produce severe anxiety reactions (Gainotti 1972). Moreover, Gur et al. (1987) showed a linear decrease in cortical metabolic rate (i.e., lower cortical metabolism) with increased anxiety. Thus these findings as well as the findings in poststroke anxiety suggest that the integrity of subcortical structures may be necessary for the generation and/or expression of anxious features in depressed patients with cortical lesions and that abulia and apathy are the clinical outcome when the basal ganglia structures are damaged (Starkstein et al. 1990a).

Poststroke Mania

Although mania occurs less frequently than depression, a manic syndrome may be precipitated by brain injury. Starkstein et al. (1988a) compared patients who met DSM-III criteria (American Psychiatric Association 1980) for an organic affective syndrome, manic type, and who developed mania after a stroke, traumatic brain injury, or tumors, with patients with functional (i.e., no known neuropathology) mania. Both groups of patients showed similar frequencies of elation, pressured speech, flight of ideas, grandiose thoughts, insomnia, hallucinations, and paranoid delusions. Thus the symptoms of mania that occur after brain damage (secondary mania) appear to be the same as those found in mania without brain damage (primary mania).

Lesion location.   Several studies (Robinson et al. 1988; Starkstein et al. 1990b) of patients with brain damage have found that patients who develop secondary mania have a significantly greater frequency of lesions in the right hemisphere than patients with depression or no mood disturbance. The right-hemisphere lesions that lead to mania tend to be in specific right-hemisphere structures that have connections to the limbic system. The right basotemporal cortex appears to be particularly important because direct lesions as well as distant hypometabolic effects (diaschisis) of this cortical region are frequently associated with secondary mania.

Risk factors.   The relatively rare occurrence of mania after stroke suggests that there are premorbid risk factors that impact on the expression of this disorder. Studies thus far have identified two such factors. One is a genetic vulnerability for affective disorder (Robinson et al. 1988); the other is a mild degree of subcortical atrophy. Starkstein et al. (1987a) compared patients with secondary mania to patients with no mood disturbance who were matched for size, location, and etiology of brain lesion. The groups were also compared with patients with primary mania and control subjects. No significant between-group differences were found either in demographic variables or neurological evaluation. Patients with secondary mania, however, had significantly greater degree of subcortical atrophy, as measured by the bifrontal and the third ventricular to brain ratio. Moreover, of the patients who developed secondary mania, those who had a positive family history of psychiatric disorders had significantly less atrophy than those without such a family history, suggesting that genetic predisposition to affective disorders and brain atrophy may be independent risk factors.

Mechanism of secondary mania.   Although the mechanism of secondary mania remains unknown, both lesion studies and metabolic studies suggest that the right basotemporal cortex may play an important role. A combination of biogenic amine system dysfunction and release of tonic inhibitory input into the basotemporal cortex and lateral limbic system may lead to the production of mania.

Several studies have demonstrated that the amygdala (located in the limbic portion of the temporal lobe) has an important role in the production of instinctive reactions and the association between stimulus and emotional response (Gloor 1986). The amygdala receives its main afferents from the basal diencephalon (which in turn receives psychosensory and psychomotor information from the reticular formation) and the temporopolar and basolateral cortices (which receive main afferents from heteromodal association areas) (Beck 1949; Crosby et al. 1962). The basotemporal cortex receives afferents from association cortical areas and the orbitofrontal cortex and sends efferent projections to the entorhinal cortex, hippocampus, and amygdala. By virtue of these connections, the basotemporal cortex may represent a cortical link between sensory afferents and instinctive reactions (Goldar and Outes 1972).

The orbitofrontal cortex may be subdivided into two regions: a posterior one, which is restricted to limbic functions and should be considered part of the limbic system, and an anterior one, which exerts a tonic inhibitory control over the amygdala by means of its connection through the uncinate fasciculus with the basotemporal cortex (Nauta 1971). Thus the uncinate fasciculus and the basotemporal cortex may mediate connections between psychomotor and volitional processes generated in the frontal lobe and vital processes and instinctive behaviors generated in the amygdala (Starkstein and Robinson 1992).

It may be hypothesized that, through orbito-temporo-amygdala connections, cognitive functions may influence limbic activity. Thus a lesion in the orbitofrontal cortex, uncinate fasciculus, or basotemporal cortex may release the tonic inhibition exerted by the frontal lobe on the amygdala, which in turn results in emotional disinhibition. The loss of frontolimbic connections may release emotions from intellectual control, and this dissociation results in the cluster of symptoms we identify as secondary mania (Goldar and Outes 1972).

As discussed above, most of the patients with secondary mania have lesions of the right hemisphere. In a rat model of focal brain injury, Starkstein et al. (1988b) found that right, but not left frontolateral cortical lesions produced locomotor hyperactivity as well as bilateral increases in dopaminergic turnover in the nucleus accumbens. Thus it is possible that in the presence of specific risk factors for secondary mania (e.g., subcortical atrophy) increases in biogenic amine turnover produced by right- but not left-hemisphere lesions may play an important role in the production of secondary mania. This biogenic amine dysfunction may also be most pronounced in the basotemporal cortex, which is one of the cortical regions with the highest concentration of serotonergic terminals from the raphe nuclei.

Treatment of secondary mania.   Although no systematic treatment studies of secondary mania have been conducted, Bakchine et al. (1989) suggested several potentially useful treatment modalities. In a single patient with secondary mania, clonidine (600 μg/day) rapidly reversed the manic symptoms, whereas carbamazepine (1200 mg/day) was associated with no mood changes, and levodopa (375 mg/day) was associated with an increase in manic symptoms. Other treatment modalities, such as anticonvulsants (valproate and carbamazepine), neuroleptics, and lithium therapy, have been reported to be useful in treating secondary mania (Starkstein et al. 1988a).

Poststroke Bipolar Disorder

Although some patients have one or more manic episodes after brain injury, other manic patients also have depression after brain injury. In an effort to examine which factors are crucial in determining which patients have bipolar as compared with unipolar disorder, Starkstein et al. (1991) examined 19 patients with the diagnosis of secondary mania. The bipolar (manic-depressive) group consisted of patients who, after the brain lesion, met the DSM-III-R criteria (American Psychiatric Association 1987) for organic mood syndrome, manic, followed or preceded by organic mood syndrome, depressed. The unipolar mania (mania only) group consisted of patients who met the criteria for mania described above, not followed or preceded by depression.

No significant between-group differences were observed in the type or frequency of manic symptoms. The bipolar group, however, showed significantly greater intellectual impairment as measured by Mini-Mental State Exam (MMSE; Folstein et al.

1975) scores. Almost half of the bipolar patients had recurrent episodes of depression, whereas recurrent episodes of mania occurred in approximately one-fourth of patients in both the unipolar and bipolar groups.

Six of the seven bipolar patients had subcortical lesions, and one had a cortical-subcortical lesion. On the other hand, nine of the unipolar patients had cortical lesions, one had a cortical lesion with subcortical extension, and two had subcortical lesions. Patients with unipolar mania also had significantly larger lesion volumes than the patients in the bipolar group.

Subcortical lesions may play a role in the mechanism that causes bipolar disease. Subcortical lesions have been reported to produce hypometabolic effects in widespread regions including contralateral brain areas (i.e., crossed-hemisphere and crossed-cerebellar diaschisis) (Pappata et al. 1987). Thus it is possible that subcortical lesions may have induced metabolic changes in left frontocortical regions, which are associated with depression. Mania may develop at a later stage, when these metabolic changes become restricted to the orbitofrontal and/ or basotemporal cortices of the right hemisphere.

CONCLUSIONS

Depression occurs in about 40% of patients with acute stroke lesions, and its natural evolution is from 1 to 2 years, although patients with subcortical or brain stem lesions may show shorter duration depressions. Both intrahemispheric and interhemispheric lesion location appear to contribute to the development of depression. Major depression is significantly more frequent among patients with left-hemisphere lesions involving anterior cortical (frontal) or subcortical (basal ganglia) regions than any other lesion location. On the other hand, depressions following right-hemisphere lesions are usually associated with a genetic vulnerability and frontal and parietal lobe damage. Finally, an important risk factor for the development of PSD is the presence of subcortical atrophy before the stroke lesion.

Generalized anxiety disorder in the absence of other psychiatric problems is a rare complication of stroke lesions and is frequently associated with a prior history of alcohol abuse. On the other hand, almost 50% of patients with major PSD also meet DSM-III criteria for generalized anxiety disorder. Patients with both major depression and generalized anxiety disorder tend to have cortical lesions, whereas patients with major PSD without anxiety tend to have subcortical lesions.

Mania that develops after brain injury has a phenomenology similar to that of mania without known neuropathology. Secondary mania, however, is almost always the consequence of lesions in the right hemisphere, involving cortical (orbitofrontal or basotemporal) or subcortical (head of the caudate or thalamus) limbic-related regions. Among these areas, dysfunction of the basotemporal cortex seems to be particularly important to the development of secondary mania, and basotemporal dysfunction may be produced by direct or indirect (diaschisis) damage.

REFERENCES

American Psychiatric Association: Diagnostic and Statistical Manual of Mental Disorders, 3rd Edition. Washington, DC, American Psychiatric Association, 1980

American Psychiatric Association: Diagnostic and Statistical Manual of Mental Disorders, 3rd Edition, Revised. Washington, DC, American Psychiatric Association, 1987

Bakchine S, Lacomblez L, Benoit N, et al: Manic-like state after orbitofrontal and right temporoparietal injury: efficacy of clonidine. Neurology 39:777–781, 1989

Barry S, Dinan TG: Alpha-2 adrenergic receptor function in post-stroke depression. Psychol Med 20:305–309, 1990

Beck E: A cytoarchitectural investigation into the boundaries of cortical areas 13 and 14 in the human brain. J Anatomy 83:145–157, 1949

Benson DF: Psychiatric aspects of aphasia. Br J Psychiatry 123:555–566, 1976

Bolla-Wilson K, Robinson RG, Starkstein SE, et al: Lateralization of dementia of depression in stroke patients. Am J Psychiatry 146:627–634, 1989

Carroll BJ, Feinberg M, Gredent JF: A specific laboratory test for the diagnosis of melancholia: standardization, validation and clinical utility. Arch Gen Psychiatry 38:15–22, 1981

Crosby E, Humphrey T, Lauer E: Correlative Anatomy of the Nervous System. New York, Macmillan, 1962

Cummings JL, Benson DF: Dementia: A Clinical Approach, 2nd Edition. Stoneham, MA, Butterworth-Heineman, 1992

Eastwood MR, Rifat SL, Nobbs H, et al: Mood disorder following cerebrovascular accident. Br J Psychiatry 154:195–200, 1989

Fedoroff UP, Starkstein SE, Parikh RM, et al: Are depressive symptoms non-specific in patients with acute stroke? Am J Psychiatry 148:1172–1176, 1991

Finset A: Depressed mood and reduced emotionality after right hemisphere brain damage, in Cerebral Hemisphere Function in Depression. Edited by Kinsbourne M. Washington, DC, American Psychiatric Press, 1988, pp 49–64

Folstein MF, Folstein SE, McHugh PR: "Mini-Mental State": a practical method for grading the cognitive state of patients for the clinician. J Psychitr Res 12:189–198, 1975

Gainotti G: Emotional behavior and hemispheric side of the brain. Cortex 8:41–55, 1972

Gloor P: Role of the human limbic system in perception, memory and affect: lessons for temporal lobe epilepsy, in The Limbic System: Functional Organization and Clinical Disorders. Edited by Doane BK, Livingstone KE. New York, Raven, 1986, pp 159–169

Goldar JC, Outes DL: Fisiopatologia de la desinhibicion instintiva. Acta Psiquiatrica y Psicologica de America Latina 18:177–185, 1972

Goldstein K: The Organism: A Holistic Approach to Biology Derived from Pathological Data in Man. New York, American Books, 1939

Graff-Radford NR, Eslinger PJ, Damasio AR: Nonhemorrhagic infarction of the thalamus: behavioral, anatomic and physiologic correlates. Neurology 34:14–23, 1984

Gur RC, Gur RE, Resnick SM, et al: The effect of anxiety on cortical cerebral blood flow and metabolism. J Cereb Blood Flow Metab 7:173–177, 1987

Hamilton M: Rating depressive patients. J Clin Psychiatry 41:21–24, 1960

Lipsey JR, Robinson RG, Pearlson GD, et al: Nortriptyline treatment for post-stroke depression: a double-blind trial. Lancet 1:297–300, 1984

Lipsey JR, Robinson RG, Pearlson GD: Dexamethasone suppression test and mood following strokes. Am J Psychiatry 142:318–323, 1985

Lipsey JR, Spencer WC, Rabins PV, et al: Phenomenological comparison of poststroke depression and functional depression. Am J Psychiatry 143:527–529, 1986

Mayberg HS, Robinson RG, Wong DF, et al: PET imaging of cortical S_2, serotonin receptors after stroke: lateralized changes and relationship to depression. Am J Psychiatry 145:937–943, 1988

Morris PLP, Robinson RG, Raphael B: Lesion characteristics and post-stroke depression: evidence of a specific relationship in the left hemisphere. Neuropsychiatry, Neuropsychology and Behavioral Neurology 5:75–82, 1992

Morrison JH, Molliver ME, Grzanna R: Noradrenergic innervation of the cerebral cortex: widespread effects of local cortical lesions. Science 205:313–316, 1979

Murray GB, Shea V, Conn DK: Electroconvulsive therapy for poststroke depression. J Clin Psychiatry 47:258–260, 1987

Nauta WJH: The problem of the frontal lobe: a reinterpretation. Journal of Psychological Research 8:167–187, 1971

Olsson T, Astrom M, Eriksson S: Hypercortisolism revealed by the dexamethasone suppression test with acute ischemic stroke. Stroke 20:1685–1690, 1989

Oradei DM, Waite NS: Group psychotherapy with stroke patients during the immediate recovery phase. Am J Orthopsychiatry 44:386–395, 1974

Pappata S, Dinh ST, Baron JC, et al: Remote metabolic effects of cerebrovascular lesions: magnetic resonance and positron tomography imaging. Neuroradiol 29:1–6, 1987

Parikh RM, Robinson RG, Lipsey JR, et al: The impact of poststroke depression on recovery in activities of daily living over a 2-year follow-up. Arch Neurol 47:785–789, 1990

Rabins PV, Starkstein SE, Robinson RG: Risk factors for developing atypical (schizophreniform) psychosis following stroke. Journal of Neuropsychiatry and Clinical Neurosciences 3:6–9, 1991

Robinson RG: Differential behavioral and biochemical effects of right and left hemispheric cerebral infarction in the rat. Science 205:707–710, 1979

Robinson RG, Benson DF: Depression in aphasic patients: frequency, severity and clinical pathological correlations. Brain Lang 14:282–291, 1981

Robinson RG, Price TR: Poststroke depressive disorders: a follow-up study of 103 patients. Stroke 13:635–641, 1982

Robinson RG, Kubos KL, Starr LB, et al: Mood changes in stroke patients: relationship to lesion location. Compr Psychiatry 24:555–566, 1983a

Robinson RG, Starr LB, Kubos KL, et al: A two-year longitudinal study of poststroke mood disorders: findings during the initial evaluation. Stroke 14:736–741, 1983b

Robinson RG, Kubos KL, Starr LB, et al: Mood disorders in stroke patients: importance of lesion location. Brain 107:81–93, 1984

Robinson RG, Bolduc PL, Price TR: Two-year longitudinal study of post-stroke mood disorders: diagnosis and outcome at one and two years. Stroke 18:837–843, 1987

Robinson RG, Boston JD, Starkstein SE: Comparison of mania with depression following brain injury causal factors. Am J Psychiatry 145:172–178, 1988

Ross ED, Mesulam MM: Dominant language functions of the right hemisphere: prosody and emotional gesturing. Arch Neurol 36:144–148, 1979

Sinyor D, Amato P, Kaloupek P: Poststroke depression: relationship to functional impairment, coping strategies, and rehabilitation outcome. Stroke 17:1102–1107, 1986a

Sinyor D, Jacques P, Kaloupek DG: Post-stroke depression and lesion location: an attempted replication. Brain 109:537–546, 1986b

Starkstein SE, Robinson RG: Aphasia and depression. Aphasiology 2:1–20, 1988

Starkstein SE, Robinson RG: The role of the frontal lobes in affective disorder following stroke, in Frontal Lobe Function and Injury. Edited by Levin HS, Eisenberg HM. Oxford, England, Oxford University Press, 1992, pp 288–303

Starkstein SE, Pearlson GD, Boston JD, et al: Mania after brain injury: a controlled study of causative factors. Arch Neurol 44:1069–1073, 1987a

Starkstein SE, Robinson RG, Price TR: Comparison of cortical and subcortical lesions in the production of post-stroke mood disorders. Brain 110:1045–1059, 1987b

Starkstein JE, Boston JD, Robinson RG: Mechanisms of mania after brain injury: 12 case reports and review of the literature. J Nerv Ment Dis 176:87–100, 1988a

Starkstein SE, Moran TH, Bowersox JA, et al: Behavioral abnormalities induced by frontal cortical and nucleus accumbens lesions. Brain Res 473:74–80, 1988b

Starkstein SE, Robinson RG, Berthier ML, et al: Depressive disorders following posterior circulation compared with middle cerebral artery infarcts. Brain 111:375–387, 1988c

Starkstein SE, Robinson RG, Price TR: Comparison of patients with and without post-stroke major depression matched for size and location of lesion. Arch Gen Psychiatry 45:247–252, 1988d

Starkstein SE, Robinson RG, Price TR: Comparison of spontaneously recovered versus non-recovered patients with poststroke depression. Stroke 19:1491–1496, 1988e

Starkstein SE, Robinson RG, Honig MA, et al: Mood changes after right-hemisphere lesions. Br J Psychiatry 155:79–85, 1989

Starkstein SE, Cohen BS, Fedoroff P, et al: Relationship between anxiety disorders and depressive disorders in patients with cerebrovascular injury. Arch Gen Psychiatry 47:246–251, 1990a

Starkstein SE, Mayberg HS, Berthier ML, et al: Mania after brain injury: neuroradiological and metabolic findings. Ann Neurol 27:652–659, 1990b

Starkstein SE, Fedoroff P, Berthier ML, et al: Manic-depressive and pure manic states after brain lesions. Biol Psychiatry, 29:149–158, 1991

Stravakaki C, Vargo B: The relationship of anxiety and depression: a review of the literature. Br J Psychiatry 149:7–16, 1986

Thompson SC, Sobolew-Shobin A, Graham MA, et al: Psychosocial adjustment following a stroke. Soc Sci Med 28:239–247, 1989

Watziawick P, Coyne JC: Depression following stroke: brief, problem-focused family treatment. Family Treatment 19:13–18, 1980

Wells CE: Pseudodementia. Am J Psychiatry 136:895–900, 1979

Wolf PA, Dawber TR, Thomas HE, et al: Epidemiology of stroke, in Advances in Neurology, Vol 16. Edited by Thompson RA, Green JR. New York, Raven, 1977, pp 5–19

Chapter 18

Neuropsychiatric Aspects of Brain Tumors

Trevor R. P. Price, M.D.
Kenneth L. Goetz, M.D.
Mark R. Lovell, Ph.D.

With an annual incidence of 30 per 100,000 and a point prevalence of 80 per 100,000 people, brain tumors account for an estimated 10% of all neoplasms and 2% of cancer-related deaths (Kurtzke 1984). Eighty percent of brain tumors in adults are primary and 20% are metastatic, with the reverse being the case in children. Seventy percent are supratentorial, whereas 30% are infratentorial with distribution by lobe as indicated in Figure 18–1. This distribution is influenced to some degree by tumor histology (Figure 18–2). Gliomas and meningiomas are the most common histological types of primary brain tumors; the most common metastatic lesions are from lung and breast primaries. A substantial proportion of central nervous system (CNS) tumors are associated with psychiatric symptomatology and/or neuropsychological deficits.

Large-scale studies carefully examining correlations between clinical phenomenology and various tumor parameters have not as yet been done. Thus our knowledge of the neuropsychiatric and neuropsychological aspects of brain tumors is based on a relatively small number of clinical case reports and larger, uncontrolled case series from the older neurological and neurosurgical literature.

FREQUENCY OF NEUROPSYCHIATRIC SYMPTOMS IN PATIENTS WITH BRAIN TUMORS

Keschner et al. (1938) noted psychiatric symptoms in 78% of their 530 cases, and Schlesinger (1950) found behavioral changes in 51% of his series of 591 patients with brain tumors. Although complex neuropsychiatric symptoms may occur in conjunction with focal neurological signs and symptoms, frequently they may be the first clinical indication of a tumor.

Minski (1933) studied patients with cerebral tumors and reported that the psychiatric symptomatology of 25 of these patients simulated "functional psychoses." Nineteen of these patients attributed the onset of their behavioral symptoms to various

The authors wish to acknowledge the assistance of Olga Petruska in the preparation of this manuscript.

361

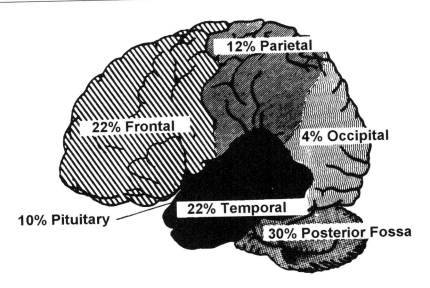

Figure 18–1. Relative frequency of intracranial brain tumors according to location in the adult.
Source. Reprinted from Lohr JB, Cadet JL: "Neuropsychiatric Aspects of Brain Tumors," in *American Psychiatric Press Textbook of Neuropsychiatry.* Washington, DC, American Psychiatric Press, 1987, p. 355. Used with permission.

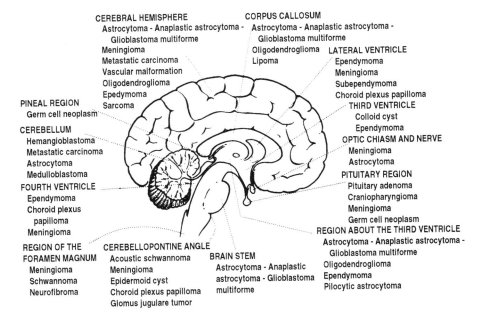

Figure 18–2. Topographic distribution of intracranial tumors in the adult.
Source. Reprinted from Burger PC, Scheithauer BW, Vogel FS: *Surgical Pathology of the Nervous System and Its Coverings,* 3rd Edition. New York, Churchill Livingstone, 1991, p. 195. Copyright 1991 by Churchill Livingstone. Used with permission.

sources of stress, underscoring the difficulty clinicians face in making accurate early diagnoses. Fortunately, the risk of an occult neoplasm presenting with purely psychiatric complaints is low. One survey found that only 34 of approximately 17,000 patients had been diagnosed as having "psychosis due to brain tumor" (Remington and Robert 1962). Ten of those 34 patients were known to have had tumors on admission; the other 24 were initially hospitalized for psychiatric complaints.

Selecki (1965) summarized autopsy data of institutionalized psychiatric patients (among whom the incidence of brain tumors ranged from 1% to 13.5%) and noted that, on average, 55% of brain tumors went unrecognized before the patient's death. Klotz (1957) found that 2.1% of 44,000 psychiatric patients had brain tumors on autopsy, 45% of which had been unrecognized before death. These high rates of undiagnosed tumors, and the fact that the prevalence of brain tumors is higher than among the general population, means that mental health professionals must be keenly aware of the neuropsychiatric manifestations of brain tumors.

GENERAL NEUROPSYCHIATRIC AND NEUROPSYCHOLOGICAL CONSIDERATIONS

General Neuropsychiatric Considerations

CNS tumors can present with behavioral symptoms identical to those of the major psychiatric disorders. Although clinicians and researchers have sought a predictable relationship between tumor location and psychiatric symptoms, this association does not appear to be strong. Studies evaluating psychiatric symptoms in patients with brain tumors (Keschner et al. 1938; Selecki 1965) concluded that behavioral changes did not have localizing value, and that no mental symptoms were indicative of lesions involving specific areas of the brain.

The factors that most significantly influence symptom formation appear to include the extent of tumor involvement, the rapidity of its growth, and its propensity to cause increased intracranial pressure (ICP). Additionally, the patient's premorbid psychiatric history, level of functioning, and characteristic psychological defense mechanisms may play a significant contributing role in determining the nature of the particular symptoms the patient manifests.

In a study of patients who developed mania after a variety of brain lesions, Starkstein et al. (1988) concluded that the unifying aspect was the interconnection of the involved structures with the orbitofrontal cortex. Increased ICP is a consequence of CNS tumors and has been implicated in behavioral changes such as apathy, depression, irritability, agitation, and changes in consciousness. Allen (1930) concluded that the majority of mental changes were due to increases in ICP rather than to focal effects of the tumors themselves.

Another factor is the patient's premorbid level of functioning. Tumors frequently cause an exaggeration of the individual's previous predominant character traits and coping styles. Once a brain tumor has been discovered, the behavioral changes may represent a combination of premorbid psychiatric status, tumor-associated organic mental symptoms, and adaptive psychological responses to the stress associated with diagnosis. In addition, rapidly growing tumors are commonly associated with severe, acute psychiatric symptoms, while slow-growing tumors are more likely to present with vague personality changes, apathy, or depression, without cognitive changes. Multiple tumor foci produce behavioral symptoms with greater frequency.

The relationship between tumor type and neuropsychiatric symptoms is unclear. Several large studies (e.g., Keschner et al. 1938) have noted no association between histological type of tumor and behavioral symptoms. Lishman (1978), however, found that gliomas may be more likely than benign tumors to produce behavioral changes, either because of the rapidity of growth or the multiplicity of tumor sites. Patton and Sheppard (1956), on the other hand, noted a greater incidence of meningiomas among psychiatric patients. Because of their location and slow growth, meningiomas may produce few focal signs and less obvious symptomatology, tend to be neurologically silent, and therefore are associated with an increased likelihood that the patient will first present to a psychiatrist.

Although lesion location does not appear to play an important role in determining the occurrence of specific types of neuropsychiatric symptoms, some research has suggested that brain lesions in certain locations may be associated with an increased frequency of certain kinds of psychiatric symptoms. For example, although Keschner et al. (1936) noted no difference in the types of symptoms found in association with frontal and temporal lobe tumors, they did find that complex visual and auditory hallucinations were more common among patients with temporal lobe tumors and "facetiousness" was more frequently found among those with frontal lobe tumors. Mental changes were twice as likely to occur among patients with supratentorial as compared with infratentorial lesions (Keschner et al. 1938). Likewise, mental changes tended to be early symptoms in 18% of the patients with supratentorial tumors but in only 5% of those with infratentorial tumors.

Psychotic symptoms tend to occur more commonly in patients with tumors of the temporal lobes and pituitary gland and less commonly in those with occipital and cerebellar tumors. Bilateral tumors and those with multifocal involvement appear to be frequently associated with neuropsychiatric symptoms.

General Neuropsychological Considerations

Brain tumors can have a wide range of effects on cognitive functioning, and patients with brain tumors rarely present with a circumscribed cognitive deficit in one area without more diffuse dysfunction elsewhere (Lezak 1983). The nature and severity of neuropsychological dysfunctions that accompany tumors are determined by several factors (Bigler 1984).

The histological type of tumor and rate of growth may affect the expression of symptoms. A rapidly growing tumor is likely to result in obvious cognitive dysfunction, whereas patients with slower-growing tumors may demonstrate subtle personality changes but no obvious cognitive changes or focal neurological deficits. This may be due to the individual's ability to compensate better for less severe, more gradually developing cognitive deficits (Golden 1983). With slower-growing tumors, the degree to which cognitive deficits will be clinically apparent is affected by the individual's premorbid level of intelligence. Thus patients with higher IQs tend to have a broader range of coping and adaptive skills, which allows them to compensate for and conceal emerging cognitive impairment. Younger patients are likely to manifest less striking cognitive and behavioral deficits than are older patients (Bigler 1984).

The size of the tumor is likely to have a significant impact on the expression of cognitive dysfunction. Larger tumors give rise to more clinically apparent, focal cognitive abnormalities directly reflecting the anatomical location of the lesion and more diffuse, nonspecific manifestations secondary to cerebral edema, compression of adjacent brain tissue, or elevation of ICP.

Other factors may result in cognitive deficits that do not reflect the anatomic location of the tumor. According to Lezak (1983), several types of "distance effects" may be important in determining the types of deficits found on neuropsychological testing. *Diaschisis* refers to the depression of neural activity in a functionally related but distant region of the brain. *Disconnection* of a region of the brain from a more distant region by a structural lesion can also affect the cognitive expression of the symptom, as has been dramatically demonstrated in patients who have undergone surgical sectioning of the corpus callosum as a treatment for intractable seizures (Sperry 1974). Although, as stressed above, the cognitive sequelae of tumors may not reflect the site of the tumor, the cognitive deficit demonstrated may have some localizing value.

Laterality of Brain Tumors and Clinical Manifestations

Although many older, larger studies reported no consistent differences in the psychiatric and behavioral symptoms associated with left- and right-sided tumors, Flor-Henry (1969) proposed that schizophrenia-like psychoses are more common with left-hemisphere lesions, and affective psychoses with right-hemisphere lesions. More recent work with unilateral frontal tumors (Belyi 1987) suggests that left frontal tumors are more commonly associated with akinesia and depression, whereas right frontal tumors often present with euphoria and denial. Studies reviewing cases of mania secondary to CNS lesions, including tumors, have found a preponderance of right-hemisphere lesions (Cummings and Mendez 1984; Starkstein et al. 1988). This research suggests that lesion laterality may have a larger impact on symptom formation than previously thought. It also implies a need to reevaluate tumor location and its implications for neuropsychiatric and neuropsychological symptomatology and provides a theoretical framework from which to begin to study the psychopathology associated with brain tumors.

NEUROPSYCHIATRIC AND NEUROPSYCHOLOGICAL SYMPTOMATOLOGY AND BRAIN TUMOR LOCATION

Frontal Lobe Tumors

Tumors of the frontal lobe are frequently associated with neuropsychiatric symptoms, with some studies reporting mental changes in as many as 90% of cases (Strauss and Keschner 1935). In the study by Strauss and Keschner (1935), 43% of 85 patients with frontal lobe tumors manifested behavioral changes early in the course of their illnesses. This is not surprising considering the higher level "executive" and cognitive functions carried out by this region of cortex.

Injuries to the frontal lobes have been associated with three different clinical syndromes (Cummings 1985) (Table 18–1). Most patients with frontal lobe tumors present with a mixture of symptoms. This is because frontal tumors are rarely confined to a single subregion of the frontal lobes and may have effects on other areas through pressure effects and edema, as well as diaschisis and disconnection.

The orbitofrontal syndrome is characterized by behavioral disinhibition with emotional lability, irritability, and socially inappropriate behavior. Cognitively, patients with this syndrome often demonstrate poor judgment and a lack of insight into their behavior. These patients have been referred to as *pseudopsychopathic* (McAllister and Price 1987).

Patients with injuries to the frontal convexities, the so-called convexity syndrome, often present with apathy, indifference, and psychomotor retardation. Cognitively, such patients demonstrate difficulty initiating or persisting in behavioral activities, have problems with sustained attention and/or sequencing, or may demonstrate perseverative behavior (Goldberg 1986). These latter deficits usually become obvious on more specific tests of executive functioning, such as the Wisconsin Card Sorting Test (Goldberg 1986). This syndrome has been referred to as the *pseudodepressed* state (McAllister and Price 1987). Finally, patients with a medial frontal syndrome are predominantly akinetic, with frequent mutism and failure to respond to commands.

Affective symptoms are common in patients with frontal lobe tumors and include depression, irritability, apathy, and euphoria. Frequently psychomotor retardation, with aspontaneity, hypokinesia or akinesia, or inertia is present. In one study of 25 patients with frontal lobe tumors (Direkze et al. 1971), 20% presented to psychiatric units with mood disturbances. Strauss and Keschner (1935) reported affective disturbances in 63% of 85 patients, 30% with euphoria and 4% with hypomania. Although these authors found no correlation between clinical presentation and lesion laterality, Belyi (1987) noted a tendency for right frontal lesions to present with euphoria and left frontal lesions to present with akinesia, abulia, and depressed affect.

Table 18–1.   Clinical characteristics of the three principal frontal lobe syndromes

Orbitofrontal syndrome (disinhibited)	Motor programming deficits
Disinhibited, impulsive behavior (pseudopsychopathic)	Three-step hand sequence
	Alternating programs
Inappropriate jocular affect and euphoria	Reciprocal programs
Emotional lability	Rhythm tapping
Poor judgment and insight	Multiple loops
Distractibility	Poor word-list generation
Frontal convexity syndrome (apathetic)	Poor abstraction and categorization
	Segmented approach to visuospatial analysis
Apathetic (pseudodepressed)	**Medial frontal syndrome (akinetic)**
Occasional brief angry or aggressive outbursts common	Paucity of spontaneous movement and gesture
Indifference	Sparse verbal output (repetition may be preserved)
Psychomotor retardation	
Motor perseveration and impersistence	Lower extremity weakness and loss of sensation
Loss of set	
Stimulus boundedness	Incontinence
Discrepant motor and verbal behavior	

Source.   Reprinted from Cummings JL: *Clinical Neuropsychiatry.* Orlando, FL, Grune & Stratton, 1985, p. 58. Used with permission of Allyn and Bacon.

Changes in personality have been found in 70% of patients with frontal lobe tumors (Strauss and Keschner 1935). They include irresponsibility, childishness, facetiousness, disinhibition, and indifference toward others, as well as inappropriate sexual behavior. Although these behaviors are consistent with the orbitofrontal syndrome, similar "frontal lobe" personality changes have been described in patients with both temporal lobe and diencephalic lesions.

Psychotic symptoms also may occur in patients with frontal lobe tumors (Strauss and Keschner 1935). Reported psychotic manifestations include delusions, hallucinations, vague paranoid ideation, and ideas of reference. Hypersomnolence has also been reported (Frazier 1935). Careful evaluation may be needed to differentiate this symptom from the lethargy and fatigue in patients with major depression.

Patients with tumors of the frontal and prefrontal regions may present with behavioral changes in the absence of intellectual decline or focal neurological dysfunction. Previously acquired cognitive skills are often preserved and patients may perform adequately on formal intelligence testing. However, more sophisticated neuropsychological assessments often reveal profound deficits in the ability to organize, initiate, and direct personal behavior (Teuber 1972). Tumors of the frontal lobes can also result in significant deficits in attentional function (Luria 1973). Additionally, posterior frontal lobe tumors can lead to expressive (Broca's) aphasia when the lesion is localized to the dominant hemisphere, or aprosody when localized to the nondominant hemisphere.

Temporal Lobe Tumors

It is important to distinguish ictal from interictal phenomena when discussing the neuropsychiatry of temporal lobe tumors. Ictal phenomena are discussed in Chapter 15; here we discuss interictal phenomena associated with temporal lobe tumors.

A high likelihood of schizophrenic-like illness has been noted with temporal lobe tumors (Malamud 1967; Selecki 1965), although one must note that since these studies predate the DSM-III-R diagnostic criteria (American Psychiatric Association 1987) they tend to overdiagnose schizophrenia. In fact, patients with temporal lobe dysfunction tend to present with psychotic symptoms atypical for classical schizophrenia. Frequently they present with episodic mood swings, suicidal ideation or suicide attempts, and visual, olfactory, and tactile hallucinations, as well as with the typical auditory hallucinations seen in schizophrenia (Tucker et al. 1986). Patients with temporal lobe disease often complain of "spells" or report "staring" or "dazed feelings" (Tucker et al. 1986). Unlike schizophrenic patients who have flat or inappropriate affect and markedly diminished capacity to relate to others, patients with temporal lobe diseases often retain appropriate, broad affect and interact interpersonally in a relatively normal fashion.

Personality changes have been described in more than half of temporal lobe tumor patients and may be an early manifestation of a previously unsuspected tumor (Keschner et al. 1936). Bear and Fedio (1977) suggested that characteristic interictal personality traits occur in patients with temporal lobe epilepsy and that the presence or absence of certain traits depends on whether the seizure focus is right or left sided. However, others (Mungas 1982; Rodin and Schmaltz 1984) have not confirmed these findings. Frequently, patients present with an intensification of their previous character traits, predominant coping mechanism, or adaptive styles, or with symptoms similar to those seen with frontal lobe tumors. Organic personality syndromes with episodic behavioral dyscontrol and/or affective instability are also frequent.

Anxiety symptoms are commonly associated with temporal lobe tumors. Mulder and Daly (1952) noted anxiety in 36% of their 100 patients. Two cases of panic attacks in patients with right temporal lobe tumors have been reported (Drubach and Kelly 1989; Ghadirian et al. 1986).

Tumors of the temporal lobe can also result in neuropsychological and cognitive deficits. Verbal and nonverbal memory may be affected. Dominant temporal lobe dysfunction is often associated with deficits in the patient's ability to learn and remember information of a verbal nature, whereas nondominant temporal lobe dysfunction is often associated with deficits in acquiring and retaining nonverbal (i.e., visuospatial) information (Butters 1979). Tumors of the dominant temporal lobe may result in receptive (Wernicke's) aphasia, whereas nondominant tumors may lead to disruption of the discrimination of nonspeech sounds (Spreen et al. 1965).

Cognitive dysfunction may result from the occurrence of tumor-associated seizure activity, which may induce dysfunction in other areas of the brain, due to the administration of anticonvulsants, especially when used in high doses, for long time periods, or in multidrug regimens.

Parietal Lobe Tumors

Tumors of the parietal lobe generally cause few behavioral changes. Schlesinger (1950) found affective symptomatology in only 16% of 31 patients with parietal lobe tumors. Affective symptoms in these patients reflected predominantly depression and apathy, rather than euphoria or mania. Psychotic symptoms appear to be less common in parietal lobe tumor patients.

Tumors localized in the parietal lobes are likely to result in cognitive as opposed to psychiatric symptoms. Tumors of the anterior parietal lobe may result in abnormalities of sensory perception in the contralateral hand. Inability to recognize objects placed in the hand (astereognosis) is common. Difficulty in the recognition of shapes, letters, and numbers drawn on the hand (agraphesthesia) is also seen; apraxias may be present. Tumors of the parietal lobe may also affect the patient's ability to decipher visuospatial information, particularly when the tumor is localized to the nondominant hemisphere (Warrington and Rabin 1970).

Dominant parietal lobe tumors may lead to dysgraphia, acalculia, finger agnosia, and right-left confusion (Gerstmann's syndrome) and may often affect reading and spelling. Individuals with parietal lobe tumors may present with a lack of awareness or even denial of their neurological and/or neuropsychiatric difficulties, even in the face of rather obvious organic dysfunction (Critchley 1964a). Because of the often bizarre neurological complaints and atypical symptoms that may accompany tumors in this area, such patients are frequently initially diagnosed as having either a conversion disorder or some other type of somatization disorder (Critchley 1964b).

Occipital Lobe Tumors

Occipital lobe tumors may present with psychiatric symptoms but, like tumors involving the parietal lobes, they appear less likely to do so than tumors of the frontal or temporal lobes (Keschner et al. 1938). However, Allen (1930) found psychiatric symptoms in 55% of 40 such patients. In fact, in 17% of these patients, behavioral symptoms were the presenting complaint. The most characteristic finding appears to have been visual hallucinations, present in 25%. Other changes included agitation, irritability, suspiciousness, and fatigue

Tumors of the occipital lobe cause difficulties in cognitive and perceptual functions. A typical finding in patients who have neoplasms localized to the occipital lobe is a homonymous hemianopsia, the loss of one-half of the visual field in each eye. Inability to recognize items visually (visual agnosia) may also be seen (Lezak 1983). Inability to recognize familiar faces, prosopagnosia, may also accompany lesions in the occipital lobes, particularly when there is bilateral involvement (Meadows 1974).

Diencephalic Tumors

Tumors of deep midline structures, such as the thalamus, hypothalamus, and the areas surrounding the third ventricle, involve regions that are contiguous with the limbic system. These lesions are frequently associated with psychiatric symptoms. For example, Cairns and Mosberg (1951) reported "emotional instability" and psychosis in patients with colloid cysts of the third ventricle. Hypothalamic tumors have been associated with disorders of eating behavior, including hyperphagia and symptoms indistinguishable from anorexia nervosa (Climo 1982; Coffey 1989). Additionally, lesions of the hypothalamus can present with hypersomnia and daytime somnolence.

Neoplasms of subcortical brain regions have their most dramatic effect on memory, resulting in impairments in new learning, whereas other aspects of cognitive functioning may remain intact (Lishman 1978). Tumors in this area may lead to diffuse, generalized cognitive dysfunction by interfering with the normal circulation of cerebral spinal fluid, thereby causing hydrocephalus.

Corpus Callosum Tumors

Tumors of the corpus callosum have been associated with behavioral symptoms in up to 90% of patients (Selecki 1964). Such symptoms appear to be most common with tumors of the genu and splenium (Schlesinger 1950). A broad array of behavioral changes has been found, ranging from depression and apathy to psychotic symptoms, as well as organic personality features similar to those seen with frontal lobe tumors.

Pituitary Tumors

Pituitary tumors frequently present with behavioral changes resulting from upward extension of the tumor into the diencephalon. This may be most common with craniopharyngiomas, which sometimes present with disorders of sleep or temperature regulation, clinical phenomena otherwise seen with tumors of the hypothalamus. Tumors of the pituitary can result in endocrine disturbances, which can produce neuropsychiatric symptoms. Basophilic adenomas are commonly associated with Cushing's syndrome, which is frequently associated with affective lability, depression, or psychosis. Acidophilic adenomas frequently present with acromegaly, which has been associated with both anxiety and depression (Avery 1973).

As with most brain tumors, the whole gamut of psychiatric symptoms from depression and apathy to paranoia has been reported with pituitary tumors. In Russell and Pennybacker's study (1961), 33% of 24 patients had mental disturbances severe enough to dominate their clinical picture, and 13% had initially presented to psychiatric hospitals for diagnosis and treatment.

Posterior Fossa Tumors

Infratentorial tumors present only infrequently with psychiatric symptoms. Virtually every behavioral change described with supratentorial tumors has also been reported with infratentorial lesions. In fact, mental symptoms have been found in as many as 76% of such patients and have included paranoid delusions and affective disorders (Wilson and Rupp 1946). Cases of mania have also been noted (Greenberg and Brown 1985). Posterior fossa tumors have been associated with irritability, apathy, and hypersomnolence. Auditory hallucinations have also been reported (Cairns 1950).

CLINICAL DIAGNOSIS AND TREATMENT

For the clinician, the early diagnosis of a brain tumor rests on an awareness of the many clinical manifestations such tumors may produce. The most characteristic aspect of CNS tumors is that they cause focal neurological signs and symptoms, as well as neuropsychiatric symptoms, such as personality changes, changes in affect or sensorium, and neuropsychological deficits. Neurological signs and symptoms commonly associated with brain tumors include headaches (25%–35%), nausea and vomiting (33%), seizures (20%–50%), and visual changes including field cuts, diplopia, and papilledema. Focal motor and sensory changes are helpful in localizing the tumor (Table 18–2).

When to Suspect a Brain Tumor in a Psychiatric Patient

Although recognition of a brain tumor presenting with focal neurological signs and symptoms should not be problematic, one presenting with predominantly psychiatric and behavioral symptoms may be difficult to diagnose. The occurrence of one or more of the five following complaints in a known psychiatric patient or in a patient presenting for the first time with psychiatric symptoms should heighten the clinician's index of suspicion of a possible brain tumor:

1. Seizures: especially if new and partial; seizures may be the initial neurological manifestation of a tumor in as many as 50% of cases.
2. Headaches: especially if generalized; dull; of new onset; of increasing severity and/or frequency; or if positional, nocturnal, or present on awakening.
3. Nausea and vomiting: especially if occurring in conjunction with headaches.
4. Sensory changes: visual changes such as loss or diminution of vision, visual field defects, or diplopia; auditory changes such as tinnitus or hearing loss, especially unilateral; vertigo.

5. Other focal neurological signs and symptoms: localized weakness, sensory loss, paresthesias or dysesthesias, ataxia, and incoordination.

The Diagnostic Evaluation

A careful history of the nature and time course of both psychiatric and neurological signs and symptoms is the cornerstone of diagnosis. This must be supplemented by physical and neurological examinations, brain imaging and electrodiagnostic studies, and formal neuropsychological testing.

Table 18–2. Neurological and neuropsychological findings that have localizing value

Brain region	Neurological and neuropsychological findings
Frontal lobes	
Prefrontal	Contralateral grasp reflex, executive functioning deficits (inability to formulate goals, to plan, and to effectively carry out these plans), decreased oral fluency (dominant hemisphere), decreased design fluency (nondominant hemisphere), motor perserveration or impersistence, and inability to hold set
Posterior	Contralateral hemiparesis, decreased motor strength, speed and coordination, and Broca's aphasia
Temporal lobes	Partial complex seizures, contralateral homonymous inferior quadrantanopsia, Wernicke's aphasia, decreased learning and retention of verbal material (dominant hemisphere), decreased learning and retention of nonverbal material (nondominant hemisphere), amusia (nondominant hemisphere), and auditory agnosia
Parietal lobes	Partial sensory seizures, agraphesthesia, astereognosis, anosognosia, Gerstmann's syndrome (acalculia, agraphia, finger agnosia, and right-left confusion), ideomotor and ideational apraxia, constructional apraxia, agraphia with alexia, dressing apraxia, prosopagnosia, and visuospatial problems
Occipital	Partial sensory seizures with visual phenomena, homonymous hemianopsia, alexia, agraphia, prosopagnosia, color agnosia, and construction apraxia
Corpus callosum	Callosal apraxia
Thalamus	Contralateral hemisensory loss and pain
Basal ganglia	Contralateral choreoathetosis, dystonia, rigidity, motor perseveration, and parkinsonian tremor
Pituitary and hypothalamus	Bitemporal hemianopia, optic atrophy, hypopituitarism, and diabetes insipidus
Pineal	Loss of upward gaze (Parinaud's syndrome)
Cerebellum	Ipsilateral hypotonia, ataxia, dysmetria, intention tremor, and nystagmus toward side of tumor
Brain stem	
Midbrain	Pupillary and extraocular muscle abnormalities and contralateral hemiparesis
Pons	Sixth and seventh nerve involvement (diplopia and ipsilateral facial paralysis)

Source. Reprinted from Lohr JB, Cadet JL: "Neuropsychiatric Aspects of Brain Tumors," in *The American Psychiatric Press Textbook of Neuropsychiatry.* Washington, DC, American Psychiatric Press, 1987, p. 354. Used with permission.

All psychiatric patients should have full physical, neurological, and mental status examinations. Brain tumor patients often manifest focal neurological findings as well as abnormalities in cognitive functioning. Table 18–2 highlights some of the important localizing neurological findings that occur with brain tumors in various locations. However, some brain tumors are not clinically apparent until late in their course. Such tumors frequently involve the anterior frontal lobes, the corpus callosum, the nondominant parietal and temporal lobes, and posterior fossa: so-called silent regions. Thus despite negative neurological examinations, other diagnostic studies are necessary to rule out conclusively the presence of a tumor.

CT scans.   In the 1970s, the computed tomography (CT) scan largely replaced plain skull films, radioisotope brain scans, electroencephalography (EEG), echoencephalography, and pneumoencephalography in the diagnosis of brain tumors because of the greater resolution in the delineation of anatomic brain structures. The CT scan's capacity to detect neoplasms can be further enhanced with intravenous contrast material. In addition, CT scans can reveal calcifications, cerebral edema, obstructive hydrocephalus, a shift in midline structures, or other changes in the ventricular system. CT scans may not reveal very small tumors, tumors in the posterior fossa, tumors that are isodense with respect to brain tissue and/or cerebrospinal fluid, or tumors diffusely involving the meninges (i.e., carcinomatosis).

MRI scans.   Magnetic resonance imaging (MRI) is superior to CT scanning in the diagnosis of brain tumors and other soft tissue lesions of the brain because of a higher degree of spatial resolution. In addition, MRI does not entail exposure to radiation. The chief drawbacks are its cost and the fact that it does not adequately image calcified lesions. It also cannot be used in patients in whom ferrometallic foreign objects are present. Enhancement of MRI scans with gadolinium further increases their diagnostic sensitivity.

Cisternography.   CT cisternography is used to evaluate the ventricular system, subarachnoid spaces, and basilar cisterns, which may be helpful in the differential diagnosis of intraventricular and pituitary tumors, as well as hydrocephalus. This technique has largely replaced pneumoencephalography, which was poorly tolerated.

Skull films.   Plain skull films are no longer routinely used in the diagnosis of brain tumors, although tomographs of the sella turcica may be helpful in the diagnosis of pituitary tumors, craniopharyngiomas, and the so-called *empty sella syndrome*.

Cerebral angiography.   In certain circumstances cerebral angiography may be helpful in delineating the vascular supply to a tumor before surgery.

Lumbar puncture.   Lumbar punctures (LPs) are used much less frequently in the diagnosis of brain tumors than in the past. Brain tumors may be associated with elevated cerebrospinal fluid protein and increased ICP, but these findings are diagnostically nonspecific. With certain types of neoplastic diseases of the CNS, such as meningeal carcinomatosis and leukemia, an LP may be helpful when other neurodiagnostic studies have been unrevealing.

EEG.   EEG in patients with brain tumors may reveal nonspecific electrical abnormalities, such as spikes and slow waves, diffuse or focal, paroxysmal or continuous. However, since the EEG is often normal, it is neither a specific nor sensitive test for brain tumors.

Others.   Single photon emission computed tomography (SPECT), positron-emission tomography (PET), and brain electrical activity mapping (BEAM) are newly emerging, quantitative, computer-based techniques for evaluating various aspects of brain structure, as well as brain metabolic and electrical functioning. At present, none of these appears to have major advantages over the standard diagnostic approaches.

TREATMENT OF PSYCHIATRIC AND BEHAVIORAL SYMPTOMS ASSOCIATED WITH CEREBRAL TUMORS

Because psychiatric and behavioral symptoms may sometimes be eliminated with complete removal of the cerebral tumor, this is the first goal of treatment. When this is not possible, decreasing the size or slowing the growth of the tumor through surgery, chemotherapy, or radiation therapy (alone, in combination, or sequentially) may ameliorate the behavioral symptoms. Improvement may be dramatic with treatments that diminish increased ICP or relieve hydrocephalus associated with a brain tumor.

When neuropsychiatric or behavioral symptoms persist after surgical and nonsurgical interventions, psychopharmacological, psychotherapeutic, and psychosocial interventions become a major focus. Working closely with the attending neurosurgeon, the consulting psychiatrist may contribute significantly to the patient's level of functioning and quality of life. Ameliorating the dysphoria and anergia of a severe depression, alleviating the distress of anxiety, or simply providing support to patients and their families may make a difference. Often such interventions can also lead to increased patient motivation and improved compliance.

Although patients with cerebral tumors frequently have psychiatric symptoms, only some of these are a direct manifestation of the organic mental syndrome caused by the tumor. The consulting psychiatrist must differentiate as precisely as possible among symptoms that are tumor related; those that result from preexisting, primary psychiatric disorders; and those that are reactive in nature and secondary to stress. Optimal pharmacological and psychotherapeutic interventions are often quite different for each.

Pharmacological Management of Preexisting Primary Psychiatric Disorders

The psychopharmacological management of patients with preexisting primary psychiatric illnesses with cerebral tumors should follow the same general principles that apply to tumor-free patients with similar disorders. The psychiatrist should be cognizant of the potential need to make reductions in medication dose and to use drugs that are less likely to cause delirium in brain tumor patients, especially those in the immediate postoperative period or those who are receiving chemotherapy or radiation therapy. Lithium, low-potency antipsychotic drugs, tertiary amine tricyclic antidepressants (TCAs), and antiparkinsonian agents all have significant, dose-related deliriogenic potential when given alone or with other deliriogenic agents. It may be necessary to substitute haloperidol, carbamazepine, valproate, and/or a benzodiazepine such as lorazepam or clonazepam for lithium in a brain tumor patient with mania, a "newer generation" heterocyclic or secondary amine TCA for a tertiary amine TCA in a brain tumor patient with depression, or a high-potency for a low-potency neuroleptic in a brain tumor patient with schizophrenia.

Another concern is the potential for precipitating seizures when using these drugs in brain tumor patients. Neuroleptics, antidepressants, and lithium all can lower seizure threshold, to variable degrees. Molindone, fluphenazine, and haloperidol are among the antipsychotic drugs believed to carry the lowest risk for seizures. Among the antidepressants, maprotiline and bupropion appear to have the greatest seizure-inducing potential, but it is unclear which antidepressants carry the least risk. In acutely manic brain tumor patients, for whom lithium would otherwise be the drug of choice, carbamazepine, valproic acid, lorazepam, or clonazepam might be preferable. The psychiatrist should also bear in mind that brain tumor patients with psychiatric disorders who are taking anticonvulsants for a known seizure diathesis should be monitored carefully for the adequacy of their anticonvulsant blood levels; the dose of the anticonvulsant should be adjusted as indicated when psychotropic agents are added.

Psychotherapeutic Management of Syndromes Associated With Brain Tumors

Supportive psychotherapy geared to the patient's functional status, cognitive capacities, and emotional needs is an important element in treatment. The stress of undergoing treatment for a brain tumor can trigger recurrences of a primary psychiatric disorder as well as reactive psychiatric symptoms as the patient attempts to cope. In either case, supportive psychotherapy can be beneficial. Some patients who have been completely cured may also manifest anxiety, fear, and depression and may benefit from psychotherapy.

Psychotherapy ideally involves both the patient and the family and revolves around concrete, reality-based, cognitive, and psychoeducational issues such as diagnosis and prognosis, impact of the illness on the patient's functional status, its effect on the family, coping with actual or anticipated disability, and dealing with anticipatory grief related to potential losses and eventual death. Patients with cerebral tumors worry about changes in mental and intellectual functioning, physical incapacity, and ultimately death. Patients vary widely in their capacity to deal with the potentially devastating consequences of brain tumors; the success of their adjustment depends largely on the adaptiveness of their previous coping styles.

Denial as a coping mechanism is common and may be effective in helping patients allay their fears, especially in the early stages of illness. On the other hand, during later stages, it can result in the failure of patients or their families to comply with optimal treatment measures or to handle legal, family, or other reality-based issues. The clinician may need to directly encourage the patient and family who are in denial to address such issues as increasing disability, incapacity, or death. While there are no clear-cut guidelines for discussions of prognosis with brain tumor patients, most clinicians believe that they and their families should be given realistic prognostic information in a time frame that will allow them to make well-considered decisions and appropriate plans. Such information should be conveyed by the physician as sensitively as possible.

Psychodynamically focused, insight-oriented psychotherapy may be contraindicated in psychiatrically ill patients with brain tumors. This is because such patients often have impairment of cognitive and abstracting abilities as a result of the tumor or neurosurgery, chemotherapy, or radiotherapy. When such impairments are present, psychodynamically oriented therapies may actually cause distress when patients are confronted with mental tasks and cognitive demands they can no longer handle.

Somatic Treatment of Organic Mental Disorders

As with primary psychiatric disorders, the psychopharmacological treatment of behavioral symptoms secondary to organic mental syndromes caused by cerebral tumors, whether characterized by psychotic, affective, anxiety, or cognitive disturbances, follows the same general principles as those of phenomenologically similar symptoms resulting from primary functional psychiatric illnesses.

Patients with psychiatric symptoms that are a direct consequence of a brain tumor, like other patients with organic brain disorders, may require and tolerate significantly lower doses of psychotropic medication. Thus the side effect profiles of psychotropic drugs need to be carefully evaluated with regard to sedative, extrapyramidal, delirioficient, and epileptogenic effects, as well as drug-drug interactions.

Drug Treatment of Tumor-Associated Organic Psychoses

Standard antipsychotic medications may be effective in treating hallucinations, delusions, and thought disturbances secondary to tumor-associated organic psychotic syndromes. High-potency agents, which have fewer nonneurological side effects, are generally preferable to lower-potency antipsychotics, even though they frequently cause extrapyramidal symptoms. In organic psychotic disorders the therapeutically effective dose is often lower than that required for the treatment of primary functional psychoses, especially for the elderly, for whom effective neuroleptic doses are 25%–50% lower than for younger patients.

Antiparkinsonian agents such as benztropine, trihexyphenidyl, and orphenadrine are effective in the treatment of extrapyramidal side effects resulting from the use of neuroleptics in brain tumor patients. However, these agents are likely to cause or contribute to anticholinergic delirium when used with low-potency neuroleptics and/or tertiary amine TCAs. Thus their use should be avoided unless there is a clear-cut indication, and when they are used the dose should be minimized. Diphenhydramine or amantadine for dystonic and parkinsonian symptoms and benzodiazepines for akathisia are effective alternatives and have less delirioficient potential.

Treatment of Organic Mood Syndromes

Antidepressant medications are effective in the treatment of organic mood syndromes of the depressed type in brain tumor patients. Standard TCAs are useful, though the newer-generation heterocyclic or secondary amine TCAs are used preferentially because of their lesser anticholinergic activity and sedating effects. Methylphenidate has also been shown to be effective in depression secondary to brain tumors. It is generally well tolerated and does not lower the seizure threshold. Monoamine oxidase inhibitors (MAOIs) may be effective when other antidepressants are not. However, the clinician must bear in mind that the cognitive impairment in such patients may interfere with their ability to maintain a tyramine-free diet.

If single antidepressant medication regimens are ineffective, various combination regimens may work, and when pharmacological treatments have failed, electroconvulsive therapy (ECT) should be given serious consideration. Previously, brain tumors were thought to be an absolute contraindication to ECT, especially when associated with increased ICP. However, Zwil et al. (1990) reviewed cases of refractory depression associated with brain tumors that were treated with ECT without associated evidence of increased ICP.

Treatment of Organic Anxiety Syndromes

Anxiety symptoms associated with brain tumors should not be treated with neuroleptics unless psychotic features are present for the reasons noted previously and because neuroleptics are generally not effective with nonpsychotic anxiety and often result in dysphoria in nonpsychotic patients. The benzodiazepines are effective and have the added benefit of possessing anticonvulsant properties. However, these drugs (particularly long-acting types) may induce delirium in patients with organic brain disease when used in high doses, for long periods of time, and in older age groups. Other disadvantages of benzodiazepines include their abuse potential and the occasional propensity to cause paradoxical reactions.

Buspirone is an alternative to the benzodiazepines. Its main drawbacks are its delayed onset and modest degree of anxiolytic action. Vistaril, or low doses of tertiary amine TCAs such as doxepin or amitriptyline, may also have beneficial anxiolytic effects in some patients. Finally, panic attacks associated with temporal lobe tumors may respond to carbamazepine, valproate, or primidone, as well as to the usual antidepressant and antianxiety drugs.

Treatment of Delirium

Delirium in brain tumor patients may be associated with a wide variety of psychiatric symptoms as well as cognitive impairments. Hallucinations and delusions often respond to symptomatic treatment with low doses of haloperidol or other high-potency neuroleptics while the underlying causes of the delirium are being sought.

Treatment of Organic Personality Syndromes

Mood lability may be a manifestation of an organic personality disorder due to a brain tumor and may respond to lithium or carbamazepine. Some patients with tumor-associated frontal lobe syndromes respond to carbamazepine, as do some patients with temporal lobe tumors who present with interictal aggression and violent behavior. Brain tumor patients with impulse dyscontrol and explosiveness may respond to anticonvulsants, such as carbamazepine, as well as to lithium, β-blockers, high-potency neuroleptics, and/or stimulants.

Cognitive Rehabilitation

In addition to psychopharmacological and psychotherapeutic treatments, cognitive rehabilitation may be helpful for patients whose tumors, or whose treatments for these tumors, have produced behavioral or cognitive sequelae. Cognitive rehabilitation strategies can be developed to address deficits in intellectual, language, visuospatial, and memory functioning resulting from a brain tumor. (For a more detailed discussion see Chapter 28.)

CONCLUSIONS

Brain tumors are frequently associated with a broad range of psychiatric and/or neuropsychological symptoms. The differential diagnosis of any patient who displays acute or progressive changes in behavior, personality, or cognitive function, should include a brain tumor, especially if there are any associated focal neurological signs and symptoms. The nature, frequency, and severity of psychiatric symptoms observed with brain tumors depend on the type, location, size, rate of growth, and malignancy of the tumor. Although frontal, temporal, and diencephalic tumors appear to be most commonly associated with psychiatric and behavioral symptoms, the variation in symptoms that may occur with each is exceedingly broad. In general, correlations between particular neuropsychiatric symptoms and anatomic locations of the causative brain tumors are not very robust.

Optimal treatment of tumor-associated psychiatric, neuropsychiatric, and neuropsychological dysfunctions should be multidimensional and requires the coordinated interventions of a multidisciplinary treatment team. With well-planned integration and coordination of therapeutic approaches, both the quantity and quality of the brain tumor patient's life may be substantially enhanced.

REFERENCES

Allen IM: A clinical study of tumors involving the occipital lobe. Brain 53:194–243, 1930

American Psychiatric Association: Diagnostic and Statistical Manual of Mental Disorders, 3rd Edition, Revised. Washington, DC, American Psychiatric Association, 1987

Avery TL: A case of acromegaly and gigantism with depression. Br J Psychiatry 122:599–600, 1973

Bear DM, Fedio P: Quantitative analysis of interictal behavior in temporal lobe epilepsy. Arch Neurol 34:454–467, 1977

Belyi BI: Mental impairment in unilateral frontal tumors: role of the laterality of the lesion. Int J Neurosci 32:799–810, 1987

Bigler ED: Diagnostic Clinical Neuropsychology. Austin, TX, University of Texas Press, 1984

Burger PC, Scheithauer BW, Vogel FS: Surgical Pathology of the Nervous System and Its Coverings, 3rd Edition. New York, Churchill Livingstone, 1991

Butters N: Amnestic disorders, in Clinical Neuropsychology. Edited by Heilman KM, Valenstein E. New York, Oxford University Press, 1979, pp 439–474

Cairns H: Mental disorders with tumors of the pons. Folia Psychiatrica Neurologica Neurochirurgica 53:193–203, 1950

Cairns H, Mosberg WH: Colloid cysts of the third ventricle. Surg Gynecol Obstet 92:545–570, 1951

Climo LH: Anorexia nervosa associated with hypothalamic tumor: the search for clinical-pathological correlations. Psychiatric Journal of the University of Ottawa 7:20–25, 1982

Coffey RJ: Hypothalamic and basal forebrain germinoma presenting with amnesia and hyperphagia. Surg Neurol 31:228–233, 1989

Critchley M: The problem of visual agnosia. J Neurol Sci 1:274–290, 1964a

Critchley M: Psychiatric symptoms and parietal disease: differential diagnosis. Proceedings of the Royal Society of Medicine 57:422–428, 1964b

Cummings JL: Clinical Neuropsychiatry. Orlando, FL, Grune & Stratton, 1985

Cummings JL, Mendez MF: Secondary mania with focal cerebrovascular lesions. Am J Psychiatry 141:1084–1087, 1984

Direkze M, Bayliss SG, Cutting JC: Primary tumors of the frontal lobe. Br J Clin Pract 25:207–213, 1971

Drubach DA, Kelly MP: Panic disorder associated with a right paralimbic lesion. Neuropsychiatry, Neuropsychology, and Behavioral Neurology 2:282–289, 1989

Flor-Henry P: Schizophrenic-like reactions and affective psychoses associated with temporal lobe epilepsy etiological factors. Am J Psychiatry 126:400–404, 1969

Frazier CH: Tumor involving the frontal lobe alone: a symptomatic survey of 105 verified cases. Archives of Neurology and Psychiatry 35:525–571, 1935

Ghadirian, AM, Gauthier S, Bertrand S: Anxiety attacks in a patient with a right temporal lobe meningioma. J Clin Psychiatry 47:270–271, 1986

Goldberg E: Varieties of perseverations: comparison of two taxonomies. J Clin Exp Neuropsychol 6:710–726, 1986

Golden CJ: Cerebral tumors, in Clinical Neuropsychology: Interface With Neurologic and Psychiatric Disorders. Edited by Golden CJ, Moses JA, Coffman JA, et al. New York, Grune & Stratton, 1983, pp 3–20

Greenberg DB, Brown GL: Mania resulting from brain stem tumor: single case study. J Nerv Ment Dis 173:434–436, 1985

Keschner M, Bender MB, Strauss I: Mental symptoms in cases of tumor of the temporal lobe. Archives of Neurology and Psychiatry 35:572–596, 1936

Keschner M, Bender MB, Strauss I: Mental symptoms associated with brain tumor: a study of 530 verified cases. JAMA 110:714–718, 1938

Klotz M: Incidence of brain tumors in patients hospitalized for chronic mental disorders. Psychiatr Q 31:669–680, 1957

Kurtzke JF: Neuroepidemiology. Ann Neurol 16:265–277, 1984

Lezak MD: Neuropsychological Assessment. New York, Oxford University Press, 1983

Lishman WA: Organic Psychiatry: The Psychological Consequences of Cerebral Disorder. New York, Oxford University Press, 1978

Lohr JB, Cadet JL: Neuropsychiatric aspects of brain tumors, in The American Psychiatric Press Textbook of Neuropsychiatry. Washington, DC, American Psychiatric Press, 1987, pp 351–364

Luria AR: The Working Brain: An Introduction to Neuropsychology. New York, Basic Books, 1973

McAllister TW, Price TRP: Aspects of the behavior of psychiatric inpatients with frontal lobe damage: some implications for diagnosis and treatment. Compr Psychiatry 28:14–21, 1987

Malamud N: Psychiatric disorder with intracranial tumors of limbic system. Arch Neurol 17:113–123, 1967

Meadows JC: The anatomical basis of prosopagnosia. J Neurol Neurosurg Psychiatry 37:489–501, 1974

Minski L: The mental symptoms associated with 58 cases of cerebral tumor. Journal of Neurology and Psychopathology 13:330–343, 1933

Mulder DW, Daly D: Psychiatric symptoms associated with lesions of temporal lobe. JAMA 150:173–176, 1952

Mungas D: Interictal behavior abnormality in temporal lobe epilepsy: a specific syndrome or non-specific psychopathology? Arch Gen Psychiatry 39:108–111, 1982

Patton RB, Sheppard JA: Intracranial tumors found at autopsy in mental patients. Am J Psychiatry 113:319–324, 1956

Remington FB, Robert SL: Why patients with brain tumors come to a psychiatric hospital: a thirty-year survey. Am J Psychiatry 119:256–257, 1962

Rodin E, Schmaltz S: The Bear-Fedio personality inventory and temporal lobe epilepsy. Neurology 34:591–596, 1984

Russell RW, Pennybacker JB: Craniopharyngioma in the elderly. J Neurol Neurosurg Psychiatry 24:1–13, 1961

Schlesinger B: Mental changes in intracranial tumors and related problems. Confinia Neurologica 10:225–263, 1950

Selecki BR: Cerebral mid-line tumours involving the corpus callosum among mental hospital patients. Med J Aust 2:954–960, 1964

Selecki BR: Intracranial space-occupying lesions among patients admitted to mental hospitals. Med J Aust 1: 383–390, 1965

Sperry RW: Lateral specialization in the surgically separated hemispheres, in The Neurosciences: 3rd Study Program. Edited by Worden OF, Worden FG. Cambridge, MA, MIT Press, 1974, pp 5–19

Spreen O, Benton A, Fincham R: Auditory agnosia without aphasia. Arch Neurol 13:84, 1965

Starkstein SE, Boston JD, Robinson RG: Mechanisms of mania after brain injury: 12 case reports and review of the literature. J Nerv Ment Dis 176:87–100, 1988

Strauss I, Keschner M: Mental symptoms in cases of tumor of the frontal lobe. Archives of Neurology and Psychiatry 33:986–1005, 1935

Teuber HL: Unity and diversity of frontal lobe functions. Acta Neurobiol Exp 32:615–656, 1972

Tucker GJ, Price TRP, Johnson VB, et al: Phenomenology of temporal lobe dysfunction: a link to atypical psychosis: a series of cases. J Nerv Ment Dis 174:348–356, 1986

Warrington EK, Rabin P: Perceptual matching in patients with cerebral lesions. Neuropsychologia 8:475–487, 1970

Wilson G, Rupp C: Mental symptoms associated with extra medullary posterior fossa tumors. Transactions of the American Neurological Association (New York) 71:104–107, 1946

Zwil AS, Bowring MA, Price TRP, et al: ECT in the presence of a brain tumor: case reports and a review of the literature. Convulsive Therapy 6:299–307, 1990

Chapter 19

Effects of Human Immunodeficiency Virus on the Central Nervous System

John C. Markowitz, M.D.
Samuel W. Perry, M.D.

This chapter provides an overview of the spectrum of neuropsychiatric disorders associated with the acquired immunodeficiency syndrome (AIDS) and its etiological agent, human immunodeficiency virus (HIV). Neuropsychiatric deficits may be *primary* (directly induced by HIV), *secondary* (as when immunodeficiency leads to opportunistic infections or tumors systemically or within central nervous system [CNS]), or *iatrogenic* (resulting from treatment of HIV or its sequelae).

HUMAN IMMUNODEFICIENCY VIRUS

Epidemiology

HIV has been spreading in the United States since the 1970s. The blood-borne virus is transmitted through unprotected sexual contact, use of blood-contaminated needles or other drug paraphernalia, receiving tainted blood or blood product transfusions, or intrauterine infection. The course of HIV infection is highly variable but generally chronic, with a mean duration of roughly 10 years between inoculation and the development of physical symptoms. Most of the estimated one million adults in the United States infected by HIV are currently asymptomatic, and their serological status is generally unreported even when known.

The majority of adults with AIDS are homosexual or bisexual men (62%), but the percentage of infected intravenous-drug abusers continues to rise (27% versus 13%–17% in the early 1980s). Also increasing have been the percentage of female and heterosexual cases (4%) and the number of children with AIDS. AIDS is the leading cause of death among intravenous-drug abusers and hemophiliac patients (Heyward and Curran 1988).

This chapter is dedicated to the memory of Samuel W. Perry, M.D., whose untimely death in March 1994 deprived the field of neuropsychiatry of further important work in this area.
Supported in part by Grants MH-19069, 42277, and 46250 from the National Institute of Mental Health.

Neuropsychiatric Effects

HIV attacks the CNS (Price et al. 1988) as well as the immune system (Fauci 1988). AIDS, being a syndrome rather than a discrete disorder, involves complex, multietiological mental changes resulting both from HIV itself and from the host of secondary disease states it unleashes.

It is believed (Price et al. 1990) that HIV invades the brain shortly after systemic infection, when macrophages bearing HIV cross the blood-brain barrier. Release of virus within the CNS causes an acute or subclinical meningoencephalitis. Newly infected patients, not yet having been immunocompromised by chronic destruction of T4 lymphocytes, can generally contain this initial infection. As immunocompetence wanes over months or years, viral replication within the CNS escapes the mastery of immune defenses. Progressive multifocal leukoencephalopathy may occur. Different strains of HIV and constitutional and environmental cofactors may explain differences in CNS pathology.

Histopathology

HIV most prominently affects subcortical areas, including central white matter and deep gray structures such as the basal ganglia, thalamus, and brain stem. The cerebral cortex is relatively spared: hence the term *subcortical dementia.* White matter pallor may be accompanied by astrocytic reaction and marked atrophy, or there may be few inflammatory changes and little pallor.

When encephalitis exists, reactive infiltrates of multinucleated cells, parenchymal and perivascular foamy macrophages, lymphocytes, and microglia are found. Oligodendrocytes and neurons are generally preserved. The minimal neuronal lysis suggests that neurotoxicity results either from an autoimmune response, from HIV synergy with other pathogens, or from release of toxic substances from the viral genes themselves or from adjacent infected cells. Spinal cord involvement usually consists of "vacuolar myelopathy" due to swelling of myelin sheaths.

Psychiatric Differential Diagnosis

Organic mental disorders (OMDs) occur frequently among hospitalized patients with AIDS (Price and Brew 1988), may occur in the absence of systemic symptomatology (Marotta and Perry 1989), and may mimic functional psychiatric disorders. Psychiatrists should consider HIV-spectrum disease in the differential diagnosis of patients with high-risk behaviors and in cases with atypical presentations.

PRIMARY NEUROPSYCHOLOGICAL IMPAIRMENT BY HIV

HIV Staging

Many investigators are researching early neuropsychological impairment among diverse groups of HIV-seropositive adults who have yet to develop other AIDS-related symptoms. Most studies use the staging system for HIV infection developed by the Centers for Disease Control (CDC; 1987) (Table 19–1).

The CDC classification discards "AIDS-related complex" and "pre-AIDS," imprecise clinical terms that might correspond to stages III, IV-A, and milder opportunistic infections now classified under stage IV-C2. The CDC staging does not describe prognosis or severity. Patients in stages I through IV-A sometimes deteriorate rapidly. By contrast, patients with "frank AIDS" (stages IV-B through IV-E) may have relatively mild Kaposi's sarcoma or have recovered long ago from an opportunistic infection and may live for years with minimal physical debility. Longevity and chronicity of the syndrome have increased since the advent of early therapeutic intervention and chemoprophylaxis with maintenance medications such as zidovudine (AZT) and pentamidine (Markowitz and Perry 1990).

Neuropsychological Impairment and Clinical Diagnosis

DSM-III-R (American Psychiatric Association 1987) defines OMDs as disorders due to a specific and known brain dysfunction, in distinction to disorders that are responses to psychological or social factors (e.g., adjustment disorders) and those where a specific organic factor has not yet been clearly established (e.g., schizophrenia) (Perry and Markowitz 1988; also see Chapter 9). Organic etiologies may be multiple in an individual, with manifestations ranging from dementia, delirium, delusions, and hallucinosis to subtle but clinically significant changes in cognitive functioning, mood, personality, and impulse control.

Neuropsychological impairment is a test result, **not** a diagnosis. "Impairment" implies that scores are abnormal (assuming normative data exist) or fall beneath a

Table 19–1. Centers for Disease Control (CDC) staging for human immunodeficiency virus (HIV) infection

CDC stage	Description
I	Acute HIV infection Asymptomatic Viral syndrome Meningoencephalitis
II	Latent infection
III	Chronic lymphadenopathy
IV-A	Constitutional symptoms Weight loss Fever Chronic diarrhea
IV-B	HIV-induced neuropathology Dementia Myelopathy Peripheral neuropathy
IV-C	Opportunistic infections
IV-C1	Secondary infectious diseases, including Pneumocystis carinii pneumonia, toxoplasmosis, and cryptococcosis
IV-C2	Other secondary infectious diseases, including oral hairy leukoplakia, multidermatomal herpes zoster, tuberculosis, and oral candidiasis (thrush)
IV-D	HIV-associated tumors
IV-E	Other conditions, including chronic lymphoid interstitial pneumonitis

Source. Adapted from Centers for Disease Control 1987.

cutoff (usually two standard deviations below the sample mean), but the results of neuropsychological testing are not disease specific. In general, the more sensitive the test, the more likely it lacks specificity. The relationship among neuropsychological impairment, OMD, and social and vocational function remains unclear for HIV-seropositive individuals (Marotta and Perry 1989). Test batteries may find neuropsychological impairment in patients who do not meet criteria for a DSM-III-R OMD; conversely, OMD may coexist with a normal neuropsychological examination.

AIDS Dementia Complex

The relationship between AIDS dementia complex and OMD according to DSM-III-R also bears examination. Neurologists invented the former term to describe medical inpatients with AIDS whose loss of mentation and motor function was not attributable to CNS tumors, opportunistic infection, or systemic disease (Navia et al. 1986). The population originally studied had advanced neurological symptoms including significant intellectual deficits—hence "dementia"—as well as a "complex" of motoric and behavioral manifestations including poor ambulation and co-ordination, agitation, and hallucinations. Studying a wider range of patients at different stages of HIV infection indicates that patients may have HIV-related mental status changes before developing AIDS. Early cognitive and behavioral changes tend not to predominantly involve higher cortical function and are therefore not characteristic of "dementia." And the "complex" triad of cognitive, motor, and behavioral impairment is not invariably present (Perry and Tross 1984).

Studies of Primary Neuropsychological Impairment

By 1987, a variety of evidence suggested that organic mental changes at least oc-casionally preceded physical signs and symptoms of HIV infection. Case reports (Marotta and Perry 1989) indicated that some HIV-seropositive adults who had not yet developed AIDS experienced subjective mental slowing, forgetfulness, apathy, lethargy, social withdrawal, avoidance of complex tasks, and personality change. Although these symptoms initially appeared to be "functional," thorough clinical evaluation suggested a "subcortical dementia" (Cummings and Benson 1984). Other HIV-seropositive patients initially presented with acute psychosis (Perry and Jacobsen 1986), delirium (Levy et al. 1985), amnesia (Beresford et al. 1986), depression (Navia and Price 1987), or mania (Kermani et al. 1985).

McArthur et al. (1988) found HIV in the cerebrospinal fluid (CSF) of asymptom-atic homosexual men with 6–24 months of known seropositivity. Early presence of HIV, pleocytosis, and elevated protein in CSF, as well as isolation of HIV from neural tissue (Gabuzda et al. 1986), implied that HIV could affect the CNS before any phys-ical manifestations of disease. HIV-specific antigens and immunoglobulins were also discovered in spinal fluid of both symptomatic and asymptomatic infected patients (Brew et al. 1989).

Brain abnormalities appeared on computed tomography (CT), magnetic reso-nance imaging (MRI), and electroencephalogram (EEG) of patients with AIDS and AIDS-related complex in the absence of CNS opportunistic infections and malignan-cies. CT scans showed marked atrophy and enlarged ventricles, MRI showed scat-tered parenchymal lesions and calcification (Olsen et al. 1988), and EEG showed slow alpha rhythms and diffuse theta waves (Koppel et al. 1985). Neuropathological studies (Gray et al. 1988) described subcortical involvement consistent with subtle, non-cognitive mental changes, which could explain vague, seemingly psychological symptoms in the absence of intellectual (cortical) impairment.

Of 31 studies published or presented at medical symposia, 18 reported neuropsychological impairment before the onset of systemic AIDS, but 13 did not find meaningful early impairment (Perry 1990). These studies, however, varied broadly in site of recruitment, sample selection, size, design, extent of neuropsychological testing, data analysis, and interpretation of results. The largest studies to date derive from the Multicenter AIDS Cohort Study of homosexual and bisexual men. Visscher et al. (1989) administered a neuropsychological battery to 838 subjects with CDC stages II and III and to 767 seronegative subjects. No significant differences were found between the two groups.

By contrast, studies using more exhaustive neuropsychological test arrays on generally smaller patient samples (Grant et al. 1987; Perry et al. 1989; Tross et al. 1988) have found HIV-seropositive subjects with CDC stages II and III scoring below cutoffs on subtests at higher rates than seronegative control subjects. These results have been interpreted (Grant et al. 1987; Perry et al. 1989) as evidence that a small subgroup may have HIV-induced neuropsychological impairment before developing AIDS. Others (Tross et al. 1988) contend that such inference is premature given the absence of appropriate statistical correction for multiple test comparisons.

Overall, a review of research indicates that, although dementia as a late sequela is not uncommon, it is rarely the initial presentation of HIV infection. Most HIV-seropositive subjects do **not** meet diagnostic criteria for or show overt signs of dementia. According to the CDC (Stern et al. 1989), only 3.0% of 38,666 adults and 3.3% of 666 children presented with HIV encephalopathy as the first manifestation of AIDS. These epidemiological data corroborate clinical studies that found that 6%–14% of HIV-seropositive patients present to medical clinics with dementia as their initial problem (Navia and Price 1987).

DIAGNOSING EARLY HIV-INDUCED OMD

Since early mental status changes can be subtle, emotional, behavioral, and personality changes may be misdiagnosed as functional disorders or attributed to the stress of living with an incurable, stigmatizing infection. No single clinical finding, neuropsychological test, or procedure has proven sensitive and specific to diagnose neuropsychological impairment. As with other organic mental disorders (Perry and Markowitz 1988), diagnosis usually depends on clinical judgment (see Chapter 9). The patient's complaint, mental status examination, physical examination, and laboratory measures have been found to contribute imperfectly to detection of early neuropsychological impairment and HIV-induced OMD (HIV-OMD) in seropositive patients.

Subjective Complaints of Cognitive Impairment

Several studies have corroborated early clinical impressions (Perry et al. 1989) that HIV-seropositive patients do not reliably report presence or absence of early neuropsychological impairment. Temoshok et al. (1989) found that severity of cognitive complaints reported by 102 homosexual men with at least one HIV-related physical symptom did not correlate highly with neuropsychological impairment. Herns et al. (1989) reported that 77 homosexual men in CDC stages II or III had more subjective complaints about cognitive functioning than did 32 seronegative control subjects, but no greater actual neuropsychological impairment. Kocsis et al. (1989) found that 75 patients with AIDS perceived their deterioration in cognitive performance inaccurately although caregiving partners provided more valid ratings.

One explanation for the poor correspondence between subjective complaints and measurable impairment is that seropositive patients develop situational anxiety that impairs their concentration and memory and which they attribute to HIV. Correlation of measures of distress with perceived cognitive complaints (Herns et al. 1989; Kocsis et al. 1989; Temoshok et al. 1989) supports this hypothesis. Alternatively, some patients may correctly recognize mental deterioration. Their apparently exaggerated complaints might reflect insensitivity of the instruments with which they were tested or lack of premorbid baseline ratings to demonstrate actual decline from a superior to a normal range.

Mental Status Examination

Studies have suggested that standardized mental status examinations are insufficiently sensitive to early neuropsychological impairment. Dilley et al. (1989) administered the Mini-Mental State Exam (MMSE; Folstein et al. 1975) to 50 hospitalized patients with AIDS. Although 78% of the subjects had abnormal scores, only 8% were below the standard cutoff. Another study of a smaller group of patients corroborated the instrument's lack of sensitivity (Van Gorp et al. 1989). Similarly, the Neurobehavioral Cognitive Status Examination (Northern California Neurobehavioral Group 1988) indicated that 31 patients with AIDS had greater neuropsychological impairment than 39 control subjects, but scores did not reliably correlate with dysfunction (Kobayashi et al. 1989).

Distinction From Mood Disorder

Several authors have warned that HIV-OMD may be misdiagnosed as "functional" depression (Perry and Marotta 1987), yet research suggests the processes are usually clinically distinct. Only one study has uncovered even a weak correlation between neuropsychological impairment and depressive measures (Herns et al. 1989), and most have found none at all (Grant et al. 1989a; Perry et al. 1989). These results are limited by low depression scores: few subjects scored in the range associated with clinical depression. Furthermore, the research failed to distinguish cognitive from noncognitive impairment. These results support the perception (Navia and Price 1987) that neuropsychological impairment due to early HIV-OMD—apathy, mental slowing, avoidance of complex tasks, and social withdrawal—is clinically distinguishable from the poor self-esteem, irrational guilt, pessimism, and other symptoms of depression.

Individuals at risk for AIDS have high rates of lifetime mood disorders (Atkinson et al. 1988; Perry et al. 1990a). The clinician must always consider that mood disorders and HIV-OMD may be concomitant. Although advances in neurochemistry may eventually explain the phenomenological overlap between comorbid "subcortical dementia" and depression (Cummings and Benson 1984), the two studies to date are contradictory (Britton et al. 1989; Keilp et al. 1989).

Neurological Examination

Neurological findings are not pathognomonic of HIV-OMD. Peripheral neuropathies or vacuolar myelopathy due to HIV may produce motor weakness and sensory abnormalities yet cause no clinically significant mental status changes (Berger 1988; Cornblath and McArthur 1988). Ataxia (Fauci 1988; Navia et al. 1986), motor slowing (Fitzgibbon et al. 1989), and autonomic dysfunction with orthostatic hypotension (Cohen and Laudenslager 1989) are other indications of HIV-related neurological impairment that can occur in the absence of cognitive and psychological changes. Conversely, mental status changes may precede focal neurological signs (Navia and Price 1987; Price and Brew 1988).

Laboratory Measures

CSF levels.   Various studies have correlated CSF abnormalities with serum immunosuppression (McArthur et al. 1989b) and CSF p24 antigen levels with neurological signs (Portegies et al. 1989), but not CSF abnormalities with neuropsychological impairment. On the contrary, physically asymptomatic seropositive individuals frequently have CSF pleocytosis, elevated protein, immunoglobulins, and HIV antibodies and antigens (Appleman et al. 1988). Thus CSF measures cannot diagnose HIV-OMD. Nonetheless, lumbar puncture is indicated for any HIV-seropositive patient whose change in mental status could reflect meningoencephalitis.

Lymphocyte studies.   Neuropsychological impairment has been associated with lymphocyte cell subsets in some studies (Perry et al. 1989; Price and Brew 1988), but not others (Fernandez et al. 1989a). Even positive studies have generally found only weak correlations. Reduced total T4 lymphocyte count does not reliably indicate neuropsychological impairment and should not be used to screen for vocational competence (Perry et al. 1989).

Electrophysiological measures.   EEG abnormalities have been found in 21%–44% of patients with CDC stage II (Arendt et al. 1989), stages III and IV-A (Riedel et al. 1989), and stages IV-B through IV-E (Koppel et al. 1985). Yet slowed alpha rhythms and diffuse theta waves often appear in the absence of clinical signs (Parisi et al. 1989). Seropositive patients without AIDS also have abnormalities on computed eye tracking (Otto et al. 1988), auditory (Otto et al. 1988) and somatosensory (Smith et al. 1988) evoked potentials, vibratory threshold (Franzblau et al. 1989), perception of transcutaneous stimulation (Katims et al. 1989), centrally mediated motor dysfunction (Arendt et al. 1989), and cortical stimulation (Moglia et al. 1989).

Imaging.   Many studies (Navia et al. 1986; Olsen et al. 1988) have described MRI and CT abnormalities in patients with AIDS, but their correlation with clinical pathology is frequently low (Janssen et al. 1988; McArthur et al. 1989a). Mild cerebral atrophy on CT did not correlate with neuropsychological impairment (Aronow et al. 1989); sulcal widening on MRI was not associated with neurological and CSF abnormalities (Koralnik et al. 1989). Of 107 patients with HIV-induced CNS disease, 31 (29%) had normal CT and MRI scans (Henkes et al. 1989). Arendt et al. (1989) reported that EEG was more sensitive than MRI in detecting HIV pathology of the CNS. As with EEG, CNS imaging is indicated in HIV-seropositive patients to explore the differential diagnosis of OMD due to treatable opportunistic infections or tumors, not to assess HIV-OMD.

Mild cerebral atrophy on CT and lucent areas on MRI bear no consistent relationship to clinical findings (Jarvik et al. 1988). When organic mental syndrome is suspected and both CT and MRI are unremarkable, either enhanced MRI (Henkes et al. 1989) or single photon emission computed tomography (SPECT) (Pigorini et al. 1989) may be more sensitive and specific in detecting a lesion. In a longitudinal study (Grant et al. 1989b), development of neuropsychological impairment was predicted by initial MRI findings of high cortical fluid levels and subcortical hyperdensities. This result is consistent with the neuropsychological and laboratory findings discussed above: various tests indicating CNS involvement may be harbingers of later development of HIV-OMD.

PROGRESSION OF HIV-OMD

Case reports (Morgan et al. 1988) have described rapid mental decline in some HIV-seropositive subjects, whereas others have a protracted and fluctuant course (Berger and Mucke 1988). Sidtis et al. (1989) found that of 132 patients initially diagnosed as having equivocal or subclinical AIDS, about 25% developed clinically significant dementia within 9 months, and another 25% did so within a year.

Many investigators have noted that risk of neuropsychological impairment increases with disease progression (Chave et al. 1989; Tross et al. 1988). However, others have not confirmed this. The largest longitudinal study (Selnes et al. 1990) found no decline in neuropsychological performance among 238 men remaining in CDC stages II and III for approximately 1 year, although the analysis excluded 50 subjects who developed AIDS-related complex or AIDS. Longitudinal studies of progressive neuropsychological impairment must consider concurrent systemic disease, opportunistic infections and malignancies of the CNS, and side effects of medications, all of which can cause OMD not directly caused by HIV itself. The development of any CNS complication markedly decreases survival time (Wilson et al. 1989).

TREATMENT

Treatment of HIV-OMD must be tailored to each patient. Strategies include psychoeducation, psychosocial support, evaluation of suicide potential, and pharmacotherapy (Faulstich 1987; Perry and Markowitz 1986).

Psychoeducation should begin before patients develop neuropsychological impairment or HIV-OMD. This provides them the opportunity to make informed decisions about their lives while they still possess time, competence, and judgment to do so. Neuropsychological impairment should not be explained in an alarming manner.

The clinician can assert that HIV-related mental changes are not inevitable and are unlikely to be dramatic unless the patient has become severely ill. It is important to differentiate HIV-neuropsychological impairment and OMD from Alzheimer's dementia. Sexual partners and family members may also be counseled about the risk of cognitive changes.

Psychosocial treatments for patients with severe neuropsychological impairment include measures generally undertaken for dementia: titration of external stimuli, repeated correction of misperceptions and distortions, maintenance of a familiar environment, and structuring of the environment to prevent impulsive behavior, including HIV transmission (Ostrow et al. 1988; also see Chapter 24). Interpersonal support can dramatically aid patients and those surrounding them, who often feel isolated by this stigmatizing illness and have limited resources for problem solving.

Assessment of suicidal risk is a necessary component of treating AIDS-related OMD. Marzuk et al. (1988) found the odds ratio for suicide in 20- to 50-year-old male New Yorkers who had AIDS to be 36 times that of those without AIDS. Since knowledge of HIV infection does not seem to increase suicidal intent (Perry et al. 1990b), increased rates may be related to premorbid mood disorders or substance abuse (Atkinson et al. 1988), psychosocial stressors (Faulstich 1987), systemic illness (Whitlock 1986), depression and delirium secondary to medication (Marzuk et al. 1988), or the development of HIV-OMD. The lower levels of CSF serotonin metabolites found in some HIV-seropositive subjects have been associated with impulsive violent behavior, including suicide (Mann et al. 1986).

Pharmacotherapy for HIV-OMD includes antiviral and symptomatic neurological, analgesic, and psychotropic medication. Patients with OMD often have decreased pain tolerance and may express their discomfort through disruptive behavior. Analgesia alleviates agitation, irritability, and anger in both patients and their caretakers (Perry and Marotta 1987).

Psychopharmacology for secondary mood and behavioral disorders is under study. Psychostimulants have demonstrated efficacy in treating the apathy, lethargy, and withdrawal of patients with AIDS (Fernandez et al. 1988). Depressed subjects with AIDS-related complex responded better to antidepressants than those with AIDS (Fernandez et al. 1989b). High-potency neuroleptics appear more likely to produce severe dystonia and neuroleptic malignant syndromes (Swenson et al. 1989) in patients with HIV-related delirium and psychosis; lower-potency neuroleptics or benzodiazepines may be more effective in producing acute sedation. Electroconvulsive therapy (ECT) has been safely used with AIDS patients (Schaerf et al. 1989).

SECONDARY CNS DISEASE IN HIV-SEROPOSITIVE PATIENTS

As HIV progressively cripples the immune response to infection, patients become vulnerable to infection both from without and within. Usually nonpathogenic organisms in the external environment and harmless internal flora have the "opportunity" to attack the defenseless patient. Previously suppressed syphilitic or tubercular infections may recrudesce. In the absence of immune surveillance, HIV-infected patients are much more susceptible to a wide array of malignancies; more than one opportunistic infection, cancer, or neurological disorder may arise simultaneously. Treatments for these illnesses are often themselves toxic. As relapses

are common, internists struggle to balance prophylaxis of infection with minimizing the toxicity of medications. The following outline of common infections and
tumors is hardly exhaustive (Table 19–2).

Pneumocystis Carinii Pneumonia (PCP)

Pneumocystis is a commensal organism residing in alveoli. PCP is a hallmark of
AIDS, the initial opportunistic infection in 60% of cases and a complication in
more than 80% overall (Glatt et al. 1988). PCP often begins with apparently benign
symptoms: an unproductive cough and mild dyspnea on exertion. It may take several weeks before fever, weight loss, and respiratory distress require hospitalization. Chest roentgenogram may be unremarkable, but usually shows a diffuse
granular infiltrate radiating symmetrically from the hilum. Diagnosis is confirmed
by bronchoscopic washings or biopsy.

Treatment of PCP has improved considerably: hospitalizations are shorter and
survival rates higher, increasing overall life expectancy of patients with AIDS. Common medications are trimethoprim and sulfamethoxazole (Bactrim), diaminodi-
phenylsulfone (Dapsone), α-difluromethylornithine (DFMO), and intravenous
pentamidine isethionate. Seropositive individuals, even if asymptomatic or without
history of PCP, are often prophylactically given aerosolized pentamidine, Bactrim, or
Dapsone; pentamidine appears least toxic (Montgomery et al. 1987).

Zidovudine decreases recurrence of PCP. Zidovudine inhibits reverse trans-
criptase, the retroviral enzyme crucial for HIV replication. In double-blind (Fischl et
al. 1987) and open (Creagh-Kirk et al. 1988) trials, the drug increased longevity and
quality of life for patients with AIDS and provided some protection against opportunistic infections; it may also improve HIV-induced mental changes, at least in children
(Pizzo et al. 1988).

Zidovudine has significant side effects, particularly macrocytic anemia and gran-
ulocytopenia (Richman et al. 1987). Administering zidovudine in conjunction with
dideoxycytidine (Yarchoan et al. 1988), another viral enzyme blocker, may maximize
antiviral effect with less toxicity. Zidovudine itself can cause fatigue and a depression-
like syndrome that is often difficult to distinguish from psychological factors, direct
effects of HIV, and secondary illnesses.

Toxoplasma Gondii

Toxoplasma gondii is a protozoan that principally affects the CNS by causing an
encephalitis with headache, fever, delirium, and coma (Luft et al. 1984), or mass
lesions in the brain that produce seizures, mental changes, and focal neurological
findings. Mass lesions can be diagnosed either by CT or MRI. Treatment requires
pyrimethamine and sulfadiazine for at least 6–8 weeks (Wong et al. 1984). HIV-
infected patients should avoid handling raw meat and cat litter boxes, prime
sources of *Toxoplasma*.

Cryptococcus

Cryptococcus is a fungus that can cause fulminant and multisystemic infection.
Encephalitic patients may present with subtle mental changes, including depres-

sion, in the absence of meningeal signs or focal findings (Dismukes 1988). Diagnosis is made by lumbar puncture. Amphotericin B is the principal treatment, with flucytosine added if the patient does not have bone marrow suppression. Treatment generally takes more than 6 weeks (Zuger et al. 1986).

Candida

This fungus often causes a discomfiting albeit not dangerous oral thrush (candidiasis), enveloping the tongue and oral cavity in white. Often an early sign of immune dysfunction, thrush responds to topical nystatin, clotrimazole troches, or oral

Table 19–2. Common secondary human immunodeficiency virus (HIV)-associated disease

Etiology	Neuropsychiatric symptoms	Treatments
Pneumocystis carinii pneumonia (PCP)	Cough, dyspnea, fever, and weight loss	Pentamidine Trimethoprim and sulfamethoxazole Diaminodiphenylsulfone
Toxoplasma gondii	Headache, fever, delirium, and coma; seizures, mental status changes, and focal neurological findings	Pyrimethamine Sulfadiazine
Cryptococcus	Encephalitis, organic mood disorder, and mental status change	Amphotericin B Flucytosine Fluconazole

Candida	Thrush and systemic infection	Local
		  Nystatin
		  Ketoconazole
		  Clotrimazole troches
		Systemic
		  Ketoconazole
		  Amphotericin B

Gastrointestinal *Fiosospora Cryptosporidium*	Diarrhea	Symptomatic
Cytomegalovirus (CMV)	Meningoencephalitis; pneumonia, retinitis, and colitis	Dihydroxypropoxymethylguanine (DHPG)
Herpes zoster virus	Multidermatomal shingles	Acyclovir
Herpes simplex virus	Encephalitis; mucocutaneous ulceration	Acyclovir
Atypical mycobacteria	Cough, fever, weight loss, and night sweats	(Antitubercular medication until *Mycobacterium tuberculosis* has been ruled out)
Kaposi's sarcoma	Violaceous lesions of skin and internal organs	Cosmetics Topical cryo- or radiotherapy α-Interferon and chemotherapy for advanced lesions
Central nervous system lymphoma	Focal neurological findings; mental status changes	Chemotherapy; surgery

ketoconazole, which is continued for life. Candidal infection of the esophagus, trachea, bronchi, lungs, and systemic dissemination are more worrisome. Systemic involvement is confirmed by biopsy and treated with ketoconazole or amphotericin B.

Gastrointestinal Pathogens

Unrecognized as human pathogens before the AIDS epidemic, *cryptosporidium* and *Fiosospora* cause severe, chronic, watery, and ultimately fatal diarrhea. There are no effective treatments. Symptomatic management consists of hydration, electrolyte replacement, and opiate control of bowel motility. Management is often further complicated when *Giardia lamblia,* amoebae, or other protozoans are present, as may frequently occur in sexually active gay men.

Viral Pathogens

More than 95% of homosexual men are seropositive for cytomegalovirus (CMV) (Felsenstein et al. 1985). In HIV-infected patients CMV can cause pneumonia, meningoencephalitis, and retinitis leading to blindness. CMV retinitis and colitis show some response to dihydroxypropoxymethylguanine (DHPG), although the drug causes marrow suppression and relapse is common (Felsenstein et al. 1985).

Herpes zoster virus can cause severe, multidermatomal "shingles." Even the usually milder herpes simplex virus (HSV) may produce gastrointestinal and CNS disease. Local mucocutaneous HSV lesions may progress to chronic, enlarging perianal ulcers, particularly in homosexual males with AIDS. Oral acyclovir effectively treats mucocutaneous lesions and has relatively few side effects; used for prophylaxis, it may help prevent HIV immune impairment (Strauss et al. 1984).

Other Pathogens

HIV-infected patients may have reactivation of previously treated *Mycobacterium tuberculosis* (MTB). Early symptoms such as cough, fatigue, weight loss, fevers, and night sweats may be misattributed to HIV or PCP before pulmonary or miliary spread make secondary MTB infection evident. For this reason, skin testing of HIV-infected patients is advisable, perhaps followed by isoniazid prophylaxis (Pitchenik et al. 1986). HIV-infected patients are also susceptible to infection with atypical mycobacteria, most commonly *Mycobacterium avium cellulare* (MAI). Because prodromal symptoms of fever, weight loss, and malaise mimic HIV and other infections, MAI may be missed until severe abdominal pain, diarrhea, and malabsorption occur. The toxicity of standard antitubercular drugs is high and their effectiveness doubtful (Hawkins et al. 1986). Yet patients with mycobacterial infections should be treated at least until the organism is subtyped, because MTB is responsive to isoniazid, rifampin, ethambutol, and other medications.

Patients with a history of documented, adequate treatment for syphilis may have recurrence with immunosuppression, developing the otherwise rare stigmata of secondary and tertiary lues. Other pathogens include *Coccidioides* and *Histoplasma* (especially in endemic geographic regions), *Salmonella septicemia,* and, in children, the agent causing lymphoid interstitial pneumonitis.

HIV-Related Malignancies

Various types of malignancies have been reported in association with HIV, of which two are especially noteworthy to psychiatrists. Kaposi's sarcoma (KS), a previously rare disorder that had comprised only 0.02% of all malignancies in the United States (Robbins and Cotran 1979), was among the first clinical markers identifying AIDS to physicians. KS associated with HIV is aggressive and disseminated; skin lesions are easily diagnosed by their characteristic purplish color and absence of blanching when pressed. Smaller early skin lesions or suspected lung lesions require biopsy for diagnosis. KS has occurred almost exclusively among seropositive gay men and has decreased in incidence from nearly half of all early cases of AIDS to roughly 16% of the current United States caseload.

KS alone is not usually lethal and may linger chronically before suddenly increasing internal and external lesions produce severe disfigurement and respiratory compromise. Vincristine and other highly toxic oncotherapeutic regimens are then employed. α-Interferon and other agents have been approved for palliative treatment (Kaplan et al. 1987). The second neoplasm relevant to psychiatry is lymphoma of the brain, which can cause mental changes before diagnosis. Prognosis for these tumors is worse than that for cancer patients without HIV infection.

CONCLUSIONS

HIV is responsible either directly or indirectly for a complex, symptomatically overlapping series of disorders. Most HIV-seropositive individuals are physically asymptomatic, and it is unclear how prevalent and significant neuropsychiatric impairment is in this population. No single clinical or laboratory finding is pathognomonic either of HIV-induced neuropsychiatric impairment or of OMD directly caused by HIV itself. The clinician assessing patients who are seropositive or at risk for HIV must keep in mind the great variability of presentations and comorbidities accompanying the virus.

REFERENCES

American Psychiatric Association: Diagnostic and Statistical Manual of Mental Disorders, 3rd Edition, Revised. Washington, DC, American Psychiatric Association, 1987

Appleman ME, Marshall DW, Brey RL, et al: Cerebrospinal fluid abnormalities in patients without AIDS who are seropositive for the human immunodeficiency virus. J Infect Dis 158:193–199, 1988

Arendt G, Hefter H, Elsing C, et al: Motor dysfunction and cognitive disturbances in 50 clinically asymptomatic HIV-infected patients with normal MRI scans, in Abstracts of the Fifth International Conference on AIDS. Montreal, Quebec, International Development Research Centre, 1989, p 460

Aronow H, Keilp JG, Krol G, et al: Cerebral atrophy in HIV-1 infected patients: relationship to neurological and neuropsychological measures, in Abstracts of the Fifth International Conference on AIDS. Montreal, Quebec, International Development Research Centre, 1989, p 458

Atkinson JH, Grant I, Kennedy J, et al: Prevalence of psychiatric disorders among men infected with human immunodeficiency virus. Arch Gen Psychiatry 45:859–864, 1988

Beresford TP, Blow FC, Hall RCW: AIDS encephalitis mimicking alcohol dementia and depression. Biol Psychiatry 21:394–397, 1986

Berger JR: The neurological complications of HIV infection. Acta Neurol Scand 116:40–76, 1988

Berger JR, Mucke L: Prolonged survival and partial recovery in AIDS-associated progressive multifocal leukoencephalopathy. J Neurol 38:1060–1065, 1988

Brew BJ, Bhalla RB, Fleisher M, et al: Cerebrospinal fluid beta 2 microglobulin in patients infected with human immunodeficiency virus. Neurology 39:830–834, 1989

Britton CB, Kranzler S, Naini A, et al: Serotonin metabolite deficiency in HIV infection and AIDS, in Abstracts of the Fifth International Conference on AIDS. Montreal, Quebec, International Development Research Centre, 1989, p 453

Centers for Disease Control: Revision of the CDC surveillance case definition for acquired immunodeficiency syndrome. MMWR 36 (suppl 1):1S–15S, 1987

Chave JP, Thuillard F, Assal G, et al: Neuropsychological manifestations of HIV infection: a prospective study, in Abstracts of the Fifth International Conference on AIDS. Montreal, Quebec, International Development Research Centre, 1989, p 451

Cohen JA, Laudenslager M: Autonomic nervous system involvement in patients with human immunodeficiency virus infection. Neurology 39:1111–1112, 1989

Cornblath DR, McArthur JC: Predominantly sensory neuropathy in patients with AIDS and AIDS-related complex. J Neurol 38:794–796, 1988

Creagh-Kirk T, Doi P, Andrews E, et al: Survival experience among patients with AIDS receiving zidovudine. JAMA 260:3009–3015, 1988

Cummings JL, Benson DF: Subcortical dementia: review of an emerging concept. Arch Neurol 41:874–879, 1984

Dilley JW, Boccellari A, Davis A: The use of the Mini-Mental State Exam as a cognitive screen in patients with AIDS, in Abstracts of the Fifth International Conference on AIDS. Montreal, Quebec, International Development Research Centre, 1989, p 384

Dismukes WE: Cryptococcal meningitis in patients with AIDS. J Infect Dis 157:624–628, 1988

Fauci AS: The human immunodeficiency virus: infectivity and mechanisms of pathogenesis. Science 239:617–622, 1988

Faulstich ME: Psychiatric aspects of AIDS. Am J Psychiatry 144:551–556, 1987

Felsenstein D, D'Amico DJ, Hirsch MS, et al: Treatment of cytomegalovirus retinitis with O-[2-hydroxy-1(hydroxymethyl) ethoxymethyl] guanine. Ann Intern Med 103:377–380, 1985

Fernandez F, Adams F, Levy JK, et al: Cognitive impairment due to AIDS-related complex and its response to psychostimulants. Psychosomatics 29:38–46, 1988

Fernandez F, Levy JK, Pirozzolo FP: Neuropsychological and immunological abnormalities in advanced HIV infection, in Abstracts of the Fifth International Conference on AIDS. Montreal, Quebec, International Development Research Centre, 1989a, p 384

Fernandez F, Levy JK, Mansel PWA: Response to antidepressant therapy in depressed persons with advanced HIV infection, in Abstracts of the Fifth International Conference on AIDS. Montreal, Quebec, International Development Research Centre, 1989b, p 383

Fischl MA, Richman DD, Grieco MH, et al: The efficacy of azidothymidine (AZT) in the treatment of patients with AIDS and AIDS-related complex. N Engl J Med 317:185–191, 1987

Fitzgibbon ML, Cella DF, Mumfleet G, et al: Motor slowing in asymptomatic HIV infection. Percept Mot Skill 68:1331–1338, 1989

Folstein MF, Folstein SE, McHugh PR: Mini-Mental State: a practical method for grading the cognitive state of patients for the clinician. J Psychiatr Res 12:189–198, 1975

Franzblau A, Letz RE, Hershman D, et al: Quantitative vibration threshold testing and computer-based neurobehavioral testing of persons infected with HIV, in Abstracts of the Fifth International Conference on AIDS. Montreal, Quebec, International Development Research Centre, 1989, p 462

Gabuzda DH, Ho DD, de la Monte SM, et al: Immunohistochemical identification of HTLV-III antigen in brains of patients with AIDS. Ann Neurol 20:289–295, 1986

Glatt AE, Chirgwin K, Landesman SH: Treatment of infections associated with human immunodeficiency virus. N Engl J Med 318:1439–1448, 1988

Grant I, Atkinson JH, Hesselink JR, et al: Evidence for early central nervous system involvement in AIDS and other HIV infections. Ann Intern Med 107:828–836, 1987

Grant I, Olshen R, Atkinson H, et al: Discriminating depression from cognitive impairment in HIV illness, in Abstracts of the Fifth International Conference on AIDS. Montreal, Quebec, International Development Research Centre, 1989a, p 390

Grant I, Heaton RK, Jernigan T, et al: Neuropsychological changes in CDC II, III, and IV persons after 6 to 12 months: evidence for decline, in Abstracts of the Fifth International Conference on AIDS. Montreal, Quebec, International Development Research Centre, 1989b, p 459

Gray F, Gherardi R, Keohane C, et al: Pathology of the central nervous system in 40 cases of acquired immunodeficiency syndrome (AIDS). Neuropathol Appl Neurobiol 14:365–380, 1988

Hawkins CC, Gold JMW, Whimbey E, et al: Mycobacterium avium complex infections in patients with acquired immunodeficiency syndrome. Ann Intern Med 105:184–188, 1986

Henkes H, Schorner W, Jochens R, et al: MR imaging of intracranial manifestations of AIDS: unenhanced and GD-DTPA enhanced studies, in Abstracts of the Fifth International Conference on AIDS. Montreal, Quebec, International Development Research Centre, 1989, p 215

Herns M, Newman S, McAllister R, et al: Mood state, neuropsychology and self-reported cognitive deficits in HIV infection, in Abstracts of the Fifth International Conference on AIDS. Montreal, Quebec, International Development Research Centre, 1989, p 382

Heyward WL, Curran JW: The epidemiology of AIDS in the U.S. Sci Am 259(4):72–81, 1988

Janssen RS, Saykin AJ, Kaplan JE, et al: Neurological complications of human immunodeficiency virus infection in patients with lymphadenopathy syndrome. Ann Neurol 23:49–55, 1988

Jarvik JG, Hesselink JR, Kennedy C, et al: Acquired immunodeficiency syndrome: magnetic resonance patterns of brain involvement with pathologic correlation. Arch Neurol 45:731–736, 1988

Kaplan LD, Wofsy CB, Volberding PA: Treatment of patients with acquired immunodeficiency syndrome and associated manifestations. JAMA 257:1367–1373, 1987

Katims JJ, Taylor DN, Wallace JI, et al: Current perception threshold in HIV positive patients, in Abstracts of the Fifth International Conference on AIDS. Montreal, Quebec, International Development Research Centre, 1989, p 463

Keilp JG, Brew BJ, Heyes M, et al: Tryptophan levels are unrelated to disturbances of mood in HIV-1 infected patients, in Abstracts of the Fifth International Conference on AIDS. Montreal, Quebec, International Development Research Centre, 1989, p 384

Kermani EJ, Borod JC, Brown PH, et al: New psychopathologic findings in AIDS: case report. J Clin Psychiatry 46:240–241, 1985

Kobayashi J, Heaton R, Thompson L, et al: A comparison of neuropsychological testing and mental status exam in AIDS patients, in Abstracts of the Fifth International Conference on AIDS. Montreal, Quebec, International Development Research Centre, 1989, p 382

Kocsis AE, Church J, Vearnals S, et al: Personality, behavior, and cognitive changes in AIDS as rated by patients and their careers and as related to neuropsychological test results, in Abstracts of the Fifth International Conference on AIDS. Montreal, Quebec, International Development Research Centre, 1989, p 385

Koppel BS, Wormer GP, Tuchman AJ, et al: Central nervous system involvement in patients with acquired immune deficiency syndrome (AIDS). Acta Neurol Scand 71:337–353, 1985

Koralnik I, Beaumanoir A, Hausler R, et al: Abnormalities of EEG and otoneurologic tests in asymptomatic HIV infected homosexuals: a prospective controlled study, in Abstracts of the Fifth International Conference on AIDS. Montreal, Quebec, International Development Research Centre, 1989, p 462

Levy RM, Bredesen DE, Rosenblum ML: Neurological manifestations of the acquired immunodeficiency syndrome (AIDS): experience at UCSF and review of the literature. J Neurosurg 62:475–495, 1985

Luft BJ, Brooks RG, Conley FK, et al: Toxoplasmic encephalitis in patients with the acquired immunodeficiency syndrome. JAMA 252:913–915, 1984

McArthur JC, Cohen BA, Farzedegan H, et al: Cerebrospinal fluid abnormalities in homosexual/bisexual men with and without neuropsychiatric findings. Ann Neurol 23 (suppl):S34–S37, 1988

McArthur JC, Cohen BA, Selnes OA, et al: Low prevalence of neurological and neuropsychological abnormalities in otherwise healthy HIV-1-infected individuals: results from the Multicenter AIDS Cohort Study. Ann Neurol 26:601–611, 1989a

McArthur JC, McArthur JH, Herman C, et al: Increasing CSF abnormalities in HIV-1 infected individuals with declining systemic immune status, in Abstracts of the Fifth International Conference on AIDS. Montreal, Quebec, International Development Research Centre, 1989b, p 463

Mann JJ, Stanley M, McBride PA, et al: Increased serotonin-2 and beta-adrenergic receptor binding in the frontal cortices of suicide victims. Arch Gen Psychiatry 43:954–959, 1986

Markowitz J, Perry S: AIDS: a medical overview for psychiatrists, in American Psychiatric Press Review of Psychiatry, Vol 9. Edited by Tasman A, Goldfinger SM, Kaufmann CA. Washington, DC, American Psychiatric Press, 1990, pp 574–592

Marotta R, Perry S: Early neuropsychological dysfunction caused by the human immunodeficiency virus. Journal of Neuropsychiatry and Clinical Neurosciences 1:225–235, 1989

Marzuk PM, Tierney H, Tardiff K, et al: Increased risk of suicide in patients with AIDS. JAMA 259:1333–1337, 1988

Moglia A, Zandrini C, Alfonsi E, et al: Electrophysiological investigation of central and peripheral nervous system in HIV-infected patients, in Abstracts of the Fifth International Conference on AIDS. Montreal, Quebec, International Development Research Centre, 1989, p 215

Montgomery AB, Debs RJ, Luce JM, et al: Aerosolised pentamidine as sole therapy for pneumocystis carinii pneumonia in patients with acquired immunodeficiency syndrome. Lancet 2:480–483, 1987

Morgan MK, Clark ME, Hartman WL: AIDS-related dementia: a case report of rapid cognitive decline. J Clin Psychiatry 44:1024–1028, 1988

Navia BA, Price RW: The acquired immunodeficiency syndrome dementia complex as the presenting or sole manifestation of human immunodeficiency virus infection. Arch Neurol 44:65–69, 1987

Navia BA, Jordan BD, Price RW: The AIDS dementia complex, I: clinical features. Ann Neurol 19:517–524, 1986

Northern California Neurobehavioral Group: Test Booklet for the Neurobehavioral Cognitive Status Examination. Fairfax, CA, Northern California Neurobehavioral Group, 1988

Olsen WL, Longo FM, Mills CM, et al: White matter disease in AIDS: findings at MR imaging. Radiology 169:445–448, 1988

Ostrow D, Grant I, Atkinson H: Assessment and management of the AIDS patient with neuropsychiatric disturbances. J Clin Psychiatry 49:S14–S22, 1988

Otto D, Hudnell K, Boyes W, et al: Electrophysiological measures of visual and auditory function as indices of neurotoxicity. Toxicology 49:205–218, 1988

Parisi A, Di Perri G, Strosselli M, et al: Usefulness of computerized electroencephalography in diagnosing, staging, and monitoring AIDS-dementia complex. AIDS 3:209–213, 1989

Perry SW: Organic mental disorders caused by HIV: update on early diagnosis and treatment. Am J Psychiatry 147:696–710, 1990

Perry SW, Jacobsen P: Neuropsychiatric manifestations of AIDS-spectrum disorders. Hosp Community Psychiatry 37:135–142, 1986

Perry SW, Markowitz J: Psychiatric interventions for AIDS-spectrum disorders. Hosp Community Psychiatry 37:1001–1006, 1986

Perry SW, Markowitz J: Organic mental disorders, in The American Psychiatric Press Textbook of Psychiatry. Edited by Talbott JA, Hales RE, Yudofsky SC. Washington, DC, American Psychiatric Press, 1988, pp 279–311

Perry S, Marotta R: AIDS dementia: a review of the literature. Alzheimer Dis Assoc Disord 1:221–235, 1987

Perry SW, Tross S: Psychiatric problems of AIDS inpatients at The New York Hospital: a preliminary report. Public Health Rep 99:200–205, 1984

Perry S, Belsky-Barr D, Barr WB, et al: Neuropsychological function in physically asymptomatic, HIV-seropositive men. Journal of Neuropsychiatry and Clinical Neurosciences 1:296–302, 1989

Perry S, Jacobsberg LB, Fishman B, et al: Psychiatric diagnosis before serological testing for the human immunodeficiency virus. Am J Psychiatry 147:89–93, 1990a

Perry S, Jacobsberg L, Fishman B: Suicidal ideation and HIV testing. JAMA 263:679–682, 1990b

Pigorini F, Pau FM, Galgani S, et al: Single photon emission computed tomography findings in HIV infection, in Abstracts of the Fifth International Conference on AIDS. Montreal, Quebec, International Development Research Centre, 1989, p 458

Pitchenik AE, Burr J, Cole CH: Tuberculin testing for persons with positive serologic studies for HTLV-III (letter). N Engl J Med 314:447, 1986

Pizzo PA, Eddy J, Falloon J, et al: Effect of continuous infusion of zidovudine (AZT) in children with symptomatic HIV infection. N Engl J Med 319:889–896, 1988

Portegies P, Epstein LG, Hun ST, et al: Human immunodeficiency virus type 1 antigen in cerebrospinal fluid: correlation with clinical neurologic status. Arch Neurol 46:261–264, 1989

Price RW, Brew BJ: The AIDS dementia complex. J Infect Dis 158:1079–1083, 1988

Price RW, Brew B, Sidtis J, et al: The brain in AIDS: central nervous system HIV-1 infection and AIDS dementia complex. Science 239:586–591, 1988

Price RW, Brew BJ, Rosenblum M: The AIDS Dementia Complex and HIV-1 brain infection: a pathogenic model of virus-immune interaction, in Immunological Mechanisms in Neurological and Psychiatric Disease. Edited by Waksman BH. New York, Raven, 1990

Richman DD, Fischl MA, Grieco MH, et al: The toxicity of azidothymidine (AZT) in the treatment of patients with AIDS and AIDS-related complex. N Engl J Med 317:191–197, 1987

Riedel RR, Clarenbach P, Bulau P, et al: Neurological and neuropsychological deficits in 240 HIV-seropositive hemophiliacs in WR2-6, in Abstracts of the Fifth International Conference on AIDS. Montreal, Quebec, International Development Research Centre, 1989, p 210

Robbins SL, Cotran RS (eds): Pathologic Basis of Disease. Philadelphia, PA, WB Saunders, 1979

Schaerf FW, Miller RR, Lipsey JR, et al: ECT for major depression in four patients infected with human immunodeficiency virus. Am J Psychiatry 146:782–784, 1989

Selnes OA, Miller E, McArthur J, et al: HIV-1 infection: no evidence of cognitive decline during the asymptomatic stages. Neurology 40:204–208, 1990

Sidtis JJ, Thaler H, Brew BJ, et al: The interval between equivocal and definite neurological signs and symptoms in the AIDS dementia complex, in Abstracts of the Fifth International Conference on AIDS. Montreal, Quebec, International Development Research Centre, 1989, p 215

Smith T, Jakobsen J, Gaub J, et al: Clinical and electrophysiological studies of human immunodeficiency virus-seropositive men without AIDS. Ann Neurol 23: 295–297, 1988

Stern Y, Sano M, Goldstein S, et al: Neuropsychological manifestations of HIV infection in gay men, in Abstracts of the Fifth International Conference on AIDS. Montreal, Quebec, International Development Research Centre, 1989, p 383

Strauss SE, Seidlin M, Takiff H, et al: Oral acyclovir to suppress recurring herpes simplex virus infections in immunodeficient patients. Ann Intern Med 100:522–524, 1984

Swenson JR, Erman M, Labell J, et al: Extrapyramidal reactions: neuropsychiatric mimics in patients with AIDS. Gen Hosp Psychiatry 11:248–249, 1989

Temoshok L, Canick JP, Sweet DM: Cognitive dysfunction and psychosocial factors in symptomatic seropositive men, in Abstracts of the Fifth International Conference on AIDS. Montreal, Quebec, International Development Research Centre, 1989, p 385

Tross S, Price RW, Navia B, et al: Neuropsychological characterization of the AIDS dementia complex: a preliminary report. AIDS 2:81–88, 1988

Van Gorp W, Miller E, Satz P, et al: Neuropsychological performance in HIV-1 immunocompromised patients, in Abstracts of the Fifth International Conference on AIDS. Montreal, Quebec, International Development Research Centre, 1989, p 464

Visscher BR, Miller E, Satz P, et al: Neuropsychological followup of 1,787 participants in the Multicenter AIDS Cohort Study, in Abstracts of the Fifth International Conference on AIDS. Montreal, Quebec, International Development Research Centre, 1989, p 449

Whitlock FA: Suicide in physical illness, in Suicide. Edited by Roy A. Baltimore, MD, Williams & Wilkins, 1986, pp 151–170

Wilson MJ, Lemp GF, Neal D, et al: The epidemiology of AIDS-related neurologic diseases, in Abstracts of the Fifth International Conference on AIDS. Montreal, Quebec, International Development Research Centre, 1989, p 449

Wong B, Gold JWM, Brown AE, et al: Central nervous system toxoplasmosis in homosexual men and parenteral drug abusers. Ann Intern Med 100:36–42, 1984

Yarchoan R, Mitsuya H, Broder S: AIDS therapies. Sci Am 259(4):110–119, 1988

Zuger A, Louie E, Holzman RS, et al: Cryptococcal disease in patients with the acquired immunodeficiency syndrome. Ann Intern Med 104:234–240, 1986

Chapter 20

Neuropsychiatric Features of Endocrine Disorders

Morris B. Goldman, M.D.

In this chapter I review those hormonal deficiencies and excesses most clearly associated with neuropsychiatric syndromes. The gonadal axis is not addressed. Releasing factors and anterior pituitary trophic hormones are discussed with their prime target hormones; panhypopituitarism is discussed in the section on adrenal insufficiency (which it frequently mimics).

Neuropsychiatric symptoms are prominent in many endocrine disorders, and in some cases the first medical contact may be the psychiatrist. In most cases, prompt treatment of the endocrinopathy leads to resolution of the neuropsychiatric signs and symptoms. To promote expedient diagnosis, psychiatrists should familiarize themselves with the characteristic symptoms and signs (Table 20–1) and the preliminary screening studies.

Although the neuropsychiatric features vary both within and between the different endocrinopathies, endocrinopathies of similar severity and duration tend to share similar neuropsychiatric features. Thus mild to moderately severe abnormalities lasting weeks to months often manifest a combination of affective and anxiety symptoms (Table 20–2). Most patients with such abnormalities have mild cognitive impairments. By contrast, longstanding mild to moderately severe endocrinopathies are more likely to present with personality changes characterized by apathy or dementia (Table 20–3).

Acute severe disease, or longstanding disease that progresses to a severe disorder, is likely to induce an acute delirium, which may herald a catastrophic outcome (Table 20–4). In some cases the delirium is clearly linked to secondary metabolic disturbances. Psychotic symptoms most often occur with delirium. Some severe (and occasionally moderate) endocrinopathies induce automatisms, depersonalization, or heightened sensory awareness. In these cases, the patient may be incorrectly diagnosed with temporal lobe epilepsy or somatoform disorder.

The suspicion of an underlying endocrinopathy should be high in treatment-resistant atypical affective or anxiety syndromes in which vegetative or cognitive complaints appear out of proportion to the other symptoms. Also late-onset personality disorders characterized by apathy, "neurasthenia," depersonalization, or automatisms warrant an endocrine assessment. Finally, treatment-resistant or atypical

The author wishes to acknowledge Jeff Bennett for assistance in preparing this chapter; Mary B. Dratman, Daniel J. Luchins, and Ned Weiss for their constructive reviews; and Lela Louis for secretarial assistance.

psychotic patients and all patients presenting with dementia should have an endocrine disorder excluded. Table 20–5 summarizes the endocrinopathies that should be considered in the differential diagnosis of common primary psychiatric disorders. The screening tests for each are uncomplicated, except for that for hypocortisolism.

THYROID HORMONE

The term *hyperthyroidism* is sometimes limited to excessive hormone production by the thyroid gland, but it is used here to mean thyrotoxicosis of any etiology. Lithium interferes with hormone biosynthesis and release and may accelerate autoimmune thyroiditis. Hypothyroidism occurs in about 10% of patients on lithium and is more common in those with diminished thyroid reserve, particularly women

Table 20–1. Nonpsychiatric symptoms and signs of endocrinopathies

Endocrinopathy	Symptoms	Signs
Hyperthyroidism	Diaphoresis	Tachycardia
	Heat intolerance	Tremor
	Oligomenorrhea	Proptosis
Hypothyroidism	Cold intolerance	Goiter
	Menorrhagia	Reflex delay
	Muscle cramps	Myxedema
Hypercortisolism	Oligomenorrhea	Hirsutism
	Easy bruising	Moon facies
	Weakness	Hypertension
Hypocortisolism	Nausea	Hypotension
	Weakness	Hyperpigmentation
Panhypopituitarism[a]	Nausea	Hypotension
	Weakness	
Hyperparathyroidism	Nausea	Hypertension
	Polyuria	
	Abdominal pain	
Hypoparathyroidism	Muscle spasms	Choreiform movements
	Paresthesias	
Hyperinsulinism	Diaphoresis	Tachycardia
	Hunger	
Hypoinsulinism	Polydipsia	Neuropathy
	Polyuria	
	Polyphagia	
Excessive vasopressin	Nausea	Ataxia
	Headache	Tremor
	Weakness	Weight gain
Deficient vasopressin	Polydipsia	Fever dehydration
	Polyuria	
Hyperprolactinemia	Galactorrhea[b]	Gynecomastia
	Amenorrhea	Osteoporosis
	Impotence[c]	

[a]Function of affected hormones.
[b]In females.
[c]In males.

and rapid cyclers. It can occur early or after several years of therapy (Erhardt and Goldman 1991). Lithium has been associated with hyperthyroidism, but the link may be coincidental (Yassa et al. 1988).

Table 20–2. Symptoms of mild or moderate endocrinopathies lasting weeks to months

Endocrinopathy	Anxious	Depressed	Impaired cognition[a]	Mimics psychiatric disorder
Hyperthyroidism	++	+	C, M	++
Hypothyroidism	+	++	C, M	++
Hypercortisolism	++	++	C, M, H	++
Hypocortisolism	+	++		++
Panhypopituitarism[b]	+	++		++
Hyperparathyroidism	+	++	M	++
Hypoparathyroidism	++	+	?	++
Hyperinsulinism	++		H, C	++
Hypoinsulinism			C	
Excessive vasopressin			C, M	+[c]
Deficient vasopressin			M	+[d]
Hyperprolactinemia	+	++[e]		+

Note. + = sometimes; ++ = often.
[a]C = concentration; M = memory; H = higher order functions (e.g., abstract thinking).
[b]Function of affected hormones.
[c]May mimic psychotic exacerbation in psychiatric patient.
[d]Psychogenic polydipsia.
[e]Females more than males.

Table 20–3. Symptoms of mild or moderately severe longstanding endocrinopathies

Endocrinopathy	Apathy	Dementia	Other personality changes[a]	Cyclical course
Hyperthyroidism	++		L	
Hypothyroidism	++	+		
Hypercortisolism				+
Hypocortisolism	+	+	P	
Panhypopituitarism[b]	+	+		
Hyperparathyroidism	++	++[c]	I	
Hypoparathyroidism	?	+++		
Hyperinsulinism	++	+	D,L	+
Hypoinsulinism		?		
Excessive vasopressin	+			
Deficient vasopressin				
Hyperprolactinemia	+[d]			

Note. + = usually mild; ++ = usually moderate; +++ = usually prominent.
[a]L = labile; P = paranoia; D = dementia; I = irritable.
[b]Function of affected hormones.
[c]Predominantly elderly; may be of short duration.
[d]Males.

Hyperthyroidism

Diagnostic issues.   About 10% of psychiatric inpatients (regardless of diagnosis) show transient elevations of total serum triiodothyronine (T-3), thyroxine (T-4), and free (unbound) T-4 index, apparently because of pituitary or hypothalamic stimulation (Rose 1985). Thus psychiatric inpatients who have elevated thyroid hormone levels on admission should have tests repeated 2 weeks later. Acute drug intoxication, particularly with psychostimulants, can closely mimic hyperthyroidism and may also produce transient hyperthyroidism.

Patients with hyperthyroidism may be distinguished from those with primary anxiety disorders by warm rather than cold skin, increased appetite, and a reported inability to associate anxiety to specific ideas or concerns (Jefferson and Marshal 1981). Hyperthyroidism can usually be distinguished from mania by decreased energy and activity levels. On the other hand, hyperthyroidism in bipolar patients is easily missed, because hyperthyroidism may precipitate mania, and subsequent lithium treatment may lead to a partial response (by its antithyroid and antimanic actions).

Details of neuropsychiatric features.   Pervasive anxiety, insomnia, and tense dysphoria are common. Patients may be tearful and crying and baffled about why. Depression may occur but is rarely prominent in younger patients. Psychological testing, although confirming the presence of increased anxiety and depression, rarely fits prescribed patterns of psychiatric illnesses (Bauer et al. 1987). The elderly, however, who are often apathetic, may exhibit classic melancholia.

Diminished concentration and memory are frequent complaints in all hyperthyroid patients and can be confirmed by standard psychological batteries. Many of these symptoms are seen in control subjects given thyroid hormone (Bauer et al. 1987). Psychosis is occasionally seen as part of a delirium and may herald the potentially

Table 20–4.   Other neuropsychiatric features of severe endocrinopathies

Endocrinopathy	Psychosis plus delirium	Psychosis without delirium	Other[a]
Hyperthyroidism	+		
Hypothyroidism	++		I
Hypercortisolism	++		D, I
Hypocortisolism	++		H
Panhypopituitarism[b]	++		H
Hyperparathyroidism	++	++	
Hypoparathyroidism	++		A
Hyperinsulinism	++		A, D
Hypoinsulinism	+		
Excessive vasopressin	+		
Deficient vasopressin	+		
Hyperprolactinemia			

Note.   + = sometimes present; ++ = often present.
[a]H = heightened sensory acuity; I = impaired sensory acuity; A = automatisms; D = depersonalization.
[b]Function of affected hormones.

fatal thyroid storm. Psychosis was diagnosed more frequently in the past, perhaps because of a higher prevalence of severe endocrinopathy or overly zealous use of the term *psychosis.*

Treatment. Neuropsychiatric symptoms (including the putative personality syndrome) usually reverse with antithyroid treatment, but a year may be needed for complete recovery (Bauer et al. 1987). Psychosis may occur or be exacerbated by antithyroid medication, and haloperidol and perphenazine may induce a syndrome resembling thyroid storm and neuroleptic malignant syndrome in psychotic hyperthyroid patients (Bauer et al. 1987). Available evidence suggests low-potency neuroleptics are tolerated in hyperthyroid patients and thus should be prescribed if indicated.

Hypothyroidism

Diagnostic issues. Patients with primary hypothyroidism have been divided into three groups corresponding to grades of severity of symptoms and hormone deficiency. Patients with mild ("subclinical") hypothyroidism (i.e., grade III) may present

Table 20–5. Endocrinopathies resembling primary psychiatric disorders

Anxiety disorders	Hyperthyroidism[a]
	Hypercortisolism
	Panhypopituitarism
	Hypoparathyroidism
	Hyperinsulinism
Affective disorders	Hyperthyroidism[b]
	Hypothyroidism
	Hypocortisolism
	Hypercortisolism
	Panhypopituitarism
	Hyperparathyroidism
	Hyperprolactinemia[a]
Anorexia nervosa	Hypocortisolism
	Panhypopituitarism
Somatoform disorder	Hypothyroidism
	Hypercortisolism
	Hypoparathyroidism
	Hyperinsulinism
Psychotic disorders	Hypothyroidism
	Hypercortisolism
	Hypocortisolism[a]
	Panhypopituitarism[a]
	Hyperparathyroidism
	Hypoparathyroidism[a]
	Hyperinsulinism[a]
Dementia	Hypothyroidism
	Hyperparathyroidism[b]
	Hypoparathyroidism[a]
	Hyperinsulinism[a]

[a]Can usually be distinguished from primary psychiatric disturbance by careful history.
[b]In elderly.

solely with psychiatric symptoms (Extein and Gold 1988). Grade III hypothyroidism can only be diagnosed by measuring the thyrotropin (TSH) response to thyrotropin-releasing hormone (TRH) because thyroid hormone levels and TSH are normal. Generally, TSH is obtained as the routine screening test for hypothyroidism. Although total T-4 is diminished in severe cases of hypothyroidism, it may be normal in moderate cases, which still require thyroid replacement (i.e., grade II).

Because moderate hormone deficiency can closely mimic primary anxiety and depression (and particularly postpartum disorders), it is reasonable routinely to order TSH levels in these instances. Routine TRH testing (to rule out grade III hypothyroidism) in patients with affective disorders cannot be recommended until the incidence and significance of these mild disturbances and the benefits of thyroid replacement therapy (or any treatment different from standard antidepressant regimens) have been more clearly established.

Details of neuropsychiatric features.   Acute and especially longstanding hypothyroidism are associated with changes in cognition and affective state. Changes in cognition may occur alone and seem more pervasive than mood disturbances (Loosen 1986). Affective disturbances ranging from mild depression to psychosis and suicidality occur in more than one-half of patients with grade I hypothyroidism (Bauer et al. 1987). Depression, and to a lesser extent anxiety, may occur as early as 3 weeks after the onset of hypothyroidism, particularly in patients with histories of affective disorders (Denicoff et al. 1990). Marked irritability, emotional lability, and insomnia are frequently seen. Patients have a reduced amount of stage 3 and stage 4 sleep, similar to that seen in depression. Psychosis occurs in about 10% of patients with grade I hypothyroidism, but may rarely be seen in milder cases. The quality of the psychosis is nonspecific and usually is part of a delirium.

Changes in concentration may be apparent as early as 3 weeks after the onset of the hypothyroid state, before other cognitive functions are altered (Denicoff et al. 1990). A progressive slowing of mental processing follows, characterized by diminished initiative and impaired memory and concentration (easily identified by asking the patient to perform serial subtractions) (Jefferson and Marshal 1981). Many patients report losing things and making "stupid" mistakes. Although initially very frustrated, ultimately the patient becomes indifferent. Longstanding disease induces marked dementia (Bauer et al. 1987).

Treatment.   Nearly complete recovery of cognitive and affective deficits can be anticipated with thyroid replacement in adult patients with grade I hypothyroidism. Neuropsychiatric symptoms may be the first to resolve, with patients recovering completely over the course of a few days with just thyroid hormone replacement, although complete recovery can take up to 6 months. Moderate doses of neuroleptics (e.g., 2–4 mg of haloperidol) are usually well tolerated, although patients who become psychotic may not fully recover. Many believe that affective symptoms are resistant to treatment with antidepressants alone.

Thyroid hormone relieves physical symptoms in patients with grade II hypothyroidism. However, definitive studies have not yet established whether affective disorders associated with grade II or grade III hypothyroidism preferentially respond either to thyroid hormone alone or in combination with standard antidepressant therapy.

Hypothyroidism must be corrected slowly because acute cardiac or neuropsychiatric decompensation (Bauer et al. 1987) can occur with rapid replacement, particularly in the elderly. Finally, hypothyroidism in patients receiving lithium may spontaneously resolve. If it does not, replacement therapy with T-4 should be instituted, and T-4 and TSH should be monitored to exclude both excessive and inadequate treatment.

CORTISOL

Cushing's syndrome may present as an organic mood, anxiety, or personality syndrome or with delirium. Iatrogenic Cushing's syndrome, and occasionally other causes of Cushing's syndrome, can induce an organic delusional syndrome or organic hallucinosis. Neuropsychiatric changes, particularly depression or personality changes, may be the exclusive presenting symptoms.

Adrenal insufficiency may be accompanied by an organic personality or mood syndrome. Delirium may presage adrenal crisis. In both hypercortisolism and adrenal insufficiency, periods of neuropsychiatric symptoms may be punctuated by return to premorbid function.

Hypercortisolism

Diagnostic issues. Patients with Cushing's syndrome may look similar to persons with alcoholism, who, on the other hand, may have all the physical and biochemical signs of Cushing's syndrome. Because the depression in Cushing's syndrome may be cyclical (Reus 1987) and occur in the absence of physical symptoms (Starkman et al. 1986b), it can closely resemble a primary affective disease.

The similarities of hypercortisolism and depression have led investigators to posit a fundamental link between the two disorders. A popular hypothesis, that excess corticotropin-releasing factor (CRF) causes hypercortisolism and depression in primary psychiatric illness could not, however, account for the neuropsychiatric symptoms in Cushing's disease because CRF is presumably suppressed.

Corticosteroid abuse cannot be diagnosed by measuring basal steroid levels (because endogenous production is suppressed, and the oral agents are present in small quantities), but it can be suspected if the patient shows no evidence of adrenal insufficiency yet has a diminished cortisol response to adrenocorticotropic hormone (ACTH) stimulation.

Details of neuropsychiatric features. Depression and anxiety (with or without panic attacks) are seen in about half the patients with Cushing's syndrome. Cognitive changes (most marked in spatial and visual ideation) are equally common, though less pronounced, and may be a consequence of depression (Starkman et al. 1986b).

Patients usually emphasize sadness, decreased libido, insomnia, somatic preoccupation, depersonalization, and impaired concentration (Reus 1987). Unlike most patients with primary major affective disorders, though, many Cushing's syndrome patients note mood lability and deny anhedonia, inappropriate guilt, and hopelessness (Starkman et al. 1986a). Pure mania or hypomania is infrequent (except with oral corticosteroids), and instead the picture resembles that of a mixed manic and depressed state. Suicidal preoccupation or action is not unusual (Jefferson and Marshal

1981). The severity of depression has been related to levels of steroid production (Starkman et al. 1986a).

Psychosis occurs in up to 20% of cases. A delirium is often present and may be a result of electrolyte disturbances, congestive heart failure, hypertensive encephalopathy, or uncontrolled diabetes. Either manic or depressive symptoms may accompany paranoia, auditory and visual hallucinations, and disorientation. Patients frequently complain of sensory flooding and may become mute.

Neuropsychiatric symptoms may occur in patients treated with prednisone (Reus 1987) and are related to dose and duration of treatment. Acute response seen in most patients includes a mild euphoria, increased appetite, insomnia, irritability, and restlessness. Patients may become depressed on steroid withdrawal, leading to continued elicit use. Psychosis, with or without altered consciousness and cognition, has been reported in up to 20% of patients receiving prednisone 80 mg/day or more and may be more common in women.

Treatment.   Neuropsychiatric symptoms improve in parallel with normalization of urinary free cortisol, although complete recovery may take months to years (Starkman et al. 1986a). Diminished libido lags behind the recovery of other symptoms.

The treatment of neuropsychiatric symptoms in patients with iatrogenic Cushing's syndrome is often challenging because of the likelihood of relapse of the underlying condition on steroid withdrawal and the frequent difficulty of identifying the cause of neuropsychiatric exacerbations. If possible, patients should be on alternative-day therapy, receiving medication in the morning to simulate the diurnal pattern and to minimize insomnia.

Tricyclic antidepressants may exacerbate depression secondary to hypercortisolism, particularly if the patient is psychotic. The optimal treatment of depression has not been determined, though electroconvulsive therapy may help. Lithium carbonate and neuroleptics appear to be effective in preventing or treating mania (Reus 1987).

Hypocortisolism

Diagnostic issues.   Weakness, anorexia, nausea, vomiting, and weight loss are the classic presenting symptoms of adrenal insufficiency. Patients may have hypotension and hyperpigmentation. "Chronic fatigue syndrome," characterized by at least 6 months of fatigue, fever, myalgias, arthralgias, and depression after an acute infection, has also recently been linked in preliminary reports to adrenal insufficiency (Demitrack et al. 1990).

Panhypopituitarism often presents with signs and symptoms of adrenal insufficiency (except for easy tanning). It is usually caused by pituitary or hypothalamic damage and less frequently by ischemic necrosis (e.g., postpartum), aneurysms, or radiation. Although apathy and weakness are usually the prominent symptoms, the disorder may present as hypogonadism or hypothyroidism (Smith et al. 1972).

Patients with adrenal insufficiency may very closely resemble patients with major depression or anorexia nervosa, and the correct diagnosis is easily missed. Recent onset of easy, prolonged tanning; gastrointestinal distress; hypotension; other medical disorders (e.g., tuberculosis, amyloidosis, and carcinoma); and particularly autoimmune diseases may be helpful clues.

Details of neuropsychiatric features. Fluctuating anxiety, depression, and suspiciousness are seen in about half of the patients with hypocortisolism. In almost all cases of anxiety, depression is also present. The patient may have anorexia nervosa, and the voice may be weak and whiny (Jefferson and Marshal 1981). Intellectual function has not been carefully assessed. Occasionally the history is that of a progressive dementia. Patients often show (but rarely are aware of) heightened sensory acuity, which has been linked to diminished latency of the evoked responses (Reus 1987). Such changes may contribute to the occasional diagnosis of somatoform disorder. Diminished slow-wave sleep (stages 3 and 4) has been documented. Finally, frank psychosis usually occurs in the context of a delirium, with visual hallucinations, paranoia, bizarre posturing, and catatonia described (Jefferson and Marshal 1981).

Treatment. The use of psychotropic drugs and the normalization of affective state following glucocorticoid replacement have not been adequately studied (Jefferson and Marshal 1981). Persistence of neuropsychiatric symptoms may indicate other concurrent endocrinopathies (e.g., hypothyroidism) (Johnstone et al. 1990). In some cases the neuropsychiatric symptoms, particularly psychosis, can be attributed to secondary metabolic impairments; however, complete recovery does not occur until glucocorticoids have been replaced (Reus 1987).

Patients with hypocortisolism are notoriously sensitive to central nervous system (CNS) depressants and are particularly susceptible to drugs that induce hypotension. Lithium may alter the requirements for mineralocorticoid replacement, and it may be difficult to maintain stable lithium levels.

PARATHYROID AND SERUM CALCIUM REGULATION

Hypercalcemia can present as an organic personality or mood syndrome, dementia, or delirium. It is more likely than other endocrinopathies to present with an organic delusional syndrome. As with hypothyroidism, hypercortisolism, and hypocortisolism, neuropsychiatric changes occur early on and may be the only prominent symptoms. This is particularly true in the elderly, in whom minimal changes can induce reversible dementia. Hypocalcemia may be a chronic disorder with prominent neuropsychiatric, but minimal neuromuscular symptoms. Lithium induces mild increases in parathyroid hormone (PTH) in about 80% of patients within the first month of treatment, but significant increases may occur and are related to dose and duration of treatment (Mallette and Eichhorn 1986).

Hyperparathyroidism and Hypercalcemia

Diagnostic issues. The normal range of PTH varies with the assay. Because hypercalcemia is common and can mimic many neuropsychiatric conditions and because calcium levels are inexpensive and easily obtained, the disorder should be excluded in most psychiatric diagnostic evaluations.

Details of neuropsychiatric features. Neuropsychiatric symptoms are found in 66% of hyperparathyroid patients in prospective studies (G. G. Brown et al. 1987). Fatigue, apathy, diminished appetite, concentration, and depression occur in about half the patients. Suicidality is not uncommon, and several completed suicides have occurred. A personality change may occur over the course of years, and a previously active and sociable person may become progressively withdrawn, incapacitated, and depressed. The symptoms are similar in quality, but diminished in intensity, to those of primary depression (Linder et al. 1988). Cognitive testing reveals impaired verbal memory, although it is unclear if this is related to depression or other effects of hypercalcemia (G. G. Brown et al. 1987).

Acute psychotic paranoid states, with or without depression, have occurred with clear sensorium. Patients may become extremely violent and homicidal (R. S. Brown et al. 1987). Delirium with prominent hallucinations and delusions occurs with high levels of serum calcium (Petersen 1968). The elderly are very sensitive to hypercalcemia and may develop dementia with very mild increases in serum calcium (Joborn et al. 1986). Electroencephalographic (EEG) changes are not a sensitive diagnostic tool (Cooper and Schapira 1973).

Treatment.   If the disorder is not chronic, cognitive and affective symptoms are generally reversed by normalizing serum calcium. In particular, elderly patients with dementia who also have hyperparathyroidism usually show considerable improvement if surgery is done within the first 2 years of the illness (Joborn et al. 1986). Improvement is evident within a matter of days and appears to plateau by 3–6 months.

Appropriate treatment of middle-aged, mildly hypercalcemic, "asymptomatic" hyperparathyroid patients is controversial, although most would operate on younger, healthy patients based on the inconvenience of lifetime monitoring. Clearly, if patients complain of fatigue and muscle weakness they are likely to benefit from surgery. The response of other symptoms, such as depression and anxiety, is not predictable (Heath 1989; McAllion and Paterson 1989). Several cases of a delayed, self-limited, postparathyroidectomy psychosis with altered consciousness have been described (Mikkelsen and Reider 1979) and related to the rapid drop in serum calcium that occurs in patients with hypercalcemia and secondary bone disease.

Patients on lithium who become hypercalcemic should first have a lithium level obtained, to rule out lithium toxicity (the two cations are handled similarly by the kidney). If asymptomatic, the patient may be followed, or given another antimanic agent. In either case, calcium levels should be rechecked because lithium may induce, or accelerate, the growth of parathyroid adenomas. Lithium may be restarted after parathyroidectomy (Mallette and Eichhorn 1986).

Hypoparathyroidism and Hypocalcemia

Diagnostic issues.   Serum calcium and inorganic phosphorous should be obtained in suspected cases of hypocalcemia and followed up with ionized calcium and PTH if further workup is indicated. Referral of patients with undiagnosed mild cases of hypocalcemia (partial parathyroid insufficiency) to psychiatrists for treatment-resistant anxiety is not unusual. Anxious hypocalcemic patients may have panic disorder, causing them to hyperventilate and develop tetany (Fourman et al. 1967). Thus hypocalcemia should be excluded in all cases of hyperventilation-induced tetany. Rarely the picture resembles bipolar disorder (Denko and Kaelbling 1962).

Hypocalcemic patients who exhibit choreiform movements, paresthesias, and atypical seizures may be referred to psychiatry for "histrionic behavior." These patients may exhibit no symptoms of tetany, and the EEG may be normal (Fonseca and Calverley 1967).

Details of neuropsychiatric features.   The neuropsychiatric features of hypocalcemia have not been as carefully studied as those of other endocrinopathies. Neuropsychiatric symptoms, particularly anxiety and dementia, are common. In addition, patients may appear depressed, parkinsonian, or have choreiform movements. Typical and atypical seizures are frequent. Progressive intellectual decline is particularly common in hereditary hypoparathyroidism and pseudohypoparathyroidism.

Treatment.   Patients with mild hypocalcemia and no symptoms other than anxiety and depression may have "partial parathyroid insufficiency," which benefits from calcium supplementation (Fourman et al. 1967). With severe hypocalcemia, delirium may take 1–3 months to clear and may recur periodically during the recovery period despite "normocalcemia." Because serum calcium is usually maintained in the low-normal range (to prevent kidney stones), the recurrences may actually be secondary to hypocalcemia. Dementia tends to respond poorly.

Seizures and anxiety respond poorly to anticonvulsant and antianxiety agents, respectively (Carlson 1986). Hypocalcemic patients are reported to be more susceptible to the development of extrapyramidal syndrome (EPS) when given neuroleptic medication, although calcium levels (within the normal range) do not appear to influence EPS (Pratty et al. 1986).

INSULIN

The neuropsychiatric effects of hyperinsulinism include organic anxiety, personality, amnestic, or delusional syndrome; delirium and dementia; and other organic mental syndromes characterized by dissociative symptoms and automatisms. Hyperglycemia may predispose to subtle deficits in higher cognitive functions. The two major metabolic complications of diabetes mellitus (diabetic ketoacidosis [DKA] and nonketotic hyperosmolar syndrome) induce delirium and coma.

Premature neonates are also frequently hypoglycemic. Several fatal cases of hypoglycemia have occurred in anorexia nervosa (Rich et al. 1990), and irreversible complications occurred not infrequently in schizophrenic patients who received insulin shock therapy. If the hypoglycemia occurs abruptly (as in postsurgical situations and the controversial idiopathic postprandial syndrome), adrenergic symptoms of anxiety, tremor, diaphoresis, and tachycardia tend to predominate, along with hunger and weakness. In cases of chronic hypoglycemia (e.g., insulinoma), "neuroglyclopenic" symptoms, including loss of concentration, confusion, emotional lability, automatisms, and amnesia, are more prominent.

Hyperinsulinism and Hypoglycemia

Diagnostic issues.   The diagnosis of hypoglycemia requires 1) demonstration of hypoglycemia with fasting or after meals similar to those inducing symptoms (if postprandial); 2) the presence of symptoms consistent with hypoglycemia; and 3) improvement with normalization of glucose levels.

Many hypoglycemic patients seek medical advice because of postprandial adrenergic symptoms and are found to have an "abnormal" (i.e., blood glucose <50 mg/dl) 5-hour glucose tolerance test. These patients may be given a diagnosis of hypoglycemia even though they never become hypoglycemic with normal meals, and many nonhypoglycemic subjects have similar glucose levels but no symptoms. Psychological testing suggests that many of these patients have a somatoform disorder (Jefferson and Marshal 1981).

Factitious hypoglycemia caused by surreptitious administration of insulin occurs most frequently in medical personnel, family members of diabetic patients, or the diabetic patients themselves. In the first two groups, the diagnosis can be made with depressed C peptide levels. However, diagnosis can be difficult in diabetic patients (Grunberger et al. 1988). Case reports suggest that these patients usually have serious personality disturbances (Toth 1990) and respond poorly to psychotherapy (Grunberger et al. 1988).

On the other hand, patients with hypoglycemia may be mistakenly diagnosed as hysteric, epileptic, or intoxicated because they exhibit a combination of dissociative states, automatisms, and rage (Jefferson and Marshal 1981). In many cases hypoglycemic patients have appeared assaultive and paranoid and hence given a primary psychiatric diagnosis. In retrospect, however, these patients had clear signs of delirium: either waxing consciousness or disorientation (Steinberg and Mackenzie 1989). In instances of recurrent episodic hypoglycemia, diagnosis may be challenging.

Many patients with abrupt onset of hypoglycemia due to insulin treatment have anxiety attacks that are difficult for the patient and physician to distinguish from a primary anxiety disorder. Furthermore, patients with diabetes seem prone to develop anxiety disorders because of the stress of the illness and as a "conditioned" response to prior episodes of hypoglycemia (Steel et al. 1989).

Details of neuropsychiatric features.   Unchecked lowering in blood glucose may cause excitement, overactivity, automatisms, muscular spasms, and finally decerebrate rigidity. In control subjects, neurophysiological changes (increased latency of the P300 component of the event-related brain potential) and subtle cognitive impairment are apparent at plasma glucose levels in the range of 45–70 mg/dl and increase in proportion to further reduction in blood glucose levels (Table 20–6) (Blackman et al. 1990). Attention and memory seem less impaired than do higher order cognitive functions (Widom and Simonson 1990).

The neuropsychiatric response of patients with diabetes mellitus (whether or not they are in good glycemic control) is similar to that of nondiabetic individuals. In particular, even though basal glucose levels modulate the threshold for the adrenergic and other hormones involved in the counterregulatory response to hypoglycemia (i.e., lower the threshold for hormone release for those in tight control and raise it for those who are hyperglycemic), the neuroglycopenic threshold is unrelated to basal glucose (Widom and Simonson 1990).

Many diabetic patients lose the adrenergic behavioral response entirely, or it may occur at progressively lower blood glucose levels (Widom and Simonson 1990). Thus these patients may depend on neuroglycopenic signals to identify hypoglycemia. If, however, confusion is the primary symptom, the patient may be unable to react appropriately. Elderly patients, and perhaps those with chronic mental disorders

(Fishbain and Rotundo 1988), also appear to lose their adrenergic behavioral response. Recurring episodes of moderate hypoglycemia may produce irreversible neurophysiological and cognitive changes in neonates (Lucas et al. 1988), in children, and to a lesser extent in adults (Ryan 1988).

Treatment. Although recovery from moderate levels of hypoglycemia is usually complete (except for amnesia for the incident), recovery from the so-called medullary phase (i.e., blood glucose ≤ 10 mg/dl) is often prolonged and incomplete. Chronic hypoglycemia and multiple episodes of symptomatic hypoglycemia cause irreversible deficits. In modest hypoglycemia, full cognitive recovery lags reestablishment of euglycemia by about 1 hour (Blackman et al. 1990).

Hypoinsulinism and Hyperglycemia

Diagnostic issues. The diagnosis of hyperglycemia is generally not difficult to make, but the physician must remain alert. In particular, symptoms of polyuria or polyphagia in psychiatric patients should not be attributed to medication side effects or psychogenic polydipsia until diabetes mellitus has been excluded.

Details of neuropsychiatric features. In adults, a history of poorly controlled diabetes (as assessed by retinopathy or glycosylated hemoglobin values) appears to impair learning, but the impairment is usually of little clinical significance (Ryan 1988). Longstanding disease is associated with micro- and macrocerebrovascular changes, which can cause multiple neuropsychiatric deficits. The severe metabolic complications of diabetes mellitus are DKA and hyperosmolar coma. Both present as a delirium, progressing to coma. Patients with hyperosmolar coma frequently convulse and may exhibit focal neurological signs.

VASOPRESSIN

Arginine vasopressin, the antidiuretic hormone, is secreted by the posterior pituitary (neurohypophysis) in response to increases in plasma sodium concentration

Table 20–6. Neuropsychiatric response to hypoglycemia

Blood glucose (mg/dl)	P300[a]	Cognition	Attention	Amnesia	Activity	Automatism	Decorticate
45–70	Increase						
30–45	Increase	Decrease					
20–30	NM	Decrease[b]	Decrease	+	Increase		
10–20	NM	Decrease[b]	Decrease[b]	+	Increase or decrease[b]	Increase	
10	NM	(coma)	(coma)	+	Decrease[b]		+

Note. NM = not measurable; + = present.
[a]Latency of P300 component of evoked potential.
[b]Markedly decreased.

and plasma osmolality. The hormone acts on the distal nephron to increase water reabsorption and is the major means by which the body regulates water content. The regulatory centers for vasopressin secretion and thirst appear to lie adjacent to each other in the hypothalamus.

Excessive vasopressin may induce hyponatremia and water intoxication; whereas vasopressin deficiency causes polyuria and a secondary polydipsia. If water intake does not keep up with water loss, the patient becomes hypernatremic and delirious. Studies have shown that 3%–5% of chronic psychiatric patients have elevated vasopressin levels (Illowsky and Kirch 1988). Impaired water excretion in other psychiatric patients is often attributable to antidepressant-induced hypotension (particularly in the elderly) (Emsley et al. 1990). Current evidence suggests that neuroleptics rarely play a role (Raskind et al. 1987).

Excessive Vasopressin and Hyponatremia

Diagnostic issues.   Many times the diagnosis of hyponatremia is missed and psychiatric patients with seizures secondary to water intoxication are erroneously given the diagnosis of idiopathic epilepsy and maintained on anticonvulsant medication (which probably does not reduce the incidence of seizures) (Erhardt and Goldman 1991; Illowsky and Kirch 1988). Water intoxication (along with other secondary causes) should always be excluded after diagnosing a seizure disorder in a psychotic patient, particularly if the seizure is followed by a massive diuresis or the patient has a history of polydipsia, vomiting, or prior alcohol abuse (Ripley et al. 1989).

Because patients may be normonatremic between episodes, the diagnosis may require measuring diurnal weight changes over a 1- to 2-week period (Godleski et al. 1989) and taking a careful history focusing on latent symptoms of water intoxication (Goldman 1991). Special care should be taken to exclude lung cancer because psychiatric patients are usually heavy smokers and lung cancer frequently causes the syndrome of inappropriate antidiuresis (SIAD).

Details of neuropsychiatric features.   Moderate acute hyponatremia (120–130 mEq/L) impairs cognition but does not produce affective disturbances or psychosis (Gehi et al. 1981). In psychiatric patients, however, aggression may occur as a result of hyponatremia (Koczapski and Millson 1989). Signs and symptoms of hyponatremia develop as a function of the rapidity of the fall of serum sodium. Thus a drop in sodium level of 10 mEq/L over a few hours may produce symptoms (Koczapski and Millson 1989), whereas markedly diminished levels (i.e., 30 mEq/L below normal) produce no obvious symptoms if they occur over days or weeks. Symptoms may progress with an acute fall in sodium level, or the patient may be asymptomatic but then convulse suddenly. Asymmetrical neurological findings have been described (Fraser and Arieff 1987).

Treatment.   Patients on antidepressants should have orthostatic blood pressure determined and, if indicated, should be switched to another structural class not associated with orthostatic hypotension. Patients requiring treatment for hypertension should be switched from thiazide diruretics to another agent, such as a calcium channel blocker. Patients on carbamazepine may show spontaneous resolution of hyponatremia, or resolution, if the dose is lowered or lithium is added (because it blocks vasopressin's actions). Nicotine, a potent stimulant for arginine vasopressin release, contributes to some cases of hyponatremia (Allon et al. 1990), and thus regulating smoking may help. Patients on thorazine may do better when switched to another neuroleptic with less potential to induce orthostasis.

In some cases of asymptomatic or episodic mild hyponatremia, the clinician may do nothing more than educate the patient and family about early signs and symptoms of water intoxication. Voluntary water restriction may work in medical patients with symptomatic hyponatremia but rarely succeeds with psychiatric patients. If reversible factors are not present, water intoxication in psychiatric inpatients can be prevented by monitoring acute changes in body weight and imposing fluid restriction if weight precipitously increases.

Deficient Vasopressin and Hypernatremia

Diagnostic issues.   Although 24-hour urine collections are the ideal means of diagnosing polyuria, they are often unreliable in psychiatric patients. Preliminary evidence suggests that polyuria can be inferred by obtaining afternoon urine creatinine concentrations, which are highly correlated to 24-hour urine volumes (Goldman et al. 1992). Vasopressin deficiency (versus psychogenic polydipsia or nephrogenic diabetes insipidus; see below) can usually be diagnosed by imposing a fluid restriction. After urine osmolality has become stabilized, the patient receives a subcutaneous injection of vasopressin. Patients with psychogenic polydipsia may take a long time after restriction is imposed to attain a stable urine osmolality, but generally increase their urine osmolality above plasma levels and then show little further increase with vasopressin.

It may be difficult to determine whether the polyuria in psychiatric patients is from psychogenic polydipsia, central diabetes insipidus, or (in certain instances) lithium-induced nephrogenic diabetes insipidus, which may take over a year to resolve after the drug is discontinued. "Psychogenic" polydipsia is exceedingly common among psychiatric patients, occurring in all diagnostic classes and up to 70% of chronic psychotic patients. Because central diabetes insipidus is much less common than primary polydipsia in psychiatric patients, clinicians normally assume the polydipsia is not secondary to a defect in vasopressin secretion. However, the clinician's index of suspicion should be raised if 1) the patient does not have a serious psychiatric disorder, or polyuria is present when other psychiatric symptoms are in complete remission; 2) the serum is hypertonic; 3) the patient has a history of head trauma, CNS surgery, or infection; 4) the patient has a family history of polyuria or diabetes insipidus; 5) the water intake or output seems to vary little day-to-day; or 6) the patient has anorexia nervosa.

Details of neuropsychiatric features.   Hypernatremia in control subjects induces extreme thirst, weakness, and impaired cognition. Impaired consciousness may occur late. The symptoms are rarely confused with a psychiatric disturbance.

Treatment.   Lithium-induced nephrogenic diabetes insipidus usually responds to lowering the lithium dose, changing to a single daily dose, or adding amiloride with or without a thiazide diuretic (Erhardt and Goldman 1991). Care should be taken to reduce the lithium dose if a diuretic is added.

Vasopressin deficiency rarely is responsible for the polyuria in psychiatric patients. If a trial of vasopressin is considered, extreme caution must be used to prevent water intoxication. There are no effective treatments for psychogenic polydipsia, although several interventions have been tried (Goldman 1991). Although the anticholinergic properties of the various psychotropic medications do not appear to make a large contribution to the polydipsia (via dry mouth), polydipsic patients should be treated with drugs with minimal anticholinergic effects.

PROLACTIN

Hyperprolactinemia in women may induce an organic mood syndrome; in men it can induce apathy. The most common cause of hyperprolactinemia in psychiatric patients is neuroleptic medication. Even low doses of neuroleptic drugs can produce the full syndrome of hyperprolactinemia (Erhardt and Goldman 1991).

Diagnostic issues.   Hyperprolactinemia should be based on at least two levels in the absence of stress or pregnancy. Hyperprolactinemia may mimic depression, but symptoms of prolactin excess are nearly always present. Neuroleptics rarely raise prolactin levels above 100 ng/dl. Higher levels suggest the presence of a prolactin-secreting adenoma.

In patients taking neuroleptic medication who consistently show elevated levels, a drug holiday should be employed, if possible, to assess whether prolactin levels fall. One report (Gangbar and Swinson 1983) suggested that 4 days off noninjectable neuroleptic is adequate for drug-induced elevations to normalize.

Details of neuropsychiatric features.   Women with hyperprolactinemia tend to be depressed, with symptoms of increased hostility, anxiety, and diminished self-esteem (Koppelman et al. 1987). Although the severity of these symptoms on self-reports may be severe (Kellner et al. 1984), patients rarely seek psychiatric treatment (Koppelman et al. 1987). Men often present with more advanced disease, complaining of headache and visual field defects (Cohen et al. 1984). Apathy is the predominant neuropsychiatric symptom, which may contribute to the delay in seeking treatment.

Treatment.   Depression is ameliorated with bromocriptine (Koppelman et al. 1987). The salutary effects are apparent within 4 weeks, are maintained over long periods, and are unrelated to recurrence of menses; depression reoccurs with drug withdrawal (Mattox et al. 1986). Both amantadine and bromocriptine are effective in treating symptoms of hyperprolactinemia caused by neuroleptics (Erhardt and Goldman 1991). Psychotic exacerbations are rare as long as the patient is maintained on an antipsychotic. Because of lower cost and fewer side effects, amantadine is preferred.

REFERENCES

Allon M, Allen HM, Deck LV, et al: Role of cigarette use in hyponatremia in schizophrenic patients. Am J Psychiatry 147:1075–1077, 1990

Bauer MS, Droba M, Whybrow PC: Disorders of the thyroid and parathyroid, in Handbook of Clinical Psychoneuroendocrinology. Edited by Nemeroff CB, Loosen PT. New York, Guilford, 1987, pp 41–70

Blackman JD, Towle VL, Lewis GF, et al: Hypoglycemic thresholds for cognitive dysfunction in humans. Diabetes 39:828–835, 1990

Brown GG, Preisman RC, Kleerekoper M: Neurobehavioral symptoms in mild primary hyperparathyroidism: related to hypercalcemia but not improved by parathyroidectomy. Henry Ford Hospital Medical Journal 34:211–215, 1987

Brown RS, Fischman A, Showalter CR: Primary hyperparathyroidism, hypercalcemia, paranoid delusions, homicide, and attempted murder. J Forensic Sci 32:1460–1463, 1987

Carlson RJ: Longitudinal observations of two cases of organic anxiety syndrome. Psychosomatics 27:529–531, 1986

Cohen LM, Greenberg DB, Murray GB: Neuropsychiatric presentation of men with pituitary tumors (the "four A's"). Psychosomatics 25:925–928, 1984

Cooper AF, Schapira K: Case report: depression, catatonic stupor, and EEC changes in hyperparathyroidism. Psychol Med 3:509–515, 1973

Demitrack MA, Dale JK, Laue L, et al: Hypothalamic-pituitary-adrenal activity in patients with chronic fatigue syndrome. Neuroendocrinology Letters 12:343, 1990

Denicoff KD, Joffe RT, Lakshmanan MC, et al: Neuropsychiatric manifestations of altered thyroid state. Am J Psychiatry 147:94–99, 1990

Denko JD, Kaelbling R: The psychiatric aspects of hypoparathyroidism. Acta Psychiatr Scand 38 (suppl 164):1–70, 1962

Emsley RA, Van Der Meer H, Aalbers C, et al: Inappropriate antidiuretic state in long-term psychiatric inpatients. S Afr Med J 77:307–308, 1990

Erhardt VR, Goldman MB: Drug-induced endocrine dysfunction, in Drug-Induced Dysfunction in Psychiatry: Diagnosis and Management. Edited by Keshavan MS, Kennedy J. Washington, DC, Hemisphere Publications, 1991, pp 295–310

Extein IL, Gold MS: Thyroid hormone potentiation of tricyclics. Psychosomatics 29:166–174, 1988

Fishbain DA, Rotundo D: Frequency of hypoglycemic delirium in a psychiatric emergency service. Psychosomatics 29:346–348, 1988

Fonseca OA, Calverley JR: Neurological manifestations of hypoparathyroidism. Arch Intern Med 120:202–206, 1967

Fourman P, Rawnsley K, Davis RH, et al: Effect of calcium on mental symptoms in partial parathyroid insufficiency. Lancet 2:914–915, 1967

Fraser CL, Arieff AL: Metabolic encephalopathy associated with water, electrolyte, and acid-base disorders, in Clinical Disorders of Fluid Electrolyte Metabolism. Edited by Maxwell MH, Kleeman C, Narins R. New York, McGraw-Hill, 1987, pp 1153–1196

Gangbar R, Swinson RP: Hyperprolactinemia and psychiatric illness. Am J Psychiatry 140:790–791, 1983

Gehi MM, Rosenthal RH, Fizette NB, et al: Psychiatric manifestations of hyponatremia. Psychosomatics 22:739–743, 1981

Godleski LS, Vieweg WVR, Hundley PL, et al: Day-to-day case of chronic schizophrenic patients subject to water intoxication. Annals of Clinical Psychiatry 1:179–185, 1989

Goldman MB: A rational approach to disorders of water balance in psychiatric patients. Hosp Community Psychiatry 42:488–494, 1991

Goldman MB, Marks RC, Blake L, et al: Estimating daily urine volume in psychiatric patients: empiric confirmation. Biol Psychiatry 31:1228–1231, 1992

Grunberger G, Weiner JL, Silverman R, et al: Factitious hypoglycemia due to surreptitious administration of insulin. Ann Intern Med 108:252–257, 1988

Heath DA: Primary hyperparathyroidism. Endocrinol Metab Clin North Am 18:631–646, 1989

Illowsky BP, Kirch DG: Polydipsia and hyponatremia in psychiatric patients. Am J Psychiatry 145:675–683, 1988

Jefferson JJ, Marshal JR: Endocrine disorders, in Neuropsychiatric Features of Medical Disorders. New York, Plenum, 1981, pp 133–177

Joborn C, Hetta J, Frisk P, et al: Primary hyperparathyroidism in patients with organic brain syndrome. Acta Med Scandanavia 219:91–98, 1986

Johnstone PA, Rundell JR, Esposito M: Mental status changes of Addison's disease. Psychosomatics 31:103–107, 1990

Kellner R, Buckman MT, Fava GA, et al: Hyperprolactinemia, distress, and hostility. Am J Psychiatry 141:759–763, 1984

Koczapski AB, Millson RC: Individual differences in serum sodium levels in schizophrenic men with self-induced water intoxication. Am J Psychiatry 146:1614–1615, 1989

Koppelman MCS, Parry BL, Hamilton JA, et al: Effect of bromocriptine on affect and libido in hyperprolactinemia. Am J Psychiatry 144:1037–1041, 1987

Linder J, Brismar K, Granberg PO, et al: Characteristic changes in psychiatric symptoms, cortisol and melatonin but not prolactin in primary hyperparathyroidism. Acta Psychiatr Scand 78:32–40, 1988

Loosen PT: Hormones of the hypothalamicpituitary thyroid axis: a psychoneuroendocrine perspective. Pharmacopsychiatry 19:401–415, 1986

Lucas A, Morley R, Cole TJ: Adverse neurodevelopmental outcome of moderate neonatal hypoglycaemia. Br Med J 297:1304–1308, 1988

McAllion SJ, Paterson CR: Psychiatric morbidity in primary hyperparathyroidism. Postgrad Med J 65:628–631, 1989

Mallette LE, Eichhorn E: Effects of lithium carbonate on human calcium metabolism. Arch Intern Med 146: 770–776, 1986

Mattox JH, Buckman MT, Bernstein J, et al: Dopamine agonists for reducing depression associated with hyperprolactinemia. J Reprod Med 31:694–698, 1986

Mikkelsen EJ, Reider AA: Post-parathyroidectomy psychosis: clinical and research implications. J Clin Psychiatry 40:352–358, 1979

Petersen P: Psychiatric disorders in primary hyperparathyroidism. Journal of Clinical Endocrinology 28:1491–1495, 1968

Pratty JS, Ananth J, O'Brien JE: Relationship between dystonia and serum calcium levels. J Clin Psychiatry 47:418–419, 1986

Raskind MA, Courtney N, Murburg MM, et al: Antipsychotic drugs and plasma vasopressin in normals and acute schizophrenic patients. Biol Psychiatry 22:453–462, 1987

Reus VI: Disorders of the adrenal cortex and gonads, in Handbook of Clinical Psychoneuroendocrinology. Edited by Nemeroff CB, Loosen PT. New York, Guilford, 1987, pp 71–84

Rich LM, Caine MR, Findling JW, et al: Hypoglycemic coma in anorexia nervosa. Arch Intern Med 150:894–895, 1990

Ripley TL, Millson RC, Koczapski AB: Self-induced water intoxication and alcohol abuse. Am J Psychiatry 146:102–103, 1989

Rose RM: Psychoendocrinology, in Williams Textbook of Endocrinology, 7th Edition. Edited by Wilson JD, Foster DW. Philadelphia, PA, WB Saunders, 1985, pp 653–681

Ryan CM: Neurobehavioral complications of type 1 diabetes. Diabetes Care 11:86–93, 1988

Smith CK, Barish J, Correa MD, et al: Psychiatric disturbance in endocrinologic disease. Psychosom Med 34:69–86, 1972

Starkman MN, Schteingart DE, Schork MA: Cushing's syndrome after treatment: changes in cortisol and ACTH levels, and amelioration of the depressive syndrome. Psychiatry Res 19:177–188, 1986a

Starkman MN, Schteingart DE, Schork MA: Correlation of bedside cognitive and neuropsychological tests in patients with Cushing's syndrome. Psychosomatics 27:508–511, 1986b

Steel JM, Masterton G, Patrick AW, et al: Hyperventilation or hypoglycaemia? Diabetic Med 6:820–821, 1989

Steinberg PI, Mackenzie R: A patient with insulinoma presenting for psychiatric assessment. Can J Psychiatry 34:68–69, 1989

Toth EL: Factitious hypoglycemia and the multiple personality disorder (letter). Ann Intern Med 112:76, 1990

Widom B, Simonson DC: Glycemic control and neuropsychologic function during hypoglycemia in patients with insulin-dependent diabetes mellitus. Ann Intern Med 112:904–912, 1990

Yassa R, Saunders A, Nastase C, et al: Lithium-induced thyroid disorders: a prevalence study. J Clin Psychiatry 49:14–16, 1988

Chapter 21

Neuropsychiatric Aspects of Poisonous and Toxic Disorders

Lawrence S. Gross, M.D.
Robert M. Nagy, M.D.

In modern society we are exposed to a variety of substances with potential neurotoxic effects. *Toxins* have been defined as substances derived from the tissues of a plant, animal, or microorganism that have a deleterious effect on another plant or animal; *poisons* are substances that, in relatively small amounts, produce death or serious dysfunction of tissues or organs (Russell 1980). In this chapter we use the terms interchangeably and address selected industrial toxicities with prominent neuropsychiatric symptomatology.

METAL POISONING

Although many metals are ubiquitous in nature, their presence in toxic forms and concentrations in the environment has increased significantly since the Industrial Revolution. The neurotoxic effects of certain heavy metals are well documented and are summarized in Table 21–1. Other metals have been less prominently associated with neurotoxicity and are listed in Table 21–2.

Lead

Lead accumulates in the human body throughout life after exposure, which may occur from a variety of environmental sources. The abnormal oral ingestion (pica) of lead-based paints from old houses is a common cause of lead intoxication in children; 70%–90% of children with serious lead poisoning have a history of pica (Feldman 1986). In addition, ingestion of other lead-containing objects as well as contaminated food, water, air, dust, and soil can contribute to pediatric lead toxicity (Chisolm and Barltrop 1979). Adults are most commonly exposed to lead via inhalation in occupations where lead is used in manufacturing and processing. Nonoccupational sources of lead poisoning include ingestion of home-distilled whiskey, eating from unfired pottery, retention of bullets, and gasoline sniffing (Louria 1988).

Adults absorb 5%–10% of an ingested lead load, whereas children have increased gastrointestinal absorption (almost 40%). Absorption after inhalation is 50%–70% if the particle size is small enough to reach the alveoli. Inorganic lead does not pass

Table 21–1. Selected metals with prominent neurotoxic effects

Metal	Delirium	Dementia	Mood changes	Psychosis	Personality changes	Seizures	Peripheral neuropathy	Comments
Aluminum		X			X	X	X	Dialysis dementia; association with Alzheimer's disease, amyotrophic lateral sclerosis, and parkinsonism— dementia (Guam).
Arsenic	X	X	X	X	X	X	X	Large acute arsenic ingestions and acute arsine gas poisoning are frequently fatal.
Lead	X	X	X	X	X	X	X	Subtle subclinical changes.
Lithium	X					X	X	Parkinsonian syndrome, movement disorders, tremor, paralysis, stupor, coma; symptoms may appear at therapeutic as well as toxic levels.
Manganese	X	X	X	X	X			"Manganese madness"; parkinsonism.
Mercury	X	X	X		X	X	X	Intention tremor, ataxia, visual field disturbances; organic mercurials quite neurotoxic.
Thallium	X	X	X	X		X	X	Acute ingestions frequently fatal.

through the skin, but organic lead gasoline additives, such as tetraethyl lead, may be absorbed through intact skin as well as through the lungs.

In the circulation, 95% of lead is in the red blood cells, but, because of distribution into soft tissue or bone stores, blood levels may not reflect the total body lead burden. Ninety percent of total body lead is contained in bone, where lead is principally stored and has a half-life of 20–30 years (Ellenhorn and Barceloux 1988).

Action. Lead interferes with enzyme systems throughout the body, which leads to diffuse effects. In children, severe central nervous system (CNS) symptomatology is thought to be due to lead's easier passage through the blood-brain barrier and disruption of mitochondrial function (Ellenhorn and Barceloux 1988).

Neuropsychiatric manifestations. Lead toxicity in adults may involve both the CNS and the peripheral nervous system. Early manifestations are often nonspecific. Encephalopathy is rare among adults, with most of the reported cases associated with the ingestion of illicit whiskey. Seizures are the most commonly reported symptom (75%), but obtundation, confusion, focal motor dysfunction, papilledema, headaches, and optic neuritis are also described. Cerebrospinal fluid (CSF) changes include elevated opening pressure, increased protein, and slight pleocytosis (Cullen et al. 1983).

In contrast to adults, children are more likely to develop acute lead encephalopathy, the most severe clinical manifestation of lead poisoning. As in adults, early CNS symptoms are often nonspecific ones such as anorexia, apathy, irritability, abdominal pain, vomiting, headache, emotional lability, incoordination, sleep disturbance, and memory lapses. Persistent exposure leads to the rapid development of signs of en-

Table 21–2.   Selected metals with reported neurotoxic effects

Metal	Neuropsychiatric symptoms
Barium	Progressive flaccid paralysis
Copper	Lethargy and coma with severe toxicity
Gold	Encephalopathy with gold therapy
Iron	Lethargy, coma and seizures in severe toxicity
Magnesium	Central nervous system depression, paralysis, and hyporeflexia
Phosphorus	
Yellow phosphorus	Lethargy, stupor, coma, restlessness, hypotension, and shock
Phosphine gas	Headache, fatigue, paresthesias, ataxia, intention tremor, weakness, and diplopia
Platinum	
Cisplatin	Peripheral neuropathy, memory loss, and intention tremor
Potassium	Weakness, paresthesias, hyporeflexia, and paralysis
Selenium	Fatigue, irritability, hyperreflexia, muscle tenderness, and tremor
Tin	
Organic tin compounds	Headache, paresthesias, visual disturbances, tinnitus, deafness, memory loss, disorientation, aggressive behavior, psychosis, movement disorder, and coma
Zinc	Lethargy, ataxia, and writing difficulty

Source.   Ellenhorn and Barceloux 1988.

cephalopathy such as disorientation, psychosis, ataxia, syncope, focal neurological signs, delirium, and lethargy progressing to stupor, seizures, blindness, and coma. Pathologically, the syndrome is characterized by massive cerebral edema with associated vasculopathy.

Chelation therapy has reduced the mortality to less than 5%, but when the therapy is begun after the symptoms of acute encephalopathy appear 25%–50% of patients show permanent neuropsychiatric sequelae such as seizures, blindness, hemiparesis, and mental retardation (Chisolm and Barltrop 1979).

Peripheral nerve involvement occurs much more often in adults than in children; peripheral neuropathy is the most common neurological manifestation of lead toxicity in adults. The neuropathy is typically motor with wrist drop and foot drop seen most frequently. The appearance of clinical neuropathy seems to be related to the magnitude and duration of lead exposure (Cullen et al. 1983).

Psychiatric symptomatology, such as organic affective illness, has been associated with lead intoxication (Schottenfeld and Cullen 1984). Signs of chronic lead intoxication may be confused with depression (Cullen et al. 1983). Organic lead intoxication from inhaling gasoline fumes may cause insomnia, irritability, nervousness, euphoria, delusions, hallucinations, and seizures.

There is increasing evidence of "subclinical" nervous system effects of lead in both children and adults who are found to have increased lead absorption but display no symptoms or only mild nonspecific symptoms of lead intoxication. It has been estimated that between 3 and 4 million American children have blood lead levels above 15 μg/dl, a level previously considered to be safe. Prenatal and postnatal exposure to lead at this level has been associated with undesirable health effects in young children (Agency for Toxic Substances and Disease Registry 1988). Effects include reduced gestational age, reduced birth weight, and impaired neurobehavioral development (Davis and Svendsgaard 1987); slowed motor nerve conduction velocity (Schwartz et al. 1988); and disturbances in attention, learning, and classroom behavior in school children (Needleman 1983). Mean reductions in IQ scores of 4–7 points have been demonstrated in children exposed to lead compared with control groups (Needleman 1989)l; 11-year follow-up of children exposed to lead has shown academic and cognitive deficits persisting into young adulthood (Needleman et al. 1990).

Subclinical CNS effects in adults with increased lead absorption include nonspecific symptoms such as fatigue, irritability, insomnia, nervousness, headache, and weakness along with abnormalities in neuropsychological testing (Cullen et al. 1983). Some subclinical lead-induced neuropsychiatric deficits may be reversible with reduced exposure (Baker et al. 1985; Yokoyama et al. 1988).

Diagnosis. Often the most important diagnostic information is the identification of a history of lead exposure. The whole blood lead level is the best measure of recent exposure. In children, a whole blood level of 25 μg/dl is considered evidence of increased lead absorption (Centers for Disease Control 1985). This threshold level is the result of downward revision in recent years as symptomatology has been demonstrated at progressively lower levels. For adults, a whole blood level of more than 40 μg/dl indicates excessive absorption. Blood concentration of 60 μg/dl or more is indicative of definite lead poisoning in children (Louria 1988); symptoms of lead intoxication appear at slightly higher blood levels in adults. The current allowable industrial concentration is 50 µg/dl; levels above this require removal from the work place until they decrease to below 40 µg/dl (Ellenhorn and Barceloux 1988).

Elevated blood lead levels are accompanied by increases in urinary δ-aminolevulinic acid and coproporphyrin levels. Measurement of blood levels of free erythrocyte protoporphyrin (FEP) is the best screening for chronic lead intoxication. Asymptomatic increased body lead burdens can be detected by measuring urinary lead excretion after administration of calcium disodium edetate (CaNa$_2$EDTA mobilization test) (Ellenhorn and Barceloux 1988).

Treatment and prognosis.   Patients must be removed from the source of lead exposure. Parenterally administered chelating agents dimercaprol (also known as British anti-lewisite; BAL) and CaNa$_2$EDTA are usually administered in combination to bind lead and promote tissue excretion in symptomatic poisoning. Penicillamine is a commercially available oral chelating agent, but its use in lead poisoning remains investigational (Ellenhorn and Barceloux 1988). The U.S. Food and Drug Administration (FDA) has approved an oral chelator succimer, 2,3-dimercaptosuccinic acid (DMSA), for the treatment of lead poisoning in children with blood lead levels above 45 µg/dl (McNeil Consumer Products Company 1991). DMSA appears to be safe, effective, and simple to administer (Graziano et al. 1988). Initial clinical improvement from the reduction of blood lead levels may be followed by reemergence of symptoms requiring further chelation therapy as lead is mobilized from bone. Treatment response of neuropsychiatric manifestations is often slow and incomplete.

Mercury

Mercury has been used for centuries in medicine and industry. The historical use of mercurials for medicinal purposes (e.g., as diuretics and cathartics and in the treatment of syphilis) has largely been discarded. Industrialization has led to increased environmental exposure to mercury via mining, smelting, and the burning of fossil fuels. Mercury is used in dental amalgams and in a variety of industries.

Mercury exists in three forms: elemental mercury, inorganic mercury, and organic mercury. Occupational exposure to elemental and inorganic mercury occurs among miners, smelters, jewelers, photographers, dentists, dental assistants, and makers of mirrors, batteries, and instruments (Landrigan 1982). Mercury from industrial waste and environmental sources usually settles in the aquatic environment and is concentrated in the food chain. Organic mercury compounds, used as fungicides and pesticides, have been associated with occupational exposure but more extensively with community outbreaks of poisoning from eating contaminated fish or grains (Landrigan 1982).

Action.   The toxicity of mercury is thought to result from its high affinity for sulfhydryl groups leading to inhibition of various enzymes and disruption of membrane functions (Landrigan 1982). Methyl mercury inhibits choline acetyltransferase, the enzyme that catalyzes the final step in the synthesis of acetylcholine (Elhassani 1983).

Neuropsychiatric manifestations.   Acute toxic exposure to elemental mercury vapor results primarily in encephalopathy; rarely, seizures occur (Ellenhorn and

Barceloux 1988). Mild exposure to inhaled elemental mercury vapor is associated with subtle symptomatology such as insomnia, nervousness, mild tremor, headache, emotional lability, fatigue, decreased sexual drive, depression, and impaired judgment, coordination, and cognition; these early manifestations have been referred to as *micromercurialism* (Louria 1988).

Toxic symptoms from chronic occupational exposure to elemental mercury involve problems in the oral cavity (e.g., gingivitis, salivation, and stomatitis); tremor (intention tremor that disappears with sleep); and neuropsychological changes (e.g., emotional lability, shyness, and loss of sleep, appetite, and memory) (Ellenhorn and Barceloux 1988). Workers exposed to elemental mercury vapors have shown prolonged motor and sensory distal latencies on nerve conduction testing (Levine et al. 1982).

Toxicity from chronic inorganic mercury exposure is usually occupational and clinically resembles that from chronic inhalation of mercury vapor. The symptoms include dermatitis, gingivitis, stomatitis, tremor, and neuropsychiatric dysfunction termed *erethism*, which is a syndrome consisting of irritability, pathological shyness, and impairment of memory, attention span, and intellect (Landrigan 1982).

Methyl mercury is the most neurotoxic of the short-chain alkyl mercury compounds and serves as the model for organic mercury poisoning. Early symptoms include paresthesias of the limbs, nose, and lips. Motor incoordination, ataxic gait, and loss of position sense are accompanied by dysarthria, constriction of visual fields, hearing defects, and muscle rigidity or spasticity with hyperreflexia. Neuropsychiatric symptoms that have been reported include headache, sleep disturbances, dizziness, irritability, emotional instability, mania, and depression (Elhassani 1983). Methyl mercury easily crosses the blood-brain barrier, exerting a permanent effect on the nervous system, particularly the cerebellum. It also passes through the placenta; established embryotoxic effects include microcephaly and cerebral palsy (Elhassani 1983).

Diagnosis.   Classic findings on physical examination and a history of exposure are often sufficient to identify cases of mercury poisoning, but determining the type and level of mercury in samples of blood, urine, hair, and food will help confirm the diagnosis. Normal concentration of mercury in the blood is less than 3–4 µg/dl; concentrations greater than 4 µg/dl are considered abnormal in adults. Normal urinary mercury excretion is less than 25 µg/L (Klaassen 1985a).

Treatment and prognosis.   After acute inorganic and organic mercury ingestion, treatment should be initiated with the induction of emesis or gastric lavage along with the administration of activated charcoal and cathartics. The use of chelating agents such as dimercaprol (BAL), BAL derivatives, and penicillamine has been helpful in elemental and inorganic mercury poisoning, but these agents have little or no effect in organic intoxication. Dimercaprol is contraindicated in the treatment of organic mercury poisoning because it increases methyl mercury levels in laboratory animals; polythiol resins may be more effective than penicillamine in removing methyl mercury compounds from the body (Klaassen 1985a).

Hemodialysis may be helpful in treating acute inorganic mercury poisoning in patients with renal impairment. Conventional hemodialysis is of little use in the treatment of methyl mercury intoxication, but L-cysteine has been effective in complexing methyl mercury into a more dialyzable form (Klaassen 1985a). Diaphoresis has been used for centuries in the therapy of mercury poisoning (Sunderman 1988). Mercury is sequestered in lysosomal dense bodies in neurons and persists in the brain for long periods of time (Cavanagh 1988). Damage to the central and peripheral nervous systems appears to be permanent, but physical therapy has been associated with clinical improvement in less severely poisoned patients. Administration of neostigmine has been reported to improve motor strength in patients with methyl mercury intoxication (Elhassani 1983).

Arsenic

Infamous for its long history as a homicidal poison, arsenic is a tasteless, odorless metal found naturally in the environment and used in a variety of industries. Previously used to treat a number of infectious bacterial and parasitic illnesses, arsenic compounds have largely been eliminated from modern medicine.

Arsenic is used in pesticides, herbicides, rodenticides, ant paste, glassware, paints, metal alloys, pigments, wood preservatives, and cosmetics (Ellenhorn and Barceloux 1988; Zaloga et al. 1985). Workplace exposure occurs in the above industries and has been reported among chemical workers, pesticide formulators, pesticide applicators, and carpenters working with treated woods. Community exposure has resulted through airborne emissions from smelters and from well water contaminated by natural arsenic deposits (Landrigan 1982). Transformation by microorganisms leads to accumulation in seafood (Ellenhorn and Barceloux 1988). Significant amounts of arsenic are found in natural and processed foods. The average daily ingestion of arsenic has been estimated to be about 1 mg (Schoolmeester and White 1980).

Arsenic is present in three toxic forms in the environment: pentavalent salts, trivalent salts, and arsine gas. The pentavalent form (arsenate) is found in the earth's crust and in most foods and is water soluble, rapidly absorbed through mucous membranes, and less toxic than the trivalent form (arsenite) which is more lipid soluble, has greater skin absorption, and accumulates in the body (Louria 1988; Schoolmeester and White 1980). Fine powders have more effective gastrointestinal absorption than do coarser forms. Inhalation of arsenic compounds can result in significant absorption. Colorless, odorless arsine gas used in the semiconductor industry is released when acid is added to arsenic compounds and is extremely toxic (Ellenhorn and Barceloux 1988).

After absorption, arsenic in the bloodstream is initially localized in erythrocytes and bound to proteins with minimal penetration of the blood-brain barrier. Within 24 hours, arsenic redistributes mainly into liver, kidney, heart, and lungs with lesser amounts in muscle and nervous tissue; 2–4 weeks after ingestion, deposition of arsenic begins in the sulfhydryl-rich keratin of hair, skin, and nails where it remains for years. Long-term incorporation also takes place into bones and teeth.

Action. The most clinically significant toxic effect is thought to be the reversible combination of arsenic with sulfhydryl groups. This leads to the inhibition of many enzyme systems. Blockage of the Krebs cycle and interference with oxidative phosphorylation lead to depletion of cellular energy stores, disruption of multiple metabolic systems, and cell death. A secondary mechanism disrupting oxidative phosphorylation is termed *arsenolysis,* in which arsenic is substituted for phosphate (Schoolmeester and White 1980).

Neuropsychiatric manifestations.   Ingestion of large amounts of arsenic in homicide or suicide attempts frequently results in acute intoxication. Initial symptoms of a metallic taste and garlic breath odor begin within 30 minutes to several hours after ingestion and progress to profound gastrointestinal inflammation and varying degrees of circulatory collapse from generalized vasodilation. CNS symptoms include drowsiness, headache, vertigo, stupor, encephalopathy, delirium, convulsions, and coma (Landrigan 1982; Zaloga et al. 1985). Neuropathologically, it is thought that capillary damage leads to cerebral edema and focal microhemorrhages (Schoolmeester and White 1980) with multiple symmetrical foci of hemorrhagic necrosis present in both the gray and white matter (Klaassen 1985a). In severe arsenic exposures, death usually occurs within 1–4 days from circulatory collapse (Ellenhorn and Barceloux 1988).

A symmetrical sensorimotor polyneuropathy is the most prominent feature after the first week of acute intoxication (Louria 1988). The lower extremities are affected first. Sensory symptoms predominate initially and include paresthesias, numbness, and pain in a stocking-glove distribution. Motor involvement may progress from weakness to muscle atrophy with loss of reflexes to paralysis in prolonged poisoning. Microscopically, demyelination and axonal degeneration progress to nerve atrophy and perineural fibrosis in chronic poisoning (Schoolmeester and White 1980).

Cranial nerves are usually spared in chronic arsenic intoxication, but visual changes, optic neuritis, vestibular toxicity, and facial nerve palsy have been reported (Schoolmeester and White 1980; Zaloga et al. 1985). Encephalopathy may be a rare initial presentation of chronic poisoning; headache, personality changes, seizures, or coma may occur but are much more common in acute intoxication. Neurosis or psychosis may be present, and the encephalopathy may resemble the Wernicke-Korsakoff syndrome secondary to arsenic's interference with thiamine metabolism (Schoolmeester and White 1980).

Acute arsine gas poisoning is frequently fatal from hemolysis and/or renal failure. Associated neuropsychiatric features may include headache, paresthesias, and encephalopathy characterized by agitation and disorientation (Klaassen 1985a; Louria 1988). Survivors may develop signs of chronic arsenic intoxication.

Diagnosis.   A history of arsenic exposure and recognition of clinical signs are extremely important. Severe abdominal pain with bloody diarrhea, albuminuria, and a garlic breath odor are commonly seen in acute arsenic poisoning. Chronic intoxication is often insidious and overlooked diagnostically; it should be considered in patients with combinations of neuropathy, skin rash, and gastrointestinal and blood disturbances (Schoolmeester and White 1980).

Aldrich-Mee's lines are transverse whitish bands from arsenic deposits in fingernails and may be seen in acute and chronic poisoning. Because of arsenic's short half-life in blood, blood levels may be helpful only for same-day exposure. Urine levels are more accurate for recent exposures (1–2 days); dietary contamination of foods with arsenic must be ruled out. Urine levels between 100 µg/L and 200 µg/L suggest arsenic intoxication, and levels greater than 200 µg/L indicate significant exposure (Ellenhorn and Barceloux 1988).

Treatment and prognosis. If the patient presents within the first few hours after acute arsenic ingestion, attempts should be made to remove arsenic by emesis, gastric lavage, activated charcoal, and a cathartic; hemodialysis may be helpful as an adjunct only in the presence of renal failure and is otherwise not indicated (Schoolmeester and White 1980). Exposed skin surfaces should be thoroughly cleaned. Care must be taken to maintain intravascular volume with intravenous fluids; pressor agents may be added if necessary.

Topical dimercaprol may be helpful in dermal exposures. Chelation with parenteral dimercaprol is indicated in symptomatic acute arsenic exposures except for arsine gas and should be administered as early as possible to minimize systemic toxicity. The benefit of dimercaprol in chronic poisoning is unclear; it may be helpful for hematologic disturbances, but it usually does not affect the neurological symptoms (Schoolmeester and White 1980). Penicillamine is used adjunctively in serious acute intoxications, but oral penicillamine alone may be sufficient after chronic arsenic exposure (Klaassen 1985a).

In arsine gas poisoning, initial decontamination and supportive measures are followed by exchange transfusions and forced alkaline diuresis. Dimercaprol has not been shown to be effective (Klaassen 1985a).

Aluminum

Aluminum is one of the most abundant elements in the earth's crust, and healthy persons are at little risk for developing aluminum toxicity. Aluminum is poorly absorbed through the gastrointestinal tract and once absorbed is bound to protein. Accumulation of aluminum in the body tends to occur when either the gastrointestinal absorption barrier is bypassed (e.g., parenteral introduction) or renal excretion is impaired; patients with renal failure are particularly at risk. Medical sources of aluminum exposure include aluminum-containing antacids and phosphate-binding gels, as well as contaminated dialysis solutions, total parenteral nutrition (TPN) solutions, and human serum albumin used in plasmapheresis (Monteagudo et al. 1989). Occupational exposure occurs in the aluminum production industry.

Action. The exact mechanism for aluminum neurotoxicity is unknown. Aluminum has been shown to alter the function of the blood-brain barrier by affecting membrane function, and it has been postulated that many of aluminum's effects on the CNS and peripheral tissues can be explained by its actions as a membrane toxin (Banks and Kastin 1989).

Neuropsychiatric manifestations. Intraneuronal aluminum accumulation has been demonstrated in patients with amyotrophic lateral sclerosis (ALS) and parkinsonism dementia of Guam, an area with unusually high incidences of these disorders (Perl et al. 1982). Senile dementia of the Alzheimer type (SDAT) is associated with the intranuclear presence of aluminum in neurons with neurofibrillary changes but not in adjacent normal appearing neurons (Perl and Brody 1980). Total body aluminum levels appear to be normal in Alzheimer's patients (Alfrey 1983). Despite the association between the presence of aluminum and these degenerative nervous system disorders, no etiologic role for aluminum has been established.

Dialysis dementia is a progressive encephalopathy described in patients on long-term renal dialysis. Initial symptoms include speech difficulties and electroencephalographic (EEG) changes; these are followed by the development of dyspraxia, asterixis, tremor, myoclonus, memory loss, and personality changes. In the late stages, seizures and progressive deterioration of speech and motor coordination are frequently followed by death, which usually occurs within 6–9 months (Wisniewski and Sturman 1989).

Increased aluminum in the brain gray matter of patients who died of this syndrome led Alfrey et al. (1976) to propose aluminum intoxication as the etiology. This remains the commonly accepted theory resulting from exposure to aluminum-containing dialysis solutions and phosphate-binding gels. Unlike Alzheimer's dementia, patients dying from dialysis encephalopathy do not demonstrate neurofibrillary degeneration; aluminum accumulates in the cytoplasm and lysosomes of histologically normal-appearing neurons throughout the central gray matter, and brain and total body aluminum levels are markedly increased (Alfrey 1983; Wisniewski and Sturman 1989).

Diagnosis. Identifying a history of exposure in patients at risk (e.g., those with renal failure) is extremely important. Because aluminum is highly protein bound, serum levels may not reflect total body burden. Average serum aluminum levels are less than 10 µg/ml; asymptomatic dialysis patients may have levels up to 50 µg/ml. Levels greater than 60 µg/ml are indicative of increased absorption. Toxicity may appear at levels above 100 µg/ml, and serum aluminum concentrations greater than 200 µg/ml are usually associated with clinical symptoms (Ellenhorn and Barceloux 1988).

Treatment and prognosis. The management of aluminum toxicity begins with identifying the source of aluminum exposure and eliminating it if possible. Removing aluminum from water used for dialysis has reduced the incidence and morbidity of dialysis encephalopathy. Elimination or reduction of aluminum-containing medications and phosphate-binding gels should be attempted if the patient's clinical situation will permit. Calcium carbonate may be substituted as it has been shown to effectively bind phosphate in both adults and children with chronic renal failure (Monteagudo et al. 1989). Chelation of aluminum with deferoxamine has been helpful in the treatment of dialysis dementia, but the best mode of administration, optimum dose, and duration of treatment are not clearly established (Monteagudo et al. 1989). Successful renal transplantation early in the course of dialysis encephalopathy has been associated with gradual although often incomplete recovery. Because transplantation late in the course of the disease does not halt the downhill progression, diagnosis at an early, potentially reversible stage is essential (Parkinson et al. 1981).

Manganese

Manganese is an essential trace element used in the production of metal alloys, dry-cell batteries, and various chemicals. It is found in paints, ceramics, glass, inks, dyes, matches, pigments, welding rods, fungicides, fertilizers, and antiknock gasoline additives. Toxic exposure is strictly occupational, with most cases reported in the mining and processing of manganese ores; intoxication has also been reported in metal workers and persons working in fertilizer preparation and the dry-cell battery industry (Emara et al. 1971; Hine and Pasi 1975; Wang et al. 1989). Due to the low solubility of inorganic manganese, gastrointestinal absorption and dermal absorption are negligible. Toxicity results from chronic inhalation of dust and fumes containing mainly manganese dioxide. Symptoms usually follow months to years of exposure.

Action. The exact mechanism of manganese neurotoxicity is unknown.

Neuropsychiatric manifestations. Chronic manganese intoxication (manganism) begins insidiously, often with complaints of anorexia, apathy, sleep disturbance, and impaired motor performance. Manganese miners may present with a transient psychiatric disturbance characterized by psychomotor agitation, hallucinations, emotional lability, compulsions, and aberrant behavior; this syndrome has been termed *manganese madness* and lasts from 1 to 3 months whether the miner is removed from the mine or not (Huang et al. 1989).

Neurological signs in chronic poisoning include bradykinesia, gait disturbance, postural instability, impaired arising ability, masked facies, disordered speech, rigidity, tremor, micrographia, and dystonia. Psychiatric abnormalities also occur, such as depression, anxiety, emotional lability, compulsive acts, inappropriate affect, pathological laughter, and impaired memory and calculation ability (Cook et al. 1974; Hine and Pasi 1975).

The extensive extrapyramidal symptomatology described above results in a clinical picture of parkinsonism. However, unlike in Parkinson's disease, neuropathological changes in autopsy specimens of patients with manganese intoxication have shown degeneration of the medial segment of the globus pallidus, frequently of the caudate nucleus and the putamen, and rarely of the substantia nigra (Huang et al. 1989).

Diagnosis. The diagnosis of chronic manganese intoxication depends on the presence of clinical signs and symptoms along with a positive history of manganese exposure. There are no specific diagnostic tests, although elevated manganese levels in blood and urine may confirm an increased level of exposure. Normal manganese levels are 2–8 μg/dl in blood and 0.1–0.8 μg/dl in urine (Hine and Pasi 1975).

Treatment and prognosis. Manganese workers who develop symptoms and signs of intoxication should be removed from further exposure. If this is done early in the course of the illness, some signs may slowly resolve. In most cases the disability stabilizes after removal, but occasionally the symptoms progress. Speech deficits and tremor may improve with time; gait disturbances show little change (Cook et al. 1974). Chronic psychosis has been reported (Emara et al. 1971). Young patients and those with shorter durations of exposure have a better prognosis, with reports of complete recovery (Hine and Pasi 1975). Treatment with levodopa (L-dopa) and CaNa$_2$EDTA have been associated with some improvement, but their therapeutic benefit remains inconsistent and controversial (Cook et al. 1974; Hine and Pasi 1975; Huang et al. 1989).

ORGANOPHOSPHATES

Organophosphates are anticholinesterases that were used first as insecticides and later for chemical warfare (nerve gas). Generally, exposure occurs via contact with pesticides. Occupational exposure, which can be chronic, is commonly dermal or pulmonary. In suicidal or homicidal presentations, exposure is usually by oral ingestion (Taylor 1985). It has been estimated that less than 1% of cases of work-related illness secondary to pesticides are actually reported (Kahn 1976).

Action.   Organophosphates bind to the anticholinesterase enzyme, creating a stable, generally irreversible, inactive compound that leads to accumulation of acetylcholine in the neuronal gap. Acute intoxication is due to muscarinic, nicotinic, and CNS effects.

Neuropsychiatric manifestations.   In a study of 236 patients (Lerman et al. 1984), 40% presented with CNS symptoms. These included giddiness, subjective tension, anxiety, restlessness, labile mood, insomnia, headache, tremor, nightmares, increased dreaming, apathy, withdrawal and depression, drowsiness, confusion, slurred speech, ataxia, generalized weakness, and coma with absence of reflexes.

Onset of action can be quite sudden (5 minutes) in massive ingestion. Usual presentation is 4–12 hours after exposure. Exceptions are the highly lipophilic organophosphates, which have mild initial symptoms followed by severe cholinergic symptoms 48 hours later. Duration depends on severity of exposure; mild to moderate acute symptoms usually resolve within 1 month.

Chronic effects include both polyneuropathies and neurobehavioral changes. The polyneuropathies include delayed sensorimotor peripheral neuropathies that occur 8–14 days after exposure and are not necessarily preceded by acute cholinergic symptoms (Barret and Oehme 1985). Persistent neuropsychiatric symptoms include drowsiness, lability, depression, fatigue, anxiety, and irritability (Tabershaw and Cooper 1966). Most of the persistent symptoms that develop from acute exposure resolve in less than a year.

Diagnosis.   Diagnosis is usually made by obtaining a history of exposure to pesticides. A garlic odor from either the patient or the container can sometimes aid in the diagnosis. Inhibition of acetylcholinesterase is a confirming test in conjunction with history of exposure. The red blood cell cholinesterase is the preferred marker because it measures the same enzyme active in nervous tissue. With acute exposure, there can be a 50% decrease in baseline cholinesterase levels. In mild to moderate exposure, there is return to normal levels in several weeks (Ellenhorn and Barceloux 1988).

Treatment and prognosis.   The first response must be to stabilize any vital sign abnormalities. Decontamination procedures include removing contaminated clothing and washing exposed skin surfaces. Because of possible potentiation of the organophosphates, the use of phenothiazines, antihistamines, tricyclics, and anticholinergics should be avoided; CNS depressants can increase the possibility of respiratory depression. Full resolution is expected of acute CNS symptoms if appropriate and prompt treatment is rendered. However, persistent CNS effects (irritability, fatigue, lethargy, poor memory, depression, and psychosis) have been seen in a few survivors (Ellenhorn and Barceloux 1988).

ORGANIC SOLVENTS

Organic solvents are found in a variety of substances. Selected solvents with neuropsychiatric toxicities are listed in Table 21–3. Toluene is found in plastic cement, airplane model cement, lacquer thinner, ink, liquid shoe polish, cleaning fluid, and other industrial solvents; it is also used as a replacement for benzene. Acetone is contained in fingernail polish remover and plastic cement (Ellenhorn and Barceloux 1988).

Most of the halogenated hydrocarbons such as carbon tetrachloride, trichlorethylene, and trichloroethane are lipid soluble and metabolically stable. Thus they are easily absorbed via the gastrointestinal tract, skin, or respiratory surfaces. Most of the aliphatic hydrocarbons act as CNS depressants (Klaassen 1985b).

Of the alcohol solvents, isopropyl alcohol (isopropanol) is prominent for universality in industrial and home settings. It is found in large concentrations in such items as frost remover, windshield washer solvent, antifreeze, rubbing alcohol, dog repellent, rust preventive, and gasket cement (Lacouture et al. 1983). Poisoning occurs from ingestion and inhalation. The toxic oral dose of isopropyl alcohol in adults is 1 ml/kg body weight, but symptoms are possible at 0.5 ml/kg body weight (Ellenhorn and Barceloux 1988). Isopropyl alcohol is a CNS depressant, and its metabolite acetone is believed to contribute to the symptoms.

Methyl alcohol (methanol) is found in 95% concentration in antifreeze and 35%–95% in windshield washer fluid. Methyl alcohol itself has CNS depressant effects, and poisoning occurs when its metabolites formaldehyde and formic acid are created. The level of toxicity correlates best with the production of formic acid (Ellenhorn and Barceloux 1988).

Neuropsychiatric manifestations. Symptoms of toluene exposure include headache, dizziness, vertigo, syncope, sensorimotor neuropathy, cerebellar signs, hallucinations, emotional lability, personality changes, lethargy, and coma (Ellenhorn and Barceloux 1988).

Table 21–3. Selected organic solvents with neuropsychiatric toxicities

Alcohols	**Glycols**
Isopropanol	Ethylene glycol
Methanol	Propylene glycol
Aliphatic hydrocarbons	**Halogenated hydrocarbons**
Hexane	Carbon tetrachloride
	Trichloroethane
Aromatic hydrocarbons	Trichloroethylene
Benzene	**Ketones**
Toluene	Acetone
Xylene	

Mild acute exposure to benzene presents with dizziness, weakness, euphoria, and headache, whereas severe acute exposure can cause blurred vision, tremor, and unconsciousness. Chronic exposure leads to loss of appetite, drowsiness, and nonspecific anxiety (Klaassen 1985b).

Acetone and xylene exposure can lead to initial CNS excitement. With acetone this is often followed by lethargy, stupor, or coma. Chronic xylene exposure can cause cerebral and cerebellar degeneration.

Ethylene glycol has a three-stage presentation of intoxication, the first of which has prominent neuropsychiatric symptoms. Within the first 12 hours after ingestion, transient excitation occurs followed by convulsions, myoclonic jerks, nystagmus, and ophthalmoplegia. Further CNS depression is caused by cerebral edema (Ellenhorn and Barceloux 1988). Propylene glycol, besides acting as a CNS depressant, can also cause seizures and hypoglycemia (Demey et al. 1984).

Various visual symptoms have been described in methyl alcohol poisoning, including blurred vision and photophobia as well as signs such as retinal edema, fixed pupils, and constricted visual fields (Swartz et al. 1981). Mild intoxication can cause headache, vertigo, lethargy, and confusion. Higher levels can lead to coma and convulsions via cerebral edema. Putamen necrosis and a permanent Parkinson-like syndrome have also occurred (Ellenhorn and Barceloux 1988).

Treatment and prognosis.   Stabilization and supportive care are the primary treatment goals. The solvent must be identified, and metabolic complications associated with that solvent must be assessed. Electrolyte disturbances and acute tubular necrosis require aggressive treatment. With isopropyl alcohol ingestions, gut decontamination, elimination enhancement via dialysis, and supportive care can quickly reduce the effects. The primary antidote for methyl alcohol poisoning is ethyl alcohol, which inhibits the enzyme alcohol dehydrogenase from creating formaldehyde and formic acid. Folic acid is given as a cofactor to facilitate the conversion of formic acid to carbon dioxide (Ellenhorn and Barceloux 1988). Despite prompt therapy, 25% of visual defects do not resolve (Swartz et al. 1981).

With both ethylene glycol and propylene glycol intoxications, supportive care and decontamination are the mainstays for treatment. Ethyl alcohol infusion is used with ethylene glycol poisoning to block the enzymatic formation of toxic metabolites (Gabow et al. 1986). The cofactors pyridoxine and thiamine are given to promote the conversion of ethylene glycol to nontoxic products (Ellenhorn and Barceloux 1988).

CARBON MONOXIDE

Carbon monoxide is a colorless, tasteless, and generally undetectable gas that is formed from incomplete combustion of organic matter. It is the leading cause of poisoning deaths in the United States (Ellenhorn and Barceloux 1988). From 15% to 40% of persons with serious nonlethal carbon monoxide poisoning develop neuropsychiatric symptoms, which can appear after apparent recovery (Ginsburg and Pomano 1976).

The average concentration of carbon monoxide in the atmosphere is about 0.1 parts per million (ppm). An automobile can produce concentrations of up to 115 ppm, with underground garages and tunnels having levels greater than 100 ppm for extended periods of time. Catalytic converters have decreased carbon monoxide emissions considerably (Klaassen 1985b).

Cigarette smoking is another significant source of carbon monoxide. Endogenous production of carbon monoxide results in a blood carboxyhemoglobin (COHb) level of 0.4%–0.7%. A one-pack-a-day smoker has a COHb level of 5%–6%, whereas a two to three-pack-a-day smoker has a COHb level of 7%–9% (Ellenhorn and Barceloux 1988). Passive inhalation of carbon monoxide can occur (with secondhand smoke).

Heating equipment such as charcoal grills, kerosene space heaters, and hibachis can give off carbon monoxide in closed spaces. Paint removers can be another source of carbon monoxide from in vivo conversion of methylene chloride. COHb levels of up to 50% have been recorded after methylene chloride exposure (Fagin et al. 1980). Any survivor of a fire is especially at risk for carbon monoxide exposure.

Action.   Carbon monoxide combines with hemoglobin to form COHb. Hemoglobin in this form cannot perform its primary function of carrying oxygen. The affinity of hemoglobin for carbon monoxide is more than 200 times greater than that for oxygen. This high affinity makes carbon monoxide potent and very dangerous. The increased metabolic activity of children makes them more susceptible than adults to the effects of carbon monoxide.

Neuropsychiatric manifestations.   The presentation can look very similar to that of hypoxia. High concentrations of carbon monoxide may give no warning before producing loss of consciousness; however, there are often preliminary signs of transient weakness and dizziness.

At 20% COHb, there is headache with throbbing temples. This headache is characteristically bandlike. At 30% COHb, there is irritability, disturbed judgment, fatigue, dizziness, and dimming of vision. At 40%–50% COHb, there is increasing confusion and collapse. At 60%–70% COHb, the patient can present with unconsciousness, convulsions, and death if exposure is prolonged (Winter and Miller 1976). The severe headache following exposure to carbon monoxide is believed to be caused by cerebral edema and increased intracranial pressure from excessive transudation across capillaries. Gross pathological changes in the brain show congestion and/or edema, petechiae, hemorrhagic focal necrosis, and perivascular infarct. Bilateral necrosis of the globus pallidus is the characteristic lesion of carbon monoxide toxicity. Other vulnerable gray matter areas include the substantia nigra, hippocampus, cerebral cortex, and cerebellum (Ginsberg 1985).

After initial recovery from carbon monoxide exposure, patients may develop neurological symptoms of apathy, mutism, amnesia, irritability, personality changes, confusion, memory loss, and visual changes within 2–4 weeks of exposure (Myers et al. 1985). Cerebellar signs are unusual.

Diagnosis.   Laboratory tests are generally not helpful. Clinical features are at best roughly correlative with COHb levels. Abnormal EEG findings are common and can reflect the progression of hypoxic encephalopathy. Common EEG findings include low-voltage waves and diffuse slow waves.

Treatment and prognosis. The first step should be transfer from the contaminated environment to fresh air. Control of airway, support of breathing with high oxygen concentration (preferably 100%), and cardiac monitoring should also be initiated. Supplemental oxygen should be continued until COHb is significantly reduced (Ellenhorn and Barceloux 1988). The use of hyperbaric oxygen is controversial (Min 1986).

Rates of complete recovery from carbon-monoxide–induced hypoxic unconsciousness are inversely related to the age of the patient (Bokorjic 1963). The level of consciousness on initial evaluation has some correlation with subsequent development of gross neuropsychiatric sequelae (Smith and Brandon 1973). However, loss of consciousness is not necessary for developing delayed neurological problems (Min 1986). Up to 75% of the neuropsychiatric sequelae, except memory deficits and gait disturbances, resolve after 1 year (Lee 1978).

REFERENCES

Agency for Toxic Substances and Disease Registry: The Nature and Extent of Lead Poisoning in Children in the United States: A Report to Congress. Atlanta, GA, U.S. Department of Health and Human Services, 1988

Alfrey AC: Aluminum. Adv Clin Chem 23:69–91, 1983

Alfrey AC, LeGendre GR, Kaehny WD: The dialysis encephalopathy syndrome, possible aluminum intoxication. N Engl J Med 294:184–188, 1976

Baker EL, White RF, Pothier LJ, et al: Occupational lead neurotoxicity: improvement in behavioural effects after reduction of exposure. Br J Ind Med 42:507–516, 1985

Banks WA, Kastin AJ: Aluminum-induced neurotoxicity: alterations in membrane function at the blood-brain barrier. Neurosci Biobehav Rev 13:47–53, 1989

Barret DS, Oehme FW: A review of organophosphorus ester induced delayed neurotoxicity. Vet Hum Toxicol 27:22–37, 1985

Bokorjic N: Stagnant anoxia and carbon monoxide poisoning. Electroencephalogr Clin Neurophysiol 21 (suppl):1–102, 1963

Cavanagh JB: Long term persistence of mercury in the brain. Br J Ind Med 45:649–651, 1988

Centers for Disease Control: Preventing Lead Poisoning in Young Children. Atlanta, GA, U.S. Department of Health and Human Services, Public Health Service, 1985

Chisolm JJ Jr, Barltrop D: Recognition and management of children with increased lead absorption. Arch Dis Child 54:249–262, 1979

Cook DG, Fahn S, Brait KA: Chronic manganese intoxication. Arch Neurol 30:59–64, 1974

Cullen MR, Robins JM, Eskenazi B: Adult inorganic lead intoxication: presentation of 31 new cases and a review of recent advances in the literature. Medicine 62:221–247, 1983

Davis JM, Svendsgaard DJ: Lead and child development. Nature 329:297–300, 1987

Demey H, Daelemans R, De Broe ME, et al: Propylene glycol: intoxication due to intravenous nitroglycerin. Lancet 1:1360, 1984

Elhassani SB: The many faces of methyl mercury poisoning. J Toxicol Clin Toxicol 19:875–906, 1983

Ellenhorn MJ, Barceloux DG: Medical Toxicology, Diagnosis and Treatment of Human Poisoning. New York, Elsevier Science, 1988

Emara AM, El-Ghawabi SH, Madkow OI, et al: Chronic manganese poisoning in the dry battery industry. Br J Ind Med 28:78–82, 1971

Fagin J, Bradley J, Williams D: Carbon monoxide poisoning secondary to inhaling methylene chloride. BMJ 281:1461, 1980

Feldman MD: Pica: current perspectives. Psychosomatics 27:519–523, 1986

Gabow PA, Clay K, Sullivan JB, et al: Organic acids in ethylene glycol intoxication. Ann Intern Med 105:16–20, 1986

Ginsberg MD: Carbon monoxide intoxication: clinical features, neuropathology and mechanisms of injury. Clinical Toxicology 23:281–288, 1985

Ginsburg R, Pomano J: Carbon monoxide encephalopathy: need for appropriate treatment. Am J Psychiatry 133:317–320, 1976

Graziano JH, Lolacono NJ, Meyer P: Drug-response study of oral 2,3-dimercaptosuccinic acid in children with elevated blood lead concentrations. J Pediatr 113:751–757, 1988

Hine CH, Pasi A: Manganese intoxication. West J Med 123:101–107, 1975

Huang CC, Chu NS, Lu CS, et al: Chronic manganese intoxication. Arch Neurol 46:1104–1106, 1989

Kahn E: Pesticide related illness in California farm workers. J Occup Med 18:693–696, 1976

Klaassen CD: Heavy metals and heavy-metal antagonists, in Goodman and Gilman's The Pharmacological Basis of Therapeutics, 7th Edition. Edited by Gilman AG, Goodman LS, Rall TW, et al. New York, Macmillan, 1985a, pp 1605–1627

Klaassen CD: Nonmetallic environmental toxicants, air pollutants, solvents, vapors, and pesticides, in Goodman and Gilman's The Pharmacological Basis of Therapeutics, 7th Edition. Edited by Gilman AG, Goodman LS, Rall TW, et al. New York, Macmillan, 1985b, pp 1628–1650

Lacouture PG, Wason S, Abrams A, et al: Acute isopropyl alcohol intoxication: diagnosis and management. Am J Med 75:680–686, 1983

Landrigan PJ: Occupational and community exposures to toxic metals: lead, cadmium, mercury, and arsenic. West J Med 137:531–539, 1982

Lee H: Clinical studies on delayed sequelae of carbon monoxide intoxication. Journal of the Korean Neuropsychiatric Association 15:374–385, 1978

Lerman Y, Hirshberg A, Shteger Z: Organophosphate and carbamate pesticide poisoning: the usefulness of a computerized clinical information system. Am J Ind Med 16:17–26, 1984

Levine SP, Cavender GD, Langolf GD, et al: Elemental mercury exposure: peripheral neurotoxicity. Br J Ind Med 39:136–139, 1982

Louria DB: Trace metal poisoning, in Cecil Textbook of Medicine, 18th Edition. Edited by Wyngaarden JB, Smith LH Jr. Philadelphia, PA, WB Saunders, 1988, pp 2385–2393

McNeil Consumer Products Company: A Summary of Pharmacological and Clinical Data for Chemet⇒ (Succimer). Fort Washington, PA, McNeil Consumer Products Company, 1991

Min SK: A brain syndrome associated with delayed neuropsychiatric sequelae following acute carbon monoxide intoxication. Acta Psychiatr Scand 73:80–86, 1986

Monteagudo FSE, Cassidy MJD, Folb PI: Recent developments in aluminum toxicology. Medical Toxicology and Adverse Drug Experience 4:1–16, 1989

Myers RAM, Synder SK, Emhoff TA: Subacute sequelae of carbon monoxide poisoning. Ann Emerg Med 14:1163–1167, 1985

Needleman HL: Lead at low dose and the behavior of children. Neurotoxicology 4:121–133, 1983

Needleman HL: The persistent threat of lead: a singular opportunity. Am J Public Health 79:643–645, 1989

Needleman HL, Schell A, Bellinger D, et al: The long-term effects of exposure to low doses of lead in childhood: an 11-year follow-up report. N Engl J Med 322:83–88, 1990

Parkinson IS, Ward MK, Kerr DNS: Dialysis encephalopathy, bone disease and anemia: the aluminum intoxication syndrome during regular hemodialysis. J Clin Pathol 34:1285–1294, 1981

Perl DP, Brody AR: Alzheimer's disease: X-ray spectrometric evidence of aluminum accumulation in neurofibrillary tangle-bearing neurons. Science 208:297–299, 1980

Perl DP, Gajdusek DC, Garruto RM, et al: Intraneuronal aluminum accumulation in amyotrophic lateral sclerosis and parkinsonism-dementia of Guam. Science 217:1053–1055, 1982

Russell FE: Snake Venom Poisoning. Philadelphia, PA, JB Lippincott, 1980

Schoolmeester WL, White DR: Arsenic poisoning. South Med J 73:198–208, 1980

Schottenfeld RS, Cullen MR: Organic affective illness associated with lead intoxication. Am J Psychiatry 141:1423–1426, 1984

Schwartz J, Landrigan PJ, Feldman RG, et al: Threshold effect in lead induced peripheral neuropathy. J Pediatr 112:12–17, 1988

Smith JS, Brandon S: Morbidity from carbon monoxide poisoning at three year follow up. BMJ 1:318–321, 1973

Sunderman FW: Perils of mercury. Ann Clin Lab Sci 18:89–101, 1988

Swartz RD, Millman RP, Billi JE, et al: Epidemic methanol poisoning: clinical and biochemical analysis of a recent episode. Medicine 60:373–382, 1981

Tabershaw IR, Cooper WC: Sequelae of acute organophosphate poisoning. J Occup Med 8:5–20, 1966

Taylor P: Anticholinesterase agents, in Goodman and Gilman's The Pharmacological Basis of Therapeutics, 7th Edition. Edited by Gilman AG, Goodman LS, Rall TW, et al. New York, Macmillan, 1985, pp 110–129

Wang JD, Huang CC, Hwang YH, et al: Manganese induced parkinsonism: an outbreak due to an unrepaired ventilation control system in a ferromanganese smelter. Br J Ind Med 46:856–859, 1989

Winter PM, Miller JN: Carbon monoxide poisoning. JAMA 236:1502–1504, 1976

Wisniewski HM, Sturman JA: Neurotoxicity of aluminum, in Aluminum and Health, A Critical Review. Edited by Gitelman HJ. New York, Marcel Dekker, 1989, pp 125–165

Yokoyama K, Araki S, Aono H: Reversibility of psychological performance in subclinical lead absorption. Neurotoxicology 9:405–410, 1988

Zaloga GP, Deal J, Spurling T, et al: Case report: unusual manifestations of arsenic intoxication. Am J Med Sci 289:210–214, 1985

Chapter 22

Alcohol-Induced
Organic Mental Disorders

John E. Franklin, Jr., M.D.
Richard J. Frances, M.D.

Alcoholism is one of the leading public health problems in the United States, directly affecting 14 million people (West et al. 1984). Robins et al. (1984) found that substance abuse disorders rank first among 15 DSM-III (American Psychiatric Association 1980) diagnoses.

Pathological neuropsychiatric findings in alcoholism are prevalent (Table 22–1). Problems range from transient organic brain syndromes during intoxication to permanent dementia and memory difficulty. Psychiatric and neuropsychological assessment is important in treatment selection and implementation. Effective recognition and treatment of signs and symptoms of alcoholism require knowledge of its major neuropathological findings.

ALCOHOL INTOXICATION

Alcohol intoxication is a common, time-limited, organic condition precipitated by varying amounts of alcohol use. Stages of intoxication range from mild inebriation to anesthesia, coma, respiratory depression, and (rarely) death. Pathological ramifications include acute delirium, seizures, pathological or idiosyncratic intoxication, and blackouts. Alcohol is a central nervous system depressant that, in low amounts, disinhibits higher cortical activity, producing clinical excitement (Adams and Victor 1981). A direct depressant action on cortical neurons produces sedation at higher blood levels.

Phenomenological presentations of intoxication depend not only on absolute blood levels but also on the rate of rise of blood alcohol level, duration of consumption, and the tolerance of the individual involved. Women have higher blood alcohol levels than do men after consuming comparable amounts of alcohol, even with allowances for differences in size. Recently, the "first pass" metabolism by gastric tissue has been found to be lower in women alcoholic patients compared with men and this may explain the increased bioavailability of alcohol in women and increased rates of hepatic injury (Frezza et al. 1990).

In nonhabituated persons, alcohol blood levels of 30 mg/dl can lead to mild euphoria, and 50 mg/dl can cause mild coordination problems. Ataxia is present at 100 mg/dl. Confusion and decreased consciousness can occur at 200 mg/dl. Blood levels of 500 mg/dl may produce anesthesia, coma, and even death (Adams and Victor

Table 22–1. Pathological neuropsychiatric signs and symptoms

Syndrome	Key signs and symptoms	Key neuropsychiatric signs and symptoms	Time of onset of syndrome	Treatment (medication)
Alcohol intoxication	Disinhibition, sedation at high doses	Acute organic brain syndrome	Rapid; depends on tolerance of individual	Time, protective environment
Alcohol idiosyncratic intoxication	Marked aggressive or assaultive behavior	Absence of focal neurological signs and symptoms	Erratic occurrence	None
Alcohol withdrawal	Tremulousness, irritability, nausea, vomiting, insomnia, malaise, autonomic hyperactivity	Transient sensory disturbances possible	Several hours; peak symptoms 24–48 hours after last drink or relative drop-in level	See Table 22–3
Alcohol seizures	Grand mal seizures in bursts of 2–6 seizures; rarely status epilepticus	Loss of consciousness, tonic-clonic movements, urinary incontinence, postictal confusion; look for focal signs	7–38 hours after cessation of alcohol	Diazepam, phenytoin; maintenance phenytoin if underlying seizure disorder is present; prevent by chlordiazepoxide detoxification
Alcohol withdrawal delirium	Confusion, disorientation, fluctuating consciousness, perceptual disturbances, autonomic hyperactivity	Marked variations in levels of consciousness and disorientation; may be fatal	Gradual onset 2–3 days after cessation of alcohol; peak intensity at 4–5 days	Chlordiazepoxide detoxification; haloperidol 2–5 mg po bid for psychotic symptomatology may be added if necessary
Alcohol hallucinosis	Vivid auditory hallucination with affect appropriate to content (often threatening)	Clear sensorium	Usually within 48 hours or less of last drink; may last several weeks	Haloperidol 2–5 mg po bid for psychotic symptoms
Wernicke's	Oculomotor disturbances, cerebellar ataxia	Mental confusion	Abrupt onset; ataxia may precede mental confusion	Thiamine 100 mg iv with MgSO4 1–2 ml in 50% solution should be given before glucose loading
Korsakoff's	Alcohol stigmata possible	Retrograde and anterograde amnesia; confabulation early; intellectual functioning generally spared	Several days following occurrence of Wernicke's	No effective treatment; institutionalization often needed
Alcohol dementia	Absence of other causes for dementia	Nonprogressing dementia if alcohol free	Associated with greater than 10-year history of drinking	None

1981). Due to tolerance, persons with chronic alcoholism consume larger quantities and reach proportionally higher blood levels without obvious signs of drunkenness.

Acute alcohol intoxication produces deficits in functions associated with prefrontal and temporal lobes (Peterson et al. 1990). Tolerance to alcohol may involve adaptive changes in membrane lipids, neuromodulators, neurotransmitter receptors, ion channels, G proteins, and intracellular second messengers that serve to counteract the short-term effects of ethanol (Charness et al. 1989).

Alcohol intake modifies γ-aminobutyric acid (GABA)-activated inhibitory neurotransmission by stimulating ion flux through chloride channels activated by GABA and dissolves into plasma membrane causing disruption of membrane lipids and proteins (Glowa et al. 1989). The N-methyl-D-aspartate (NMDA) receptor of glutamate, an excitatory neurotransmitter, may contribute to cognitive impairments associated with alcohol intoxication. Alcohol affects components of the second messengers system (i.e., adenylate cyclase [AC]) (Tabakoff and Hoffman 1987). Alcohol intoxication has also been related to release of epinephrine. Dopaminergic activity may be involved in the reinforcing properties of alcohol, and tolerance has been associated with changes in neuronal calcium channels (Dolin and Little 1989).

Inebriation can produce exhilaration, excitement, and gregariousness. Other manifestations are impaired motor performance with poor muscular control, increased risk taking, slurred speech, and ataxia. Thinking is slowed, with impaired concentration, reasoning, attention, judgment, and ability to form word associations (Lishman 1978). Fairly consistent psychophysiological symptoms occur with intoxication: an increase in heart rate, nystagmus, electromyographic (EMG) and electroencephalographic (EEG) changes, and slowed reaction times (Cohen et al. 1983).

Treatment of Intoxication

Intoxication is a time-limited condition. General management principles include decreasing threatening external stimuli, interrupting alcohol ingestion, and, when necessary, protecting individuals from damaging themselves and others. There is no effective method of hastening ethanol removal, except in potentially fatal cases, in which hemodialysis has been attempted. Several experimental amethystic agents have been suggested. These include α_2-adrenergic receptor agonists such as atipamezole (Linnoila 1989) and naloxone in reversing ethanol-induced coma and respiratory depression (Liskow and Goodwin 1987).

Zimelidine, a serotonin reuptake blocker, and ibuprofen have shown reversal in some alcohol-induced cognitive deficits, and lithium has attenuated the subjective sense of intoxication. The inverse benzodiazepine receptor agonist Ro 15-4513 has been shown to antagonize specific biochemical and behavioral effects of alcohol (Liebowitz et al. 1990), but because it causes anxiety and seizures, it is unlikely to be clinically useful. Fluvoxamine, fluoxetine, citalopram, and buspirone have shown promise in reducing alcohol consumption (Collins and Myers 1987; Naranjo et al. 1986).

Blackouts

Alcohol blackouts are transient episodes of amnesia that accompany varying degrees of intoxication. These phenomena are characterized by relatively dense retrograde amnesia for events and behavior during periods of intoxication. Behavior during these episodes may be relatively benign or grossly abnormal. Blackouts can occur in isolated episodes of drinking in persons who never become alcoholic as well as at any time in the course of the disease of alcoholism (Adams and Victor 1981). In general, blackouts occur relatively late in the course of the illness and are directly correlated with severity and duration (Goodwin et al. 1969).

Explanations of pathogenesis range from psychological repression to organic etiologies such as deep seizures and problems in capacity for laying down long-term memory during these episodes (Ballenger and Post 1984; Lishman 1978). Recent theories have proposed decreased central serotonin neurotransmission and disruption at excitatory neurotransmitter synapses (Tabakoff et al. 1990). Low plasma tryptophan levels and blackouts in male alcoholic patients suggest a specific relationship between memory problems and serotonergic activity (Branchey et al. 1985).

ALCOHOL IDIOSYNCRATIC INTOXICATION

Alcohol idiosyncratic intoxication (DSM-III-R; American Psychiatric Association 1987), or pathological intoxication, has been a controversial concept that is associated with blind unfocused assaultive and destructive behavior with intoxication. DSM-III-R defines alcohol idiosyncratic intoxication as a marked aggressive or assaultive behavioral change, with drinking, that is not typical of the person when sober. In susceptible individuals, this reaction occurs with small amounts of alcohol ingestion, insufficient to induce intoxication in most people. Differentiation of idiosyncratic intoxication from severe intoxication, frank epileptic phenomena, delirium tremens (DTs), compromised brain function from trauma, or hysterical phenomena may be difficult. There may be certain individuals with a genetic vulnerability and possible subclinical epileptic focus, but these phenomena have not been well studied and cases are anecdotal. Workup includes an EEG and a computed tomography (CT) scan if focal neurological signs or symptoms are present.

ALCOHOL WITHDRAWAL SYMPTOMS

Alcohol withdrawal symptoms can occur after cessation of alcohol in patients with chronic alcoholism or secondary to a relative drop in blood levels. Therefore, clear-cut withdrawal symptoms may be present during a period of continuous alcohol consumption. Alcohol withdrawal proper (DSM-III-R) may precede or accompany more pathological withdrawal phenomena such as DTs, seizures (rum fits), and alcohol hallucinosis. A pattern of pathological use of alcohol, which can include withdrawal or tolerance symptoms, has been defined in DSM-III-R as alcohol dependence. Increased duration of drinking and binge patterns of alcohol ingestion are clearly tied to an increase in withdrawal phenomena. By far, the most common and earliest symptoms are tremulousness, general irritability, nausea, and vomiting occurring several hours after the last drink or, frequently, the next morning. Peak symptoms occur 24–48 hours after the last drink and, in uncomplicated cases, subside in 5–7 days, even without treatment, although mild irritability and insomnia may last 10 days or longer.

The generalized tremor is coarse, of low frequency, usually observed when the tongue or hands are extended, and can worsen with motor activity or emotional stress. Patients manifest malaise and autonomic hyperactivity, tachycardia, increased blood pressure, sweating, and orthostatic hypotension. Careful attention should be given to vital signs in patients suspected of having alcoholism. Individuals may complain of disturbed sleep with nightmares, transitory illusions, or hallucinations.

Alcohol Withdrawal Seizures

Seizures are associated with cessation of long-term use of alcohol. Ninety percent of such seizures occur 7–38 hours after last use, with peak incidence somewhat greater than 24 hours (Adams and Victor 1981; Holloway et al. 1984). In some series (Espir and Rose 1987), 10% of patients with chronic alcoholism have recurrent seizures, and a considerably higher number have solitary seizures.

Seizures can be precipitated during a short bout of drinking by lowering seizure threshold. These alcohol-precipitated seizures usually occur after the period of acute intoxication (Adams and Victor 1981). Ng et al. (1988) concluded, however, that alcohol in a dose-related fashion can independently induce seizures outside the normal withdrawal period. Devetag et al. (1983) found that patients with alcohol withdrawal seizures had increased amounts and years of drinking. Alcohol-induced epilepsy can occur with less than 5 years of steady drinking (Brennan and Lyttle 1987).

EEG findings in nonepileptic individuals can be abnormal during withdrawal, with occurrences of brief periods of dysrhythmia that usually result in a normal EEG with clearance. Two studies of alcoholic seizure patients (Feussner et al. 1981; Tarter et al. 1983) reported that 50% had abnormal CT scans. In a study of patients with no other indication of a major intracranial process (Earnest et al. 1988), 16% had significant intracranial lesions on CT. Feussner et al. (1981) found that 39% had generalized cerebral atrophy and 15% had focal structural lesions. Focal neurological signs were found in 30% of those with a focal deficit on CT scan versus 6% of those without a focal deficit. A careful neurological examination may predict those who may need a CT scan.

Hypomagnesemia, respiratory alkalosis, hypoglycemia, and increased intracellular sodium have been associated with alcohol seizures, and the seizures may be the result of hyperexcitability of the neuronal systems caused by these conditions (Victor and Wolfe 1973). Approximately one-third of patients with generalized seizures secondary to alcohol withdrawal go on to develop alcoholic withdrawal DTs (Adams and Victor 1981).

Alcohol Withdrawal Delirium (DTs)

Alcohol's association with DTs was first described in the 18th century, but it was not until 1955 that Isbell related it specifically to sudden withdrawal from alcohol (Isbell et al. 1955). DTs are distinguished from uncomplicated withdrawal symptoms by a characteristic delirium. Confusion, disorientation, fluctuating or clouded consciousness, and perceptual disturbances may all be present. The syndrome includes delusions, vivid hallucinations, agitation, insomnia, mild fever, and marked autonomic arousal that can appear suddenly, but more usually appear gradually, 2–3 days after cessation of drinking, with peak intensity on the fourth or fifth day.

Terror, agitation, and primarily visual hallucinations of insects, small animals, or other perceptual distortions are classic, although a wide variation in presentation can occur.

The clinical picture can vary from quiet confusion, agitation, and peculiar behavior lasting several weeks to marked abnormal behavior, vivid terrifying delusions, and hallucinations. Hallucinations may be auditory and of a persecutory nature, or they may be kinesthetic, such as a tactile sensation of crawling insects. Hallucinations may be systematized or unsystematized. The level of consciousness may fluctuate widely.

Approximately one-half of cases present in an atypical manner (Victor and Adams 1953). The syndrome is often modified by illness, therapeutic medications such as sedatives or analgesics, or trauma. Patients may show similar patterns of behavior each time they withdraw from alcohol (Turner et al. 1989). During the height of delirium, the rhythms show moderate increases in fast frequencies or EEGs in the normal range. In most cases, the DTs are benign and short lived. Most cases subside after 3 days of full-blown DTs, although DTs may last as long as 4–5 weeks. Deaths due to DTs may be related to infections, fat emboli, or cardiac arrhythmia associated with hyperkalemia, hypokalemia, hyponatremia, hypophosphatemia, alcoholic keto-acidosis, hyperpyrexia, poor hydration, rhabdomyolysis, and hypertension. Other complications include pancreatitis, gastritis, upper gastrointestinal bleeds, and hepatitis.

DTs generally occur in alcoholic individuals with 5–15 years of heavy drinking who decrease their blood alcohol levels and who have a major physical illness, such as infection, trauma, liver disease, or metabolic disorders. Useful predictors of DTs include a past history of DTs or seizures (Cushman 1987). Only 1%–10% of alcoholic patients hospitalized for detoxification develop DTs (Holloway et al. 1984).

Alcohol Hallucinosis

Alcohol hallucinosis is described in DSM-III-R as a vivid auditory hallucination, occurring shortly after the cessation or reduction of heavy ingestion of alcohol. Differential diagnoses include DTs, withdrawal syndrome, paranoid psychosis, other drug abuse, and borderline transient psychotic episodes. Withdrawal-induced hallucinosis is not a predictor of DTs (Holloway et al. 1984). In contrast to delirium, the hallucinations usually occur in a clear sensorium. A paucity of autonomic symptoms also differentiates the syndrome from withdrawal syndrome. The hallucinations may range from sounds such as clicks, roaring, humming, ringing bells, or chanting to frank voices of friends or enemies (Lishman 1978). Patients usually respond with fear, anxiety, and agitation.

These symptoms may resemble paranoid schizophrenia (Surawicz 1980). However, the diagnosis is usually made on the basis of heavy alcohol use, lack of formal thought disorder, and lack of schizophrenia or mania in past or family history. The onset is classically after cessation of drinking, but onset during drinking bouts has been reported. In the great majority of cases, the symptoms recede in a few hours to days, with patients fully realizing that the voices were imaginary. A small percentage of patients may proceed to develop a quiet, chronic paranoid delusional state or frank schizophrenia (Sellers and Kalant 1976).

Treatment of the Withdrawal Syndrome

Treatment and prevention of complications from the cessation of alcohol use in an alcohol-dependent individual depend on recognition of patterns of alcohol abuse and a careful evaluation of the stage of the illness, complicating medical problems, and flexibility in the use of treating medications. A high index of suspicion is needed to treat target symptoms in individuals undergoing withdrawal. Denial is a major defense mechanism in alcoholism, and the magnitude of an individual's drinking may not be evident until withdrawal phenomena appear.

Inpatient versus outpatient treatment. The choice of setting for treatment of withdrawal symptoms depends on the severity of symptoms, medical complications, the use of other substances, and the patient's cooperation, ability to follow instructions, social support systems, and past history. Patients with organic brain syndrome, low intelligence, Wernicke's encephalopathy, dehydration, history of trauma, neurological symptoms, medical complications, psychopathology that may require psychotropic medications, DTs, alcoholic seizures, or alcoholic hallucinosis are probably best treated in an inpatient setting. A past history of withdrawal seizures, DTs, or poor compliance also warrants withdrawal in an inpatient setting. Concomitant use of other substances (e.g., barbiturates and benzodiazepines) may complicate alcohol withdrawal. Concomitant opiate addiction may require cautious use of more than one agent for detoxification.

For the majority of people with mild withdrawal symptoms, an outpatient medical detoxification is possible. Close follow-up, including daily visits, is essential to assure adequate sedation and observation for complications. This method has the advantages of leaving the patients in their own work and social settings and of fostering a positive therapeutic alliance with the treating outpatient therapist.

General management of inpatient treatment. If inpatient treatment is deemed necessary, an atmosphere that avoids overstimulation and that is well structured is preferable. A good medical history and physical and neurological examinations are required. Standard laboratory tests are listed in Table 22–2.

Table 22–2. Medical workup for alcohol withdrawal

Medical history and complete physical examination	Magnesium
	Albumin with total protein
Routine laboratory tests	Hepatitis B surface antigen
Complete blood count with differential	B_{12} folic acid levels
Serum electrolytes	Stool guaiac
Liver function tests (including bilirubin)	Urinalysis
Blood urea nitrogen	Urine drug and alcohol screen
Creatinine	Chest X ray, electrocardiogram
Fasting blood glucose	**Ancillary tests**
Prothrombin time	Electroencephalogram
Cholesterol	Head computed tomography
Triglycerides	Gastrointestinal series
Calcium	

Patients with alcoholism are often nutritionally deficient. Deficiencies in thiamine, vitamin B_{12}, and folic acid levels are commonly found. Magnesium sulfate should be given to any individual with a past history of alcohol withdrawal seizures. In severe cases where autonomic hyperarousal, sweating, and fever cause considerable dehydration, careful rehydration and attention to electrolyte replacement should be done with medical supervision.

In mild uncomplicated cases of withdrawal, nonpharmacological withdrawal can be attempted. Many alcoholic patients have had the experience of stopping alcohol rather suddenly and tolerating withdrawal symptoms without complication. Several studies have reported supportive care being sufficient for the vast majority of withdrawing alcoholic patients (Shaw 1981; Whitfield et al. 1978).

Pharmacological treatment.   The rationale for pharmacological treatment of withdrawal symptoms is to relieve discomfort secondary to autonomic symptoms and to prevent complications such as seizures and DTs. An ideal medication, although currently unavailable, would produce adequate sedation, abort autonomic hyperarousal, be easy to administer, provide a good therapeutic safety index, be without primary liver metabolism, and be nonaddicting.

Numerous medications have been reported to be effective for uncomplicated withdrawal symptoms, such as alcohol, paraldehyde, chloral hydrate, antihistamines, barbiturates, chlormethiazole, major tranquilizers, phenytoin, propranolol, piracetam, and benzodiazepines. Cross-tolerance with alcohol and sedation has been the main rationale for the medications used; the major advantage of cross-tolerance being the prevention of seizure activity during withdrawal. Moskowitz et al. (1983) reviewed 81 therapeutic trials in 2,313 randomized patients and found only four deaths. No definite conclusion other than the efficacy of benzodiazepines could be ascertained.

Propranolol can decrease anxiety, tremor, mild hypertension, tachycardia, and subjective symptoms. In severe withdrawal, propranolol may decrease tremor but provides no protection from seizures or DTs (Sellers and Kalant 1976). A randomized clinical trial of atenolol (a β-blocker) during alcohol withdrawal (Horowitz et al. 1989) showed beneficial effects compared with placebo; atenolol also seemed to be associated with a reduction in craving. Major tranquilizers do produce sedation but are not cross-tolerant with alcohol: they have the disadvantages of causing hypotension and lowering seizure threshold.

Carbamazepine is an anticonvulsant, antikindling drug that has demonstrated efficiency in treating withdrawal (Malcolm et al. 1989) and may have a role in treating psychiatric sequelae of repeated withdrawal. Clonidine has been reported to be as effective as chlordiazepoxide in relieving the subjective symptoms of withdrawal and more effective in reducing systolic blood pressure and heart rate (Baumgartner and Rowen 1987). Lofexidine (an α_2-adrenergic agonist) also had successful clinical trials (Cushman et al. 1985). Successful use of high-potency antipsychotics in controlling the agitated psychotic symptoms associated with delirium has been reported (Holloway et al. 1984).

Barbiturates and benzodiazepines are both cross-tolerant. Barbiturates have had a decreased popularity in recent years, secondary to high incidence of respiratory depression and a low therapeutic safety index compared with those of benzodiazepines. In the presence of severe liver disease, oversedation is a danger with the use of barbiturates because of their decreased liver metabolism. Longer-acting barbiturates such as phenobarbital are preferable over short-acting medications and can be used with equivalent doses of benzodiazepines.

Benzodiazepines are clearly the medication of choice for withdrawal symptoms because of a relatively high therapeutic safety index, oral and intravenous administration, anticonvulsant properties, and good prevention of DTs. Disadvantages include poor intramuscular absorption (except for lorazepam), primary liver metabolism, high cost, and abuse potential. There are no clear advantages to any one benzodiazepine, although special circumstances may favor one over another. Short-acting benzodiazepines such as triazolam should generally be avoided. Rapidly fluctuating blood levels may promote withdrawal seizures. In patients with severe liver disease and in the elderly, intermediate-acting benzodiazepines such as lorazepam or oxazepam can be used. Oxazepam has the added advantage of renal versus liver excretion.

Diazepam and chlordiazepoxide, longer-acting benzodiazepines, are comparable in length of action, with half-lives of 24–36 hours. The onset of action is slow, thus rapid loading doses are often needed. Chlordiazepoxide and diazepam have the advantage of smooth induction and gradual decline in blood levels so that there are fewer symptoms on discontinuation of low dosages. Chlordiazepoxide may be preferable because of its greater sedation. In severe withdrawal cases with a history of seizures, and in cases of cross-addiction with other depressant drugs, diazepam is used because of its greater anticonvulsant effect. Diazepam 10 mg is the eqivalent of chlordiazepoxide 25 mg.

For inpatient withdrawal, generally 100–400 mg of chlordiazepoxide is given the first day in quarterly divided dosages (Table 22–3). This generally provides adequate sedation and control of autonomic symptoms, although chlordiazepoxide may not take away all the subjective discomforts of withdrawal. If some sedation is not achieved 1 hour after the first dose, chlordiazepoxide can be prescribed hourly until the patient is sedated. Sellers and Kalant (1976) suggested that higher levels of chlordiazepoxide may be necessary for cigarette smokers.

Single withdrawal seizures do not require anticonvulsant medication. Alcohol withdrawal seizures are generally self-limited and only require supportive care.

Treatment of status epilepticus. Status epilepticus is a major neurological emergency. Diazepam usually aborts status epilepticus; however, phenytoin may be necessary. Patients with abnormal EEGs repeated 2–3 weeks after withdrawal may

---

Table 22–3. Standard treatment regimen for alcohol withdrawal

Outpatient
Chlordiazepoxide 25–50 mg po qid on first day; 20% decrease in dose over a 5-day period
Daily visits to assess symptoms

Inpatient
Chlordiazepoxide 25–100 mg po qid on first day; 20% decrease in dose over 5–7 days
Chlordiazepoxide 25–50 mg po qid prn for agitation, tremors, or change in vital signs
Thiamine 100 mg po qid
Folic acid 1 mg po qid
Multivitamin one per day
Magnesium sulfate 1 g im every 6 hours for 2 days (if status postwithdrawal seizures)

require maintenance phenytoin. Calcium channel blocking agents may play a role in management of withdrawal seizures (Koppi et al. 1987).

Treatment of DTs.   The best care for DTs is preventive treatment. There is evidence that once DTs occur the course may not be significantly altered by available treatment (Victor and Wolfe 1973). The chief aims are sedation and supportive care. Diazepam can be used, but oversedation should be avoided. In less extreme agitation benzodiazepine can be used. Restraints should be used only if necessary; in paranoid patients they may increase agitation. Correction of metabolic derangements and vitamin supplementation are parts of the supportive care. High-potency neuroleptics such as haloperidol may be helpful in patients who are psychotic with marked perceptual changes.

Treatment of alcohol hallucinosis.   Patients with alcohol hallucinosis should receive the same basic appropriate withdrawal treatment. For those patients with hallucinosis and extreme agitation, a potent antipsychotic such as haloperidol successfully decreases symptoms. Medication should not be continued indefinitely and reassessment should take place shortly after cessation of symptoms.

WERNICKE-KORSAKOFF SYNDROME

Wernicke-Korsakoff syndrome is a spectrum neurological disorder associated with thiamine deficiency. It is most often associated with alcoholism, but can occur in any condition that causes thiamine deficiency (e.g., malabsorption syndrome, severe anorexia, hemodialysis). Repeated bouts of marginal thiamine deficiency could lead to the same pathological changes induced by a single episode of severe thiamine deficiency (Harper 1983).

Wernicke's Encephalopathy

Classically, Wernicke's encephalopathy has an abrupt onset with oculomotor disturbances, cerebellar ataxia, and mental confusion. Several authors (e.g., Brew 1986) have suggested that the diagnosis of Wernicke's encephalopathy should not rely on the presence of all three criteria and that the presence of two of the three criteria is suggestive of limited forms of the disorder. Autopsy studies (Harper et al. 1986) confirm that there is a high rate of mental confusion (82%), but lower rates of ataxia (23%) and oculomotor disturbances (29%). The oculomotor disturbances range from various types of nystagmus to complete gaze palsy. The ataxia is truncal, and these conditions may precede the mental confusion by days. A general confusional state with disorientation, in addition to slow response, may proceed to frank stupor and coma.

Wernicke's encephalopathy should be suspected in any unexplained case of coma. It has a 17% mortality rate and should be considered a medical emergency. Thiamine deficiency produces a diffuse decrease in the use of glucose, and the neurotoxicity may be due to release of excitatory neurotransmitters such as glutamic acid. If a patient does not respond quickly to treatment, the development of Korsakoff's psychosis (also known as Korsakoff's syndrome or Korsakoff's disease) is likely.

Alcohol Amnestic Disorder (Korsakoff's Psychosis)

Korsakoff's psychosis is classically a chronic condition, with both retrograde and anterograde amnesia. The period of retrograde amnesia may cover up to a few years before the onset of the illness. Confabulation may be typical in the early stages, but it is not always present. Korsakoff's psychosis can also show changes in behavior indicative of frontal lobe damage (e.g., apathy, inertia, and loss of insight). Numerous studies have outlined neuropathological aspects of the disorder. Selzer and Benson (1974) confirmed the classic Korsakoff memory problem in which recent, well-known public events were poorly remembered compared with remote events. Sensory, motivational, and visuospatial difficulties have also been found in Korsakoff's psychosis, but intellectual functioning is generally spared.

Structural and neurochemical findings have characterized Wernicke-Korsakoff syndrome. Punctate lesions in the periventricular, periaqueductal regions of the brain stem and diencephalon have been found on brain autopsy (Victor et al. 1989). Periventricular lesions of the thalamus, hypothalamus, mammillary bodies, the reticular activating system, periaqueductal areas of the midbrain, and floor of the fourth ventricle have been found and may relate to the memory problems and various states of consciousness (Victor et al. 1989). Magnetic resonance imaging (MRI) brain images demonstrate loss of tissue in the area of the mammillary bodies (Charness and DeLaPaz 1987). Edema has been found in the mammillary bodies around the third ventricle and the aqueductal floor of the fourth ventricle (Mensing et al. 1984).

Weingartner et al. (1983) suggested that the memory pathology in Korsakoff's psychosis may be based on a disruption of the functional anatomic linkages between the reward-reinforcement and memory systems. Because patients may have access to semantic memory, unlike Alzheimer's disease patients, psychobiological mechanisms have been proposed. Decreases in CSF levels of norepinephrine, dopamine, and serotonin have been found (McEntee and Mair 1978). The hypothesis is that norepinephrine systems are selectively damaged in Korsakoff's psychosis, producing memory deficits but not global dementia. Butters (1985) reported deficits in the acetylcholine system, suggesting a milder form of damage to the basalis of Meynert compared to what is found in Alzheimer's disease. Direct alcohol neurotoxicity to the basalis of Meynert may also play a role (Arendt et al. 1988). Cholinergic blockade produces anterograde amnesia similar to the pattern seen in Alzheimer and Korsakoff patients (Kopelman and Corn 1988).

Abnormalities in the metabolism of thiamine have been postulated as a contributory factor in the development of severe thiamine deficiency. Transketolase activity in the muscle fibroblasts of Wernicke-Korsakoff patients has been found to be decreased, but the expression of the syndrome may not become evident unless there is a thiamine-deficient diet (Blass and Gibson 1977).

Treatment

Wernicke's encephalopathy is a life-threatening condition; treatment should be considered a medical emergency. Treatment consists of parenteral thiamine; resistance to thiamine replacement may result from hypomagnesemia because magnesium is a cofactor for thiamine transketolase. Magnesium sulfate should be administered. Ophthalmoplegia usually responds fairly quickly, but truncal ataxia may persist.

Korsakoff's psychosis can be a devastating illness that often requires institutionalization. Korsakoff's psychosis and alcoholic dementia may occur in combination and may be difficult to separate clinically. Clonidine has been reported to improve recent memory and recall, perhaps as a result of hypothesized damage to the ascending norepinephrine-containing neurons in the brain stem and diencephalon (McEntee et al. 1981). Propranolol has been used for rage attacks in Korsakoff's psychosis (Yudofsky et al. 1984). Fluvoxamine has shown some promise in reducing memory deficits, hypothesized to occur through its serotonergic effects (Martin et al. 1989).

ALCOHOL DEMENTIA

Alcohol dementia is dementia presumably caused by long-term alcohol use. Because it may be difficult to separate the effects from subacute Wernicke-Korsakoff syndrome, trauma, and hepatic encephalopathy, careful exclusion criteria may decrease the reported incidence of this entity. Impaired neuropsychological testing is evident in 50%–70% of sober alcoholic patients (Charness et al. 1989). Cala and Mastaglia (1981) reviewed the literature on CT scans in patients with chronic alcoholism. There is positive evidence for cortical shrinkage but no direct correlation between CT atrophy and neuropsychological deficits, except in the frontal lobe areas. This accompanies findings in Alzheimer's disease in which cortical atrophy does not necessarily predict level of dementia. Reversal of cortical atrophy can follow a prolonged period of abstinence, suggesting that neuronal fallout is not the only factor responsible for alcohol brain atrophy. Advances in the use of positron-emission tomography (PET) scans now provide a potential for further study of alcohol's functional metabolic effect on the brain.

OTHER NEUROLOGICAL COMPLICATIONS

Hepatic encephalopathy is a reversible neurological deficit often caused by severe alcohol liver disease. Clinical symptoms range from mild confusion, decreased attention, and irritability to coma. Simple cognitive exams, like a trail making test, can detect early stages. There is generally good correlation between clinical stage of hepatic encephalopathy and degree of abnormality of the EEG; however, there is not a good correlation between ammonia levels and degree of hepatic encephalopathy. Behavioral and electrophysiological manifestations of hepatic encephalopathy may be due to functional increase in GABAergic tone in the brain (Gammal and Jones 1989).

Acquired (non-Wilsonian) hepatocerebral degeneration is a chronic, largely irreversible hepatocerebral syndrome frequently developing after several episodes of hepatic coma. Symptoms may include tremor, dysarthria, ataxia, choreoathetosis, and dementia, usually in the context of classic signs of cirrhosis. The syndrome may resemble Wilson's disease; however, there are no Kayser-Fleischer rings, and cerebral lesions tend to be more cortical.

Trauma-induced acute and chronic subdural hematoma are not uncommon in alcoholic patients who are exposed to falls and blunt head injury. Acute subdural hematomas are often confused with cerebral contusion and laceration. CT scans are particularly effective in diagnosis. Chronic subdural hematomas may reveal little in the way of focal signs. Disturbances in mentation, concentration, mood, or thought processes are more common.

Alcohol cerebellar degeneration is a slowly evolving condition encountered along with long-standing history of excessive alcohol use. It affects the cerebellar midline structures and produces truncal ataxia and gait disturbance. The exact course is unknown, but typical symptoms, alcoholic history, and supporting CT findings may make the diagnosis. Etiology may be related to thiamine deficiency or electrolyte abnormalities but is not correlated with alcohol consumption.

Central pontine myelinolysis, Marchiafava-Bignami disease, and nutritional amblyopia are rare neurological conditions associated with chronic alcoholism. Pontine dysfunction evident in central pontine myelinolysis is of unknown etiology and often causes death. Signs and symptoms include paraparesis and quadriparesis, dysarthria, dysphagia, and "locked in" syndrome. Marchiafava-Bignami disease is a rare demyelinating disease of the corpus callosum, whose etiology is totally unknown. The course may be acute or chronic and is associated with dementia, spasticity, and gait disturbance (Victor et al. 1989). A nutritional amblyopia is associated with alcohol and tobacco use and is treated with B complex vitamins.

Alcoholism is also associated with an increased risk of stroke, possibly due to hyperlipidemia, hypertension, or blood flow abnormalities. There is a positive correlation between moderate alcohol consumption and hemorrhagic stroke and possible excess risk of ischemic stroke at high levels of alcohol consumption and protection from ischemic stroke at moderate levels of use (Gorelick 1989).

CONCLUSIONS

Alcohol can have acute and chronic effects that can lead to neuropsychiatric impairment, making diagnosis difficult. Intoxication, withdrawal, and temporary and lasting brain effects require careful history taking, mental status evaluation, selective laboratory testing, and treatment planning. Frequently these problems become complicated by interactions of alcohol-related organic brain syndromes with psychiatric, medical, and neurological conditions. Further research (using approaches such as PET scanning and tools for study of neurotransmitters, receptor sites, ion channels, and second messenger systems) is needed to establish the specific pathogenesis of these neuropsychiatric problems. Ultimately, prevention and early diagnosis are the best ways to minimize the devastating consequences of alcohol abuse and dependence.

REFERENCES

Adams RD, Victor M: Principles of Neurology. New York, McGraw-Hill, 1981

American Psychiatric Association: Diagnostic and Statistical Manual of Mental Disorders, 3rd Edition. Washington, DC, American Psychiatric Association, 1980

American Psychiatric Association: Diagnostic and Statistical Manual of Mental Disorders, 3rd Edition, Revised. Washington, DC, American Psychiatric Association, 1987

Arendt T, Allen Y, Sinden J, et al: Cholinergic-rich brain transplants reverse alcohol-induced memory deficits. Nature 332:448–450, 1988

Ballenger JC, Post RM: Carbamazepine in alcohol withdrawal syndromes and schizophrenic psychoses. Psychopharmacol Bull 20:572–584, 1984

Baumgartner GR, Rowen RC: Clonidine vs. chlordiazepoxide in the management of acute alcohol withdrawal syndrome. Arch Intern Med 147:1223–1226, 1987

Blass JP, Gibson GE: Abnormality of a thiamine requiring enzyme in patients with Wernicke-Korsakoff syndrome. N Engl J Med 297:1367–1370, 1977

Branchey L, Branchey M, Zucker D, et al: Association between low plasma tryptophan and blackouts in male alcholic patients. Alcoholism 9:393–395, 1985

Brennan FN, Lyttle JA: Alcohol and seizures: a review. J R Soc Med 9:571–573, 1987

Brew BJ: Diagnosis of Wernicke's encephalopathy. Aust N Z J Med 16:676–678, 1986

Butters N: Alcoholic Korsakoff's syndrome: some unresolved issues concerning etiology: neuropathology and cognitive deficits. J Clin Exp Neuropsychol 7:181–210, 1985

Cala LA, Mastaglia FL: Computerized tomography in chronic alcoholics. Alcoholism (NY) 5:283–294, 1981

Charness ME, DeLaPaz RL: Mamillary body atrophy in Wernicke's encephalopathy: antemortem identification using magnetic resonance imaging. Ann Neurol 22:595–600, 1987

Charness ME, Simon RP, Greenberg DA: Ethanol and the nervous system. N Engl J Med 321:442–454, 1989

Cohen MJ, Schandler SL, Naaliboff BD: Psychophysiological measures from intoxicated and detoxified alcoholics. J Stud Alcohol 44:271–282, 1983

Collins DM, Myers RD: Buspirone attenuates volitional alcohol intake in chronically drinking monkey. Alcohol 4:49–56, 1987

Cushman P Jr: Delirium tremens: update on an old disorder. Postgrad Med 82(5):117–122, 1987

Cushman P Jr, Forbes R, Lerner W, et al: Alcohol withdrawal syndromes: clinical management with lofexidine. Alcoholism (NY) 9:103–108, 1985

Devetag F, Mandich G, Zaiotte G, et al: Alcoholic epilepsy: review of a series and proposed classification and etiopathogenesis. Ital J Neurol Sci 3:275–284, 1983

Dolin SJ, Little HJ: Are changes in neuronal calcium channels involved in ethanol tolerance. J Pharmacol Exp Ther 250:985–991, 1989

Earnest MP, Feldman F, Marx JA, et al: Intracranial lesions shown by CT scans in 259 cases of first alcohol-related seizures. Neurology 38:1561–1565, 1988

Espir ML, Rose FC: Alcohol, seizures, and epilepsy. J R Soc Med 9:542–543, 1987

Feussner J, Linfus E, Blessing C, et al: CAT scanning in ETOH withdrawal syndromes: value of the neurological exam. Ann Intern Med 94:519–522, 1981

Frezza M, Di Padova G, Pozzato G, et al: High blood alcohol levels in women: the role of decreased gastric alcohol dehydrogenase activity and first-pass metabolism. N Engl J Med 322:95–99, 1990

Gammal SH, Jones EA: Hepatic encephalopathy. Med Clin North Am 73:793–813, 1989

Glowa JR, Crawley J, Suzdak PD, et al: Ethanol and the GABA receptor complex: studies with the partial inverse benzodiazepine receptor agonist RO 15-4513. Pharmacol Biochem Behav 3:767–772, 1989

Goodwin DW, Crane JB, Guze SB: Alcoholic blackouts: a review and clinical study of 100 alcoholics. Am J Psychiatry 126:174–177, 1969

Gorelick PB: The status of alcohol as a risk factor for stroke. Stroke 20:1607–1610, 1989

Harper C: The incidence of Wernicke's encephalopathy in Australia: a neuropathological study of 131 cases. J Neurol Neurosurg Psychiatry 46:593–598, 1983

Harper CG, Giles M, Finlay-Jones R: Clinical signs in the Wernicke-Korsakoff complex: a retrospective analysis of 131 cases diagnosed at necropsy. J Neurol Neurosurg Psychiatry 49:341–345, 1986

Holloway HC, Hales RE, Wantanabe HK: Recognition and treatment of acute alcohol withdrawal syndrome. Psychiatr Clin North Am 7:729–743, 1984

Horowitz RI, Gottlieb LD, Kraus ML: The efficacy of atenolol in the outpatient management of the alcohol withdrawal syndrome. Arch Intern Med 149:1089–1093, 1989

Isbell H, Fraser HG, Winkler A, et al: An experimental study of the etiology of "rum fits" and delirium tremens. Quarterly Journal of the Study of Alcohol 16:1–13, 1955

Kopelman MD, Corn TH: Cholinergic "blockade" as a model for cholinergic depletion. Brain 111:1079–1110, 1988

Koppi S, Eberhardt G, Haller R, et al: Calcium-channel blocking agent in the treatment of acute alcohol withdrawal: cavoreine versus meprobamate in a randomized double-blind study. Neuropsychobiology 17: 49–52, 1987

Liebowitz NR, Kranzler HR, Meyer RE: Pharmacologic approaches to alcoholism treatment, in Alcohol and Health (Seventh Special Report to the U.S. Congress from the Secretary of Health and Human Services). Washington, DC, U.S. Department of Health and Human Services, 1990, pp 144–153

Linnoila M: Alcohol withdrawal syndrome and sympathetic nervous system function. Alcohol Health and Research World 13:355–357, 1989

Lishman WA: Organic Psychiatry. Philadelphia, PA, JB Lippincott, 1978

Liskow BI, Goodwin DW: Pharmacological treatment of alcohol intoxication, withdrawal and dependence: a critical review. J Stud Alcohol 48:356–370, 1987

McEntee WJ, Mair RG: Memory impairment in Korsakoff's psychosis: a correlation with brain norepinephrine activity. Science 202:905–907, 1978

McEntee WJ, Mair RG, Langlais PJ: Clonidine in Korsakoff disease: pathophysiologic and therapeutic implications. Prog Clin Biol Res 71:211–223, 1981

Malcolm R, Ballenger JC, Sturgis ET, et al: Double-blind controlled trial comparing carbamazepine to oxazepam treatment of alcohol. Am J Psychiatry 146:617–621, 1989

Martin PR, Adinoff B, Eckardt MJ, et al: Effective pharmacotherapy of alcoholic amnestic disorder with fluvoxamine. Arch Gen Psychiatry 46:617–621, 1989

Mensing JW, Hoogland PH, Slooff JL: Computed tomography in the diagnosis of Wernicke's encephalopathy: a radiological-neuropathological correlation. Ann Neurol 16:363–365, 1984

Moskowitz G, Chalmers TG, Sacks HS, et al: Deficiencies of clinical trials of alcohol withdrawal. Alcoholism (NY) 7:42–46, 1983

Naranjo CA, Sellers EM, Lawrin MO: Modulation of ethanol intake by serotonin uptake inhibitors. J Clin Psychiatry 47 (Apr suppl):16–22, 1986

Ng SKC, Hauser WA, Brust JCM, et al: Alcohol consumption and withdrawal in new-onset seizures. N Engl J Med 319:666–673, 1988

Peterson JB, Rothfleisch J, Zelazo PD, et al: Acute alcohol intoxication and cognitive functioning. J Stud Alcohol 51:114–122, 1990

Robins LN, Helzer JE, Weissman MM, et al: Lifetime prevalence of specific psychiatric disorders in three sites. Arch Gen Psychiatry 41:949–958, 1984

Sellers EM, Kalant H: Alcohol intoxication and withdrawal. N Engl J Med 294:757–762, 1976

Selzer B, Benson DF: The temporal pattern of retrograde amnesia in Korsakoff's disease. Neurology 24:527–530, 1974

Shaw JM: Development of optimal treatment tactics for alcohol withdrawal. J Clin Psychopharmocol 1:382–389, 1981

Surawicz FG: Alcoholic hallucinosis: a missed diagnosis: differential diagnoses and management. Can J Psychiatry 1:57–63, 1980

Tabakoff B, Hoffman PL: Biochemical pharmacology of alcohol, in Psychopharmacology: The Third Generation of Progress. New York, Raven, 1987, pp 1521–1526

Tabakoff B, Hoffman PL, Peterson RC: Advances in neurochemistry, in Alchohol and Health (Seventh Special Report to the U.S. Congress from the Secretary of Health and Human Services). Washington, DC, U.S. Department of Health and Human Services, 1990, pp 109–160

Tarter RE, Goldstein G, Alterman A, et al: Alcoholic seizures: intellectual and neuropsychological sequelae. J Nerv Ment Dis 171:123–125, 1983

Turner RG, Lichstein PR, Peden JG, et al: Alcohol withdrawal syndromes: a review of pathophysiology, clinical presentation and treatment. J Gen Intern Med 4:432–444, 1989

Victor M, Adams RD: The effect of alcohol on the nervous system. Res Publ Assoc Res Nerv Ment Dis 32:526–573, 1953

Victor M, Wolfe SM: Causation and treatment of the alcohol withdrawal syndrome, in Alcoholism: Progress in Research and Treatment. Edited by Bourne PG, Fox R. New York, Academic, 1973, pp 137–166

Victor M, Adams RD, Collins GH: The Wernicke-Korsakoff Syndrome and Related Neurologic Disorders Due to Alcoholism and Malnutrition (Contemporary Neurology Series, Vol 3). Philadelphia, PA, FA Davis, 1989

Weingartner H, Groifman J, Boutelle W, et al: Forms of memory failure. Science 221:380–383, 1983

West LJ, Maxwell DS, Noble EP, et al: Alcoholism. Ann Intern Med 100:405–416, 1984

Whitfield GL, Thompson G, Lamb A, et al: Detoxification of 1,024 alcoholic patients with psychoactive drugs. JAMA 239:1409–1410, 1978

Yudofsky SC, Stevens L, Silver J, et al: Propranolol in the treatment of rage and violent behavior associated with Korsakoff's psychosis. Am J Psychiatry 141:114–115, 1984

Chapter 23

Neuropsychiatric Aspects of Degenerative Dementias Associated With Motor Dysfunction

Peter J. Whitehouse, M.D., Ph.D.
Robert P. Friedland, M.D.
Milton E. Strauss, Ph.D.

The degenerative dementias associated with motor system dysfunction are a diverse group of disorders that present a particular challenge to the neuropsychiatrically oriented clinician. In this chapter, Huntington's disease (HD), Parkinson's disease (PD), and other rarer degenerative conditions characterized by dementia and movement disorders are reviewed (Table 23–1). The dementias included in this chapter are characterized by gradual loss of function caused by progressive loss of neurons in specific regions of the brain associated with pathological hallmarks that are characteristic of the individual diseases. The specific etiologies of these diseases are often unknown, and biological interventions are limited in effectiveness.

Many attempts have been made to define subtypes of dementia. One attempt to develop a classification based on an understanding of biology has been the development of the concept of cortical and subcortical dementia (McHugh and Folstein 1975). Alzheimer's disease (AD) and Pick's disease are thought to represent cortical dementias in which the predominant pathology is found in the neocortex and the clinical symptoms are believed to reflect this cortical pathology (e.g., aphasia, apraxia, and agnosia).

It has been suggested that the clinical picture of the dementias considered in this chapter is due to primary pathology in subcortical structures and includes dysfunction in affect, speed of processing, and memory (Cummings 1990). Many authors have come to the conclusion that all dementias cannot be classified easily into these two large categories and, for example, that the dementias of HD and PD are as clinically different from one another as they are different from AD (Brown and Marsden 1988; Cummings 1990).

HUNTINGTON'S DISEASE

HD is a genetically transmitted, progressive neuropsychiatric disorder that can appear at any time in life. The peak period of onset is in the fourth and fifth decade.

Table 23–1. Degenerative dementias associated with motor system dysfunction

Extrapyramidal diseases	Cerebellar diseases
Parkinson's disease	Olivopontocerebellar atrophy
Huntington's disease	Friedreich's ataxia
Progressive supranuclear palsy	**Motor neuron diseases**
Thalamic dementias	Motor neuron disease with dementia
Wilson's disease	Amyotrophic lateral sclerosis/
Hallervorden-Spatz disease	parkinsonism-dementia complex
Fahr's disease	**Other**
	Normal-pressure hydrocephalus

Because of their clinical prominence, dyskinesias, particularly chorea, are usually considered the first sign of the disease. However, clinical presentation is quite variable in early stages of HD, and cognitive and psychiatric symptoms are often evident well before the movement disorder begins (S. E. Folstein 1989). Depression, irritability, and impulsive or erratic behavior are the most common psychiatric symptoms. Memory and concentration difficulties are cognitive symptoms that appear early (S. E. Folstein 1989; Martin and Gusella 1986).

Epidemiology

HD is an autosomal dominant disorder with variable age at onset. Presentation differs in juvenile-onset and adult-onset cases. Chorea is the cardinal motor symptom in adult-onset HD. In the 3%–9% of cases in which onset occurs before adolescence, rigidity, myoclonus, or dystonic movements are characteristic. In adult-onset cases, death usually occurs after 16–20 years (S. E. Folstein 1989). Rate of decline may be slower in patients with onset after the fifth decade of life (Martin and Gusella 1986). Estimates of the prevalence of HD vary widely. S. E. Folstein (1989) concluded that the best estimate of point prevalence among Caucasians is 5–7 cases per 100,000, although rates are much higher among some isolated pockets of European populations.

Etiology

The gene for HD is as yet unknown, but genetic linkage analysis has identified its location as at the distal end of the short arm of chromosome 4 (Gusella et al. 1983). The uniformity of the linkage among unrelated families of different ethnic and/or racial background and with varying clinical presentations suggests a single genetic locus for the disease. The mutation rate in HD is very low. The persistence of the disease is due to its onset typically after the peak period of reproduction (S. E. Folstein 1989).

Because of the complete penetrance of the HD gene, there has been considerable interest in identifying preclinical indicators of the disease in persons at genetic risk. Genetic testing for HD in the family members of affected persons is now possible in many cases because of the development of multiple genetic linkage markers for the HD gene (Gilliam et al. 1987; Wasmuth et al. 1988). However, because the test is for genetic linkage rather than for the gene itself, available tests may be inconclusive for presymptomatic testing.

Diagnosis and Clinical Features

Nearly half of HD cases initially present with emotional or cognitive symptoms. These can be very diverse and include depression, irritability, hallucinations, and apathy. Motor symptoms, if present, may be mild rigidity, restlessness, or ticlike jerks that are easily attributable to another disorder (S. E. Folstein 1989). Conditions such as PD, Sydenham's chorea, ataxias, cerebrovascular disease, other dementias, schizophrenia, affective disorder, thyroid disease, acanthocytosis, and alcoholism are also considerations in the differential diagnosis. However, when there is a positive family history, HD is a very likely explanation of these symptoms. S. E. Folstein (1989) suggested that a second reason the diagnosis of HD may be missed is the failure to take an adequate family history. It is difficult to make the diagnosis unequivocally during life without family history because of the variety of presentation and course (Martin and Gusella 1986).

Neurobiology

The most obvious gross pathology in HD occurs in the basal ganglia. The striatum is consistently affected in this disease, with degeneration beginning in the medial caudate and proceeding laterally to the putamen and then occasionally to the globus pallidus (S. E. Folstein 1989). γ-Aminobutyric acid (GABA), the most abundant neurotransmitter of the spiny output neurons, and acetylcholine, the principal neurotransmitter of Type I aspiny interneurons, are especially affected in this disease (S. E. Folstein 1989; Martin and Gusella 1986). The alterations in absolute neurotransmitter concentrations and relative balance among different systems may account for some of the symptoms of HD (S. E. Folstein 1989).

Degree of caudate atrophy correlates with cognitive dysfunction including intelligence, memory, and visuospatial deficits (Sax et al. 1983). Caudate atrophy is generally more robustly correlated than measures of frontal atrophy, with "executive" functions typically considered to be evidence of prefrontal cortical pathology (Starkstein et al. 1988).

Motor Abnormalities

Both involuntary movements and abnormal voluntary movements occur in HD (S. E. Folstein 1989) (Table 23–2). The earlier name of the disease in the United States, Huntington's chorea, emphasized the prominence of sudden jerky movements of the limbs, face, or trunk. These are less abrupt and of longer duration and involve more muscle groups than Sydenham's chorea. Unlike tics, choreic movements in HD are not repetitive or periodic. They can occur while the patient is at rest or in the course of planned movement (e.g., walking and reaching), although they appear to be absent during sleep.

Motor restlessness may occur before chorea and dystonia, in the absence of chorea, and is frequent in juvenile-onset (Westphal variant) cases (S. E. Folstein 1989). Abnormalities in voluntary motor movements are universal in HD, even in the absence of chorea. Abnormalities exist in initiation and inhibition of eye movements, coordination of limb movements, and articulation.

Cognitive Abnormalities

Cognitive deficits appear early in the course of HD and are progressive (Caine et al. 1977) (Table 23–2). If of sufficient severity, they can be detected and coarsely evaluated in brief, formal mental status testing, such as with the Mini-Mental State Exam (MMSE; M. F. Folstein et al. 1975). Detailed neuropsychological evaluation of patients with HD is often useful because of the range of deficits that may be encountered and the variability in the course of this dementia.

Very early in the disease, intelligence may be normal, but deficits in memory and verbal fluency can be detected on neuropsychological testing (Butters et al. 1978). Intellectual impairment is a major contribution to disability even early in the illness (Mayeux et al. 1986b). Dementia of the same clinically assessed level of severity (e.g., by MMSE) may be due to different disabilities in different illnesses. Brandt et al. (1988) demonstrated that at any given level of dementia the pattern of failure for specific items is different in HD as compared with AD. Object naming is relatively preserved on the MMSE even in advanced stages of HD (Brandt et al. 1988). Naming and other language functions appear to be relatively preserved in HD (Cummings and Benson 1988), but not invariably.

The cognitive deficits of HD include—in addition to those of memory and verbal fluency—difficulties in tasks requiring sustained concentration (e.g., mental arithmetic) and visuospatial skills. HD patients also have difficulty identifying or using their position in space relative to some fixed point (S. E. Folstein et al. 1990).

Planning, organizing, and mental flexibility—the "executive" functions that are typically impaired in patients with pathology of the frontal cortex—have been studied in HD as well. Such deficits are seen early in HD (Brandt and Butters 1986; Caine et al. 1978), but the "frontal" or "executive" dysfunctions of HD patients are less severe than in AD or Korsakoff's disease (KD; also known as Korsakoff's psychosis) patients

---

Table 23–2.   Clinical features of Huntington's disease

Motor symptoms	Verbal fluency
Involuntary movement abnormalities	Visuospatial skills
Chorea, consisting of nonrepetitive,	Sustained concentration
nonperiodic, jerky movements of	Executive functions (i.e., mental planning,
limbs, face, or trunk	organization of sequential actions, and
Exacerbated by stress	mental flexibility)
Absent during sleep	Language functions relatively preserved
May be consciously suppressed only	**Psychiatric features**
for short periods	Common symptoms
Voluntary movement abnormalities	Apathy
Initiation and inhibition of eye	Irritability
movements	Dysphoria
Coordination of limb movements	Anxiety
Articulation	Common syndromes
Neuropsychological deficits	Mood disorders (especially
Declarative memory, with greater	symptomatic major depression and
impairment for retrieval of	bipolar disorder)
information from memory than	Intermittent explosive disorder
in recognition	Schizophreniform disorder
Procedural memory	Atypical psychosis

(Butters 1985). These cognitive deficits of HD patients are most prominent in tasks that require keeping track of several things at once, discovering rules, or frequently changing mental set (Bylsma et al. 1990; Starkstein et al. 1988).

Psychiatric Abnormalities

Psychiatric symptomatology is common in HD and is often the first sign of the disorder. Insanity with a tendency to suicide was one of the three cardinal features of the disease noted by Huntington (1872). A schizophrenia-like syndrome was thought to be the most common psychiatric manifestation of HD (Garron 1973), although mood disorders were emphasized by some early workers as well (McHugh and Folstein 1975). More recent research, using explicit diagnostic criteria and more standardized methods, has suggested that a symptomatic affective disorder and intermittent explosive disorder are the more prevalent psychiatric conditions in HD (S. E. Folstein 1989; S. E. Folstein et al. 1990).

In earlier decades of this century, many HD patients were referred to state hospitals, and, still today, HD patients' initial contact with physicians is often a psychiatric consultation. Consequently, it is important to evaluate the incidence and distribution of psychiatric syndromes and symptoms in HD in samples of patients not specifically referred to psychiatric settings.

S. E. Folstein (1989) summarized the results of the only population-based study of psychiatric symptoms in HD as well as the experience of the research clinic for HD at Johns Hopkins Hospital. Affective disorder, meeting DSM-III criteria (American Psychiatric Association 1980), was diagnosed in nearly 40% of the 186 patients, and intermittent irritability (described as approximating the intermittent explosive disorder of DSM-III) was diagnosed in 31%. Schizophrenia, although less frequent (6%), occurred at a higher rate than would be expected in the general population. Other psychiatric symptoms are common in HD, even in the absence of diagnosable disorders. These symptoms include irritability, often precipitated by the kinds of events that previously had not provoked such reactions, and anxiety.

The dysphoria that is often seen in HD patients can be seen as an understandable reaction to the degenerative neurological disorder (Caine and Shoulson 1983). However, there are a number of lines of evidence suggesting an intrinsic association between HD and affective disorder, at least in some families. S. E. Folstein et al. (1979) found emotional disorder to precede onset of chorea in 6 of the 10 cases in which the determination could be made.

Treatment

HD is preventable but, as yet, incurable. There are no effective treatments for influencing the course of the disease (S. E. Folstein 1989; Martin and Gusella 1986). Numerous medical treatments have been used palliatively to manage concurrent psychiatric disorder and chorea.

Early in the course of the disease, chorea can be treated with low-dose neuroleptic pharmacotherapy. S. E. Folstein (1989) has recommended withholding treatment until involuntary movements become disabling because of the dysphoria and feeling of cognitive dulling that they can induce; she noted a preference for using fluphenazine because it is less likely than haloperidol to produce dysphoria. Later in the disease larger doses may be helpful, as may a combination of presynaptic and postsynaptic dopamine blockers (S. E. Folstein 1989). Treatment is not always effective (Caine and Shoulson 1983), and use of neuroleptics brings with it the risk of tardive dyskinesia (S. E. Folstein 1989).

Efforts have been made to affect the deterioration in functional capacity that occurs in HD with drugs that address specific neurotransmitter depletions. Cholinergic and GABAergic drugs have proved of no marked benefit (Martin and Gusella 1986; Nutt 1983). A recently completed trial of baclofen, thought to inhibit release of glutamate and aspartate, also proved ineffective in treating the progression of the disease (Shoulson et al. 1989).

Treatment of the emotional symptoms of HD can be more successful at times. Tricyclic antidepressants are often effective in the treatment of depressive symptoms (Caine and Shoulson 1983; S. E. Folstein 1989). Monoamine oxidase inhibitors (MAOIs) were reported useful in several cases by Ford (1986) and have been found clinically useful by Folstein's group (S. E. Folstein 1989), as has electroconvulsive therapy (ECT). Ford (1986) as well as Caine and Shoulson (1983) reported loss of therapeutic effectiveness in some cases.

Irritability and aggressive outbursts can be major problems in the management of HD patients in the home. Often irritability can be decreased by reduction in environmental complexity and the institution of unchanging routines. Neuroleptics can also be effective here (S. E. Folstein 1989). Successful treatment with the β-adrenergic blocker propranolol has been reported for three patients with aggressive outbursts who had limited response to neuroleptics (Stewart et al. 1987).

Environmental management is important in the care of HD patients, particularly to minimize incontinence and the risk of dehydration (S. E. Folstein 1989). Social support along with case management can be very important in the adaptation of the family to the diagnosis of HD and the management of the illness within the family (Shoulson 1982). Because of the inevitable progression of the disease, families need to prepare for chronic and more intensive care of patients. Referral to the Huntington's Disease Society is helpful to provide educational material and psychological support.

PARKINSON'S DISEASE

In 1817 James Parkinson described a new disorder he referred to as "paralysis agitans," which we now refer to as *idiopathic Parkinson's disease.* The cardinal neurological features of the syndrome of parkinsonism include tremor, muscle rigidity, bradykinesia, and postural instability. Neuropsychiatric symptoms, particularly dementia and depression, are frequently associated with PD.

Epidemiology

PD affects perhaps one million individuals in North America and shows dramatic age-related increases in incidence and prevalence. The prevalence of PD is approximately 150/100,000, increasing after age 65 to nearly 1,100/100,000 (Kessler 1972). Some studies (e.g., Martilla and Rinne 1980) have reported a protective effect of smoking. A low concordance rate in identical twins does not support a strong role for genetics in this disorder (Ward et al. 1983). Prevalence studies have estimated that dementia occurs in 10%–30% of patients with PD, with early studies demonstrating the highest estimates (Lieberman et al. 1979; Martilla and Rinne 1976; Sutcliffe 1985). Mayeux et al. (1988) suggested that the best overall estimate is that 10%–15% of PD patients will develop dementia (Girotti et al. 1988). Mayeux (1990) suggested that cumulative incidence of dementia in PD may be as high as 60% by age 88. The most common concomitant psychiatric condition in PD is depression, which occurs in 15%–30% of patients (Mayeux et al. 1986a).

Etiology

The primary cause of the most common form of parkinsonism, PD, is unknown. PD fits into the category of diseases referred to as *degenerative* because of its progressive clinical course in association with neuronal loss. The association between PD and arteriosclerosis has been controversial (Celesia and Wanamaker 1972; Martilla and Rinne 1976), although most authors agree that infarcts can cause parkinsonism.

The second most common cause of PD now is probably the administration of phenothiazines or related dopamine receptor blocking agents for the treatment of psychiatric symptoms. A description of PD being induced in drug abusers by the intravenous use of 1-methyl-4-phenyl-1,2,3,6-tetradropyridine (MPTP) (Langston et al. 1983) led to speculation that the idiopathic disease may result from subclinical exposure to toxic agents (Calne et al. 1986).

Neurobiology

In several brain regions, the neuronal loss in PD is accompanied by the formation of Lewy bodies, which are hyaline inclusion bodies. The loss of dopaminergic cells in the substantia nigra is thought to relate most directly to the motor abnormalities, particularly the bradykinesia and rigidity, and can be partially compensated for by the administration of levodopa (L-dopa) or dopamine agonists. Neuronal loss in the nucleus basalis of Meynert occurs to a small degree in all patients with idiopathic PD (Tagliavini et al. 1984; Whitehouse et al. 1983). Cortical cell loss also occurs and abnormalities have been reported in two neurotransmitters that are thought to be present in cortical interneurons: somatostatin (Epelbaum et al. 1983) and corticotropin-releasing factor (Whitehouse et al. 1987).

In addition to neurotransmitter concentration changes, alterations also occur in neurotransmitter receptors. Ruberg et al. (1982) reported increases in muscarinic cholinergic receptors in PD with dementia. Nicotinic cholinergic receptors are reduced (Whitehouse et al. 1988) and some types of serotonin receptors are also affected (Perry et al. 1984). Positron-emission tomography (PET) studies of dopaminergic function in PD have demonstrated reduced dopamine reuptake sites in the putamen contralateral to the most involved extremity (Tedroff et al. 1988). Reduced fluorine-18 6-fluoro-L-dopa uptake in the contralateral putamen has also been observed (Brooks et al. 1990).

Some but not all dementia patients with PD develop senile plaques and neurofibrillary tangles (Boller et al. 1980; Chui et al. 1986). Others show evidence of more widespread Lewy body formation or loss of neurons without specific stigmata. Neuronal loss occurs in cholinergic basal forebrain to a greater extent in patients who have dementia than in those who do not.

Motor Symptoms

The most disabling motor features of PD are frequently the bradykinesia and rigidity (Table 23–3). The patient has difficulty initiating movements, and when movement is started it occurs slowly. Poverty of automatic movements (such as movement of the arms when walking) is characteristic. Lack of facial expression reflects hypokinesia of facial musculature. Rigidity (which affects all muscle groups, proximal and distal, agonist and antagonist) can occur asymmetrically. Tremor is the presenting feature in most cases and is slow, often distal, and occurring most often at rest. Other tremors exacerbated by motion such as so-called action tremors also occur. Postural instability, associated with a characteristic flexion at the trunk and neck, occurs and can lead to serious falls.

Cognition

Many patients with PD show cognitive impairment even though the impairment may not be severe enough to warrant the label *dementia* (Table 23–3). In one study (Pirozzolo et al. 1982), 93% of patients with PD showed some form of cognitive impairment.

A large literature exists describing problems in visuospatial impairment including spatial capacities, facial recognition, body schema, pursuit tracking, spatial attention, visual analysis, and judgments concerning position in space (Boller et al. 1984; Levin 1990). The communication difficulties of PD are mostly due to speech abnormalities including hypophonia and dysarthria; however, language impairments can also occur and include reduced verbal fluency and naming difficulties (Matison et al. 1982). The relationships between the cognitive impairments in PD and the motor symptoms are complex. Poor performance on cognitive tests cannot be purely related to motor abnormalities.

Psychiatric Abnormalities

Affective disorder is the most common psychiatric disturbance associated with PD, with estimates ranging from 20% to 90% (Mayeux et al. 1986a; Starkstein et al.

Table 23–3. Clinical features of Parkinson's disease

Motor	Executive dysfunction (e.g., sequencing
Bradykinesia	and switching set)
Tremor	Language difficulties (e.g., naming)
Rigidity	**Psychiatric features**
Postural instability	Possible premorbid personality
Neuropsychological deficits	characteristics
Bradykinesia	Affective disorder
Verbal and visual memory	Psychosis—often medication induced
Visuospatial skills	

1989). Mayeux et al. (1986a) found that major depression and dysthymic disorder were the most frequent types. Some depression that occurs in PD, particularly early in the disorder, is believed to be reactive. However, relatively few associations between depression and disease factors such as duration of disease, degree of disability, and response to medications have been established. A higher frequency of depression has been found among patients with early-onset PD in which depression correlated with cognitive impairment and duration of disease. Mayeux et al. (1981) also found an association between depression and dementia.

Psychosis of a schizophrenic nature has been reported in PD in the absence of medication affects (Mjones 1949). However, most authors believe that the most common cause of psychosis in PD is medication. Celesia and Wanamaker (1972) observed psychotic episodes in 12% of 153 patients. Most episodes were due to drugs and occurred in patients who were cognitively impaired. Anticholinergic drugs may be particularly likely to produce delirium with psychotic features, although they are also most effective in suppressing the tremor.

Treatment

Great strides have been made in treating the motor dysfunction in PD. L-Dopa or dopamine agonists combined with anticholinergic agents can effectively treat rigidity, bradykinesia, and tremor. Postural instability is resistant to beneficial effects of drugs. Complicated motor phenomenon, such as on-off fluctuations and freezing episodes, can occur, especially later in therapy, which can be very stressful to patient and caregiver. Treatment of the neuropsychiatric symptoms involves both behavioral and biological approaches.

Treatment must begin with a careful assessment that includes not only the medical aspects of the illness, but also the effects of the illness on the patient's life and family. Nursing and social work assessments play an important role in providing a baseline for following the course of the illness. Education about the disease process and referral to lay support organizations such as the Parkinson's Foundation are important. Frequent reassessments followed by modifications of care plans are necessary.

A variety of interventions are available for the individual patient, including individual psychotherapy, particularly to deal with reactive depressions early in the illness. For patients with dementia, some authors suggest that certain forms of cognitive training or rehabilitation may be helpful (Gilmore et al. 1989.) Particularly in the dementias associated with motor problems, physical and occupational therapy may be very helpful.

The most important role for the physician in caring for patients with dementia is to prevent psychological stress that can increase the intensity of neuropsychiatric symptoms. Iatrogenic disease, usually caused by overuse of medication, needs to be monitored carefully, particularly if more than one physician is involved in care. The most effective biological interventions are probably those for the treatment of affective disorders and include the use of antidepressant medications, and, if necessary, ECT. Antidepressants or any drugs with profound anticholinergic side effects should be avoided.

OTHER DEGENERATIVE DEMENTIAS
ASSOCIATED WITH MOTOR ABNORMALITIES

Progressive Supranuclear Palsy

Progressive supranuclear palsy (PSP) is a chronic progressive disorder (also known as the Steele-Richardson-Olszewski syndrome) associated with eye movement abnormalities, parkinsonism, and dementia. It may have onset with deficient downward gaze, which causes trouble walking downstairs. The prevalence of PSP has been estimated at 1.4/100,000 (Golbe et al. 1988). Median age at onset of symptoms is approximately 63 years with a median survival of 6–10 years (Golbe et al. 1988).

Clinical features. Dementia is often not severe in early cases of PSP. It may be characterized by forgetfulness, slowing of thought processes, emotional or personality changes, and impaired ability to manipulate knowledge in the relative absence of aphasia, apraxia, or agnosia (Albert et al. 1974). PSP patients are particularly impaired on tests of frontal lobe function. Not all patients with PSP have noticeable dementia (Maher et al. 1985).

Diagnosis. The diagnosis of PSP is suggested by the presence of dementia with parkinsonism and eye movement abnormalities. There is usually extensive rigidity of the neck and spasticity of the face and extremities with bradykinesia and a parkinsonian gait. Restrictions on upward and downward gaze are present. This is most marked when tested to command (e.g., "Look up; look down"). When pursuit eye movements are tested, the deficit in vertical gaze is also apparent. However, when tested with oculocephalic maneuvers (i.e., head turning), there is relative integrity in vertical eye movements. This has led to the distinction of the eye movement abnormality in PSP as being supranuclear, because the oculocephalic reflexes demonstrate the integrity of the lower motor neuron pathways for up and down gaze.

Neurobiology. X-ray computed tomography (CT) and magnetic resonance imaging (MRI) studies show early involvement of midbrain structures with later atrophy of the pons and frontotemporal regions. PET scanning has shown reduced spiperone binding in the basal ganglia. Fluorodeoxyglucose PET studies show marked frontal and temporal hypometabolism (Maher et al. 1985). There is also decreased fluorodopa uptake in the striatum reflective of decreased striatal dopamine formation and storage (Leenders et al. 1988).

    Neuropathological findings include neuronal loss associated with gliosis and neurofibrillary tangles, most marked in the substantia nigra, basal forebrain, subthalamic nucleus, pallidum, and superior colliculus. There is extensive disruption in fibrillar proteins in subcortical neurons, with antigenic similarities between PSP and AD neurofibrillary pathology (Probst et al. 1988). The neurochemistry of PSP is characterized by massive dopamine depletion in the striatum; reduced density of dopamine, subtype 2 (D_2), receptors in caudate and putamen (Pierot et al. 1988); widespread reduction in choline acetyltransferase levels in frontal cortex, basal forebrain, and basal ganglia (Whitehouse et al. 1988); diminished nicotonic receptors in the basal forebrain; diminished serotonin receptors in the temporal lobe (Maloteaux et al. 1988); and a variable reduction in GABAergic neurotransmitter systems in certain subcortical regions.

Neuropsychiatric manifestations. PSP patients often have disturbances of sleep and depression, occasionally with schizophreniform psychoses (Aldrich et al. 1989). There is also memory loss, slowness of thought processes, changes in personality with apathy or depression, irritability, and forced inappropriate crying or laughing with outbursts of rage. PSP may also be associated with obsessive-compulsive behaviors (Destee et al. 1990). No treatment has been found to be effective in relieving the motor or cognitive deficiencies in PSP.

Dementia With Degenerative Disorders of the Cerebellum

Classification of the diseases of the cerebellum associated with cognitive impairment is difficult. Disorders of the cerebellum may involve pure cerebellar dysfunction or combinations of abnormalities in the cerebellum and brain stem, cerebellum and basal ganglia, or cerebellum and spinal cord and brain stem. Involvement of the optic nerves (optic atrophy), retina (retinitis pigmentosa), or peripheral neuropathy may also be found.

Olivopontocerebellar atrophies. The olivopontocerebellar atrophies (OPCAs) are a heterogeneous group of disorders presenting with progressive ataxia and associated with cerebellar degeneration. Dementia may be found in types III and V (Gilman et al. 1981), using the classification of Konigsmark and Weiner (1970). The occurrence of dementia in type III OPCA is controversial. In type V OPCA, there is ataxia with parkinsonism, ophthalmoplegia, and dementia. OPCA may be associated with progressive autonomic failure and parkinsonism with striatonigral degeneration.

Friedreich's ataxia. Friedreich's ataxia (FA) presents with a slow onset of progressive ataxia and may be associated with dementia. Mental function changes are often seen but have not been well characterized. In some instances, a syndrome of "generalized intellectual deterioration" has been noted; in others, specific nonverbal intellectual impairments have been identified. In other cases, a variety of psychiatric disorders, including schizophrenia-like psychoses and depression, have been felt to be the primary cognitive behavioral abnormality.

The mode of inheritance of FA is recessive. Mental deficiency may be present in approximately one-quarter of cases. Personality abnormalities may be marked and associated with juvenile delinquency and irritability. There may be excessive religiosity or mysticism. Psychotic states may also be detected including schizophrenia-like illnesses with paranoid delusions, agitated behavior, and nocturnal hallucinations.

The cerebellar ataxias may be either hereditary or sporadic. Abortive forms are common, sometimes showing little more than pes cavus or kyphoscoliosis. The cerebellar disorders are usually slowly progressive and associated with ataxia, ataxic gait, intention tremor, decreased rapid alternating movements, past pointing, loss of the ability to check rebound, and dysarthria. The ataxic disorders may not be accompanied by intellectual changes until late in the illness. Skre (1974) reported dementia in

36% of patients with autosomal dominant spinal cerebellar degeneration, 58% of those with autosomal recessive cerebellar disease, and 82% of those with autosomal recessive spinal cerebellar degeneration.

Motor Neuron Disease With Dementia

Loss of strength with diminished muscle mass (amyotrophy) and dementia may be seen in motor neuron disease, such as amyotrophic lateral sclerosis (ALS) (Mitsuyama et al. 1985). Familial motor neuron disease may be associated with other neurodegenerative conditions including HD, Pick's disease, PD, and the spinal cerebellar degenerations (Rosenberg 1982). Approximately 5% of ALS patients may demonstrate dementia or parkinsonism (Tyler 1982).

The occurrence of dementia with ALS may begin with personality changes or with motor system degeneration. There may be early personality changes in association with frontotemporal atrophy on CT and a normal electroencephalogram (EEG). Personality changes and hallucinations may occur in patients with ALS, as well as impairments in judgment, memory, abstract thinking, and calculations and anomia.

Other Conditions

Dementia may be associated with motor system impairment in a variety of other diseases of the nervous system (Table 23–1). For example, thalamic degeneration may be found rarely in isolation or in association with multisystem atrophy. Abnormal movements of the limb and trunk are seen with tremor, choreoathetosis, and occasionally myoclonus.

In Wilson's disease, the basal ganglia degenerate in association with abnormalities in liver function. Affective and behavioral changes are common in Wilson's disease and may include schizophrenia-like changes with depression or manic depressive states. Aggressive and self-destructive or antisocial acts may be noted, and schizoid hysterical or sociopathic personality traits have been reported. Intellectual deterioration in Wilson's disease is relatively mild. Pathologically, there is atrophy of the brain stem, dentate nucleus, and cerebellum with cavitary necrosis of the putamen. Wilson's disease is well treated with penicillamine and a copper-deficient diet. Neurological symptoms, including the dementia syndrome, improve with long-term therapy.

Normal-pressure hydrocephalus (NPH) is a syndrome comprised of dementia, gait disturbance, and urinary incontinence. It may be associated with a history of meningitis, intracranial bleeding, or head injury (Friedland 1989). Idiopathic cases are also seen. Gait is characterized by a wide base with slow steps. No changes occur in motor strength or tone. It is thought that this disturbance results from an obstruction to the flow of cerebrospinal fluid around the convexities in the basal cisterns. Improvement can be seen after a cerebrospinal fluid shunting procedure, but it is difficult to predict those individuals who will respond to surgery. The best results are seen in cases in which the cognitive disturbances are relatively mild with early onset of urinary incontinence and gait disturbance.

REFERENCES

Albert ML, Feldman RG, Willis AL: The "subcortical dementia" of progressive supranuclear palsy. J Neurol Neurosurg Psychiatry 37:121–130, 1974

Aldrich MS, Foster NL, White RF, et al: Sleep abnormalities in progressive supranuclear palsy. Ann Neurol 25:577–581, 1989

American Psychiatric Association: Diagnostic and Statistical Manual of Mental Disorders, 3rd Edition. Washington, DC, American Psychiatric Association, 1980

Boller F, Mizutani R, Roessmann U, et al: Parkinson's disease, dementia, and Alzheimer's disease: clinicopathologic correlations. Ann Neurol 7:329–335, 1980

Boller F, Passafiume D, Keefe NC, et al: Visuospatial impairment in Parkinson's disease. Arch Neurol 41:485–490, 1984

Brandt J, Butters N: The neuropsychology of Huntington's disease. Trends Neurosci 9:118–120, 1986

Brandt J, Folstein SE, Folstein MF: Differential cognitive impairment in Alzheimer's disease and Huntington's disease. Ann Neurol 23:555–561, 1988

Brooks DJ, Ibanez V, Sawle GV, et al: Differing patterns of striatal 18F-Dopa uptake in Parkinson's disease, multiple system atrophy, and progressive supranuclear palsy. Ann Neurol 28:547–555, 1990

Brown RE, Marsden CD: "Subcortical dementia": the neuropsychological evidence. Neuroscience 25:363–387, 1988

Butters N: Alcoholic Korsakoff's syndrome: some unresolved issues concerning etiology, neuropathology and cognitive deficits. J Clin Exp Neuropsychol 7:179–208, 1985

Butters N, Sax D, Montgomery K, et al: Comparison of the neuropsychological deficits associated with early and advanced Huntington's disease. Arch Neurol 35:585–589, 1978

Bylsma FW, Brandt J, Strauss ME: Aspects of procedural memory are differentially impaired in Huntington's disease. Archives of Clinical Neuropsychology 5:287–297, 1990

Caine ED, Shoulson I: Psychiatric symptoms in Huntington's disease. Am J Psychiatry 140(6):728–733, 1983

Caine ED, Ebert MHY, Eingartner H: An outline for the analysis of dementia: the memory disorder of Huntington's disease. Neurology 27:1087–1092, 1977

Caine ED, Hunt RD, Weingartner H, et al: Huntington's dementia: clinical and neuropsychological features. Arch Gen Psychiatry 35:377–384, 1978

Calne DB, Eisen A, McGeer E, et al: Alzheimer's disease, Parkinson's disease, and mononeurone disease: a biotropic interaction between aging and environment? Lancet II:1067–1070, 1986

Celesia GG, Wanamaker WM: Psychiatric disturbances in Parkinson's disease. Diseases of the Nervous System 33:577–583, 1972

Chui HC, Mortimer JA, Slager U, et al: Pathologic correlates of dementia in Parkinson's disease. Arch Neurol 43:991–995, 1986

Cummings JL (ed): Subcortical Dementia. New York, Oxford University Press, 1990

Cummings JL, Benson DF: Psychological dysfunction accompanying subcortical dementias. Annu Rev Med 39:53–61, 1988

Destee A, Gray F, Parent M, et al: Obsessive-compulsive behavior and progressive supranuclear palsy. Rev Neurol 146(1):12–18, 1990

Epelbaum J, Ruberg M, Moyse E, et al: Somatostatin and dementia in Parkinson's disease. Brain Res 278:376–379, 1983

Folstein MF, Folstein SE, McHugh PR: Mini-Mental State: a practical method for grading the cognitive state of patients for the clinician. J Psychiatr Res 2:189–198, 1975

Folstein SE: Huntington's Disease: A Disorder of Families. Baltimore, MD, Johns Hopkins University Press, 1989

Folstein SE, Folstein MF, McHugh PR: Psychiatric syndromes in Huntington's disease. Adv Neurol 23:281–289, 1979

Folstein SE, Brandt J, Folstein MF: Huntington's disease, in Subcortical Dementia. Edited by Cummings JL. New York, Oxford University Press, 1990, pp 87–107

Ford MF: Treatment of depression in Huntington's disease with monoamine oxidase inhibitors. Br J Psychiatry 149:654–656, 1986

Friedland RP: "Normal"-pressure hydrocephalus and the saga of the treatable dementias. JAMA 262:2577–2581, 1989

Garron DC: Huntington's chorea and schizophrenia. Adv Neurol 1:729–734, 1973

Gilliam TC, Bucan M, MacDonald ME, et al: A DNA segment encoding two genes very tightly linked to Huntington's disease. Science 238:950–952, 1987

Gilman S, Bloedel JR, Lechtenberg R, et al (eds): Disorders of the Cerebellum. Philiadelphia, PA, FA Davis, 1981

Gilmore GC, Wykle M, Whitehouse PJ: Memory, Aging, and Dementia: Theory, Testing, and Treatment. New York, Springer-Verlag, 1989

Girotti F, Soliveri P, Carella F, et al: Dementia and cognitive impairment in Parkinson's disease. J Neurol Neurosurg Psychiatry 51:1498–1502, 1988

Golbe LI, Davis PH, Schoenberg BS, et al: Prevalence and natural history of progressive supranuclear palsy. Neurology 38:1031–1034, 1988

Gusella J, Wexler NS, Conneally PM, et al: A polymorphic DNA marker genetically linked to Huntington's disease. Nature 306:234–238, 1983

Huntington G: On chorea. Adv Neurol 1:33–35, 1872

Kessler H: Epidemiological studies of Parkinson's disease, III: a community based study. Am J Epidemiol 96:242–254, 1972

Konigsmark BW, Weiner LP: The olivopontocerebellar atrophies: a review. Medicine (Baltimore) 49:227–241, 1970

Langston JW, Ballard P, Tetrud JW, et al: Chronic parkinsonism in humans due to a product of meperidine-analog synthesis. Science 219:979–980, 1983

Leenders KL, Frackowiak RS, Lees AJ: Steele-Richardson-Olszewski syndrome: brain energy metabolism, blood flow and fluorodopa uptake measured by positron emission tomography. Brain 111:615–630, 1988

Levin BE: Spatial cognition in Parkinson's disease. Alzheimer Dis Assoc Disord 4(3):161–170, 1990

Lieberman A, Dziatolowski M, Coopersmith M, et al: Dementia in Parkinson's disease. Ann Neurol 6:355–359, 1979

McHugh PR, Folstein ME: Psychiatric syndromes in Huntington's disease: a clinical and phenomenologic study, in Psychiatric Aspects of Neurologic Disease. Edited by Benson DF, Blumer D. New York, Grune & Stratton, 1975, pp 267–285

Maher ER, Smith EM, Lees AJ: Cognitive deficits in the Steele-Richardson-Olszewski syndrome (progressive supranuclear palsy). J Neurol Neurosurg Psychiatry 48:1234–1239, 1985

Maloteaux JM, Vanisberg MA, Laterre C, et al: [3H]GBR 12935 binding to dopamine uptake sites: subcellular localization and reduction in Parkinson's disease and progressive supranuclear palsy. Eur J Pharmacol 156 (3):331–340, 1988

Martilla RJ, Rinne UK: Dementia in Parkinson's disease. Acta Neurol Scand 54:431–441, 1976

Martilla RJ, Rinne UK: Smoking and Parkinson's disease. Acta Neurol Scand 62:322–325, 1980

Martin JB, Gusella JF: Huntington's disease: pathogenesis and management. N Engl J Med 20:1267–1276, 1986

Matison R, Mayeux R, Rosen J, et al: "Tip-of-the-tongue" phenomenon in Parkinson's disease. Neurology 32:567–570, 1982

Mayeux R: Dementia in extrapyramidal disorders. Current Opinion in Neurology and Neurosurgery 3:98–102, 1990

Mayeux R, Stern Y, Rosen J, et al: Depression: intellectual impairment and Parkinson's disease. Neurology 31:645–650, 1981

Mayeux R, Stern Y, Williams JBW, et al: Clinical and biochemical features of depression in Parkinson's disease. Am J Psychiatry 143:756–759, 1986a

Mayeux R, Stern Y, Herman A, et al: Correlates of early disability in Huntington's disease. Ann Neurol 20:727–731, 1986b

Mayeux R, Stern Y, Sano M, et al: The relationship of serotonin to depression in Parkinson's disease. Mov Disord 3:236–244, 1988

Mitsuyama Y, Kogo HH, Ata K: Progressive dementia with motor neuron disease: an additional case report and neuropathological review of 20 cases in Japan. Eur Arch Psychiatry Neurol Sci 235:1–8, 1985

Mjones H: Paralysis agitans: a clinical and genetic study. Acta Psychiatr Scand 54:1–195, 1949

Nutt JG: Effects of cholinergic agents in Huntington's disease: a reappraisal. Neurology 33:932–935, 1983

Perry EK, Perry RH, Candy JM, et al: Cortical serotonin-S2 receptor binding abnormalities in patients with Alzheimer's disease: comparisons with Parkinson's disease. Neurosci Lett 51:353–357, 1984

Pierot L, Desnos C, Blin J, et al: D1 and D2-type dopamine receptors in patients with Parkinson's disease and progressive supranuclear palsy. J Neurol Sci 86(2-3):291–306, 1988

Pirozzolo FJ, Hansch EC, Mortimer JA, et al: Dementia in Parkinson's disease: a neuropsychological analysis. Brain Cogn 1:71–83, 1982

Probst A, Langui D, Lautenschlager C, et al: Progressive supranuclear palsy: extensive neurophil threads in addition to neurofibrillary tangles: very similar antigenicity of subcortical neuronal pathology in progressive supranuclear palsy and Alzheimer's disease. Acta Neuropathol (Berl) 77(1):61–68, 1988

Rosenberg RN: Amyotrophy in multisystem genetic diseases, in Human Motor Neuron Diseases. Edited by Rowland LP. New York, Raven, 1982, pp 149–157

Ruberg M, Ploska A, Javoy-Agid F, et al: Muscarinic binding and choline acetyltransferase activity in parkinsonian subjects with reference to dementia. Brain Res 232:129–139, 1982

Sax DS, O'Donnell B, Butters N, et al: Computer tomographic, neurologic, and neuropsychological correlates of Huntington's disease. Int J Neurosci 18:21–36, 1983

Shoulson I: Care of patients and families with Huntington's disease, in Movement Disorders. Edited by Marsden CD, Fahn S. London, Butterworths International Medical Reviews, 1982, pp 277–290

Shoulson I, Odoroff C, Oakes D, et al: A controlled clinical trial of baclofen as protective therapy in early Huntington's disease. Ann Neurol 25:252–259, 1989

Skre H: Spino-cerebellar ataxia in Western Norway. Clin Genet 6:265–288, 1974

Starkstein SE, Brandt J, Folstein S, et al: Neuropsychologic and neuropathologic correlates in Huntington's disease. J Neurol Neurosurg Psychiatry 51:1259–1263, 1988

Starkstein SE, Berthier ML, Bolduc PL, et al: Depression in patients with early versus late onset of Parkinson's disease. Neurology 39:1441–1445, 1989

Stewart JT, Mounts ML, Clark RL: Aggressive behavior in Huntington's disease: treatment with propranolol. J Clin Psychiatry 48(3):106–108, 1987

Sutcliffe RLG: Parkinson's disease in the district of Northhampton Health Authority, United Kingdom: a study of prevalence and disability. Acta Neurol Scand 72:363–379, 1985

Tagliavini F, Pilleri G, Bouras C, et al: The basal nucleus of Meynert in idiopathic Parkinson's disease. Acta Neurol Scand 69:20–28, 1984

Tedroff J, Aquilonious SM, Hartvig P, et al: Monoamine re-uptake sites in the human brain evaluated in vivo by means of 11C-nomifensine and positron emission tomography: the effects of age and Parkinson's disease. Acta Neurol Scand 77:192–201, 1988

Tyler HR: Nonfamilial amyotrophy with dementia or multisystem degeneration and other neurological disorders, in Human Motor Neuron Diseases. Edited by Rowland LP. New York, Raven, 1982, pp 173–179

Ward CD, Duvoisin RC, Ince SE, et al: Parkinson's disease in 65 pairs of twins and in a set of quadruplets. Neurology 33:815–824, 1983

Wasmuth JJ, Hewitt J, Smith B: A highly polymorphic locus very tightly linked to the Huntington's disease gene. Nature 332:734–736, 1988

Whitehouse PJ, Hedreen JC, White CL, et al: Basal forebrain neurons in the dementia of Parkinson's disease. Ann Neurol 13:243–248, 1983

Whitehouse PJ, Vale WW, Zweig RM, et al: Reductions in corticotropin releasing factor-like immunoreactivity in cerebral cortex in Alzheimer's disease, Parkinson's disease, and progressive supranuclear palsy. Neurology 37:905–909, 1987

Whitehouse PJ, Martino AM, Marcus KA, et al: Reductions in acetylcholine and nicotine binding in several degenerative diseases. Arch Neurol 45:722–724, 1988

Chapter 24

Neuropsychiatric Aspects of Alzheimer's Disease and Other Dementing Illnesses

Jeffrey L. Cummings, M.D.

Dementing diseases are frequently accompanied by neuropsychiatric syndromes including personality alterations, mood changes, and psychosis. In this chapter, the neuropsychiatric aspects of Alzheimer's disease (AD), frontal lobe degenerations, vascular dementias, and hydrocephalus are reviewed.

DEMOGRAPHY AND DEFINITIONS

Dementia is a syndrome of acquired persistent impairment of mental function involving at least three of the following five behavioral domains: memory, language, visuospatial skills, personality or mood, and cognition (including abstraction, judgment, calculation, and executive function) (Cummings and Benson 1992). Estimates of the prevalence of dementia vary markedly, but most studies suggest that approximately 5% of persons over age 65 are severely demented and an additional 10% have mild to moderate intellectual compromise (Ineichen 1987; Jorm et al. 1987). The total financial impact of dementia on society in the United States has been estimated at approximately $30 billion annually (Hays and Ernst 1987).

ALZHEIMER'S DISEASE

AD is a progressive degenerative disorder affecting primarily the neurons of the cerebral cortex. It is the single most common dementing illness of the elderly and afflicts between two million and four million United States citizens (Katzman 1986). AD usually begins after age 55, and its incidence and prevalence rise with age; men and women are approximately equally likely to have the disease. The course is inexorably progressive, and patients survive approximately a decade from diagnosis to death.

Clinical Diagnosis

The diagnosis of AD is stratified as definite, probable, or possible according to the certainty of the available information (McKhann et al. 1984). A diagnosis of *defi-*

This project was supported by the U.S. Department of Veterans Affairs.

nite AD requires that the patient exhibit a characteristic clinical syndrome and that there be confirmatory histological evidence of AD pathology obtained from biopsy or autopsy.

The diagnosis of *probable AD* requires that the patient meet criteria for dementia based on a clinical examination, structured mental status questionnaire, and neuropsychological testing; there are deficits in at least two areas of intellectual function; there is progressive worsening of memory and other intellectual function; there is no disturbance of consciousness; the disease begins between ages 40 and 90; and there are no systemic or other brain disorders that could account for the deficits observed. *Possible AD* is diagnosed when there are variations in the onset, presentation, or course of a dementing illness that has no alternate explanation; there is a systemic illness or brain disease present that is considered not to be the cause of the dementia syndrome; or there is a single gradually progressive cognitive deficit in the absence of any other brain disorder.

The classic dementia syndrome of AD includes impairment of learning new information, poor recall of remote material, impaired naming and auditory comprehension, deterioration in constructional and visuospatial abilities, and poor calculation, abstraction, and judgment (Cummings and Benson 1986). In the final phases of the disease, there is near total abolition of intellectual function as well as progressive loss of ambulation and coordination, dysphagia, and incontinence.

Neuropsychiatric Aspects

Table 24–1 lists the principal neuropsychiatric syndromes occurring in AD (Cummings and Victoroff 1990). Personality changes are ubiquitous in AD, the most common being passivity or disengagement: patients exhibit diminished emotional responsiveness, decreased initiative, loss of enthusiasm, diminished energy, and decreased affection (Petry et al. 1988; Rubin et al. 1987). Delusions are also common in AD, affecting between 30% and 50% of patients (Cummings et al. 1987; Wragg and Jeste 1989). The most frequent delusions involve false beliefs of theft, infidelity of the spouse, abandonment, the house is not one's home, persecution,

Table 24–1. Neuropsychiatric characteristics of Alzheimer's disease

Personality alterations	Mood lability
Disengagement	**Anxiety**
Disinhibition	**Psychomotor activity disturbances**
Delusions	Agitation or combativeness
Persecutory	Wandering
Theft	Pacing
Infidelity	Purposeless activity
Capgras	**Miscellaneous**
Hallucinations	Sexual activity changes
Auditory	Decreased sexual interest
Visual	Increased sexual interest
Mood changes	Appetite changes
Depressive symptoms	Sleep disturbances
Elevated mood	Klüver-Bucy syndrome
Catastrophic reactions	

phantom boarder, and the Capgras phenomenon (Reisberg et al. 1987). Delusions do not correlate with the severity of dementia or with specific aspects of intellectual dysfunction (Flynn et al. 1991).

Hallucinations are not a common manifestation of AD; between 9% and 27% of patients have hallucinatory behavior. Visual hallucinations are most common, followed by auditory hallucinations or combined auditory and visual hallucinatory experiences. Auditory hallucinations are often persecutory and usually accompany delusions. Visual hallucinations may be indicative of a co-occurring delirium (Cummings et al. 1987).

A variety of mood changes have been observed in AD including depressive symptoms, elation, and lability. Few patients meet criteria of major depressive episodes, but elements of a depression syndrome are frequent, occurring in 20%–40% of AD patients (Cummings et al. 1987). Anxiety has been reported in approximately 40% of patients with AD (Mendez et al. 1990).

Psychomotor activity disturbances and troublesome behaviors are common in AD and become increasingly evident as the disease progresses. Wandering and pacing are pervasive behaviors in the middle and later stages of the illness. Restlessness is reported in up to 60% of AD patients, angry outbursts in 50%, and assaultive behavior in 20% (Swearer et al. 1988). Sleep disturbances with frequent interruptions of nocturnal sleep are common, occurring in 45%–70% of patients (Merriam et al. 1988; Swearer et al. 1988).

Laboratory Investigations

The results of most laboratory studies remain normal in AD. Computed tomography (CT) and magnetic resonance imaging (MRI) may reveal cerebral atrophy and help exclude intracranial processes that may imitate AD (e.g., neoplasms and subdural hematomas) but do not provide specific diagnostic information (Cummings and Benson 1992). Electroencephalography (EEG) usually reveals theta and delta slowing as the disease advances, and computed EEG studies with brain mapping demonstrate maximal abnormalities in the parietal regions of both hemispheres (Jordan et al. 1989).

Metabolic and perfusion studies offer substantial support for the diagnosis of AD. Positron-emission tomography (PET) using [^{18}F]fluorodeoxyglucose (FDG) reveals a characteristic pattern of hypometabolism (Figure 24–1). Early in the disease there is diminished glucose utilization in the parietal lobes, and the frontal lobes are affected as the disease progresses (Foster et al. 1983).

Single photon emission computed tomography (SPECT) measures cerebral blood flow. SPECT reveals diminished cerebral perfusion, most marked in the parietal and posterior temporal lobes of both hemispheres, in the majority of AD patients (Figure 24–2) (Miller et al. 1990).

Neuropathology

The major pathological alterations of AD include neuronal loss, cortical gliosis, intraneuronal cytoplasmic neurofibrillary tangles, neuritic plaques, granulovacuolar degeneration, and amyloid angiopathy of the cerebral vessels (Cummings and

Benson 1992; Katzman 1986). The pathological burden of the disease is greatest in the medial temporal, posterior cingulate, and temporal-parietal junction regions. The frontal cortex is moderately involved, and the primary motor and sensory cortices have fewer pathological abnormalities (Brun and Gustafson 1976). Neurotransmitter alterations include marked reductions of choline acetyltransferase and somatostatin, as well as more modest and variable losses of serotonin, γ-aminobutyric acid (GABA), and norepinephrine (Cummings and Benson 1992; Procter et al. 1988).

FRONTAL LOBE DEGENERATIONS

Frontal lobe degenerations (FLD) are progressive idiopathic disorders that preferentially affect the frontal lobes. In some cases, distinctive histopathological changes such as Pick cells are noted at autopsy and a diagnosis of Pick's disease is supported; in others, no specific cellular changes are found (Brun 1987).

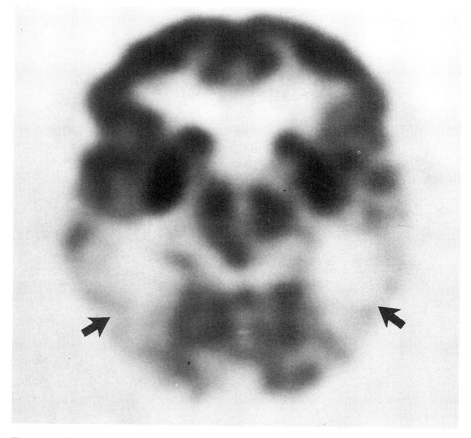

Figure 24–1.   Transaxial positron-emission tomography (PET) scan revealing decreased glucose metabolism bilaterally in the parietal lobes (*arrows*) characteristic of Alzheimer's disease.
Source.   Image courtesy of M. Mahler and D. Sultzer.

Clinical and Neuropsychiatric Features

Neuropsychiatric features dominate the presentation of FLDs. Personality alterations are often florid, and depression or psychosis may be prominent. Patients may be apathetic or disinhibited (Miller et al. 1990). Apathetic individuals exhibit social and occupational withdrawal, loss of motivation, and interpersonal disengagement. Disinhibited patients are often boisterous, prone to make vulgar or socially inappropriate remarks, exhibit undue familiarity with strangers, have poor

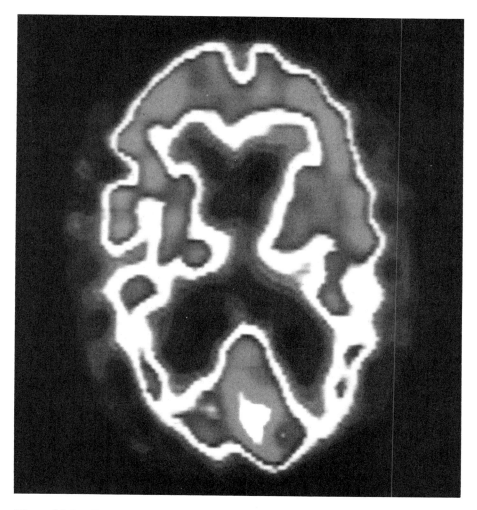

Figure 24–2. Transaxial single photon emission computed tomography (SPECT) scan of a patient with Alzheimer's disease revealing diminished cerebral perfusion in the tempoparietal regions bilaterally (red areas have normal blood flow; yellow regions have diminished perfusion).

Source. Image courtesy of I. Mena. (Please refer to page 609 of *The American Psychiatric Press Textbook of Neuropsychiatry,* Second Edition, for the full-color figure.)

judgment, and may be unusually irritable. The Klüver-Bucy syndrome or fragments of the condition may be evident in the initial phases of the disease, and patients frequently gain weight as their eating habits become less discriminating (Cummings and Duchen 1981). Stereotyped behaviors with compulsive rituals and complex repetitive acts may also be observed in the course of FLD (Gustafson 1987).

Neuropsychological deficits are less marked in FLD than in AD. Memory, visuospatial skills, and mathematical abilities are relatively spared in the early and middle stages of FLD (Cummings and Benson 1992). Patients have executive function deficits including difficulty with set shifting tasks, word list generation, divided attention, and response inhibition (Miller et al. 1991). Language may be affected relatively early in the disease. Naming deficits, impairment of auditory comprehension, and increasingly sparse verbal output are common. Speech stereotypies, echolalia, and mutism may also occur (Cummings and Benson 1992).

Laboratory Investigations

Results from routine studies of serum, urine, and cerebrospinal fluid (CSF) are normal in FLD. Neuroimaging with CT or MRI may provide supportive information if focal atrophy of the frontal or temporal lobes is revealed (Cummings and Benson 1992). More definitive diagnostic information is provided by PET or SPECT scanning. FDG-PET reveals markedly diminished frontal lobe glucose utilization, particularly in the midfrontal convexity (Kamo et al. 1987). SPECT demonstrates severely diminished cerebral perfusion in the frontal lobes and, in some cases, in the anterior temporal lobes (Figure 24–3) (Miller et al. 1991; Neary et al. 1988).

Neuropathology

The macroscopic pathology of Pick's disease includes marked atrophy of the frontal lobe anterior to the precentral sulcus and of the anterior temporal lobe (Cummings and Benson 1992). Neurons are atrophic, and there is gliosis of affected regions. Some of the remaining neurons contain intracytoplasmic argyrophilic Pick bodies (Wechsler et al. 1982). Enlarged neurons with uniformly argyrophilic cytoplasm known as *ballooned cells* may occur in affected regions. FLD patients without Pick's type pathology have nonspecific neuronal loss and gliosis in a lobar distribution (Brun 1987).

Neurochemical investigations have also been carried out in Pick's disease. Cortical choline acetyltransferase, L-glutamic acid decarboxylase, and dopamine are preserved (Yates et al. 1980). In the basal ganglia, dopamine, GABA, and substance P levels are reduced, and choline acetyltransferase levels are variably diminished (Kanazawa et al. 1988).

Differential Diagnosis

FLD can usually be distinguished from AD on the basis of contrasting clinical characteristics. In AD, memory impairment, constructional disturbances, and acalculia appear early in the clinical course, whereas these deficits are delayed until the middle or late phases of FLD. Conspicuous personality changes and executive deficits herald the onset of FLD and are more modest and delayed in AD. CT and MRI reveal generalized atrophy in AD and frontal or temporal lobar atrophy in FLD. FDG-PET and SPECT demonstrate diminished posterior temporal and parietal function in AD and decreased frontotemporal function in FLD (Cummings and Benson 1992; Miller et al. 1991). Several diseases can affect frontal lobe function in addition to FLD (Table 24–2).

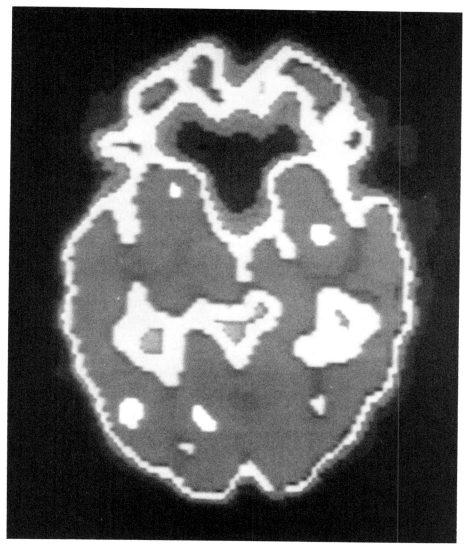

Figure 24–3.   Transaxial single photon emission computed tomography (SPECT) scan of a patient with a frontal lobe degeneration demonstrating decreased cerebral blood flow in the frontal lobes (red areas have normal blood flow; yellow regions have diminished perfusion). *Source.*   Image courtesy of I. Mena. (Please refer to page 610 of *The American Psychiatric Press Textbook of Neuropsychiatry,* Second Edition, for the full-color figure.)

Table 24–2. Principal dementia syndromes with prominent frontal lobe involvement

Disorder	Characteristic features
Pick's disease	Cortical dementia with personality changes; language alterations; memory, constructional, and arithmetic deficits delayed; and intracytoplasmic neuronal Pick bodies
Frontal lobe degeneration—non-Alzheimer type	Clinical features similar to Pick's disease and nonspecific histologic alterations
Amyotrophic lateral sclerosis	Dementia with motor neuron syndrome
Neuronal intranuclear hyaline inclusion	Dementia with aggressive behavior; some patients have choreiform movements, ataxia, or tremor; and neuronal and disease glial inclusions
Progressive supranuclear palsy	Ophthalmoplegia, parkinsonism, and dysarthria
Progressive subcortical gliosis	Clinical features similar to Pick's disease and marked subcortical and white matter gliosis
Anterior cerebral artery occlusion	Apathy and paresis and sensory loss of lower limbs
Syphilis	Grandiosity and hypomania, positive serum serology, and abnormal cerebrospinal fluid protein, cell count, and Venereal Disease Research Laboratories test results
Hydrocephalus	Gait disturbance and incontinence, enlarged ventricles, and abnormal cisternography and pressure monitoring
Depression	Marked mood change and diminished glucose metabolism or perfusion of frontal lobes

VASCULAR DEMENTIA

Vascular dementia, also known as multi-infarct dementia (MID), is a dementing condition produced by cerebral ischemic injury. In its classic form, MID is characterized by an abrupt onset, stepwise deterioration, patchy pattern of intellectual deficits, focal neurological symptoms (transient ischemic attacks), focal neurological signs, a history of hypertension, and evidence of associated cardiovascular disease (American Psychiatric Association 1987; Hachinski et al. 1975). The majority of cases are produced by hypertensive cerebrovascular disease, but MID may also occur with multiple cerebral emboli, systemic hypotension, intracerebral hemorrhage, and inflammatory and infectious vascular disease (Cummings and Benson 1992; Sulkava and Erkinjuntti 1987).

Vascular dementia is the second most common cause of dementia in the elderly, accounting for 8%–35% of dementia syndromes (Cummings and Benson 1992). MID is most common after the age of 50 and affects men more often than women. Patients survive for 6–8 years after onset; death usually results from cardiovascular disease or stroke.

Clinical and Neuropsychiatric Features

Historically, MID is characterized by an abrupt onset in concert with the occurrence of a stroke and stepwise deterioration occurring synchronously with repeated cerebrovascular events. In some cases, however, neuropsychological abnormalities accumulate gradually, imitating the course of a degenerative dementia. On examination, MID patients exhibit a combination of motor abnormalities, neuropsychological deficits, and neuropsychiatric symptoms. Motor findings may include weakness, spasticity, hyperreflexia, extensor plantar responses, bradykinesia, parkinsonism, and pseudobulbar palsy (Ishii et al. 1986). Gait abnormalities are common and may appear early in the course of the disorder.

The pattern of neuropsychological abnormalities in MID is characterized by "patchiness" with preservation of some abilities and mild to severe compromise of others. Neuropsychiatric abnormalities that occur regularly include personality changes, depression, lability of mood, and delusions, but personality changes are the most common alterations. Apathy, abulia, and aspontaneity dominate the clinical syndrome (Dian et al. 1990). Major depressive disorders occur in 25%–50% of MID patients, and up to 60% of patients evidence symptoms of a depressive syndrome (Cummings 1988). Psychosis with delusional ideation occurs in approximately 50% of MID patients (Flynn et al. 1991).

Laboratory Investigations

Serum studies of MID patients should routinely include complete blood count, erythrocyte sedimentation rate, and serum cholesterol and triglyceride levels. In the absence of a history of hypertension or other stroke risk factors, more extensive laboratory studies should be pursued including antinuclear antibodies, antiphospholipid antibodies, and lupus anticoagulant levels (Briley et al. 1989; Cummings and Benson 1992).

Neuroimaging studies provide support for the clinical diagnosis of MID. CT may reveal infarctions and evidence of periventricular ischemic changes (Aharon-Peretz et al. 1988; Erkinjuntti et al. 1987). MRI is more revealing than CT and demonstrates small subcortical infarctions and ischemic white matter changes invisible on CT (Brown et al. 1988; Hershey et al. 1987). FDG-PET and SPECT show multiple irregular areas of hypometabolism or hypoperfusion consistent with focal regions of tissue infarction (Gemmell et al. 1987).

Classification and Neuropathology

Several subtypes of MID have been identified based on the size of vessel occluded and the area of tissue injured (Cummings and Benson 1992). Atherosclerosis may lead to occlusion of carotid arteries with large hemispheric infarctions; the most marked ischemic injury is in the borderzone regions between the three principal intracranial vessels. Occlusions of the anterior, middle, or posterior cerebral arteries produce hemisphere-specific deficit syndromes with neuropsychiatric complications. Most MID is a product of sustained hypertension leading to fibrinoid necrosis of small arteries and arterioles. These vessels supply the deep gray matter nuclei including the striatum and thalamus, as well as the hemispheric white matter. Multiple small "lacunar" infarctions of the basal ganglia and thalamus produce the syndrome of lacunar state. Binswanger's disease is the syndrome characterized by extensive white matter ischemia. In most cases, lacunar state and Binswanger's disease coexist (Roman 1987).

HYDROCEPHALIC DEMENTIA

"Hydrocephalus" refers to enlargement of the cerebral ventricles with an increased amount of intraventricular CSF. Ventricular enlargement may be on an ex vacuo basis (from loss of cerebral tissue) or due to interruption of CSF flow (obstructive hydrocephalus). There are two types of obstructive hydrocephalus: noncommunicating and communicating. Noncommunicating hydrocephalus arises from obstruction of CSF flow within the ventricular system or between the ventricles and the subarachnoid space. Communicating hydrocephalus occurs with obstruction of CSF flow within the subarachnoid space, preventing absorption of the CSF into the superior saggital sinus. Communicating hydrocephalus presents as a dementia syndrome and intracranial pressure is normal, hence the alternate name *normal-pressure hydrocephalus* (NPH) (Cummings and Benson 1992).

Clinical and Neuropsychiatric Features

The classic syndrome of NPH consists of dementia, gait disturbance, and incontinence. The dementia has prominent features of frontal-subcortical dysfunction including impaired attention and mental control, poor learning, visuospatial disturbances, and impaired abstraction and judgment (Cummings and Benson 1992). The gait abnormalities of NPH are variable but commonly include shortened stride length, diminished step height, and slow speed (Sudarsky and Simon 1987). Urinary incontinence is more common than loss of bowel control.

A variety of neuropsychiatric syndromes have been described in patients with NPH including personality alterations, anxiety, mood changes, and (rarely) psychosis. Apathy, inertia, and unconcern are the typical personality alterations; aggressive outbursts have also been reported (Crowell et al. 1973; Gustafson and Hagberg 1978).

Etiologies

NPH results from impaired absorption of fluid into the superior sagittal sinus (Cummings and Benson 1992). Classic NPH follows subarachnoid hemorrhage, head trauma, encephalitis, or meningitis. Many cases are idiopathic.

Diagnosis

The diagnosis of NPH depends on a combination of neuroimaging, CSF flow, and CSF pressure observations. CT studies reveal markedly enlarged ventricles and periventricular lucencies. The ventriculomegaly is most evident anteriorly with enlarged frontal and temporal horns. MRI demonstrates the same pattern of ventricular enlargement, increased periventricular signal on T2-weighted images, and an aqueductal flow void (Cummings and Benson 1992). Routine lumbar puncture reveals normal CSF pressure, and 24-hour pressure monitoring demonstrates increased B waves (Graff-Radford et al. 1989). Cisternography provides a means of assessing the pattern of CSF flow.

EVALUATION AND TREATMENT

Evaluation of the dementia patient includes a careful history, mental status testing, and general physical and neurological examination. An assessment of past and current neuropsychiatric alterations (e.g., personality changes, anxiety, depression, mania, psychosis, and hallucinations) should be included. Appropriate laboratory studies include complete blood count, erythrocyte sedimentation rate, electrolytes, serum glucose, blood urea nitrogen, serum calcium and phosphorus levels, liver function tests, thyroid-stimulating hormone, vitamin B_{12} level, and serological test for syphilis (Cummings and Benson 1992).

Neuroimaging procedures are an important part of the evaluation of the dementia patient. CT scanning is adequate for identifying intracranial tumors, hydrocephalus, larger strokes, abscesses, or subdural hematomas. MRI is more sensitive to detection of ischemic injury and demyelination and capable of revealing more intracranial pathology than CT (Brown et al. 1988; Erkinjuntti et al. 1987). PET and SPECT, imaging cerebral metabolism and perfusion, add another important dimension to the evaluation of dementia since CT and MRI reveal only nonspecific atrophy.

There is no available therapy that ameliorates the course of AD or FLD; hydrocephalic patients have ventriculoperitoneal shunts placed; MID is currently managed with control of hypertension and administration of platelet antiaggregants (aspirin or ticlopidine) (Meyer et al. 1986). Most treatment of dementia patients is directed at control of associated behavioral disturbances rather than the underlying dementing illness. Table 24–3 lists neuropsychiatric alterations that occur in dementia syndromes

Table 24–3.   Neuropsychiatric alterations of dementia syndromes and the pharmacologic agents commonly used in their treatment

Symptom	Available agents	Usual daily dose in mg po (range)
Psychosis	Haloperidol	1 (0.5–3)
	Thioridazine	75 (30–150)
Agitation	Neuroleptics	
	Haloperidol	1 (0.5–3)
	Molindone	40 (5–100)
	Nonneuroleptics	
	Propranolol	120 (80–240)
	Trazodone	100 (100–400)
	Buspirone	15 (15–30)
	Carbamazepine	1,000 (800–1,200)
	Lorazepam	1 (0.5–6)
Depression	Nortriptyline	50 (50–100)
	Trazodone	100 (100–400)
	Fluoxetine	20 (10–40)
Anxiety	Oxazepam	30 (20–60)
	Propranolol	120 (80–240)
Insomnia	Temazepam	15 (15–30)
	Trazodone	100 (100–400)
	Thioridazine	25 (10–75)
Sexual aggression (in males)	Medroxyprogesterone	300 mg/week im

Source.   Adapted from Cummings and Benson 1992.

and the pharmacological agents most commonly used in their treatment.

In general, the drugs used in dementia are the same as those used for similar behaviors in patients without dementia, but dosages should be adjusted to reflect the fact that most dementias occur in aged individuals (Montamat et al. 1989; Thompson et al. 1983). Various nonpharmacological interventions may also be used with dementia patients in different phases of their illness including cognitive therapy, family therapy, supportive therapy, reminiscent therapy, and behavioral modification (Maletta 1988). Care of dementia patients is delivered primarily by family members and the psychological, social, and legal needs of caregivers must be assessed.

REFERENCES

Aharon-Peretz J, Cummings JL, Hill MA: Vascular dementia and dementia of the Alzheimer type: cognition, ventricular size, and leuko-araiosis. Arch Neurol 45:719–721, 1988

American Psychiatric Association: Diagnostic and Statistical Manual of Mental Disorders, 3rd Edition, Revised. Washington, DC, American Psychiatric Association, 1987

Briley DP, Coull BM, Goodnight SH Jr: Neurological disease associated with antiphospholipid antibodies. Ann Neurol 25:221–227, 1989

Brown JJ, Hesselink JR, Rothrock JF: MR and CT of lacunar infarcts. American Journal of Radiology 151:367–372, 1988

Brun A: Frontal lobe degeneration of non-Alzheimer type, I: neuropathology. Archives of Gerontology and Geriatrics 6:193–208, 1987

Brun A, Gustafson L: Distribution of cerebral degeneration in Alzheimer's disease. Archiv Psychiatrie Nervenkrankheiten 223:15–33, 1976

Crowell RM, Tew JM Jr, Mark VH: Aggressive dementia associated with normal pressure hydrocephalus. Neurology 23:461–464, 1973

Cummings JL: Depression in vascular dementia. Hillside J Clin Psychiatry 10:209–231, 1988

Cummings JL, Benson DF: Dementia of the Alzheimer type: an inventory of diagnostic clinical features. J Am Geriatr Soc 34:12–19, 1986

Cummings JL, Benson DF: Dementia: A Clinical Approach, 2nd Edition. Boston, MA, Butterworths, 1992

Cummings JL, Duchen LW: Kluver-Bucy syndrome in Pick disease: clinical and pathologic correlations. Neurology 31:1415–1422, 1981

Cummings JL, Victoroff JI: Noncognitive neuropsychiatric syndromes in Alzheimer's disease. Neuropsychiatry, Neuropsychology, and Behavioral Neurology 3:140–158, 1990

Cummings JL, Miller B, Hill MA, et al: Neuropsychiatric aspects of multi-infarct dementia and dementia of the Alzheimer type. Arch Neurol 44:389–393, 1987

Dian L, Cummings JL, Petry S, et al: Personality alterations in vascular dementia. Psychosomatics 31:415–419, 1990

Erkinjuntti T, Ketonen L, Sulkava R, et al: CT in the differential diagnosis between Alzheimer's disease and vascular dementia. Acta Neurol Scand 75:262–270, 1987

Flynn FG, Cummings JL, Gornbein J: Delusions in dementia syndromes: investigation of behavioral and neuropsychological correlates. Journal of Neuropsychiatry and Clinical Neurosciences 3:364–370, 1991

Foster NL, Chase TN, Fedio P, et al: Alzheimer's disease: focal cortical changes shown by positron emission tomography. Neurology 33:961–965, 1983

Gemmell HG, Sharp PF, Besson JAO, et al: Differential diagnosis in dementia using the cerebral blood flow agent 99mTc HM-PAO: a SPECT study. J Comput Assist Tomogr 11:398–402, 1987

Graff-Radford NR, Godersky JC, Jones MP: Variables predicting surgical outcome in symptomatic hydrocephalus in the elderly. Neurology 39:1601–1604, 1989

Gustafson L: Frontal lobe degeneration of non-Alzheimer type, II: clinical picture and differential diagnosis. Archives of Gerontology and Geriatrics 6:209–223, 1987

Gustafson L, Hagberg B: Recovery of hydrocephalic dementia after shunt operation. J Neurol Neurosurg Psychiatry 41:940–947, 1978

Hachinski VC, Iliff LD, Zilhka E, et al: Cerebral blood flow in dementia. Arch Neurol 32:632–637, 1975

Hays JW, Ernst RL: The economic costs of Alzheimer's disease. Am J Public Health 77:1169–1175, 1987

Hershey LA, Modic MT, Greenough G, et al: Magnetic resonance imaging in vascular dementia. Neurology 37:29–36, 1987

Ineichen B: Measuring the rising tide: how many dementia cases will there be in 2001? Br J Psychiatry 150:193–200, 1987

Ishii N, Nishihara Y, Imamura T: Why do frontal lobe symptoms predominate in vascular dementia with lacunes? Neurology 36:340–345, 1986

Jordan SE, Nowacki R, Nuwer M: Computerized electroencephalography in the evaluation of early dementia. Brain Topography 1:271–274, 1989

Jorm AF, Korten AE, Henderson AS: The prevalence of dementia: a quantitative integration of the literature. Acta Psychiatr Scand 76:465–479, 1987

Kamo H, McGeer PL, Harrop R, et al: Positron emission tomography and histopathology in Pick's disease. Neurology 37:439–445, 1987

Kanazawa I, Kwak S, Sasaki H, et al: Studies on neurotransmitter markers of the basal ganglia in Pick's disease, with special reference to dopamine depletion. J Neurol Sci 83:63–74, 1988

Katzman R: Alzheimer's disease. N Engl J Med 314:964–973, 1986

McKhann G, Drachman D, Folstein M, et al: Clinical diagnosis of Alzheimer's disease: report of the NINCDS-ADRDA Work Group under the auspices of Department of Health and Human Services Task Force on Alzheimer's Disease. Neurology 34:939–944, 1984

Maletta GJ: Management of behavior problems in elderly patients with Alzheimer's disease and other dementias. Clin Geriatr Med 4:719–747, 1988

Mendez MF, Martin RJ, Smyth KA, et al: Psychiatric symptoms associated with Alzheimer's disease. Journal of Neuropsychiatry and Clinical Neuroscience 2:28–33, 1990

Merriam AE, Aronson MK, Gaston P, et al: The psychiatric symptoms of Alzheimer's disease. J Am Geriatr Soc 36:7–12, 1988

Meyer JS, Judd BW, Tawakina T, et al: Improved cognition after control of risk factors for multi-infarct dementia. JAMA 256:2203–2209, 1986

Miller BL, Mena I, Daly J, et al: Temporal-parietal hypoperfusion with single-photon emission computerized tomography in conditions other than Alzheimer's disease. Dementia 1:41–45, 1990

Miller BL, Cummings JL, Villanueva-Mayer J, et al: Frontal lobe degenerations: clinical, neuropsychological and SPECT characteristics. Neurology 41:1374–1382, 1991

Montamat SC, Cusack BJ, Vestal RE: Management of drug therapy in the elderly. N Engl J Med 321:303–309, 1989

Neary D, Snowden JS, Northen B, et al: Dementia of frontal lobe type. J Neurol Neurosurg Psychiatry 51:353–361, 1988

Petry S, Cummings JL, Hill MA, et al: Personality alterations in dementia of the Alzheimer type. Arch Neurol 45:1187–1190, 1988

Procter A, Lowe SL, Palmer AM, et al: Topographical distribution of neurochemical changes in Alzheimer's disease. J Neurol Sci 84:125–140, 1988

Reisberg B, Borenstein J, Salob SP, et al: Behavioral symptoms in Alzheimer's disease: phenomenology and treatment. J Clin Psychiatry 48 (suppl 5):9–15, 1987

Roman GC: Senile dementia of the Binswanger type. JAMA 258:1782–1788, 1987

Rubin EH, Morris JC, Storandt M, et al: Behavioral changes in patients with mild senile dementia of the Alzheimer's type. Psychiatry Res 21:55–62, 1987

Sudarsky L, Simon S: Gait disturbance in late-life hydrocephalus. Arch Neurol 44:263–267,
1987

Sulkava R, Erkinjuntti T: Vascular dementia due to cardiac arrhythmias and systemic hypotension. Acta Neurol Scand 76:123–128, 1987

Swearer JM, Drachman DA, O'Donnell BF, et al: Troublesome and disruptive behaviors in
dementia. J Am Geriatr Soc 36:784–790, 1988

Thompson TL II, Moran MG, Nies AS: Psychotropic drug use in the elderly. N Engl J Med
308:134–138, 194–199, 1983

Wechsler AF, Verity A, Rosenschein S, et al: Pick's disease: a clinical, computed tomographic,
and histologic study with Golgi impregnation observations. Arch Neurol 39:287–290, 1982

Wragg RE, Jeste DV: Overview of depression and psychosis in Alzheimer's disease. Am J
Psychiatry 146:577–587, 1989

Yates CM, Simpson J, Maloney AFJ, et al: Neurochemical observations in a case of Pick's
disease. J Neurol Sci 48:257–263, 1980

Chapter 25

The Neuropsychiatry of Schizophrenia

Henry A. Nasrallah, M.D.

Schizophrenia is arguably the most serious psychiatric disorder and one that has become widely recognized as a brain disease (Nasrallah and Weinberger 1986). Evidence for the neurobiological basis of schizophrenia has been accumulating rapidly over the past two decades. The explosive advances in neuroscience research and the advent of computed brain imaging techniques have generated a windfall of new knowledge about brain structure and function in schizophrenia.

In this chapter, an overview of the neuropsychiatry of schizophrenia is presented along two main themes: 1) brain lesions that produce a schizophrenia-like psychosis (also known as *symptomatic* or *secondary* schizophrenia) and 2) neurobiological findings in *primary* schizophrenia.

STRUCTURAL AND FUNCTIONAL BRAIN LESIONS ASSOCIATED WITH SCHIZOPHRENIA-LIKE PSYCHOTIC SYNDROMES

Numerous medical conditions are known to produce psychotic symptoms that resemble schizophrenia (Cummings 1988; Nasrallah 1986). Such clinical observations have generated many hypotheses regarding the brain "dysfunction" that may elucidate the neuropsychiatry of schizophrenia.

Genetic Abnormalities

Several established genetic disorders, in addition to producing physical anomalies, are known to produce psychotic symptoms that strongly resemble schizophrenia (Propping and Friedl 1988). Table 25–1 lists genetic disorders that have been reported to present clinically with psychotic features.

Congenital (Neurodevelopmental) Disorders

Several neurological congenital anomalies have been associated with psychotic symptoms, including corpus callosum agenesis, aqueduct stenosis, arachnoid cysts, porencephaly, cerebral hamartoma, and cavum septum pellucidum. Reports of such associations (e.g., Swayze et al. 1990) lend support to the neurodevelopmental hypothesis of schizophrenia (Nasrallah 1990), which postulates that schizophrenia is associated with disruption(s) of basic neurodevelopmental processes

Table 25–1.   Genetic disorders that may present with a schizophrenia-like psychosis

1. Albinism	15. Kartagener's syndrome
2. Asperger's syndrome	16. Klinefelter karyotype
3. Ataxia, dominant type	17. Lawrence-Moon-Bardet-Biedl syndrome
4. Congenital adrenal hyperplasia	
5. Erythropoietic protoporphyria	18. Metachromatic leukodystrophy, adult type
6. Fabry's disease	
7. Familial basal ganglia calcification	19. Niemann-Pick's disease, late type
8. Glucose-6-phosphate dehydrogenase deficiency	20. Phenylketonuria
	21. Porphyria, acute intermittent type
9. Gaucher's disease	22. Porphyria variegata
10. Hemochromatosis	23. 18q or r (18) constitution
11. Homocystinuria	24. Turner's (or Noonan's) syndrome
12. Huntington's chorea	
13. Hyperasparginemia	25. Wilson's disease
14. Ichthyosis vulgaris (autosomal dominant type)	26. XXX karyotype
	27. XYY karyotype

Source.   Adapted from Nasrallah 1986.

such as neuronal proliferation, migration, and elimination during fetal life, especially during the critical second trimester (Nowakowski 1987).

Perinatal Complications

Research suggests that neurological insults resulting from pregnancy and delivery complications are associated with schizophrenic psychoses in adulthood (Lyon et al. 1989). It is postulated that perinatal complications may disrupt the brain structure and functions in a manner that facilitates the development of psychotic perceptions, thoughts, and behavior. For example, interference with neuronal migration in the hippocampus (which is especially sensitive to hypoxia in the second trimester), may result in gross hypoplasia of the hippocampal formation and aberrant histoarchitecture of pyramidal cells in parts of the hippocampus (Conrad and Scheibel 1987). Mednick et al. (1988) demonstrated that fetal exposure to influenza during the second trimester is associated with increased risk for the development of schizophrenia. Perinatal brain injury may contribute to the heterogeneous spectrum of the schizophrenic syndrome and may help explain the discordance for schizophrenia in monozygotic twins (Suddath et al. 1990) or for variations in the age at onset (Wilcox and Nasrallah 1987a) or in deficit symptoms and course (Wilcox and Nasrallah 1987b).

Neurological Disorders in Childhood and Adulthood

Many neurological disorders have been reported to be occasionally associated with psychotic signs and symptoms (Davison 1983). The following neurological disorders may present with psychosis:

1. *Epilepsy.* A higher frequency of psychosis is observed in patients with epilepsy than would be expected in the general population. This is especially true for left temporal lobe foci, an observation that led Flor-Henry (1969) to postulate a lateralized left dysfunction in schizophrenia. Roberts et al. (1990) demonstrated that even in chronic temporal lobe epilepsy, schizophrenia-like psychosis did not occur at random. Rather, psychosis a) was significantly associated with lesions that originated during fetal life, b) affected neurons in the medial temporal lobe, and c) produced first seizure at an early age.

2. *Cerebral trauma.* Many studies of psychosis subsequent to cerebral trauma have been reported (Davison and Bagley 1969). Temporal and frontal lobe traumas appear to be more likely to produce psychotic features, with left temporal lobe injury producing positive symptoms and frontal lobe injury producing mainly negative symptoms.

3. *Cerebral tumors.* Many psychotic patients who died in long-term institutions had brain tumors at autopsy; tumors in the temporal, hypophyseal, suprasellar, and supratentorial areas are particularly likely to produce schizophrenia-like features. Tumors of the third ventricle strongly resemble catatonic schizophrenia; hallucinations and delusions are more likely in temporal, frontal, and pituitary tumors (Nasrallah and McChesney 1981).

4. *Cerebral infections.* Various types of encephalitides have been associated with psychotic symptoms, such as encephalitis lethargic epidemic sequelae in the 1920s, postrheumatic Syndenham's chorea (Wilcox and Nasrallah 1988), and syphilis.

5. *Neurodegenerative disorders.* Psychotic symptoms are known to accompany or be a main feature of basal ganglia disorders as well as other neurodegenerative diseases (e.g., Alzheimer's disease, Pick's disease, and Leber's hereditary optic atrophy).

6. *Demyelinating disorders.* Up to 50% of patients with multiple sclerosis show psychiatric symptoms including psychosis.

7. *Narcolepsy.* This sleep-wake cycle disorder of rapid-eye-movement (REM) sleep (Aldrich 1990) has frequently been reported to manifest hypnagogic sleep hallucinations, which used to be regarded as a psychotic symptom.

8. *Cerebrovascular disease.* Paranoid delusions and hallucinatory experiences have been reported in conjunction with subarachnoid hemorrhage, fat embolism, bilateral carotid artery occlusion, arteriovenous malformation, stroke, and subdural hematoma (Robinson and Forrester 1987).

Systemic Diseases

Most systemic medical disorders influence brain function physiologically and/or metabolically and may produce psychotic symptoms. Physical illness has been reported to be common at the onset of catatonic psychoses (Wilcox and Nasrallah 1986). The following medical disorders may produce psychotic manifestations:

1. *Infections.* Infections that involve brain tissue may result in psychotic symptoms.
2. *Inflammatory disorders.* Inflammatory disorders, such as cerebritis, may produce psychotic symptoms.

3. *Endocrinopathies.* These include Addison's disease, hypothyroidism, hyperthyroidism, hypoparathyroidism, hyperparathyroidism, and hypopituitarism.
4. *Systemic medical diseases.* Such diseases include kidney failure and uremia, hepatic encephalopathy, hyponatremia, hypercalcemia, hypoglycemia, and myasthenia gravis.
5. *Nutritional deficiency states.* Deficiencies of thiamine (Wernicke-Korsakoff syndrome), vitamin B_{12} and folate (megaloblastic anemia), and niacin may also produce psychotic manifestations.

DRUG-INDUCED PSYCHOTIC SYNDROMES

Numerous psychotic reactions seen in the clinical setting are recognized to be associated with the use of recreational and prescription drugs. Some drug-induced psychoses are almost indistinguishable from schizophrenia (such as amphetamine and phencyclidine [PCP] psychoses), whereas others may produce nonspecific or partial psychotic syndromes, sometimes with toxic-organic features. The following classes of drugs can produce psychotic syndromes:

1. *Stimulants.* Stimulants that can produce psychotic manifestations include amphetamine, cocaine, and methylphenidate. Their mechanism of action is believed to be via dopamine release or agonist effects.
2. *Hallucinogens.* Hallucinogens, such as lysergic acid diethylamide (LSD), mescaline, psilocybin, and dimethyltryptamine, usually produce visual hallucinations and bizarre behavior.
3. *Phencyclidine.* PCP can produce a mixture of positive and negative symptoms that are indistinguishable from chronic schizophrenia.
4. *Catecholaminergic drugs.* These include levodopa (L-dopa), amantadine, and ephedrine.
5. *Anticholinergics.* Numerous psychotropic drugs have anticholinergic activity including tricyclic antidepressants (TCAs) and antiparkinsonian agents (e.g., trihexyphenidyl and benztropine).
6. *CNS depressants.* These include alcohol and benzodiazepine sedative-hypnotics.
7. *Glucocorticoids.* Glucocorticoids can exaggerate preexisting psychosis or, in sufficient doses, may produce psychotic symptoms in a nonpsychotic person.
8. *Heavy metals.* The heavy metals that can produce psychotic syndromes include lead, mercury, manganese, arsenic, and thallium.
9. *Others.* Other drugs producing psychotic manifestations include digitalis, disulfiram, cimetidine, and bromide.

NEUROBIOLOGICAL ABNORMALITIES
ASSOCIATED WITH SCHIZOPHRENIA

Many of the "psychiatric" signs and symptoms of schizophrenia are consistent with "neurological" abnormalities (Table 25–2).

In Vivo Regional Brain Abnormalities in Schizophrenia

The application of computed tomography (CT) and magnetic resonance imaging (MRI) to the in vivo study of the brain has resulted in the discovery of several regional structural abnormalities in schizophrenia. Similarly, the development and use of regional cerebral blood flow (rCBF), single photon emission computed tomography (SPECT), and positron-emission tomography (PET) have added significant new information about the functional disturbances in certain brain regions in schizophrenia. The following is a summary of the structural and/or functional pathology of various brain regions in schizophrenia.

The ventricular system.   Studies have demonstrated a significant pathological dilatation of the cerebral ventricular system in schizophrenia, particularly the lateral and third ventricles (Shelton and Weinberger 1986) (Figure 25–1). This ventricular enlargement has become one of the most established neurobiological findings in schizophrenia, implying the loss of brain tissue in periventricular regions in many but not all patients.

Clinically, ventriculomegaly is consistently shown to be unrelated to treatment(s) received or to the duration of illness (Nasrallah and Coffman 1985). Many studies have shown a correlation between ventriculomegaly and certain clinical variables including obstetric complications, poor premorbid adjustment, family history of psychosis, neuropsychological impairment, poor response to neuroleptic drugs, prominent negative symptoms, and presence of involuntary movements (Losonczy et al. 1986). However, other studies have failed to find correlations with many of those clinical variables (Nasrallah et al. 1983a).

Table 25–2.   Neurological abnormalities reported in schizophrenia

"Higher" brain function	Choreiform movements
Loss of insight re illness	Grimacing
Loss of ambition and drive	Abnormal motor tone
Loss of ability to plan	Increased blinking
Impaired judgment	Apraxia
Lack of decision-making skill	Poor hopping
Failure to abstract	Abnormal gait
Inability to initiate tasks	Abnormal finger tapping
Lack of social insight	**Sensory integration**
Gender identity confusion	Decreased pain sensation
Neurobehavioral	Decreased sense of smell
Impaired attention	Decreased temperature sensation
Impaired recognition and perception of faces	Asterognosis
Impaired perception of prosody of speech	Agraphesthesia
Decreased ability to inflect own speech	Extinction
Flat affect	Right-left confusion
Impaired memory, short-term	**Perceptual**
Impaired memory, long-term	Hallucinations
Motor function	Auditory
Abnormal smooth pursuit eye movement	Visual
Tics	Somatic
Stereotypies	Gustatory

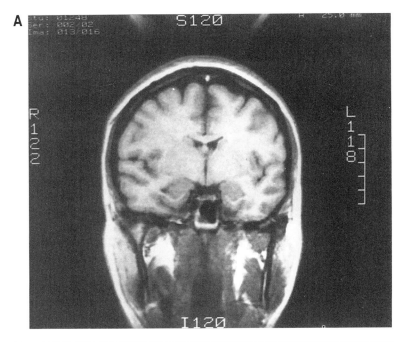

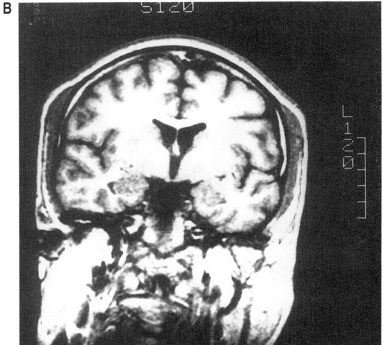

Figure 25–1.   Coronal magnetic resonance imaging (MRI) scans showing normal lateral and third ventricles in a healthy control subject (*panel A*) and enlarged lateral and third ventricles in a schizophrenic patient (*panel B*) of the same age (28 years).

Several biological correlates of ventriculomegaly in schizophrenia have also been reported, including increased blood serotonin and cerebrospinal fluid (CSF) amino acids; decreased CSF 5-hydroxyindoleacetic acid (5-HIAA), homovanillic acid (HVA), dihydroxyphenylacetic acid (DOPAC), cyclic adenosine monophosphate (cAMP), and dopamine β-hydroxylase (DBH); defective smooth pursuit eye movements; neurological soft signs; decreased slow-wave sleep; temporal attenuation of the auditory P300 wave; and lack of inverse relationship of serum prolactin with psychosis ratings (Karson et al. 1988; McCarley et al. 1989; van Kammen et al. 1988).

Although ventricular enlargement is not specific to schizophrenia, ventricular enlargement has a specific significance within schizophrenia for pathogenesis and clinical course. Research has focused on determining whether ventriculomegaly in schizophrenia is static or progressive. Nasrallah et al. (1986b) found no difference in mean ventricular size after 3 years, suggesting that ventricular dilatation is static, thus probably a neurodevelopmental lesion rather than a degenerative lesion. Although this finding was supported by others (Illowsky et al. 1988; Vita et al. 1988), recent data (Schwarzkopf et al. 1990) have demonstrated progressivity of ventricular size in at least a subgroup of schizophrenic patients.

Cerebrum and cranium. Schizophrenic patients have been shown to have smaller midsagittal craniums and cerebrums on MRI scans (Andreasen et al. 1986). Smaller brain weight in schizophrenia (a decrease of 5%–8%) has also been reported in post-mortem studies (Bruton et al. 1990). Schwarzkopf et al. (1991) found that the decrease in brain size in schizophrenia is particularly pronounced in patients with a family history of schizophrenia. Overall, the findings of smaller cerebrum and cranium in schizophrenia are consistent with a neurodevelopmental growth impairment, possibly under programmed genetic control rather than incidental environmental insult.

Sulcal widening. Studies have confirmed the presence of enlarged cortical sulci and fissures in schizophrenia (Nasrallah et al. 1982). Clinical correlates of cortical sulcal widening include cognitive impairment (Yates et al. 1990), negative symptoms, and poor response to antipsychotic therapy (Nasrallah and Coffman 1985). In addition, prefrontal sulcal prominence was found to be inversely related to response to clozapine in chronic schizophrenia (Friedman et al. 1991).

Cerebellar vermis atrophy. Studies have reported a higher frequency of what appears to be "atrophy" of the cerebellum (widening of vermal sulci, enlargement of the fourth ventricle, and cerebellar cisterns) (Nasrallah et al. 1991). Overall, about 9% of schizophrenic patients compared with about 4% of controls show these cerebellar changes, which have also been reported to be associated with third ventricular enlargement (Nasrallah et al. 1985).

Reversed cerebral asymmetries. CT studies examining cerebral hemisphere asymmetry in schizophrenia have reported abnormal structural cerebral asymmetries in schizophrenia compared with control subjects (Shelton and Weinberger 1986). The significance of this abnormality may be explained by disruption of cerebral hemisphere growth and development in schizophrenia.

Frontal lobes. Frontal lobe dysfunction has been implicated in schizophrenia. Many of the manifestations of schizophrenia, such as negative symptoms, inability to plan, poor judgment, and impaired cognition, have been attributed to frontal lobe dysfunction because of the strong similarity to the syndrome that follows damage to the frontal lobes (Mesulam 1986). However, although there is some evidence for structural abnormalities in frontal lobe MRI scans in schizophrenia (Andreasen 1986), most of the evidence for frontal lobe impairment in schizophrenic patients is that of disrupted function.

Cerebral blood flow (CBF) and PET studies have indicated a relative decrease in blood flow and glucose metabolism in the frontal lobe (Ingvar 1987), but chronicity and neuroleptic use have been implicated in this "hypofrontality" (Figure 25–2). Weinberger et al. (1986) demonstrated with xenon-133 inhalation that the rCBF in the dorsolateral prefrontal cortex (DLPFC) was significantly reduced in schizophrenic patients versus control subjects during the performance of the Wisconsin Card Sorting test (WCS; Heaton 1985), which presumably activates the DLPFC.

The frontal lobes are quite important in the neuropsychiatry of schizophrenia. However, much more needs to be learned about their structure and function (Goldman-Rakic 1984) before their role in schizophrenia is defined. Because of the extensive projections between the frontal lobes and many other brain regions, it is not possible to conclude at this time whether the impairment of frontal lobe functions in schizophrenia is related to a primary or secondary lesion.

Temporal lobes. In addition to the association between schizophrenia-like psychosis and lesions of the temporal lobe (e.g., epilepsy, tumors, trauma, and infarcts), lit-

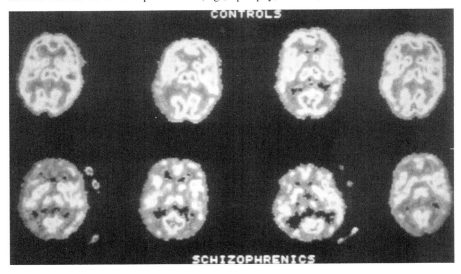

Figure 25–2. Positron-emission tomography (PET) scan in schizophrenic and healthy subjects (controls) showing the relatively reduced frontal metabolism (hypofrontality) in schizophrenia.
Source. Courtesy of M. S. Buchsbaum, Director, PET Laboratory, University of California at Irvine. (Please refer to page 630 of *The American Psychiatric Press Textbook of Neuropsychiatry,* Second Edition, for the full-color figure.)

erature on the localization of psychotic symptoms suggests that Schneiderian delusions and hallucinations, commonly seen in schizophrenia, may reflect temporal lobe pathology, especially in temporolimbic areas (Trimble 1990). The medial temporal lobe is emerging as a key structure in the neurobiology of schizophrenia because of its important connections with higher cortical areas (Roberts 1990). Gross morphological abnormalities of the temporal lobes have been revealed on CT and MRI scans in schizophrenic patients, including reduced temporal gray matter (Suddath et al. 1989), left temporal lobe size (Suddath et al. 1990), temporal horn enlargement (Crow et al. 1988), reduced limbic temporal volume (Bogerts et al. 1990), and focal temporal cortical atrophy (Yates et al. 1990). Figure 25–3 shows an example of hypoplasia of the medial temporal lobe structures (hippocampus-amygdala complex) on coronal MRI scans in a schizophrenic patient and a control subject.

Basal ganglia.   For the past quarter century, the dopamine hypothesis of schizophrenia has been a major pathophysiological model for this disorder (Carlsson 1988). Because the largest proportions of dopamine in the brain are found in the basal ganglia, it is logical to consider the basal ganglia as an important component of the neurobiology of schizophrenia. Further, basal ganglia disorders such as Huntington's chorea, which produces striatal degeneration, are known to be associated with schizophrenia-like psychosis. In addition to attributing motor abnormalities in schizophrenia to basal ganglia pathology (Manschreck 1986), other parameters such as reward, memory, attention, and higher cognitive functions have also been associated with the basal ganglia and their cortical projections (Lidsky et al. 1979). More recently, PET scan research has shown that the basal ganglia may be metabolically hyperactive in unmedicated schizophrenia (Early et al. 1987), and a possible relationship of this abnormality with thought disorder has been proposed (Early et al. 1989).

Parietal lobes.   Some reports have suggested that the parietal lobes may be impaired in schizophrenia (Mesulam and Geschwind 1983). Particular reference is made to the role of the inferior parietal lobule in selective attention (Heilman et al. 1983). Further, some symptoms of schizophrenia, such as tactile discrimination and body image distortion (Erwin and Rosenbaum 1979) and "physiognomization" of the environment and facial nonrecognition (Harrington et al. 1989) may be associated with parietal lobe dysfunction in schizophrenia.

Corpus callosum.   Since the initial study of Rosenthal and Bigelow (1972) reporting a thicker corpus callosum in postmortem brains of schizophrenic patients, there have been several postmortem (Nasrallah et al. 1983b) and in vivo MRI studies (Nasrallah et al. 1986a), some showing pathology and others not. A large literature about interhemispheric communications and integration was spawned by the possibility of an impaired callosal channel in schizophrenia (Nasrallah 1985).

Neuropathological Findings in Schizophrenia

Postmortem histopathological studies of the brain in schizophrenia produced very few consistent findings up to the 1970s, leading Plum (1972) to pessimistically label schizophrenia "the graveyard of neuropathologists." However, in the 1980s,

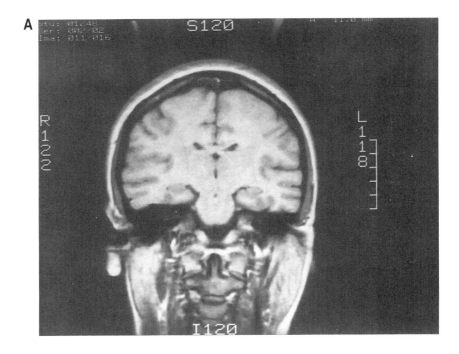

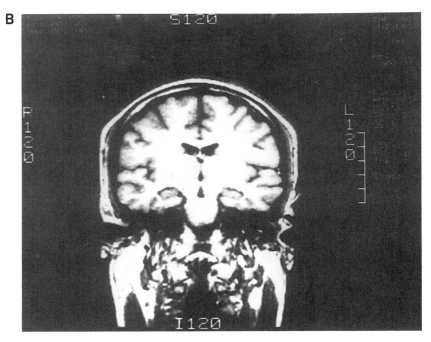

Figure 25–3.   Coronal magnetic resonance imaging (MRI) scan showing normal (*panel A*) and hypoplastic (*panel B*) medial temporal lobe tissue (hippocampus-amygdala) in a control subject and schizophrenic patient, respectively.

a remarkable consistency emerged in the neuropathological studies of schizophrenia by different investigators. These studies almost unanimously suggest that schizophrenia is associated with a neurodevelopmental disruption, probably in the second trimester, as indicated by changes in the usual histoarchitecture of brain tissue, and in failure of certain neuronal cells to migrate to their ultimate location (Altshuler et al. 1988; Conrad et al. 1991; Jakob and Beckmann 1986).

Although some neuropathological studies report increased gliosis or cellular degeneration in schizophrenia (Stevens 1982), the majority of studies do not (Roberts and Bruton 1990). Because fetal brain tissue does not react to injury with a glial response until the third trimester, it is postulated that the neuropathological lesions in schizophrenia occurred early in development (first and second trimester).

Recent findings regarding the gross and microscopic changes in the brains of schizophrenic patients point to the increasing evidence for a neurodevelopmental framework for the neurobiology and neuropsychiatry of schizophrenia. If the findings continue to be replicated, it will become more likely that the basis for the structural brain changes is mainly under genetic control, with some modulation by perinatal and other environmental factors that contribute to the heterogeneity of the schizophrenic syndrome. It is quite possible that the neurodevelopmental lesion in schizophrenia is qualitatively similar in more patients, but quantitatively different across clinical subtypes.

CONCLUSIONS

Although the exact neuropsychiatry of schizophrenia remains a mystery, neurobiological clues are accumulating at a rapid pace. Lesions practically anywhere in the brain have been associated with schizophrenia-like psychoses, with lesions of the frontal, temporal, and limbic regions more likely than others to produce psychotic features. Several lines of evidence now point to the importance of neurodevelopmental factors in schizophrenia. Many of the neurobiological findings in schizophrenia can be explained within a neurodevelopmental model. Future research should focus on neurodevelopmental factors, including genetic and environmental, in the neurobiology of schizophrenia. A particularly promising brain region at present is the limbic temporal lobe and its projections.

REFERENCES

Aldrich MS: Narcolepsy. N Engl J Med 323:389–394, 1990

Altshuler L, Casanova ME, Goldberg T, et al: Shape and area measurements of hippocampus and parahippocampal gyrus in schizophrenics, suicide, and control brains. Neuroscience Abstracts 14:247, 1988

Andreasen NC, Nasrallah HA, Dunn V, et al: Structural abnormalities in the frontal system in schizophrenia: a magnetic resonance imaging study. Arch Gen Psychiatry 43:136–144, 1986

Bogerts B, Ashtari M, Degreef G, et al: Reduced temporal limbic structure volumes on magnetic resonance images in first episode schizophrenia. Psychiatry Research: Neuroimaging 35:1–13, 1990

Bruton CJ, Crow TJ, Frith CD, et al: Schizophrenia and the brain: a prospective clinicopathological study. Psychol Med 20:285–304, 1990

Carlsson A: The current status of the dopamine hypothesis of schizophrenia. Neuropsychopharmacology 1:179–186, 1988

Conrad AJ, Scheibel AB: Schizophrenia and the hippocampus: the embryological hypothesis extended. Schizophr Bull 13:577–587, 1987

Conrad AJ, Abebe T, Austin R, et al: Hippocampal pyramidal cell disarray in schizophrenia as a bilateral phenomenon. Arch Gen Psychiatry 48:413–417, 1991

Crow TJ, Colter N, Brown N, et al: Lateralized asymmetry of temporal horn enlargement in schizophrenia. Schizophrenia Research 1:155–156, 1988

Cummings JL: Organic psychosis. Psychosomatics 29:16–26, 1988

Davison K: Schizophrenia-like psychoses associated with organic cerebral disorders: a review. Psychiatr Dev 1:1–34, 1983

Davison K, Bagley CR: Schizophrenia-like psychoses associated with organic disorders of the CNS: a review of the literature, in Current Problems in Neuropsychiatry, Part II (British Journal of Psychiatry, Special Publication No 4). Edited by Herrington E. Ashford, Headley Bros, 1969, pp 113–184

Early TS, Reiman E, Raichle ME, et al: Globus pallidus abnormality in never-medicated patients with schizophrenia. Proc Natl Acad Sci U S A 84:561–563, 1987

Early TS, Posner MI, Reiman E, et al: Left striato-pallidal hyperactivity in schizophrenia, II: phenomenology and thought disorder. Psychiatr Dev 2:109–121, 1989

Erwin BJ, Rosenbaum G: Parietal lobe syndrome and schizophrenia: comparison of neuropsychological deficits. J Abnorm Psychol 88:234–242, 1979

Flor-Henry P: Psychosis and temporal lobe epilepsy: a controlled investigation. Epilepsia 10:363–395, 1969

Friedman L, Knutson L, Shurell M, et al: Prefrontal sulcal prominence is inversely related to response to clozapine in schizophrenia. Biol Psychiatry 29:865–877, 1991

Goldman-Rakic PS: The frontal lobes: uncharted provinces of the brain. Trends Neurosci 7:425–429, 1984

Harrington A, Oepin G, Spitzer M: Disordered recognition and perception of human faces in acute schizophrenia and experimental psychosis. Compr Psychiatry 30:376–384, 1989

Heaton R: Wisconsin Card Sorting Test. Odessa, TX, Psychological Assessment Resources, 1985

Heilman KM, Watson RT, Valenstein E, et al: Localization of lesions in neglect, in Localization in Neuropsychology. Edited by Keretz A. New York, Academic, 1983, pp 471–492

Illowsky BP, Juliano DM, Bigelow LB, et al: Stability of CT scan findings in schizophrenia: results of an 8-year follow-up study. J Neurol Neurosurg Psychiatry 51:209–213, 1988

Ingvar DH: Evidence for frontal/pre-frontal cortical dysfunction in chronic schizophrenia: the phenomenon of hypofrontality reconsidered, in Biological Perspectives of Schizophrenia. Edited by Helmchen H, Henn FA. New York, John Wiley, 1987, pp 201–211

Jakob J, Beckmann H: Prenatal developmental disturbance in the limbic allocortex in schizophrenics. J Neural Transm 65:303–326, 1986

Karson CN, Coppola R, Daniel DG, et al: Alpha frequency in schizophrenia: an association with enlarged cerebral ventricles. Am J Psychiatry 145:861–864, 1988

Lidsky TI, Weinhold PM, Levin FM: Implications of basal ganglionic dysfunction for schizophrenia. Biol Psychiatry 14:3–12, 1979

Losonczy MF, Song IS, Mohs RC, et al: Correlates of lateral ventricular size in chronic schizophrenia, I: behavioral and treatment response measures. Am J Psychiatry 143:976–981, 1986

Lyon M, Barr CE, Cannon TD, et al: Fetal neural development and schizophrenia. Schizophr Bull 15:149–161, 1989

McCarley RW, Faux SF, Shenton M, et al: CT abnormalities in schizophrenia: a preliminary study of their correlation with P300/P200 electrophysiological features and positive/negative symptoms. Arch Gen Psychiatry 46:698–708, 1989

Manschreck TC: Motor abnormalities in schizophrenic disorders, in Handbook of Schizophrenia, Vol 1: The Neurology of Schizophrenia. Edited by Nasrallah HA, Weinberger DR. Amsterdam, Elsevier, 1986, pp 65–96

Mednick SA, Machon RA, Huttunen MO, et al: Adult schizophrenia following prenatal exposure to an influenza epidemic. Arch Gen Psychiatry 45:189–192, 1988

Mesulam MM: Frontal cortex and behavior. Ann Neurol 15:320–325, 1986

Mesulam MM, Geschwind N: On the possible role of neocortex and its limbic connections in the process of attention and schizophrenia. J Psychiatr Res 14:249–261, 1983

Nasrallah HA: The unintegrated right cerebral hemisphere as alien intruder: a possible mechanism for Schneiderian delusions in schizophrenia. Compr Psychiatry 26:273–282, 1985

Nasrallah HA: The differential diagnosis of schizophrenia: genetic, perinatal, neurological, pharmacological and psychiatric factors, in Handbook of Schizophrenia, Vol 1: The Neurology of Schizophrenia. Edited by Nasrallah HA, Weinberger DR. Amsterdam, Elsevier, 1986, pp 49–63

Nasrallah HA: Brain structure and function in schizophrenia: evidence for fetal neurodevelopmental impairment. Current Opinion in Psychiatry 3:75–78, 1990

Nasrallah HA, Coffman JA: Computerized tomography in psychiatry. Psychiatric Annals 15:239–249, 1985

Nasrallah HA, McChesney CM: Psychopathology of corpus callosum tumors. Biol Psychiatry 16:663–669, 1981

Nasrallah HA, Weinberger DR (eds): Handbook of Schizophrenia, Vol 1: The Neurology of Schizophrenia. Amsterdam, Elsevier, 1986

Nasrallah HA, McCalley-Whitters M, Jacoby CG: Cortical atrophy in schizophrenia and mania: a comparative CT study. J Clin Psychiatry 43:439–441, 1982

Nasrallah HA, Kuperman S, Hamra B, et al: Schizophrenia patients with and without large cerebral ventricles: a controlled clinical comparison. J Clin Psychiatry 44:407–409, 1983a

Nasrallah HA, McCalley-Whitters M, Rauscher FP, et al: A histological study of the corpus callosum in subtypes of chronic schizophrenia. Psychiatry Res 8:151–160, 1983b

Nasrallah HA, Jacoby CG, Chapman S, et al: Third ventricular enlargement on CT scans: association with cerebellar atrophy. Biol Psychiatry 20:443–450, 1985

Nasrallah HA, Andreasen NC, Coffman JA, et al: A controlled magnetic resonance imaging study of corpus callosum thickness in schizophrenia. Biol Psychiatry 21:274–282, 1986a

Nasrallah HA, Olson SC, McCalley-Whitters M, et al: Cerebral ventricular enlargement in schizophrenia: a preliminary follow-up study. Arch Gen Psychiatry 43:157–159, 1986b

Nasrallah HA, Schwarzkopf SB, Olson SC, et al: Perinatal brain injury and cerebellar vermal lobules I-X in schizophrenia. Biol Psychiatry 29:567–574, 1991

Nowakowski RS: Basic concepts of CNS development. Child Dev 58:568–595, 1987

Plum F: Prospects for research on schizophrenia, 3: neurophysiology, neuropathological findings. Neurosciences Program Bulletin 10:384–388, 1972

Propping P, Friedl W: Genetic studies of biochemical, pathophysiological, and pharmacological factors in schizophrenia, in Handbook of Schizophrenia, Vol 3: Nosology, Epidemiology, and Genetics of Schizophrenia. Edited by Tsuang MT, Simpson JC. Amsterdam, Elsevier, 1988, pp 579–608

Roberts GW: Schizophrenia: the cellular biology of a functional psychosis. Trends Neurosci 13:207–211, 1990

Roberts GW, Bruton CJ: Notes from the graveyard: neuropathology and schizophrenia. Neuropathol Appl Neurobiol 16:3–16, 1990

Roberts GW, Done DJ, Bruton C, et al: A "mock-up" of schizophrenia: temporal lobe epilepsy and schizophrenia-like psychosis. Biol Psychiatry 28:127–143, 1990

Robinson RG, Forrester AW: Neuropsychiatric aspects of cerebrovascular disease, in Textbook of Neuropsychiatry. Edited by Hales RE, Yudofsky SC. Washington, DC, American Psychiatric Press, 1987, pp 191–208

Rosenthal RLB, Bigelow LB: Quantitative brain measurements in chronic schizophrenia. Br J Psychiatry 121:259–264, 1972

Schwarzkopf SB, Olson SC, Nasrallah HA: Third and lateral ventricular volumes in schizophrenia: support for progressive enlargement of both structures. Psychopharmacol Bull 26:385–391, 1990

Schwarzkopf SB, Nasrallah HA, Olson SC, et al: Family history and brain morphology in schizophrenia: an MRI study. Psychiatry Research: Neuroimaging 40:49–60, 1991

Shelton RC, Weinberger DR: X-ray computerized tomography studies in schizophrenia: a review and synthesis, in Handbook of Schizophrenia, Vol 1: The Neurology of Schizophrenia. Edited by Nasrallah HA, Weinberger DR. Amsterdam, Elsevier, 1986, pp 207–250

Stevens JR: Neuropathology of schizophrenia. Arch Gen Psychiatry 39:1131–1139, 1982

Suddath RL, Casanova MF, Goldberg TE, et al: Temporal lobe pathology in schizophrenia: a quantitative magnetic resonance imaging study. Am J Psychiatry 146:464–472, 1989

Suddath RL, Christison GW, Torrey EF, et al: Anatomical abnormalities in the brains of monozygotic twins discordant for schizophrenia. N Engl J Med 322:789–794, 1990

Swayze VW, Andreasen NC, Ehrhardt JC, et al: Developmental abnormalities of the corpus callosum in schizophrenia. Arch Neurol 47:805–808, 1990

Trimble MR: First-rank symptoms of Schneider: a new perspective? Br J Psychiatry 156:195–200, 1990

van Kammen DP, van Kammen WB, Peters J, et al: Decreased slow-wave sleep and enlarged lateral ventricles in schizophrenia. Neuropsychopharmacology 1:265–271, 1988

Vita A, Sacchetti E, Valvassori G, et al: Brain morphology in schizophrenia: a 2- to 5-year CT scan follow-up study. Acta Psychiatr Scand 78:618–621, 1988

Weinberger DR, Berman KF, Zec RF: Physiological dysfunction of dorsolateral prefrontal cortex in schizophrenia, I: regional cerebral blood flow (CBF) evidence. Arch Gen Psychiatry 43:114–125, 1986

Wilcox JA, Nasrallah HA: Organic factors in catatonia. Br J Psychiatry 149:782–784, 1986

Wilcox JA, Nasrallah HA: Perinatal insult as a risk factor in paranoid and nonparanoid schizophrenia. Psychopathology 20:285–287, 1987a

Wilcox JA, Nasrallah HA: Perinatal distress and prognosis of psychotic illness. Neuropsychobiology 17:173–175, 1987b

Wilcox JA, Nasrallah HA: Sydenham's chorea and psychopathology. Neuropsychobiology 19:6–8, 1988

Yates WR, Swayze VW, Andreasen NC: Neuropsychological effect of global and focal cerebral atrophy in schizophrenia. Neuropsychiatry, Neuropsychology and Behavioral Neurology 3:98–106, 1990

Section V

Neuropsychiatric Treatments

Chapter 26

Psychopharmacological Treatment in Neuropsychiatry

Steven L. Dubovsky, M.D.

Psychotropic medications are used extensively in patients with neurological illnesses. In this chapter, I address the major classes of physical intervention used in psychiatry, with special attention to the neurological setting. Introductory discussions are followed by summaries of the major side effects of psychiatric and neurological uses and the important interactions.

HETEROCYCLIC ANTIDEPRESSANTS

All heterocyclic antidepressants (HCAs) are of approximately equal efficacy; their side-effect profiles, however, permit considerable flexibility in treating patients with neurological illnesses. Antidepressants currently available in the United States are summarized in Table 26–1.

Because HCAs are extensively metabolized by the liver after oral administration, conditions that affect microsomal enzyme activity can significantly alter antidepressant levels. Alcohol, anticonvulsants, barbiturates, oral contraceptives, and antidepressants themselves may stimulate liver enzymes, decreasing blood levels of the antidepressant and leading to unexpected treatment failures or relapses in compliant patients. Some substances (e.g., phenothiazines and methylphenidate) compete with HCAs for metabolizing enzymes, slowing the rate of breakdown of both the antidepressant and the other drug.

The long half-life of most HCAs makes once-daily dosing possible for all preparations except trazodone and bupropion. Inherited patterns of metabolism of HCAs probably account for two clinical phenomena. First, a patient with a blood relative who has responded to a particular medication is more likely to respond to that drug as well. Second, there is wide interindividual variation in blood levels produced by the same dose of a given drug.

Antidepressant blood levels are most appropriately used to adjust the dose of nortriptyline, desipramine, and imipramine; to investigate the reason for failure to respond to an adequate dose of other antidepressants; to evaluate slow metabolism as a cause of toxicity at low doses; and possibly to determine the correct dose of an antidepressant under urgent circumstances (American Psychiatric Association 1985). Blood levels should be measured in adults about 1 week after each dose adjustment.

Recommendations about dosage limitations for several HCAs are beginning to

Table 26–1. Heterocyclic antidepressants currently available in the United States

Drug	Trade name	Structure	Usual daily dose (mg)	Upper daily limit (mg)	Usual daily dose in elderly (mg)
Amitriptyline	Elavil	Tertiary amine[a]	150–300	300	50–100
Nortriptyline	Pamelor; Aventyl	Secondary amine[a]	75–125[b]	150[b]	25–50
Protriptyline	Vivactil	Secondary amine[a]	30–40	60	15–20
Imipramine	Tofranil	Tertiary amine[a]	150–200[b]	300	25–100
Desipramine	Norpramin; Pertofrane	Secondary amine[a]	150–250[b]	300	25–100
Trimipramine	Surmontil	Tertiary amine[a]	150–200	300	50–100
Clomipramine	Anafranil	Tertiary amine[a]	150–250	300	75–150
Doxepin	Sinequan	Tertiary amine[a]	150–250	300	25–50
Amoxapine	Asendin	Dibenzoxazepine	150–300	600	75–300
Maprotiline	Ludiomil	Tetracyclic	150–200	300	50–75
Trazodone	Desyrel	Triazolopyridine	150–400[c]	600	50–150
Fluoxetine	Prozac	Propylamine	5–40	100	5–20
Bupropion	Wellbutrin	Aminoketone	300–450[c]	450	150–300
Sertraline	Methylnaph-thalamine	Zoloft	50–200	200	25–200
Paroxetine	Phenylpiperi-dine	Paxil	20–50		10–50

[a]Tricyclic.
[b]Dosage should be adjusted according to blood level.
[c]Dose may have to be divided because of short half-life.

emerge. In the treatment of depression, doses of fluoxetine greater than 40 mg may produce no more improvement but more side effects (Wernicke et al. 1988). The long half-life of this drug, which lengthens the time to achieve a steady state, may explain why up to 8 weeks are necessary for some patients to achieve a therapeutic response to a given dosage of fluoxetine (Schweitzer et al. 1990). On the other hand, doses up to 100 mg/day of fluoxetine may be necessary to treat obsessive-compulsive disorder (OCD), bulimia, and obesity (Ayd 1990). Higher doses of chlorimipramine may also be necessary for OCD (Greist et al. 1990). Doses greater than 225 mg of maprotiline and 450 mg of bupropion should not be exceeded because of an increased risk of seizures.

Psychiatric Uses of HCAs in the Presence of Neurological Disease

HCAs have been found to be useful in the treatment of depression, panic anxiety, generalized anxiety, bulimia, posttraumatic stress disorder, OCD, and probably some symptoms associated with borderline personality disorder (Goodman and Charney 1985). Using antidepressants for psychiatric indications in neurological patients requires great skill when the psychiatric disorder is caused, obscured, or complicated by disease of the brain and when side effects of the medications can aggravate the neurological illness.

Depression and Organic Brain Disease

A number of drugs (e.g., anticonvulsants, tranquilizers, antineoplastic agents, adrenal steroids) and illnesses (e.g., stroke, HIV infection) can produce depression, which may or may not be accompanied by signs of delirium or dementia. The most appropriate approach to organically induced depression is to treat the underlying disorder or withdraw the offending drug. However, if the illness cannot be reversed immediately or if it would be unsafe to reduce the dose of medication, an antidepressant may ameliorate the depressive symptoms.

Antidepressants may also be useful for patients in whom depression mimics or is accompanied by organic brain disease, even when an obvious irreversible cause of dementia is present. A course of antidepressant therapy may be reasonable for newly diagnosed dementia patients without reversible causes on the grounds that there may be a component of depressive pseudodementia. A different problem occurs when organic disturbances that affect the right hemisphere or the balance between the hemispheres impair the ability to express emotion normally. Only a course of antidepressants or electroconvulsive therapy (ECT) may resolve the behavioral disorder, which may persist after the underlying neurological disorder has been successfully treated (Dubovsky 1986).

Because they can further impair cortical function or depress the reticular activating system, strongly anticholinergic and sedating antidepressants can be problematic for patients with organic brain syndromes. Appropriate HCAs for demented patients include desipramine, maprotiline, trazodone, or fluoxetine.

Antidepressants in the Elderly

Because organic brain syndromes and other neurological syndromes frequently occur in elderly patients, it is important to know about the differences between patients in this age group and younger patients that influence dosage and choice of antidepressants (Salzman 1985). First, there is slower demethylation of tertiary amines (which tend to produce more anticholinergic, sedative, and hypotensive side effects) to the less toxic secondary amines. The clearance of all antidepressants is slowed in the elderly, and this leads to higher blood levels and prolonged activity of all compounds. At the same time, the central nervous system (CNS) is more sensitive to the toxicity of antidepressants. For these reasons, secondary compounds are often less troublesome than are tertiary preparations, as are methylphenidate and newer antidepressants that have less anticholinergic and sedating potential.

For elderly patients, the dose of all antidepressants should be increased slowly, and the final dose should usually be lower than that for younger patients (Table 26–1). Using an antidepressant for which blood level can meaningfully be measured is a useful strategy when the clinician is unsure of the appropriate dose of these drugs. Nortriptyline has been shown to be low in hypotensive potential in the elderly, and this is probably also true of desipramine. TCAs have antiarrhythmic properties that may make it possible to discontinue or reduce the dose of other type I antiarrhythmics such as procainamide, quinidine, and disopyramide.

Antidepressants in Patients With Seizure Disorders

Particularly at higher doses, many antidepressants lower the seizure threshold in epileptic patients, and spontaneous seizures have occasionally been reported in patients without a history of epilepsy who were taking these drugs (Fiori 1977). Maprotiline in doses greater than 225 mg/day and bupropion in doses greater than 450 mg/day are the worst offenders (Pinder et al. 1977), but in lower doses the risk of seizures associated with them is not necessarily higher than that for all HCAs (Davidson 1989). The risk of seizures with bupropion is highest in patients with organic brain disease, electroencephalogram (EEG) abnormalities, brain tumors, bulimia, concomitant medications that lower seizure threshold, and high blood levels of bupropion (Davidson 1989). Doxepin and monoamine oxidase inhibitors (MAOIs) may be relatively safe for patients with epilepsy, and secondary amines may be preferable to tertiary amines.

Antidepressants and Movement Disorders

The incidence of depression is high in Parkinson's disease, and levodopa (L-dopa) may increase or produce depression in susceptible patients. From a theoretical standpoint, at least, the more anticholinergic antidepressants such as amitriptyline, protriptyline, doxepin, trimipramine, and imipramine could benefit parkinsonian patients. However, because many of these patients are elderly and are already taking anticholinergic drugs, the same side effect can prove troublesome. The dopaminergic properties of bupropion may prove useful for some parkinsonian patients. Bromocriptine, an ergot alkaloid with established antiparkinsonian properties, may also have antidepressant effects by itself and may augment antidepressants (Sitland-Marslen et al. 1990).

Because it can produce extrapyramidal syndromes (EPS), amoxapine is contraindicated in parkinsonian patients. This drug might be useful, however, for depressed patients with Tourette's syndrome. Its structural relationship to loxapine, a neuroleptic, may also make amoxapine useful in depression associated with bizarre or psychotic symptoms, which are sometimes expressed as atypical physical and neurological complaints. Fluoxetine, which may cause EPS as well as aggravate EPS caused by neuroleptics (Ciraulo and Shader 1990), should be avoided in parkinsonian patients and those taking neuroleptics.

Antidepressants and Urologic Syndromes

Some urologic complications of neurological disease require careful adjustment of antidepressant regimens. Because anticholinergic side effects can be particularly risky for uncatheterized patients with neurogenic bladder, drugs with low anticholinergic potency such as fluoxetine, trazodone, bupropion, and desipramine are preferable. Methylphenidate is even safer when urinary retention is a major concern. Desipramine, amoxapine, maprotiline, and methylphenidate seem less likely to cause erectile and orgasmic dysfunction, which can be a problem with other antidepressants, particularly highly serotonergic drugs such as fluoxetine, clomipramine, and MAOIs.

Antidepressant Withdrawal

Antidepressants are usually discontinued slowly (e.g., 25 mg/month of imipramine) to monitor for return of depression. More rapid discontinuation (25 mg every 3–5 days) is possible, but abrupt withdrawal of HCAs may result in abstinence symptoms. Withdrawal phenomena include gastrointestinal symptoms such as nausea, vomiting, and diarrhea; influenza-like syndromes; anxiety; agitation; insomnia; early-onset nightmares; parkinsonism; and hypomania. Withdrawal symptoms can be attenuated by more gradual discontinuation or, if the antidepressant must be stopped quickly, by adding 0.8 mg of atropine every 3–4 hours (Dilsaver and Greden 1984).

Neurological Uses of Antidepressants

Antidepressants have a number of actions that can be beneficial in some neurological syndromes even if depression is not present. Amitriptyline, imipramine, and doxepin appear to have analgesic effects in chronic pain (Rosenblatt et al. 1984). Amitriptyline, imipramine, and trazodone have reduced pain caused by diabetic neuropathy in a few patients (Hoogiverf 1985). Severe intractable pain of terminal cancer may be controlled by the combination of intravenous haloperidol, lorazepam, and hydromorphone (Adams 1988).

Tinnitus associated with depression is improved but not eradicated by nortriptyline (Sullivan et al. 1989). Fluvoxamine has improved memory in alcohol amnestic disorder but not alcohol dementia (Martin et al. 1989). Amitriptyline has been found to ameliorate pathological laughing and crying (pseudobulbar affect) associated with organic brain disease (Schiffer et al. 1985), and protriptyline may be helpful to some patients with sleep apnea.

Amitriptyline has been widely used as a prophylactic agent for migraine headaches (Mathew 1981); however, highly serotonergic antidepressants such as fluoxetine may make migraines worse. Histamine, subtype 2 (H_2), receptor blockade may explain the beneficial effects of trimipramine and doxepin in peptic ulcer disease (Richelson 1985b). These drugs are as effective as cimetidine, but cheaper, easier to monitor, and less toxic. Their anticholinergic effects, however, are additive with other anticholinergic drugs taken by ulcer patients.

Neurological Side Effects of HCAs

HCAs have a number of side effects that require consideration in neurological practice. Important syndromes and drugs that commonly cause these side effects are listed in Table 26–2 (Baldessarini 1985; Baldessarini and Marsh 1990; Demuth et al. 1985; Fiori 1977; Herman et al. 1990; Teicher et al. 1990).

Interactions of HCAs With Neurological Drugs

Cyclic antidepressants interact with many medications that are used in neurological and psychiatric practice. Some important interactions include the following:

Table 26–2.   Some side effects of heterocyclics

Side effect	Manifestations	Drugs
Anticholinergic	Delirium with tachycardia, warm dry skin, and mydriasis	Amitriptyline, trimipramine, protriptyline, and doxepin (especially when combined with other anticholinergic drugs)
Postural hypotension (α-adrenergic blockade)	Dizziness, unsteadiness, light-headedness, and stumbling on standing up	Tertiary amines, protriptyline, trazodone, and maprotiline
Cardiovascular	Sinus tachycardia Suppression of ventricular arrhythmias Worsening of conduction defects Cardiac depression Sinus bradycardia Worsening of ventricular arrhythmias	Especially anticholinergic compounds All but trazodone and fluoxetine Trazodone
Sedation	Oversedation, impaired cognition, and worsening of organic brain syndrome	Amitriptyline, trimipramine, trazodone, doxepin, and maprotiline
Psychomotor impairment	Impaired driving during first few weeks	Amitriptyline, imipramine, and doxepin; not fluoxetine
Auditory	Tinnitus	Imipramine, probably other TCAs
Urologic	Priapism leading to impotence Sexual dysfunction	Trazodone All antidepressants, especially MAOIs, fluoxetine, and clomipramine
Decreased seizure threshold	Spontaneous seizures or exacerbation of epilepsy	Amoxapine, maprotiline, and tertiary amines
Neuromuscular	Fine tremor and myoclonic jerks Peripheral neuropathy Proximal myopathy Phospholipid accumulation in nerve tissue	Most tricyclics, maprotiline, trazodone, and fluoxetine Amitriptyline Imipramine Imipramine
Extrapyramidal	Parkinsonism and rabbit syndrome Tremor and akathisia Tardive dyskinesia	Amoxapine, fluoxetine, imipramine, and amitriptyline in high doses Fluoxetine and amoxapine Amoxapine
Sleep changes	Increased REM latency, decreased total REM, increased stage 4, and nightmares occasionally when entire dose taken at night Insomnia	Most heterocyclics Fluoxetine and MAOIs
EEG changes	Suppressed alpha Increased synchronization at low doses Arousal in high doses	Amitriptyline Especially tertiary amines
Dermatologic	Skin rash, eosinophilia, and photosensitivity	Tricyclics and maprotiline

(continued)

Table 26–2. Some side effects of heterocyclics *(continued)*

Side effect	Manifestations	Drugs
Psychiatric	Mania and rapid cycling	Any antidepressant
	Mania in nonbipolar patients	Fluoxetine
	Anxiety, insomnia, and hyper-vigilance	Noradrenergic HCAs and fluoxetine
	Suicidal or angry obsessions	Fluoxetine
	Aggressive, assaultive, and suicidal behavior	Amitriptyline, imipramine

Note. TCAs = tricyclic antidepressants; MAOIs = monoamine oxidase inhibitors; REM = rapid eye movement; EEG = electroencephalogram; HCAs = heterocyclic antidepressants.

1. Additive anticholinergic effects with antiparkinsonian drugs, antihistamines, and neuroleptics.
2. Increase of antidepressant levels by neuroleptics, methylphenidate, amphetamine, and disulfiram.
3. Increase of neuroleptic and stimulant levels by antidepressants.
4. Decrease of antidepressant levels by alcohol, anticonvulsants (such as phenytoin), carbamazepine and barbiturates, oral contraceptives, cigarette smoking, and chloral hydrate. (Benzodiazepines [BZDs] do not have a significant effect on antidepressant metabolism.)
5. Increased antidepressant levels due to displacement of binding of antidepressants to albumin produced by aspirin, phenothiazines, phenylbutazone, aminopyrine, and scopolamine.
6. Potentiation by antidepressants of norepinephrine and amphetamine.
7. Blockade by antidepressants of substances, such as guanethidine, bethanidine, debrisoquin, and tyramine, that must actively be taken up into presynaptic nerve terminals.
8. Blockade of the central antihypertensive effect of clonidine.
9. Increased levels of TCAs, carbamazepine, and possibly neuroleptics by fluoxetine.

Alternatives to Antidepressants

When HCAs are ineffective or produce intolerable side effects in neurological patients, stimulants may ameliorate depression. Doses of 10–90 mg/day of methylphenidate or 10–60 mg/day of dextroamphetamine have been found useful in treating depression associated with a variety of neurological illnesses. Cognitive deterioration as well as depression may improve in patients with HIV encephalopathy treated with stimulants (Holmes et al. 1989). Addiction and tolerance have not been problems in medically ill patients taking this drug, which can often be discontinued after a month or two without a return of depression (Kaufman et al. 1984). Appetite and sleep often increase as depression begins to remit.

Buspirone may have antidepressant properties in doses of 40–90 mg/day (Rickels et al. 1991) and does not aggravate organic mental syndromes. Buspirone may also improve agitation in mentally retarded individuals and those with dementia. Some unipolar and more bipolar depressed patients who cannot tolerate or do not respond to antidepressants may respond to lithium or carbamazepine, with rapid cyclers perhaps responding better to carbamazepine (Ballenger 1988). ECT is an option in more severe cases, even if dementia is present.

When medications for depression cannot be tolerated and ECT is not feasible or appropriate, artificial bright light may be helpful. Bright light therapy is most effective for treatment and prophylaxis of clear-cut seasonal affective disorder but may also be helpful alone or as an adjunct to an antidepressant for depressed patients with worsening mood in the winter and some without any obvious seasonal variation (Rosenthal et al. 1985).

MONOAMINE OXIDASE INHIBITORS

Recent research has solidified the place of monoamine oxidase inhibitors (MAOIs) in the psychiatric armamentarium, especially for the treatment of depression associated with anxiety, mood reactivity, sensitivity to rejection, leaden paralysis, and reverse vegetative symptoms; chronic depression; depression resistant to other therapies; phobic-anxiety states; panic anxiety; agoraphobia; bulimia; OCD; and posttraumatic stress disorder (Baldessarini 1985; Pare 1985).

Four MAOIs are now in common psychiatric use in the United States (Table 26–3). Nonhydrazines are theoretically safer for patients with liver disease; the risk of hepatic damage is greatest with isocarboxazid. Tranylcypromine inhibits monoamine oxidase (MAO) faster than other MAOIs and may have amphetamine-like properties related to release and blockade of reuptake of norepinephrine. L-Deprenyl (selegiline), a new MAOI used to treat Parkinson's disease, is an effective antidepressant at higher doses.

MAOIs are usually given in divided doses. The last dose of an MAOI should not be taken too late in the day, or activation produced by the drug may result in insomnia. One principal route of metabolism for MAOIs other than phenelzine appears to be by acetylation in the liver (Pare 1985). About half of the physically healthy Caucasian population are "slow acetylators," which makes them more sensitive to MAOIs because of higher levels with the same dose. "Rapid acetylators," on the other hand, may not achieve therapeutic concentrations easily and may need doses that exceed the recommended range.

Located on mitochondria, MAO is a ubiquitous enzyme whose function is to inactivate biogenic amines such as norepinephrine, serotonin, dopamine, and tyra-

Table 26–3. Monoamine oxidase inhibitors (MAOIs) available in the United States

Class	Drug	Trade name	Usual daily dose (mg)	Acceptable dose limit (mg)[a]
Hydrazine	Phenelzine	Nardil	45–60	90
	Isocarboxazid	Marplan	20–30	40
Nonhydrazine	Tranylcypromine	Parnate	20–40	80
	Pargyline	Eutonyl	10–25	100
Phenylethylamine	L-Deprenyl (selegiline)	Eldepryl	10–40[b]	60

[a]Higher doses necessary for rapid metabolizers.
[b]Antiparkinsonian dose = 5–10 mg/day.

mine. The enzyme exists in two forms. MAO-A exhibits a preference for serotonin, dopamine, and tyramine and is the principal form of MAO in the lungs, intestine, and placenta. MAO-B preferentially breaks down phenylethylamine and is the principal isoenzyme in platelets and kidney. The brain and liver contain both MAO-A and MAO-B (Baldessarini 1985), although the brain may contain more MAO-B (Tabakoff et al. 1985).

MAOIs irreversibly destroy both forms of MAO, which take up to 2 weeks to regenerate themselves after the drug is stopped. For this reason, dietary restrictions should be observed for 2 weeks after drug discontinuation. Because MAO-A metabolizes tyramine in the gut and limits the amount that is absorbed, inhibition of this enzyme allows increased amounts of tyramine to enter the bloodstream. The inherent pressor effects of tyramine are augmented because more is absorbed while its inactivation by MAOI is slowed throughout the body and in sympathetic nerve terminals.

Psychiatric Uses of MAOIs in the Presence of Neurological Disease

MAOIs may be very useful in the treatment of depressed neurological patients who are not taking medications that might interact with the antidepressant. Anticholinergic MAOIs, such as phenelzine, can exacerbate confusion and memory loss in patients with dementia, and tranylcypromine may be less troublesome than the more sedating and anticholinergic of the HCAs. The principal risk in cognitively impaired patients is that they will forget to adhere to the dietary restrictions.

Phenelzine can ameliorate high blood pressure and may therefore be useful in hypertensive depressed patients. The potential hypotensive effects of MAOIs warrant slow and cautious increases in dosage in patients with marginal cerebrovascular reserve who cannot tolerate a decrease in blood pressure. Depressed patients with Parkinson's disease may be most appropriately treated with L-deprenyl; however, interactions with L-dopa could occur at higher doses of deprenyl.

Because MAOIs may have advantages in treatment of depression with prominent anxiety as well as primary anxiety states (Sheehan et al. 1980), they should probably be considered more frequently in neurological patients whose symptoms are caused or exaggerated by anxiety, especially when mixed with depression. Patients with light-headedness, dizziness, numbness, paresthesias, and other symptoms of hyperventilation, who may be misdiagnosed as having labyrinthitis, vestibular neuronitis, multiple sclerosis, or hypoglycemia, may be particularly good candidates, especially if HCAs have been ineffective or difficult to tolerate. Tolerance to antipanic and antidepressant effects may occur more frequently with MAOIs than with other antidepressants.

MAOIs in the Elderly

Lower doses and slower increments in dosage are necessary when MAOIs are prescribed for elderly patients. Elderly patients are particularly vulnerable to the effects of hypertensive reactions that can result from adverse MAOI interactions. However, hypertensive crises do not occur more frequently in older individuals than in anyone else (Jenike 1984). Some older patients, and some younger ones, become paradoxically sedated from MAOIs, but tolerance tends to develop to this side effect. Many elderly tolerate phenelzine without significant hypotension.

MAOIs in Patients With Other Neurological Syndromes

MAOIs are generally safe for use in patients with epilepsy; however, seizures have occurred in some nonepileptic patients following overdose. Interactions with anti-parkinsonian drugs can complicate the use of the anticholinergic MAOIs such as phenelzine; L-deprenyl in antiparkinsonian doses does not interact with other anti-parkinsonian drugs. Patients with carcinoid and pheochromocytoma should not receive MAOIs.

Neurological Uses of MAOIs

As already mentioned, L-deprenyl is an antiparkinsonian drug. Because they strongly suppress rapid-eye-movement (REM) sleep, MAOIs have been used to treat narcolepsy. Furazolidone, an MAOI antibiotic, may prove useful as a treatment for peptic ulcer and gastritis (Huai-Yu et al. 1985).

Neurological Side Effects of MAOIs

A serious but infrequent adverse effect of the hydrazine-type MAOIs is hepato-cellular damage, which, in rare cases, can be fatal. Hydrazines can also cause reversible peripheral neuropathy, which may be a result of direct neural toxicity or of interference with pyridoxine metabolism; treatment with pyridoxine may be helpful in the latter instances. Other MAOI side effects that are important in a neurological setting are summarized in Table 26–4 (Bernstein 1983; Lieberman et al. 1985; Meyler and Herxheimer 1968; Pare 1985).

Interactions of MAOIs With Neurological Drugs

The most dangerous interaction of an MAOI is the hypertensive reaction that can occur when the MAOI is combined with certain tyramine-containing foods and various medications. These foods include all aged cheeses, concentrated yeast extracts, sauerkraut, broad bean pods (e.g., fava beans), aged meats, salami, air-dried sausage, old chicken liver, protein extracts, spoiled protein-containing foods, and

Table 26–4. Adverse effects of monoamine oxidase inhibitors (MAOIs)

System	Manifestation
Autonomic nervous system	Orthostatic hypotension, dry mouth, constipation, and delay in micturition
Central nervous system	Toxic psychosis, insomnia, irritability, headache, and ataxia
Neuromuscular	Muscle twitching, myoclonus, motor tension, tremor, muscle and joint pain, peripheral neuropathy, carpal tunnel syndrome, and hyperreflexia
Liver	Jaundice, hepatocellular damage, and elevated liver enzymes
Genitourinary	Impotence and anorgasmia (in men and women; may respond to cyproheptadine)
Miscellaneous	Edema, skin rash, blood dyscrasia (rare), aggravation of asthma, fever, and constipation

all Chinese food and soups. Proscribed foods should not be eaten for 2 weeks after stopping MAOIs.

Headache, fever, agitation, vomiting, and chest pain signal a hypertensive crisis; these may progress to intracerebral bleeding or heart failure. A 10-mg tablet of nifedipine chewed and placed under the tongue for sublingual absorption can ameliorate hypertensive reactions with few side effects (Clary and Schweizer 1987). The definitive treatment of a severe hypertensive crisis is 2–5 mg of intravenous phentolamine.

Although hypertension, rigidity, tremor, fever, convulsions, and coma can occur when MAOIs are combined with HCAs, these two classes of drugs are frequently administered together without adverse consequences. In fact, by blocking uptake of tyramine into nerve terminals, HCAs may protect to some degree against hypertensive reactions related to ingestion of tyramine (Pare 1985). Trazodone can be used safely to treat MAOI-induced insomnia (Jacobsen 1990).

Imipramine, clomipramine, fluoxetine, and meperidine can interact with MAOIs to produce hypotension, hypothermia, seizures, coma, and fatal cardiac arrhythmias, probably due to serotonin syndrome. Because of the long elimination half-life of fluoxetine, MAOIs should not be administered within at least 6 weeks of this drug's use. The possibility of serotonin syndrome also warrants great caution combining buspirone and MAOIs. Because hydrazine and nonhydrazine MAOIs may interact severely with each other, it is advisable to wait 2 weeks before switching from one class of MAOI to another.

Because it takes 2 weeks for MAO to recover after it has been inhibited by MAOIs, most clinicians wait this length of time after completely discontinuing MAOIs before allowing the patient to take a food or medication that might lead to a hypertensive reaction. Discontinuation syndromes have occurred when MAOIs were withdrawn too rapidly. Withdrawal syndromes have included psychosis, mania, insomnia, headache, tremors, nightmares, weakness, paresthesias, and delirium (Lawrence 1985). MAOIs should therefore gradually be discontinued by decreasing the dose by one pill every few days.

In addition to hypertensive reactions and serotonin syndrome, the following are potentially dangerous interactions with MAOIs:

1. Ataxia, hyperreflexia, ankle clonus, myoclonus, nystagmus, dysarthria, paresthesias, and more severe signs of serotonin syndrome when L-tryptophan is added.
2. Potentiation of general anesthetics, sedatives, antihistamines, and narcotic analgesics. Concern about such interactions makes some physicians recommend that anesthesia for surgery or ECT be delayed until MAOIs can be discontinued; however, anesthesia has been administered safely to patients who are still taking MAOIs.
3. Potentiation of the pressor effects of amphetamine and tyramine, but not norepinephrine and epinephrine.
4. Additive anticholinergic effects with neuroleptics and antiparkinsonian drugs.
5. Potentiation of the sedative effects with neuroleptics and antiparkinsonian drugs.
6. Severe hyperpyrexia and coma with dextromethorphan.
7. Increased hypoglycemic effect of insulin.
8. Excitation with reserpine and tetrabenazine.

LITHIUM

Lithium carbonate, which is less irritating to the gastrointestinal tract than other lithium salts (Baldessarini 1985), is available in 300-mg capsules and tablets. Lithium is eliminated primarily by direct excretion by the kidney. Equilibrium between ingestion and excretion takes about 5–6 days, and the half-life of lithium in chronic administration is about 24 hours. Sustained release preparations are absorbed relatively slowly and are associated with less abrupt increases in serum levels without decreasing effectiveness (Jensen et al. 1990).

Psychiatric Uses of Lithium in the Presence of Neurological Disease

Lithium is the drug of choice for prophylaxis of recurrent mania. It is also effective in the treatment of acute mania. Because the clinical effect is not completely manifest for 1 to several weeks after lithium is initiated, neuroleptics frequently are also required during acute treatment if the patient is agitated or psychotic.

There seems little doubt about lithium's ability to prevent or attenuate antidepressant-induced mania and recurrent bipolar depression. It may be an antidepressant in cases of acute bipolar depression or affective psychoses. Whether lithium is a useful treatment or prophylaxis of acute or recurrent unipolar depression is controversial. Many clinicians have found that lithium can augment the antidepressant effect of HCAs, especially in bipolar depression and to a lesser extent in unipolar depression (Jefferson 1990). Lithium may also increase response rates in manic patients treated with carbamazepine and valproate, schizophrenic patients treated with neuroleptics, and OCD patients treated with clomipramine and fluoxetine (Jefferson 1990). Lithium may control impulsive, aggressive, and self-destructive behavior in some emotionally labile patients with brain damage and personality disorders.

Lithium and Organic Brain Disease

When a patient being treated with lithium becomes delirious, the first consideration is lithium intoxication, which may occur at therapeutic levels. Lithium should therefore be withheld until the cause of an acute organic brain syndrome is determined and the illness is treated. Hypothyroidism, which may be induced by lithium treatment itself, can aggravate lithium toxicity. Even at therapeutic levels, lithium may aggravate preexisting organic brain syndromes. However, some agitated dementia patients tolerate lithium well.

Alternatives to Lithium

Patients with dementia who require treatment for a bipolar disorder and who become more confused on lithium may benefit from one of several alternative treatments. Roughly 60%–70% of manic patients are moderately to markedly responsive to carbamazepine for the first year, but up to one-half of these patients, particularly those with an accelerating frequency of episodes, may become tolerant to carbamazepine prophylaxis (Post et al. 1990). Some lithium-resistant patients may respond better to carbamazepine. Valproate, which may be most effective when given with another antimanic drug, seems especially useful for manic patients with abnormal EEGs and possibly for patients with rapid cycling and mixed states (Chou 1991). Verapamil has been given to a small number of manic patients with dementia without adverse effects (Dubovsky et al. 1986).

Clonazepam has been found useful in reducing agitation and other acute manic symptoms, and other BZDs such as lorazepam may also be effective (Dubin 1988). Potential adverse effects in patients with organic brain disease include sedation, cerebellar signs, and paradoxical excitement or increased confusion unless lorazepam's anticonvulsant properties predominate in patients with seizure disorders. Lorazepam may also reduce agitation in acute mania. None of these drugs has been studied systematically as a mood stabilizer in patients with brain damage. ECT, on the other hand, has been found to be effective for mania.

Lithium in Patients With Other Neurological Disorders

Because lithium lowers the seizure threshold and occasionally induces seizures in nonepileptic patients (Massey and Folger 1984), increased doses of anticonvulsants may be necessary when patients with epilepsy take lithium. On the other hand, in at least one report (Shukla et al. 1988) lithium did not increase seizure frequency or anticonvulsant requirement in a small group of bipolar epileptic patients taking doses sufficient to control the mood disorder. The antiepileptic drugs carbamazepine, valproic acid, and clonazepam are logical alternatives to lithium when seizure control is difficult.

Lithium in the Elderly

Even if renal clearance is normal, a general decrease in organ reserve makes the elderly more vulnerable to confusion and other toxic effects of lithium (Table 26–5). The dose of lithium should therefore be increased more slowly in the elderly, and the final dose should be lower than in younger patients. Patients with cardiovascular disease require very close monitoring, and alternate treatment should be considered if electrocardiographic (ECG) changes occur or if adverse effects on the heart develop.

Neurological Uses of Lithium

In anecdotal reports and uncontrolled studies, lithium has been said to ameliorate cluster headaches, Huntington's disease, and spasmodic torticollis; it has also been subjected to preliminary trials in tardive dyskinesia (TD) (Baldessarini 1985). The leukocytosis induced by lithium makes it a useful therapy for leukopenia induced by chemotherapeutic agents. Lithium-induced diabetes insipidus may counteract the syndrome of inappropriate secretion of antidiuretic hormone, which can be a primary disorder or a complication of tumors and infections of the brain and lung.

Neurological Side Effects of Lithium

Lithium produces two types of side effects: those at therapeutic levels (Table 26–5) and those that are due to toxicity. Impairment of memory and concentration may be bothersome to students. Prolonged memory loss and other neurological se-

Table 26–5. Common lithium side effects unrelated to toxicity

Side effect	Manifestations	Comments
Tremor	Irregular, fine resting of fingers and hands most likely to appear after rapid increase in dose; myoclonic jerking may also occur.	May respond to decreasing the dose, adding propranolol or amantadine, switching to lithium carbonate in slow-release tablets, or bedtime doses.
Mental symptoms	Difficulty concentrating, dazed feeling, impaired memory, confusion, dizziness, and flat affect.	Can appear in normal subjects as well as in affective patients. May respond to decreasing the dose.
Polyuria and polydipsia	May be due to nephrogenic diabetes insipidus (metabolic effect) or tubular damage (structural effect).	Lithium-induced kidney disease is probably mild and clinically is insignificant. Nevertheless, renal function should be monitored regularly, and the lowest possible dose should be prescribed. Patients should be advised to avoid dehydration. Thiazide diuretics or amiloride may decrease polyuria.
Thyroid function	Hypothyroidism or enlarged thyroid with normal thyroxine but increased thyroid-stimulating hormone; decreased thyroid function may initiate rapid cycling in some bipolar patients.	Treatment with thyroxine or discontinuation of lithium usually restores normal thyroid function.
Cardiac changes	Decreased automaticity of SA node; delayed conduction through AV node.	Arrhythmias and conduction disturbances are much more common at toxic levels. A baseline ECG should be obtained if there is any suspicion of preexisting cardiac disease to compare suspected postlithium changes. Observe caution when combining with propranolol or verapamil.
EEG changes	REM suppression, high-voltage slow waves, superimposed beta, epileptiform discharges, and disorganization of background rhythm.	Seizures may occur in nonepileptic patients at therapeutic levels.
Gastrointestinal, dermatologic, metabolic, and endocrine effects	Diarrhea, indigestion, skin rash, acne, hair loss, weight gain, altered glucose hypertolerance, and parathyroidism.	Weight gain is probably due to fluid retention plus altered carbohydrate metabolism. Insulin requirement may be changed. Cataracts, depression, or renal disease on lithium should prompt serum calcium studies.
Irreversible neurological damage	Memory deficits and cerebellar symptoms.	Occasionally reported after an episode of severe toxicity.

Note.   ECG = electrocardiogram; REM = rapid eye movement; EEG = electroencephalogram; SA = sinoatrial; AV = atrioventricular.

quelae have been reported after episodes of lithium toxicity (Saxena and Maltikarjuna 1988). The onset of toxicity is heralded by a coarse tremor, ataxia, vertigo, dysarthria, disorientation, nausea, and vomiting. These signs and symptoms may progress to muscle fasciculation, gross confusion, delirium, hyperreflexia, arrhythmias, seizures, coma, irreversible brain damage, and death. Treatment of lithium intoxication involves stopping all drugs, hydration, diuresis, maintenance of electrolyte balance, and dialysis if toxicity is extreme.

Interactions of Lithium With Neurological Drugs

Lithium levels are increased by sodium-wasting diuretics, angiotensin-converting enzyme (ACE) inhibitors, and nonsteroidal anti-inflammatory drugs, but not aspirin or sulindac (Jefferson 1990; Ragheb 1990). Potassium-wasting diuretics can increase the risk of toxicity even at therapeutic levels (Bernstein 1983). A number of antibiotics, especially tetracyclines, spectinomycin, and metronidazole, may increase lithium levels, although this association has not been established definitively. Theophylline and possibly caffeine occasionally lower serum lithium concentrations (Perry et al. 1984).

Since the report by Cohen and Cohen (1974) of irreversible neurotoxicity in patients treated with lithium plus haloperidol, there has been considerable debate about the risks of combining lithium and neuroleptics, particularly with haloperidol and thioridazine, and with carbamazepine. Even though some experts feel that these combinations present no increased risk of neurotoxicity (Baldessarini 1985), reports still emerge of irreversible neurological syndromes, often following lithium intoxication (Izzo and Brody 1985). Neurotoxicity has also been reported when lithium is combined with clonazepam (Koczerinski et al. 1989), neuroleptics, carbamazepine, and calcium channel blockers (Chou 1991).

Many of these drugs, particularly neuroleptics, are often coadministered with lithium to control agitation while waiting for lithium's antimanic effect to appear. However, it is not clear that such combinations are superior in the short run to neuroleptics alone. Some authors therefore recommend using neuroleptics with or without BZDs, or carbamazepine, until the patient's behavior is controlled, at which point lithium is begun and the neuroleptic is withdrawn (Chou 1991).

ELECTROCONVULSIVE THERAPY

Electroconvulsive therapy (ECT) is usually administered under barbiturate anesthesia with succinylcholine or similar muscle relaxants to spare the patient the peripheral manifestations of major motor seizures. An anticholinergic drug such as atropine or glycopyrrolate (which does not cross the blood-brain barrier) may be administered to dry secretions and prevent bradycardia caused by central stimulation of the vagus nerve. Many psychiatrists begin ECT with unilateral nondominant electrode placement, which may minimize memory loss, and proceed to bilateral treatment if satisfactory seizures cannot be obtained or if the patient does not improve. The usual course is 6–12 treatments or 200–600 seizure seconds (Fink 1979). However, some patients require more treatment and suprathreshold stimulation, and seizure time may not be correlated with treatment response.

Psychiatric Uses of ECT in Patients With Neurological Disease

ECT is usually reserved for severely depressed patients who have not responded to medication or who are too ill to wait for antidepressants to take effect. It may also be effective in mania, catatonia, and some cases of schizophrenia (Bernstein 1983; Black et al. 1987). Space-occupying lesions in the brain (or any condition with increased intracranial pressure) have traditionally been considered to be a contraindication to ECT (Bernstein 1983). However, ECT has been administered to patients with brain tumors and with elevated intracranial pressure without ill effects (Dubovsky 1986).

Neurological Uses of ECT

According to the 1978 American Psychiatric Association (APA) Task Force Report on Electroconvulsive Therapy, most American psychiatrists "would find it strange" to use a treatment that can produce an acute organic brain syndrome in delirious patients (Dubovsky 1986). Over the years, however, a number of studies of single and small groups of patients have reported that ECT induced rapid clearing of delirious states associated with intoxication and withdrawal from numerous drugs, delirium tremens, cerebritis, meningitis, encephalitis, syphilis, uremia, pneumonia, and delirium superimposed on dementia (Dubovsky 1986).

Because repeated seizures raise the threshold for further convulsions, ECT has been used as a treatment for intractable epilepsy and as a means of clearing prolonged postictal clouding of consciousness (Dubovsky 1986). Several reports exist of improvement of Parkinson's disease and enhanced response to antiparkinsonian therapy generally lasting for weeks after ECT, even if depression was not improved (Anderson et al. 1987).

Neurological Side Effects of ECT

Confusion and memory loss are major neurological side effects of ECT. These may be proportional to the degree to which the stimulus exceeds the seizure threshold and the use of bilateral versus unilateral treatment, although the latter approach may be less effective (Sackheim et al. 1987). A small number of patients continue to complain that their memories or personalities have been permanently damaged after ECT, but objective studies have not yet provided evidence of memory loss persisting more than 6 months after treatment (Weiner 1984).

With modern anesthetic management, serious complications or death develop in fewer than 1 in 8,000 patients, making ECT one of the safest interventions that use general anesthesia (Fink 1974). Any morbidity or mortality that does occur is usually secondary to cardiovascular complications such as arrhythmia, myocardial infarction, or hypertension. The major risks are those associated with brief general anesthesia.

Interactions of ECT

Concerns that HCAs might predispose to cardiac complications and that MAOIs could potentiate pressor agents and anesthetics or could cause severe hypotension lead many clinicians to discontinue these drugs 2 weeks before beginning ECT. Although this is the safest course, research has suggested that ECT can be safe even when these antidepressants are still being taken (El-Gazour et al. 1985). Lithium may increase the severity of post-ECT confusion, memory loss, delirium, and prolonged seizures (Penney et al. 1990). To avoid these problems, it has been suggested that lithium be discontinued a week before ECT and that it be withheld for several days after ECT is completed (Small and Milstein 1990). Anticonvulsants and BZDs may make it more difficult to initiate a seizure during ECT.

ANTIPSYCHOTIC DRUGS

Neuroleptics (derived from the Greek for "to clasp the neuron") are antipsychotic drugs that control symptoms of psychosis and produce neurological side effects. All currently available antipsychotic drugs except clozapine are neuroleptics. Available antipsychotic drugs differ primarily in their anticholinergic properties, potency (i.e., effectiveness at a given dose), and tendency to produce sedation and hypotension (Table 26–6).

There are different metabolic pathways in the intestine and the liver for antipsychotic drugs (Ko et al. 1985). Chlorpromazine and thioridazine have many active metabolites, whereas butyrophenones and thioxanthenes may be metabolized only to inactive compounds. Parenteral administration avoids hepatic first-pass metabolism that occurs after oral dosage, increasing availability of the neuroleptic four to ten times (Baldessarini 1985). Some low-potency neuroleptics such as chlorpromazine and thioridazine may induce their own metabolism, resulting in decreased drug levels after a few weeks of treatment (Baldessarini 1985).

Psychiatric Uses of Antipsychotic Drugs in the Presence of Neurological Disease

Antipsychotic drugs are used to treat psychotic and agitated states. Their widest application has been in the treatment of schizophrenia, mania, and depression. Most neuroleptics ameliorate positive symptoms such as delusions, hallucinations, and agitation better than negative symptoms such as indifference, withdrawal, blunted affect, and anergia (Schooler 1986).

Clozapine is a recently introduced antipsychotic drug that appears to be more effective than traditional neuroleptics for negative schizophrenic symptoms (Ereshefsky et al. 1989). Clozapine is less likely to cause EPS, TD, or neuroleptic malignant syndrome (NMS), although these adverse effects may occur (Kane et al. 1988). Clozapine is indicated for treatment-resistant schizophrenia, schizophrenia with prominent negative symptoms, and psychotic patients with severe TD or EPS (Marder and Van Putten 1988).

Neuroleptics have been shown to reduce relapse rates in schizophrenia (Davis and Andriukaitis 1986). After initially responding, however, 20%–30% of schizophrenic patients relapse during the first 1–2 years of continuation treatment (Kane et al. 1988). Relapse rates are higher among less stable schizophrenic patients than among more stable ones (Schooler 1986). In patients with chronic schizophrenia, psychotic symptoms return an average of 4.5 months after neuroleptics are discontinued. The risk of relapse appears to be the same no matter how long patients have been taking the neuroleptic.

Some impulsive borderline patients with transient psychotic symptoms benefit

Table 26-6. Antipsychotic drugs available in the United States

Drug by class	Trade name	Usual daily oral dose (mg)	Usual single im dose (mg)	Sedative properties	Anticholinergic properties	Hypotensive effects
Phenothiazines						
Chlorpromazine	Thorazine	300–800	25–50	Very high	High	Moderate-high
Triflupromazine	Vesprin	100–150	20–60	Moderate	Moderate	Moderate
Thioridazine	Mellaril	200–700[a]	—	High	Very high	Moderate-high
Mesoridazine	Serentil	75–300	25	High	Moderate-high	Moderate
Acetophenazine	Tindal	60–120	—	Moderate	Moderate	Low
Perphenazine	Trilafon	8–40	5–10	Moderate	Moderate-low	Low-moderate
Trifluoperazine	Stelazine	6–20	1–2	Low	Low	Low
Fluphenazine	Prolixin	1–20	12.5–50	Low	Low	Low
Thioxanthenes						
Chlorprothixene	Taractan	50–400	25–50	High	High	Moderate
Thiothixene	Navane	6–30	2–4	Low-moderate	Low	Moderate
Butyrophenones						
Haloperidol	Haldol	6–20	2–5[b]	Low	Very low	Very low
Diphenylbutyl-piperidines						
Pimozide	Orap	1–10[c]	—	Moderate-high	Moderate-low	Low
Dibenzoxazepines						
Loxapine	Loxitane	60–100	12.5–50	Low-moderate	Moderate	Low
Dihydroindolones						
Molindone	Moban	50–100	—	Low-moderate	Moderate	Very low
Dibenzodiazepines						
Clozapine	Clozaril	300–450[d]	—	Very high	Moderate	Moderate-high

[a]Maximum 800 mg.
[b]Intravenous doses may be higher.
[c]Second line drug because of cardiotoxicity.
[d]Maximum 900 mg.

from the short-term use of low doses of nonsedating neuroleptics such as haloperidol. The use of neuroleptics in the treatment of organic brain syndromes is considered below. The risk of TD makes neuroleptics poor choices in nonpsychotic anxiety and most types of insomnia. Neuroleptics are necessary adjuncts in the treatment of psychotic depression and possible adjuncts to serotonergic antidepressants in treatment-resistant OCD (Jenike 1990).

Because neuroleptics produce EPS, they are usually contraindicated for patients with Parkinson's disease. Clozapine, however, appears to be well tolerated (Friedman and Lammon 1989). Theoretically, at least, another choice would be an antipsychotic drug with strong anticholinergic properties, such as thioridazine or one of the alternatives to neuroleptics described below.

Many antipsychotic drugs lower the seizure threshold, especially clozapine, loxapine, and low-potency neuroleptics such as chlorpromazine and thioridazine. This appears to be a dose-related effect, especially for clozapine (Miller 1991). Haloperidol and molindone seem safest in seizure-prone individuals (Baldessarini 1985; Fenwick 1989). The dopamine blockade produced by neuroleptics increases prolactin secretion, which is a definite problem for patients with prolactin-secreting pituitary tumors and a possible concern for patients with breast cancer.

Antipsychotic Drugs in the Elderly

As with many drugs, lower doses of neuroleptics are required in the elderly; the initial dose should be about one-third of the usual adult starting dose (Raskin 1985). Higher-potency drugs with lower anticholinergic and hypotensive potential such as haloperidol, molindone, loxapine, fluphenazine, trifluoperazine, and perphenazine are safer in older patients with heart disease (Baldessarini 1985). Thioridazine, which has been reported to cause cardiotoxicity, and chlorpromazine, which has quinidine-like myocardial depressant properties, should generally not be the first-line treatments for cardiac patients.

Alternatives to Antipsychotic Drugs in the Treatment of Psychosis

When acutely psychotic patients are in urgent need of treatment but cannot tolerate neuroleptics, several alternative strategies may be considered. If the patient has mania, alternatives such as carbamazepine, valproate, or verapamil may be useful. ECT may be effective in extreme situations, especially if the psychosis is depressive, manic, schizophreniform, or schizoaffective, and it may reduce psychotic symptoms in some schizophrenic patients (Van Valkenberg and Clayton 1983). Clonidine, clonazepam, diazepam, alprazolam, and lorazepam may augment the action of neuroleptics in ameliorating acute psychotic symptoms, thereby reducing the amount of neuroleptic needed (Bodkin 1990).

Lorazepam has been used most widely as an adjunct or alternative to neuroleptics. Lorazepam and other BZDs may be rapidly effective treatments for catatonia, as may amobarbital and ECT (Bodkin 1990; Fricchione 1989). Reserpine, baclofen, droperidol, and L-tryptophan have also been used as antipsychotic agents (Richelson 1985a). Alprazolam may occasionally augment the action of neuroleptics against negative symptoms, perhaps when panic disorder is also present, but it may induce mania or increase agitation in bipolar patients (Bodkin 1990). Short-acting barbiturates such as amobarbital (see below) may be used for emergency tranquilization and treatment of catatonia if a contraindication to their use does not exist (Bodkin 1990).

Neurological Uses of Antipsychotic Drugs

Although it has never been directly compared to intramuscular dosing, intravenous haloperidol is thought to be a more effective treatment for severe agitation and psychosis caused by delirium than oral or intramuscular dosing because rapid onset and multiple high doses are often necessary (Fernandez et al. 1988). Intravenous or oral haloperidol may be useful in reducing ictal and interictal violence associated with epilepsy (Fenwick 1989), and addition of lorazepam or any BZD would be expected to antagonize any associated reduction or seizure threshold. On the other hand, administering frequent intramuscular doses in an attempt to control psychosis rather than agitation (rapid neuroleptization) is no more effective in acute schizophrenia than are standard approaches, although it is more likely to cause EPS (Dubin 1988).

For many years, low doses of high-potency neuroleptics have been used to control recurrent agitation in patients with dementia when nonpharmacological measures such as keeping the patient oriented failed and when it was clear that intercurrent delirium was not present. Ideally, the drug should be administered intermittently to coincide with anticipated episodes of agitation. Even with this schedule, however, the risk of TD is significant in this group of patients. In addition, the primary mechanism by which neuroleptics reduce agitation in these patients may be sedation. As tolerance develops to the sedative effect, it may be necessary to escalate the dose, further increasing the risk of neurological side effects.

Propranolol is a safe and effective alternative to neuroleptics for controlling violent outbursts in patients with brain damage. Carbamazepine, fluoxetine, trazodone, and buspirone may also be useful treatments for intermittent agitation associated with organic brain disease (Silver and Yudofsky 1985; Stewart et al. 1990). Propranolol, nadolol, carbamazepine, and lithium have shown promise in the treatment of episodic dyscontrol in adults, adolescents, and children with brain damage (Stewart et al. 1990), and lithium may reduce aggression in mentally retarded children and adults (Campbell and Spencer 1988). Naltrexone has been used to control self-destructive behavior in severely mentally retarded patients (Kars et al. 1990). Stimulants may be used for aggression associated with attention-deficit hyperactivity disorder (Stewart et al. 1990). Carbamazepine is useful for the rare instances of interictal aggression associated with partial complex seizures (Stewart et al. 1990).

Most neuroleptics (except thioridazine) have antiemetic properties that make them useful treatments in low doses for nausea and vomiting induced by chemotherapy, vestibular syndromes, dysautonomia, and related physical factors (Baldessarini 1985; Richelson 1985a). A well-known use of the potent neuroleptics, especially haloperidol and pimozide, is for control of chorea and agitation in Huntington's disease and of involuntary movements and obscene vocalizations in Tourette's disorder. However, a 25% incidence of ECG changes and a risk of sudden death make pimozide a second-line drug (Teicher and Glod 1990).

Neurological Side Effects of Antipsychotic Drugs

Seizures associated with clozapine are considered above. Neuroleptics have many side effects that mimic or exacerbate neurological disease, the most familiar of which is EPS (Table 26–7). Some of the signs of parkinsonism can be mistaken for schizophrenic mannerisms and withdrawal, leading the clinician to increase the dose of medication inappropriately. Akathisia may sometimes be confused with psychotic agitation, whereas dystonia and oculogyric crises may be interpreted as psychotic posturing. Recognizing these syndromes is important because they usually call for a decrease rather than an increase in dosage. Most EPS (with the exception of akathisia) are uncommon with clozapine.

A great deal of concern exists about TD. The risk of TD may be proportional to the total amount of neuroleptic that has been taken (Ko et al. 1985). Other risk factors include being older, female, and not schizophrenic and having brain damage (Kane et al. 1985). Another possible risk factor is intermittent use of high doses (Chou 1991). Patients with a history of severe acute extrapyramidal reactions may be more likely to develop TD later, but it is not known whether aggressive treatment of these early side effects will decrease the risk of the later syndrome. Anticholinergic drugs may unmask TD, which can be temporarily suppressed but not cured by an increase in the dose of neuroleptic.

Antiparkinsonian drugs, which were once thought to reduce the risk of TD, may actually increase the risk (Dickey and Morrow 1990). Discontinuing the neuroleptic improves TD in some patients, sometimes after a delay of several years, but no specific treatment is known. The calcium channel blockers have shown some promise in animal models and a few series of patients. Clozapine is a potential treatment, but it is not known whether its capacity to suppress TD is enduring.

The most dreaded complication of neuroleptic treatment is neuroleptic malignant syndrome (NMS), which occurs in 0.5%–1.0% of patients taking neuroleptics (Guze and Baxter 1985). NMS is more likely to occur with intramuscular administration of antipsychotic drugs and may be more common with high-potency preparations, especially haloperidol, thiothixene, fluphenazine, and trifluoperazine (Mueller 1985); however, it has also been reported in patients taking chlorpromazine, promethazine, thioridazine, metoclopramide, carbidopa-levodopa, and various other drugs; in patients taking clozapine plus lithium; and after withdrawal of amantadine and carbidopa-levodopa (Mueller 1985; Pelonero et al. 1985). Patients are more vulnerable to develop NMS if they are less than 40 years old, male, unresponsive to the usual doses of neuroleptics, and debilitated or have brain damage, nonschizophrenic disorders, and neurological illnesses (Mueller 1985). Concurrent use of lithium may increase the risk of NMS (Sakkas et al. 1989).

Interactions of Neuroleptics With Neurological Drugs

Sedating neuroleptics potentiate other CNS depressants, whereas anticholinergic effects are additive with other anticholinergic drugs. Neuroleptics are sometimes used to increase the analgesic effect of narcotics, but respiratory depression may be potentiated as well. Like HCAs, chlorpromazine and other neuroleptics can interfere with the action of antihypertensive agents like guanethidine. Anticonvulsants

Table 26–7.   Neurological side effects of neuroleptic drugs and their treatment

Syndrome	Manifestations	Treatment or prevention
Akathisia	Motor restlessness and feeling of inability to remain still; may be persistent or tardive.	Propranolol, clonazepam, lorazepam, diazepam, clonidine, amantadine, or antiparkinsonian drug (e.g., benztropine).
Acute dystonia	Spasm of muscles of neck, tongue, face, eyes, or trunk.	Decrease dose of neuroleptic; diphenhydramine or antiparkinsonian drug.
Parkinsonism	Stiffness, tremor, bradykinesia, shuffling gait, and salivation.	Oral antiparkinsonian drug for 4 weeks to 3 months; decrease dose of the antipsychotic drug.
Perioral (rabbit) tremor	Perioral tremor usually appearing after long-term therapy.	Decrease dose or change to a medication in another class.
Tardive dyskinesia	Dyskinesias of tongue and face, choreoathetoid movements of neck and trunk usually, but not always, appearing after years of treatment following a reduction in dose; incidence higher in the elderly, brain damaged, non-schizophrenic patients, children and adolescents. Symptoms are worsened by antiparkinsonian drugs and masked, but not cured, by higher dose of neuroleptic.	Risk may be reduced by prescribing the least amount of drug possible for as little time as is clinically feasible, and using long drug-free holidays for patients who need to continue taking the drug. Calcium channel blockers, clonazepam, and clozapine reduce signs of tardive dyskinesia; reserpine temporarily ameliorates tardive dyskinesia but may also cause it.
Anticholinergic delirium (acute organic brain syndrome)	Psychotic symptoms, dry skin, hyperpyrexia, mydriasis, and tachycardia.	Discontinue drug; iv physostigmine for severe agitation or fever.
Neuroleptic malignant syndrome	More commonly caused by high-potency drugs; appears days to months after beginning treatment; elevated creatine phosphokinase, white blood count, and urinary myoglobin; hyperthermia, muscle rigidity, autonomic instability; parkinsonian symptoms, catatonia stupor, neurological signs; 10%–30% fatality.	Obtain serum creatine phosphokinase if altered neurological status, fever, and muscle rigidity appear; if creatine phosphokinase and urine myoglobin levels are elevated, discontinue neuroleptic and give iv dantrolene plus oral bromocriptine. Ensure hydration and cooling.
Seizures	Especially with clozapine, low potency, neuroleptics, and loxapine.	Use lower doses or coadminister anticonvulsants.
α-Adrenergic blockade	Orthostatic hypotension, more common with low-potency drugs; inhibition of ejaculation (may also be related to calcium channel blockade). Priapism, especially with chlorpromazine and thioridazine; may occur at any dose at any time.	Advise patient to stand up slowly; treat acute hypotension with norepinephrine, not epinephrine; avoid β–adrenergic stimulation; change to another medication. Do not administer to patients with a history of prolonged erections with medication.

(continued)

Table 26–7. Neurological side effects of neuroleptic drugs and their treatment *(continued)*

Syndrome	Manifestations	Treatment or prevention
Heat stroke	Decreased sweating; thirst and possible hypothalamic dysfunction cause fever, decreased sweating, and collapse.	Discontinue drug; hydrate and cool.
Behavioral toxicity	Confusion, disorganization, increased aggression, especially in children and adolescents.	Use alternative treatment for aggression.
Sedation	More common with lower-potency neuroleptics and clozapine.	Start with low dose and increase dose slowly.
Leukopenia and agranulocytosis	Sudden appearance within the first 2 months of treatment with high doses of low-potency neuroleptics; 1%–2% incidence with clozapine, usually within the first 6–18 weeks.	Advise patient to call immediately for sore throat, fever, etc., and obtain immediate blood count; discontinue drug; regular complete blood counts will usually identify clozapine-induced agranulocytosis before it becomes irreversible.
Temperature dysregulation	Transient mild hyperthermia common with clozapine.	Rule out fever secondary to infection and give antipyretics; does not progress to neuroleptic malignant syndrome.
Pigmentary retinopathy	Reported with doses of thioridazine equal to or greater than 800 mg/day.	Prescribe less than 800 mg/day of thioridazine.
Impaired psychomotor performance	May be independent of sedation.	Advise patient of risk of impaired driving.
Photosensitivity	Easy sunburning.	Advise patient to avoid strong sunlight and to use sunscreens.
Jaundice	Rare complications of low-potency phenothiazine use.	Switch to a low dose of a low-potency agent in a different class.
Hypersalivation	May be very severe with clozapine, where it is not due to extrapyramidal syndrome.	Decrease dose or add anticholinergic drug.

that induce microsomal enzyme systems (e.g., phenytoin and carbamazepine) enhance metabolism of neuroleptics, sometimes decreasing blood levels and clinical effectiveness substantially (Kahn et al. 1990; Miller 1991), whereas neuroleptics may reduce anticonvulsant effectiveness by lowering the seizure threshold (Teicher and Glod 1990). Neuroleptics raise blood levels of TCAs by as much as 500%; TCAs also raise neuroleptic levels, but the effect is not clinically significant. By interfering with gastrointestinal absorption, antiparkinsonian drugs, cimetidine, lithium, and some antacids also lower neuroleptic levels and may decrease the therapeutic efficacy of the antipsychotic drug (Ayd 1986).

ANTIANXIETY DRUGS

Since the introduction of chlordiazepoxide in 1961, the BZDs have proved to be both effective and safer than other drugs in the treatment of anxiety and insomnia.

However, these medications can produce tolerance and excessive sedation, problems that may be reduced with newer non-BZD anxiolytics such as buspirone (Table 26–8). Because blood level peaks can produce undue sedation, BZDs are often given 2–4 times a day for daytime anxiety despite half-lives of 2 days or more (Baldessarini 1985).

Psychiatric Uses of Antianxiety Drugs in the Presence of Neurological Disease

Antianxiety drugs are most appropriately used to treat time-limited anxiety or insomnia that represents response to an identifiable stress or change in sleep phase. Because generalized anxiety disorder is often episodic, intermittent treatment of this condition is often appropriate.

When chronic anxiolytic therapy is necessary, buspirone may be better tolerated by patients with organic mental syndromes; however, its delayed onset of action makes it ineffective when taken as needed. TCAs are as effective as BZDs for generalized anxiety disorder in some patients (Hoehn-Saric et al. 1988), and the sedating TCAs are often useful as hypnotics.

Alprazolam may have antidepressant properties in patients with panic disorder, but the therapeutic index of this drug is too low for use as a primary antidepressant for most patients (Borison et al. 1989). Other BZDs may also reduce depression in

Table 26–8. Commonly used antianxiety drugs

Class and medication	Trade name	Usual daily anti-anxiety dose (mg)	Onset of effect
Short half-life benzodiazepines[a]			
Alprazolam	Xanax	1.5–6.0	Intermediate
Halazepam	Paxipam	20–120	Intermediate
Lorazepam	Ativan	1.5–6.0	Intermediate
Midazolam	Versed	7.5–45	Intermediate (oral); fast (iv)
Oxazepam	Serax	45–100	Slow
Quazepam[b]	Doral	7.5–15	Fast
Temazepam	Restoril	15–30	Intermediate-slow
Triazolam	Halcion	0.125–0.25	Fast
Long half-life benzodiazepines[c]			
Chlordiazepoxide	Librium	10–100	Slow
Clonazepam	Klonopin	0.5–4.0	Intermediate-slow
Clorazepate	Tranxene	7.5–60	Fast
Diazepam	Valium	2–30	Fast
Flurazepam	Dalmane	7.5–30	Fast
Azaspirone			
Buspirone	BuSpar	15–60	Slow
Antihistamines			
Hydroxyzine	Atarax	50–200	Slow
Diphenhydramine	Benadryl	50–200	Slow
β-Adrenergic blockers			
Propranolol	Inderal	40–120	Slow

[a]Half-life 5–20 hours.
[b]Major metabolite has half-life of 50–160 hours.
[c]Half-life 20–200 hours.

mixed anxiety-depression, and these may be appropriate adjuncts when secondary anxiety does not respond to an antidepressant, particularly in epileptic patients.

Azaspirones administered in higher doses may have antidepressant properties that could make them useful as adjuncts to antidepressants or as a primary treatment for depression complicated by anxiety when the patient cannot tolerate effective doses of an antidepressant. Buspirone may also augment the antiobsessional effect of the serotonergic antidepressants.

Discontinuation Syndromes

Three syndromes may develop after abrupt discontinuation of BZDs (Busto et al. 1986; Noyes et al. 1988). Relapse occurs in 60%–80% of anxious patients, often after weeks to months. Rebound, which appears in 25%–75% of patients, is intensification of the original symptoms that usually lasts several days. Withdrawal, which may be mild to severe in 40%–100% of cases, includes autonomic and CNS symptoms that are different from those of the original disorder.

The risk of withdrawal is greatest in patients who take 40–60 mg/day of diazepam or its equivalent for more than 1 month or who take lower doses for more than 8 months (Dubovsky and Weissberg 1986).

Symptoms of withdrawal from BZDs include dysphoria, irritability, depression, anxiety, anorexia, headache, sweating, faintness, tremor, insomnia, and bad dreams. The real cause may not be apparent when acute psychosis, agitation, delirium, or a generalized seizure are secondary to BZD withdrawal, especially when the patient conceals the extent of drug use. These symptoms may not appear for some time after the patient has been admitted to the hospital if a long-acting BZD is being used or if the patient continues to take the medication after admission.

ORGANIC BRAIN SYNDROMES AND ANXIOLYTICS

When anxiety is a symptom of organic brain disease, steps should be taken to compensate for the underlying disturbance of concentration, attention, and memory while the medical or neurological disorder is being diagnosed and treated. This is accomplished by measures such as frequent orienting, keeping a light on at night, and avoiding unnecessary changes in the patient's surroundings. Although they may be useful in some forms of agitation, oral BZDs and barbiturates are often ineffective anxiolytics in patients with delirium and dementia because these medications further depress cortical and reticular activating system function, which clouds the patients' sensorium even more. Buspirone does not cloud consciousness and is a more appropriate anxiolytic for patients with dementia. Buspirone may also reduce episodic and chronic agitation in patients with dementia, as may trazodone.

Antihistamines are sometimes used to sedate patients with organic brain disease who require an EEG, because these drugs have minimal effects on the EEG. Antihistamines have also been used as sleeping pills for the elderly and patients with dementia, but their anticholinergic properties may be problematic and their antianxiety effect is unpredictable. Low doses of sedating antidepressants such as amitriptyline, doxepin, or trazodone may be useful hypnotics for dementia patients as well as for patients with insomnia induced by fluoxetine or MAOIs. Care should be taken to assess the suicide potential of such patients because antidepressants are more dangerous than BZDs when taken in overdose.

Antianxiety Drugs in the Elderly

As with other centrally acting drugs, lower doses and smaller increments in dosage are necessary for older patients. Shorter-acting BZDs such as triazolam are preferable as sleeping pills to longer-acting ones such as flurazepam. BZDs with simpler metabolic pathways such as lorazepam or oxazepam may be safer than medications with multiple active metabolites, and buspirone is probably safest. Elderly patients who complain of insomnia should not take a hypnotic unless it is clear that difficulty sleeping is not a symptom of another major disorder such as dementia, depression, gastroesophageal reflux, sleep apnea, or restless legs syndrome. Dementia and sleep apnea in particular may be aggravated by nighttime sedation.

Neurological Uses of BZDs and Related Drugs

Phenobarbital is familiar to most clinicians as a first-line anticonvulsant. Clonazepam is used to treat generalized, myoclonic, and absence epilepsy (Chouinard and Penry 1985), and may be helpful in some cases of trigeminal neuralgia and pain syndromes elsewhere in the body that are associated with paroxysmal dysesthesias, pain on stimulation or normal tissue, burning sensations, and hyperesthesia (Bouckonis and Litman 1985). Clonazepam has utility in paroxysmal choreoathetosis that might predict effectiveness in the treatment of TD (Chouinard and Penry 1985).

Neurological Side Effects of Antianxiety Drugs

The most important adverse effects of BZD use are tolerance, abstinence syndromes, sedation, and impaired psychomotor performance. Tolerance to sedation often develops within a week or so, but tolerance to psychomotor impairment takes longer and in some cases may not develop at all (Moskowitz and Smiley 1985). Patients taking BZDs often are not aware of impaired driving, but the risk of a serious accident may be increased fivefold over that for nonusers of BZDs, and even more if the patient also drinks (Dubovsky 1990). BZDs may also increase the risk of relapse of alcoholism. The risk of addiction to BZDs is low in patients without a history of substance abuse; anxious patients with such a history should be treated with buspirone or antidepressants (Dubovsky 1990). Buspirone can cause nausea, dizziness, headache, or excitement.

Paradoxical reactions to BZDs such as anxiety, irritability, aggression, agitation, and insomnia are common in children, the elderly, and patients with brain damage. Behavioral toxicity may occur in psychotic patients treated with BZDs, whereas alprazolam may induce mania (Bodkin 1990). Like the barbiturates, low doses of BZDs decrease alpha activity on the EEG and increase low-voltage fast activity (Harvey 1985). In contrast with the barbiturates, EEG changes with BZDs are more obvious in the frontal regions and are less likely to spread through the brain. Most BZDs increase stage 2 non-REM sleep and decrease stage 4 sleep, making them useful in treating some but not all nightmares (Harvey 1985). Patients with depression who have increased REM density may spend even more time in REM sleep when they take BZDs, resulting in unpleasant or vivid dreams.

Interactions of Antianxiety Drugs With Neurological Drugs

Barbiturates induce hepatic microsomal systems that metabolize many other drugs, including a number of anticonvulsants. This is not true of BZDs, but ethanol and phenytoin decrease BZD breakdown slightly (Harvey 1985). A more significant problem is the additive CNS depressant effect of most anxiolytics with other depressant drugs, including anticonvulsants. BZDs can augment respiratory depression induced by opioids other than meperidine. Buspirone has not yet been found to have any clinically significant interactions with the exception of possible serotonin syndrome with MAOIs (Ayd 1984).

PSYCHIATRIC EFFECTS OF NEUROLOGICAL DRUGS

Most drugs that affect the CNS can produce changes in thinking, emotion, and behavior that mimic primary psychiatric syndromes. The psychiatric symptoms may appear in a clear sensorium, or they may be accompanied by signs and symptoms of delirium. Antiparkinsonian drugs (e.g., trihexyphenidyl and benztropine) and some neuroleptics and antidepressants can produce anticholinergic delirium characterized by agitation, psychosis, hallucinations, tachycardia, mydriasis, fever, and warm dry skin. Common disturbances and their causes are summarized in Table 26–9 (Dubovsky and Weissberg 1986; Medical Letter 1985).

As the boundary between neurology and psychiatry continues to be explored, a number of drugs used routinely in neurological practice are proving useful for psychiatric syndromes. Some of the better studied applications, doses, and side effects are reviewed in Table 26–10.

Table 26–9. Psychiatric side effects of neurological drugs

Symptom	Medications	Comments
Depression	Amantadine	Common at usual doses
	Anticonvulsants	Usually at higher blood levels
	Corticosteroids, ACTH	More common with high doses; may occur on withdrawal
	Benzodiazepines	Depression may also decrease in anxious, depressed patients
	Barbiturates	Common side effect
	Narcotics	
	L-Dopa	Greater risk with prolonged use
	Antihypertensives	Has been reported with many preparations
	Propranolol	Can occur at usual doses
	Vinblastine	Rare
	Asparaginase	Common side effect with higher doses
	Cimetidine	

(continued)

Table 26–9. Psychiatric side effects of neurological drugs *(continued)*

Symptom	Medications	Comments
Depression *(continued)*	Oral contraceptives	In as much as 15% of all cases
	Ibuprofen	Rare
	Metoclopramide	Usual doses
Mania	Baclofen	Usually appears after sudden withdrawal
	Bromocriptine	Symptoms may continue after drug is withdrawn
	Captopril	Symptoms may continue after drug is withdrawn
	Corticosteroids, ACTH	Usually at higher doses
	Dextromethorphan	
	L-Dopa	More frequent in elderly; risk increases with prolonged use
	Antidepressants	In bipolar and some chronically depressed patients
	Digitalis	In bipolar patients with higher doses
	Cyclobenzaprine	Reported in one patient
Hallucinations	Amantadine	Rare; more common in elderly
	Anticonvulsants	Visual and auditory
	Antihistamines	Especially with higher doses
	Anticholinergics	Usually with delirium
	Corticosteroids, ACTH	See above[a]
	Digitalis	Usually at higher blood levels
	Indomethacin	Especially in elderly
	Methysergide	Occasional
	Propranolol	At usual or increased doses
	Methylphenidate	More likely in children
	L-Dopa	See above[a]
	Ketamine	Common
	Cimetidine	Usually in higher doses and in elderly
Nightmares	Antidepressants	When entire dose is taken at night
	Amantadine	Especially in elderly
	Baclofen	Usually after sudden withdrawal
	Ketamine	Also produces hallucinations, crying, changes in body image, and delirium
	L-Dopa	Often after dosage increase
	Pentazocine	During treatment
	Propranolol	See above[a]
	Digitalis	See above[a]
Paranoia	Asparaginase	May be common
	Bromocriptine	Not dose related
	Corticosteroids, ACTH	See above[a]
	Amphetamines	Even at low doses
	Indomethacin	Especially in elderly
	Propranolol	At any dose
	Sulindac	Reported in a few patients
Aggression	Bromocriptine	Not dose related; may persist
	Tranquilizers and hypnotics	A release phenomenon
	L-Dopa	See above[a]
	Phenelzine	May be separate from mania
	Digitalis	See above[a]
	Carbamazepine	In children and adolescents

Note. ACTH = adrenocorticotropic hormone.
[a]Same comments apply as for previous reactions on this drug.

Table 26–10. Psychiatric applications of some neurological drugs

Medication (usual dose in psychiatry mg/day)	Psychiatric uses	Side effects
Carbamazepine (400–2,000; blood level 8–12 µg/ml)	Mania, especially when resistant to lithium Rapid cycling Antidepressant augmentation Posttraumatic stress syndrome Adjunct to neuroleptics in schizophrenia and schizo-affective disorder Restless legs syndrome Chronic pain with dysesthesias Trigeminal neuralgia secretion	Rash (10%–15%) Bone marrow suppression (1:40,000 to 1:125,000) Hepatotoxicity Dizziness Ataxia Sedation Diplopia Dysarthria Inappropriate antidiuretic hormone Mania and aggressiveness in children Loses effectiveness when stored in humid conditions
Valproic acid (1,000–3,000; blood level 50–120 µg/ml)	Mania, especially when resistant to lithium and carbamazepine Ultra rapid cycling Usually combined with another antimanic drug	Tremor Gastrointestinal distress Weight gain Hepatotoxicity
Clonazepam (2–10)	Mania, especially as sedative or hypnotic Panic disorder Psychosis associated with epilepsy Augmentation of neuroleptics in schizophrenia Akathisia Chronic pain Tic disorders Possibly obsessive-compulsive disorder	Sedation Impaired performance Tolerance to anticonvulsant and psychotropic effects
Bromocriptine (5–200)	Neuroleptic malignant syndrome Neuroleptic-induced galactorrhea and amenorrhea Extrapyramidal syndrome Refractory depression Cocaine craving and withdrawal Restless legs syndrome	Nausea and vomiting Abdominal cramps Headaches Dizziness Delirium Psychosis Nonrecurrent syncope after first dose
Calcium channel blockers (e.g., verapamil 240–480)	Mania Adjunct in panic disorder Tourette's syndrome Tardive dyskinesia MAOI-induced hypertensive reaction	Headache Constipation Postural hypotension Increased carbamazepine and valproate levels Increased lithium toxicity Increased carbamazepine toxicity

Note. MAOI = monoamine oxidase inhibitor.

REFERENCES

Adams F: Emergency intravenous sedation of the delirious medically ill patient. J Clin Psychiatry 49(suppl):22–26, 1988

American Psychiatric Association: Tricyclic antidepressants: blood level measurements and clinical outcome: a report of the Task Force on the Use of Laboratory Tests in Psychiatry. Am J Psychiatry 142:155–162, 1985

Anderson K, Baldwin J, Gottfries CG, et al: A double-blind evaluation of electroconvulsive therapy in Parkinson's disease with "on-off " phenomenon. Acta Neurol Scand 76:191–199, 1987

Ayd F: Buspirone: a review. International Drug Therapy Newsletter 19:37–42, 1984

Ayd F: Prophylactic antiparkinsonian drug therapy: pros and cons. International Drug Therapy Newsletter 21:5–6, 1986

Ayd FJ: Fluoxetine: less seems to be more in depression? International Drug Therapy Newsletter 25:27, 1990

Baldessarini RJ: Drugs and the treatment of psychiatric disorders, in The Pharmacological Basis of Therapeutics. Edited by Gilman AG, Goodman LS, Rall TW, et al. New York, Macmillan, 1985, pp 387–445

Baldessarini RJ, Marsh E: Fluoxetine and side effects. Arch Gen Psychiatry 47:191–192, 1990

Ballenger JC: The clinical use of carbamazepine in affective disorders. J Clin Psychiatry 49 (suppl):13–19, 1988

Bernstein JG: Handbook of Drug Therapy in Psychiatry. Boston, MA, John Wright-PSG, 1983

Black DW, Winokur G, Nasrallah A: Treatment of mania: a naturalistic study of electroconvulsive therapy vs lithium in 438 pts. J Clin Psychiatry 48:132–139, 1987

Bodkin JA: Emerging uses for high-potency benzodiazepines in psychotic disorders. J Clin Psychiatry 51 (suppl):41–46, 1990

Borison RL, Siriha P, Albrecht JW, et al: Double-blind comparison of 3 and 6 mg fixed doses of alprazolam vs placebo in outpatients with major depression. Psychopharmacol Bull 25:186–189, 1989

Bouckonis AJ, Litman RE: Clonazepam in the treatment of neuralgic pain syndromes. Psychosomatics 26:933–936, 1985

Busto V, Sellers EM, Naranjo C, et al: Withdrawal reaction after long-term therapeutic use of benzodiazepines. N Engl J Med 315:854–859, 1986

Campbell M, Spencer EIK: Psychopharmacology in child and adolescent psychiatry: a review of the past five years. J Am Acad Child Adolesc Psychiatry 27:269–279, 1988

Chou JCY: Recent advances in treatment of acute mania. J Clin Psychopharmacol 11:3–21, 1991

Chouinard G, Penry JK: Neurologic and psychiatric aspects of clonazepam: an update: proceedings of a symposium. Psychosomatics 26 (suppl):1–37, 1985

Ciraulo DA, Shader RI: Fluoxetine drug-drug interactions, I: antidepressants and antipsychotics. J Clin Psychopharmacol 10:48–50, 1990

Clary C, Schweizer E: Treatment of MAOI hypertensive crisis with sublingual nifedipine. J Clin Psychiatry 48:249–250, 1987

Cohen WJ, Cohen NH: Lithium carbonate, haloperidol and irreversible brain damage. JAMA 230:1283–1287, 1974

Davidson J: Seizures and buspirone: a review. J Clin Psychiatry 50:256–261, 1989

Davis JM, Andriukaitis S: The natural course of schizophrenia and effective maintenance drug treatment. J Clin Psychopharmacol 6 (suppl 1):2S–10S, 1986

Demuth GW, Breslov RE, Drescher J: The elicitation of a movement disorder by trazodone: case report. J Clin Psychiatry 46:535–536, 1985

Dickey W, Morrow JI: Drug-induced neurological disorders. Prog Neurobiol 34:331–342, 1990

Dilsaver SC, Greden JF: Antidepressant withdrawal phenomena. Biol Psychiatry 19:237–253, 1984

Dubin WR: Rapid tranquilization: antipsychotics or benzodiazepines? J Clin Psychiatry 49 (suppl):5–11, 1988

Dubovsky SL: Using electroconvulsive therapy for patients with neurological disease. Hosp Community Psychiatry 37:819–825, 1986

Dubovsky SL: Generalized anxiety disorder: new concepts and psychopharmacologic therapies. J Clin Psychiatry 51 (suppl):3–10, 1990

Dubovsky SL, Weissberg MP: Clinical Psychiatry in Primary Care, 3rd Edition. Baltimore, MD, Williams & Wilkins, 1986

Dubovsky SL, Franks RD, Allen S, et al: Calcium antagonists in mania. Psychiatry Res 18:309–320, 1986

El-Gazour AR, Ivankovich AD, Braverman B, et al: Monoamine oxidase inhibitors: should they be discontinued preoperatively? Anesth Analg 64:592–596, 1985

Ereshefsky L, Watanabe MD, Tran-Johnson TK: Clozapine: an atypical antipsychotic agent. Clin Pharm 8:691–709, 1989

Fenwick P: The nature and management of aggression in epilepsy. Journal of Neuropsychiatry and Clinical Neurosciences 1:418–425, 1989

Fernandez F, Holmes VF, Adams F, et al: Treatment of severe refractory agitation with a haloperidol drip. J Clin Psychiatry 49:239–241, 1988

Fink M: Induced seizures and human behavior, in Psychobiology of Convulsive Therapy. Edited by Fink M, Kety S, McGaugh J, et al. Washington, DC, VH Winston, 1974, pp 1–20

Fink M: Convulsive Therapy: Theory and Practice. New York, Raven, 1979

Fiori MG: Tricyclic antidepressants: a review of their toxicology. Current Developments in Psychopharmacology 4:72–94, 1977

Fricchione G: Catasonia: a new indication for benzodiazepines? Biol Psychiatry 26:761–765, 1989

Friedman JH, Lammon MC: Clozapine in treatment of psychosis in Parkinson's disease. Neurology 39:1219–1221, 1989

Goodman WK, Charney DS: Therapeutic applications and mechanisms of action of monoamine oxidase and heterocyclic antidepressant drugs. J Clin Psychiatry 46:6–22, 1985

Greist JH, Jefferson JW, Rosenfeld R, et al: Clomipramine and obsessive compulsive disorder: a placebo-controlled double-blind study of 32 patients. J Clin Psychiatry 51:292–297, 1990

Guze BH, Baxter LR: Neuroleptic malignant syndrome. N Engl J Med 313:163–166, 1985

Harvey SC: Hypnotics and sedatives, in the Pharmacological Basis of Therapeutics, 7th Edition. Edited by Gilman AG, Goodman LS, Rall TW, et al. New York, Macmillan, 1985, pp 339–371

Herman JB, Brotman AW, Pollack MH, et al: Fluoxetine-induced sexual dysfunction. J Clin Psychiatry 51:27–29, 1990

Hoehn-Saric R, McLeod DR, Zimmerl WD: Differential effects of alprazolam and imipramine in generalized anxiety disorder. J Clin Psychiatry 49:293–301, 1988

Holmes VF, Fernandez F, Levy JK: Psychostimulant response in AIDS-related complex patients. J Clin Psychiatry 50:5–8, 1989

Hoogiverf B: Amitriptyline treatment of painful diabetic neuropathy: an inadvertent single-patient clinical trial. Diabetes Care 8:526–527, 1985

Huai-Yu, Guszhen L, Jundong G, et al: Furazalidone in peptic ulcer. Lancet 2:276–277, 1985

Izzo KL, Brody R: Rehabilitation in lithium toxicity. Arch Phys Med Rehabil 66:779–782, 1985

Jacobsen FM: Low-dose trazodone as a hypnotic when treated with MAOIs and other psychotropics. J Clin Psychiatry 51:298–302, 1990

Jefferson JW: Lithium: the present and the future. J Clin Psychiatry 51 (suppl):4–8, 1990

Jenike MA: The use of monoamine oxidase inhibitors in the treatment of elderly patients. J Am Geriatr Soc 32:571–575, 1984

Jenike MA: Approaches to the patients with treatment-refractory obsessive-compulsive disorder. J Clin Psychiatry 51 (suppl):15–21, 1990

Jensen HV, Olafsson K, Bille A, et al: Lithium every second day: a new treatment regimen? Lithium 1:55–58, 1990

Kahn EM, Schulz C, Perel JM, et al: Change in haloperidol level due to carbamazepine: a complexatory factor in combined medication for schizophrenia. J Clin Psychopharmacol 10:54–57, 1990

Kane JM, Woerner M, Borenstein M, et al: Integrating incidence and prevalence of tardive dyskinesia. Paper presented at the Fourth World Congress of Biological Psychiatry, Philadelphia, PA, September 1985

Kane JM, Honigfeld G, Singer J, et al: Clozapine for the treatment-resistant schizophrenia. Arch Gen Psychiatry 45:789–796, 1988

Kars H, Broekenia W, Glaudenmans-Gelderen I, et al: Naltrexone attenuates self-injurious behavior in mentally retarded patients. Biol Psychiatry 27:741–746, 1990

Kaufman MW, Cassem N, Murray G, et al: The use of methylphenidate in depressed patients after cardiac surgery. J Clin Psychiatry 45:82–84, 1984

Ko GN, Korpi ER, Linnoila M: On the clinical relevance and methods of quantification of plasma concentrations of neuroleptics. J Clin Psychopharmacol 5:253–262, 1985

Koczerinski D, Kennedy SH, Swinson RP: Clonazepam and lithium: a toxic combination in the treatment of mania? Int Clin Psychopharmacol 4:195–199, 1989

Lawrence JM: Reactions to withdrawal of antidepressants, antiparkinsonian drugs, and lithium. Psychosomatics 11:869–877, 1985

Lieberman JA, Kane JM, Reife R: Neuromuscular effects of monamine oxidase inhibitors. J Clin Psychopharmacol 5:217–220, 1985

Marder SR, Van Putten T: Who should receive clozapine? Arch Gen Psychiatry 45:865–867, 1988

Martin PR, Adinoff DB, Eckardt MJ, et al: Effective pharmacotherapy of alcoholic amnestic disorder with fluvoxamine: preliminary findings. Arch Gen Psychiatry 46:617–621, 1989

Massey EW, Folger WN: Seizures activated by therapeutic levels of lithium carbonate. South Med J 77:1173–1175, 1984

Mathew NT: Prophylaxis of migraine and mixed headache: a randomized controlled study. Headache 21:105–109, 1981

Medical Letter: Drugs that cause psychiatric symptoms. Med Lett Drugs Ther 26:75–78, 1985

Meyler L, Herxheimer A: Side Effects of Drugs. Baltimore, MD, Williams & Wilkins, 1968

Miller DD: Effect of phenytoin on plasma clozapine concentration in two patients. J Clin Psychiatry 52:23–25, 1991

Moskowitz H, Smiley A: Effects of chronically administered buspirone and diazepam in driving-related skills performance. J Clin Psychopharmacol 5:45–55, 1985

Mueller PS: Neuroleptic malignant syndrome. Psychosomatics 26:654–662, 1985

Noyes R, Garvey MJ, Cook BL, et al: Benzodiazepine withdrawal: a review of the evidence. J Clin Psychiatry 49:382–389, 1988

Pare CMB: The present status of monoamine oxidase inhibitors. Br J Psychiatry 146:576–584, 1985

Pelonero AL, Levenson JL, Silverman JL: Neuroleptic therapy following neuroleptic malignant syndrome. Psychosomatics 26:946–947, 1985

Penney JF, Dinwiddie SH, Zorunuski CF, et al: Concurrent close temporal administration of lithium and ECT. Convulsive Therapy 6:139–145, 1990

Perry PJ, Calloway RA, Cook BL, et al: Theophyllus-precipitated alterations of lithium clearance. Acta Psychiatr Scand 69:528–539, 1984

Pinder RM, Brogden RN, Speight TM, et al: Maprotiline: a review of its pharmacological properties and therapeutic efficacy in mental states. Drugs 13:321–352, 1977

Post RM, Leverich GS, Rosoff AS, et al: Carbamazepine prophylaxis in refractory affective disorders: a focus on long-term follow-up. J Clin Psychopharmacol 10:318–327, 1990

Ragheb M: The clinical significance of lithium-nonsteroidal anti-inflammatory drug interactions. J Clin Psychopharmacol 10:350–354, 1990

Raskin DE: Antipsychotic medication and the elderly. J Clin Psychiatry 46:36–40, 1985

Richelson E: Pharmacology of neuroleptics in use in the United States. J Clin Psychiatry 46:8–14, 1985a

Richelson E: Treatment of peptic ulcer disease with tricyclic antidepressants. International Drug Therapy Newsletter 20:21–23, 1985b

Rickels K, Amsterdam JD, Clary C, et al: Buspirone in major depression: a controlled study. J Clin Psychiatry 52:34–38, 1991

Rosenblatt RM, Reich J, Dehrung D: Tricyclic antidepressants in treatment of depression and chronic pain: analysis of the supporting evidence. Anesth Analg 63:1025–1032, 1984

Rosenthal NE, Sack DA, Carpenter CJ, et al: Antidepressant effects of light in seasonal affective disorder. Am J Psychiatry 142:163–170, 1985

Sackheim HA, Decina P, Portnoy S, et al: Studies of dosage seizure threshold and seizure duration in ECT. Biol Psychiatry 22:249–268, 1987

Sakkas P, Davis JM, Jin H: Vulnerability and presentation of NMS. Paper presented at the annual meeting of the American Psychiatric Association, San Francisco, CA, May 1989

Salzman C: Geriatric psychopharmacology. Annu Rev Med 36:217–228, 1985

Saxena S, Maltikarjuna P: Severe memory impairment with acute overdose lithium toxicity. Br J Psychiatry 152:853–854, 1988

Schiffer RB, Herndon RM, Rudide RA: Treatment of pathological laughing and weeping with amitriptyline. N Engl J Med 312:1480–1482, 1985

Schooler NR: The efficacy of antipsychotic drugs and family therapy in the maintenance treatment of schizophrenia. J Clin Psychopharmacol 6:115–195, 1986

Schweitzer E, Rickels K, Amsterdam JD, et al: What constitutes an adequate antidepressant trial for fluoxetine? J Clin Psychiatry 51:8–11, 1990

Sheehan DV, Ballenger J, Jacobson G: Treatment of endogenous anxiety with phobic, hysterical and hypochondriacal symptoms. Arch Gen Psychiatry 37:51–59, 1980

Shukla S, Mukherjee S, Decina P: Lithium in the treatment of bipolar disorders associated with epilepsy: an open study. J Clin Psychopharmacol 8:201–204, 1988

Silver JM, Yudofsky S: Propranolol for aggression: literature review and clinical guidelines. International Drug Therapy Newsletter 20:9–12, 1985

Sitland-Marslen PA, Wells BG, Froemming JH, et al: Psychiatric applications of bromocriptine therapy. J Clin Psychiatry 51:68–82, 1990

Small JG, Milstein V: Lithium and electroconvulsive therapy. J Clin Psychopharmacol 10:346–350, 1990

Stewart JT, Myers WC, Burkett RC, et al: A review of pharmacotherapy of aggression in children and adolescents. J Am Acad Child Adolesc Psychiatry 29:269–277, 1990

Sullivan MD, Sakai CS, Dobie RA, et al: Treatment of depressed tinnitus patients with nortriptyline. Ann Otol Rhinol Laryngol 98:867–872, 1989

Tabakoff B, Lee JM, De Leon-Jones L, et al: Ethanol inhibits the activity of the B form of monoamine oxidase in human platelet and brain tissue. Psychopharmacology 87:152–156, 1985

Teicher MH, Glod CA: Neuroleptic drugs: indications and guidelines for their rational use in children and adolescents. Journal of Child and Adolescent Psychopharmacology 1:33–56, 1990

Teicher MH, Glod C, Cole JO: Emergency of intense suicidal preoccupation during fluoxetine treatment. Am J Psychiatry 147:207–210, 1990

Van Valkenberg C, Clayton PJ: Electroconvulsive therapy and schizophrenia. Biol Psychiatry 20:699–700, 1983

Weiner RD: Does ECT cause brain damage? Behav Brain Res 7:1–53, 1984

Wernicke JF, Dunlop SR, Dornseif BE, et al: Low-dose fluoxetine for depression. Psychopharmacol Bull 24:183–188, 1988

Chapter 27

Psychotherapy of Patients With Neuropsychiatric Disorders

David V. Forrest, M.D.

Neuropsychiatry has potential as a paradigm for relating psychotherapy to brain function. At present, psychiatrists generally rely on their medical background to help patients understand neuropsychiatric disorders, to translate diagnostic jargon into emotionally relevant human meaning, and to help fine-tune complex treatment regimens that may include pharmacotherapy or other somatotherapy. Just as contact with patients with gross neurological impairment helps us assess neurological abnormalities in our psychiatric patients, so, too, can familiarity with the needs of more impaired psychiatric patients—especially those with schizophrenia, organic mental disorders, and substance use disorders—help us frame a psychotherapeutic approach that is tailored to the cognitive and affective needs of neurological patients.

Many of the same mechanisms overlap in neurological and psychiatric conditions. Woods and Short (1985) found that 50% of 270 newly admitted patients with major psychiatric disorders had neurological abnormalities, and Schiffer (1983) established psychiatric diagnoses in 41.9% of 241 neurology patients. Thus, in formulating an approach to neuropsychiatry, empathic medical psychotherapy techniques must be adapted to the specific neurological features of the patient.

PSYCHODYNAMIC ASPECTS OF THE MENTAL EXAMINATION

Structured examinations and formal neuropsychological testing, even those as extensive as the Halstead-Reitan battery and computerized neuropsychological tasks, do not bring out the information necessary to formulate a comprehensive treatment plan and only crudely hint at the difficulties that will be encountered as the psychiatrist adjusts the treatment to individuals. The checklists must be set aside, and a shift must be made to a psychodynamically oriented interview with ample open-ended questions that will enable the psychiatrist to appreciate the unique personality and affective qualities of each patient. Such an interview should provide an understanding of the hereditofamilial, constitutional, developmental, experiential, and interpersonal contributions to the formation of personality structure and the major traumata and conflicts the patient encountered along the way. The impact of the illness is assessed similarly and placed in the context of the person's longitudinal history. The psychiatrist goes beyond assessing the elements of function, as in physical medicine, and is interested in the operational aspects of how the patient will fare while at home and/or at work, as in rehabilitation medicine.

Employment of any structured mental examination marks a shift away from a psychotherapeutic relatedness to the patient toward an evaluative mode that always has a distancing effect and sometimes is experienced as threatening by the patient. The analogy with the physical exam is not complete because the patient's very ability to make sense of the proceedings is being questioned. This is a time for great compensatory warmth and reassurance on the part of the examiner, which pays the scientific dividend of eliciting the patient's best performance. The patient may experience emotions as strong as self-loathing and humiliation, depending on the deficits involved and the degree of investment in the integrity of those functions.

The examining psychiatrist must ensure that a methodical approach is not mistaken by the patient for scorn or that a smug supplying of the correct answers is not taken for an air of superiority. Seemingly "playing to the crowd" at the patient's expense, whether before assembled family or in front of residents and medical students, is to be scrupulously avoided. Sympathetic recognition of all deficits should be directed first to the patient. Even complex concepts such as the operationally crucial faculty of constructional ability can be evaluated empathetically. For example, the psychiatrist may ask, "Has it been difficult lately to plan your day or to grasp the overall picture in complicated situations? Have you noticed difficulty in getting things together to do something?"

Contact in Neuropsychiatric Patients

On entering the patient's room, the psychiatrist should be aware that impairments in the patient's hierarchy of capacities are likely to impede any beneficial encounter between patient and physician in specific ways that require adaptations and compensations in psychotherapeutic technique. Each capacity in Table 27–1 is dependent on the integrity of those that precede it.

Defenses: The Neuropsychodynamic Continuum

The psychiatrist who is well trained in psychodynamic psychotherapy brings to the study of defense mechanisms in neuropsychiatry a relevant but incomplete description. Defenses are psychodynamic mechanisms employed by a person in interaction with the surprises and dangers of the world and with drives and emotions from within. Traditionally, defenses have been classified on a dimension from the most mature to the most immature. The most mature defenses are viewed as the healthiest ones (such as sublimation, suppression, and laughter). Less mature defenses (such as reaction formation, rationalization, displacement, and isolation) are thought to be characteristic of a neurotic level of function. The most immature defenses (such as denial, splitting, merging, projection, and projective identification) are considered the sickest, typifying psychotic functioning. Although psychodynamic theory originally recognized a somatic contribution to the mental defenses, it did not specify which mental defenses are associated with organic impairment or how the defenses are related to organic processes.

In approaching defenses in neuropsychiatry, parallels might be sought between the mental mechanisms of defense and defensive brain (or cortical) reactions. At the very least, the confused patient and baffled family could be helped to see which de-

Table 27–1.   Hierarchy of capacities for psychotherapeutic contact that may be impaired in neuropsychiatric patients

Capacity	Adaptations in psychiatric technique
Consciousness	Adopt a reassuring manner. Avoid agitation by avoiding overstimulation. Limit time of visit. Assess changing tolerance for interventions. Keep affect positive even if patient is apparently unconscious or not fully conscious.
Attention	Eliminate distractions. Keep contacts one on one. Speak clearly and simplify language. Use brief syntax. Make sure your presence is registered. Note perceptual impairments such as field cuts or hearing deficits and position self helpfully.
Retention	Repeat from time to time. Simplify. Break down communications into simple steps. Reinforce with other channels and modalities (e.g., writing and diagrams). Practice mnemonics with patient. Identify self each visit and keep your appearance constant.
Orientation	Remind patient (as needed) of time, place, and person. Keep calendar and clock in view. Visit at the same time daily.
Recognition	Tailor approach to compensate for specific impairments of any of the many parallel brain processors, from trouble with simple geometric perceptions through facial recognition to more complex perceptual components of relationship. Adapt communication to assist and circumvent dysphasic channels (e.g., reassure with affects when verbal reception is poor).
Construction	Assist in putting together cause and effect, as well as spatial and temporal connection. Help to see how necessary activities or outing will fit into time slots of the day. Offer structures.
Emotion	Assess underlying drives of anxiety, aggressiveness, and sexuality. Do not stress patient's having difficulty with control. Identify and read out to the patient degrees of joy, fear, anger, shame, guilt, or sadness being felt by the patient. Name more specific emotions under these main headings to reduce resistance and increase the feeling of being understood.
Conation	Help patient build on fragile will and find his or her own direction in confusion. Do not be overbearing as your very presence may be commanding to the point of causing automatic obedience or opposition, echopraxia, echolalia, or cataplexy. Respect elements of prosocial intentionality in actions.
Motivation	Facilitate positive incentives by behavioral manipulation and removal of negative influences. Help patient identify latent longings for improved adaptation. Guard against helplessness.
Proposition	Accept that the first stage of proposition during recovery is usually opposition, as with a child in the "terrible twos." Respect the inherent positive energy, but set limits. Encourage half-baked initiatives and help structure only after they get going. Don't discourage the patient or complicate things.
Delineation	Help patient see origins of affects in self or from others and help him or her work on impairment in self, not project it onto world. Use projections onto the psychiatrist or onto paralyzed body parts as clues to self-concepts. Excessive blame taking may often best be handled as a failure of delineation from family anger or disappointment about the patient's not being sufficiently restored to normal.
Relation	Note quality of and changes in relations with significant others. The patient's caring about the needs of others is an extremely good sign that social function will recover and psychotherapy will be helpful. Balance looking out for the patient's needs against validating reasonable perceptions and needs of spouse and family, on whom the patient is dependent.

fensive reactions are exacerbations of characterological armor (under varying degrees of voluntary control and amenable to interpretation) and which are more primitive, automatic defenses of an injured brain that may be compensated for by tolerant understanding and environmental manipulation. Between these two extremes lie defensive formations that are rooted in both psyche and brain. Finally, one must not assume that a learning process is absent in cortical defenses, so that improvement occurs only with spontaneous recovery, or that the mental defenses have a plasticity that is completely reeducable by psychotherapy.

Certain analogical comparisons on the basis of operational principles may be made among cortical defenses, mental defenses, and a bridging area of what might be termed *neuropsychic defenses.* In Table 27–2, parallels are drawn among similar defensive structures of similar shape that are 1) mental defenses of the psyche, 2) somatopsychic or neuromental defenses clearly influenced by the neurological state, and 3) cortical neurological reactions. Potential continua among these three types of defensive structures are implied.

TECHNIQUES FROM PSYCHOTHERAPY OF SCHIZOPHRENIA

Schizophrenia is a symptom formation that is more complex than an organic deficit, but its treatment may serve as a model for psychiatric work with less familiar neurological conditions. All of the dysfunctional features previously catalogued for schizophrenia (Forrest 1983) may be variably present in the neurological patient with a brain injury (especially those with mesolimbic involvement) and require sensitive adjustments of technique by the neuropsychiatrist similar to those described for schizophrenia (Forrest 1983).

The mechanisms that occur both in schizophrenia and in neurological patients with disordered brain function include undifferentiated "catastrophic" reactions to stresses when the patient becomes overwhelmed; involuntary concreteness or metonymy (taking a part of a concept for the entire concept); incapability of moving among levels of abstraction, especially regarding interpersonal relations; fear of novel situations; segmentalization and deautomatization of previously automatic sequences of emotional response; slow habituation and extinction of reactions to stimuli; and probabilistic incapacity (poor ability to evaluate likely outcome).

Frequently there is an additional feature of language disturbance not present in schizophrenia. Although the schizophrenic person almost always exhibits an impairment of language in a larger sense, other patients with impaired brain function usually have some difficulty *accessing* language. This problem is typically absent in schizophrenia (Benson 1975). The crucial practical difference for psychotherapy is that emotions in most neurological patients are recruited to overcome cognitive and linguistic problems and to make interpersonal sense, whereas in schizophrenia cognitive and linguistic elements—often exaggerated and fanciful—are recruited to compensate for poor command of affects, and the result frustrates interpersonal sense.

The neuropsychiatrist must be crucially attuned to nuances of a patient's affect. One's own perception of affect can be calibrated against the highly reliable means of affect scoring of short videotaped interview segments by professional audiences (Forrest 1982). The six affects—joy, fear, anger, shame, guilt, and sadness—can each be rated on a scale of 0 to 4^+ like any other medical measurement. Under the general

Table 27–2. Neuropsychiatric defense continuum

Continuum	Mental defenses	Neuromental defenses	Cortical reactions
Nonrecognition	Denial of damage, avoidance, disavowal; or conscious caring for paralyzed limb	Neglect of body part or side, with preservation of the concept of a damaged limb	Hemi-inattention because of diminished cortical representation
Misdirection	Circumstantiality, tangentiality	Overinclusion, ellipsis	Inattention, distractibility
Nondenotation	Metaphor, metonymy, symptom and symbol formation, circumlocution, poetic language and logic	Rhyming, clang associations, neologism, substitution	Aphasic paraphasias, jargon, dysnomia
Nonrecall (or nongrasp)	Obsessive ordering, hysterical evasion, paranoid reductiveness, schizoid invention, sociopathic approximate answers (Ganser syndrome)	Confabulation, structure by constant talking, compensatory grandiloquence (poststroke, to prove smart), ignore what one can't structure, repeating and quoting self	Amnestic or state-dependent lapses, failure of processing with information overload
Referential loss	Delusions of reference and influence and of dementia in depression (pseudodementia)	Delusions of loss or impoverishment; metaphorical substitution of time, feces, money, or other measurable things for unacceptable and incomprehensible loss of brain function	Diminished capacity for construction, proposition, and planning
Affect application	Helplessness, hopelessness; compensation; or plaintive self-denigration with realization of deficit; schizophrenic substitutions of (sociopolitical or religiophilosophical) abstractions for interpersonal focus on emotions	Beneficence toward or degradation of self or object world without realization or recognition of deficit; parapathic substitutions of schizophrenic language for affects	Apathy, emotionalism, organic mania; flat affect in schizophrenia
Regression	Ontogenic regression to less mature states of mind, with diminished object constancy, tantrums, or catastrophic reactions to stress	Stereotypy and other complex innate primitive patterns such as mechanical repetition in stimulant abuse, touching the face in Huntington's disease, and regression to silly humor or puns (*Witzelsucht*)	Phylogenetic regression to neural reactions characteristic of lower mammalian and vertebrate predecessors (e.g., grasp and snout)

(continued)

Table 27–2. Neuropsychiatric defense continuum (*continued*)

Continuum	Mental defenses	Neuromental defenses	Cortical reactions
Kindling or temporolimbic hyperconnection (interictal)	Hypermoralism, intensified religiosity, and proselytizing; sense of urgency and mission; anger and remorse; and graphomania	Viscosity, emotional deepening, sensations of immanence, transcendence, and divine presence; thought insertion	Organic sensations of otherness or bodily intrusion; hyposexuality
Impaired worldview	"My relationship to the world has changed."	"The world is bigger, harder to deal with, more confusing," or (in schizophrenia) more aesthetically awesome	"The world has been changed, reduplicated, substituted" in patients with brain injury
Impaired view of others	Transference reactions: "It's I who changed, my perceptions differ because I'm injured"; degrees of insight; interpersonal shallowness and manipulativeness	Misidentification:"People have changed, are different, are to blame, have been replaced by impostors"; splitting and projective identification;"underlying defect" in borderline syndrome of failure of delineation	Prosopagnosia: state-dependent change in cognition of people or their relation to self
Sex object shift	Avoidance of parental object to preserve ties to family	Failure to integrate affects and sexuality	Failure to differentiate sexual object (Klüver-Bucy syndrome of bilateral hippocampal damage) or own gender
Impaired ego boundary	Creativity and regression in the service of the ego	Disturbing nightmares, other vulnerability to internal and external processes, and schizophrenia	Diminished stimulus barrier
Impairment of conation or will	Identification with the aggressor, and introjection and incorporation in health, neurosis, and depression	Made cognition, made volition, and command hallucinations in schizophrenia	Echolalia, echopraxia, and involuntary reflex activity in brain injury
Impaired movement or spatial play	Disorientation, agoraphobia, diminished sense of mastery and mobility and of bodily feedback and control, and lowered confidence in actions	Vestibular defensiveness, fear of moving, fear of falling or of whirling (twirling a soft sign in children), incoordination, and clumsiness	Vertigo, motor or proprioceptive impairment incoordination, poor eye tracking, ataxia, and tremor

affect rubrics, cognitive shadings of emotions can be specified. The most common error in treating patients with impaired brain function is not adjusting one's own projection of emotional tone to the patient's needs. For example, patients with hyperemotionalism may require us to throttle down our emotions. The challenge for most neuropsychiatrists is to increase the benevolent emotion they project toward certain patients who for various reasons are receiving signals poorly. Psychotherapy in neuropsychiatry should be eclectic, adapting elements that are helpful from various modalities (Table 27–3).

TRAUMATIC BRAIN INJURY

Childs (1985) has stated that the most difficult sequelae of head injury to treat are the psychosocial disabilities; impaired cognition is next in degree of difficulty, and impaired physical abilities are the least difficult. Also, perhaps contrary to common assumption, the patient's family suffers most severely from the disruption of emotions and object relations, next most from the intellectual impairments, and least from the physical impairments (Oddy et al. 1978). This is why psychotherapy can play a crucial role in individual and family recovery after head injury.

The emotional climate is worsened by the typical emergence of bad temper in the patient 3 or more months after the injury. The family's optimism that full recovery will occur, based on successes in physical rehabilitation, turns to disappointment when the

Table 27–3.   Modalities of psychotherapy in neuropsychiatry

Helpful aspects of the psychoanalytic approach for neuropsychiatry
1. Respect for the patient's autonomy and self-determination.
2. Theoretic concept of defense organization.
3. Most sufficient map of mental, cognitive, and emotional function.
4. Model based on conflict among mental structures.

Inappropriate aspects of the psychoanalytic approach for neuropsychiatry
1. Too passive a receptiveness rather than making affective contact.
2. Too much reliance upon free association and dreams.
3. Searching for remote causes and relationships.
4. Attribution of treatment events to abstract forces and entities in talking to the patients.
5. Overemphasis on transference versus reality issues.
6. Intentional lack of frames and structures.
7. Interpersonal relations considered as inner object relations.
8. Avoidance of direct answers or being a "blank screen" rather than being a beacon to security.

Other modalities of psychotherapy in neuropsychiatry
1. Behaviorist approaches to the patient's learning system as a black box may be helpful in structuring relearning, but they are "brainless" in their theoretical avoidance of capacities, defenses, conflicts, recruitment of affect to aid cognition, and other neuromental dynamics that are helpful in explanation.
2. Interpersonal and family approaches are surprisingly helpful communication systems despite the clear nidus of difficulty in a neuropathologically "designated patient," because of the impact on relatives and their involvement in the care of the disabilities. As there is both direct influence and imitation and a hereditary factor in neurotic, characterological, and major psychiatric disorders, the families of patients with acquired neuropsychiatric disorders may themselves be less disordered and more of a help in the treatment.

patient's impulse control worsens. The doctors often bear the transferred brunt of family anger. Interventions should aim at legitimizing family disappointment and avoiding comments that abet the splitting. Unconscious or unacknowledged family anger at the patient for being injured contributes to the patient's internalized anger within the family system and must be addressed to head off severe self-loathing or suicidal trends as the protection of denial wears off.

Regression in the patient's mental processes may parallel neurological regression, and both mental and neuromental defenses parallel pathological brain reactions. Often, borderline or other organic personality disorders result that comprise an array roughly paralleling functional personality syndromes (Childs 1985). It is important to interview family and friends to determine the premorbid personality of the patient in calculating effects of injury, which may be easier to change.

Psychotherapeutic interventions optimally begin soon after the patient is hospitalized, and management of the emotional climate is crucial to recovery. Childs (1985) has recommended placing a priority on the reestablishment of object constancy in cognitively impaired patients by staff members who are carefully selected for their lack of personal tension or anger and work one-on-one all day with each patient. This familiar and consistent other person enacts an early stage in cognitive retraining of a regressively lost relational skill. This is accomplished with a soothing voice and touch, with limitation of talk to familiar subjects and to the patient only, and the restriction of stimulation to a single channel. Later, active exercises include practice in following directions requiring progressively more sequential steps (Luria 1973), problem solving, and movement from the concrete to the abstract, retracing developmental steps and hoping for generalization of learning. Other measures the psychiatrist should consider are summarized in Table 27–4.

Language and Other Psychotherapeutic Correlates

Verbal impairment to some degree is found in all patients with closed head injuries who had been referred to a rehabilitation medicine center. Sarno (1980) found 32% of brain injury patients had classic aphasia, 38% had motor dysarthria, and 30%

Table 27–4.   Measures to assist recovery of patients with brain injury

---

1. Relate interventions to family grieving stage (denial, anger, grief resolution).
2. Structure daily events to assist patient's internalizing of routine and reestablishing circadian rhythms.
3. Establish positive rewards to reinforce responsible behavior; individualize rewards to what patient likes.
4. Approach disabilities with expectancy they will be overcome cheerfully, never as excuse for misbehavior.
5. Individualize treatment goals to patient's specific problems; for example, reward withdrawn frontal patients for conversation and aggressive patients for not reacting.
6. Break maladaptive habits by vigilance and restraint, because motivation to become involved in positive change follows elimination of irresponsible behavior.
7. Orient family extensively to structure needed before discharge to home so gains are maintained.

Note.   Adapted from Berry 1984.

had no discernible aphasic deficit in spontaneous speech but clear evidence of verbal deficit on testing. Dysarthric patients without exception showed subclinical linguistic effects. Because psychotherapy depends on the use of language with an emotional dimension, the psychiatrist should be alert to subtle evidence of dysarthria, identify any linguistic problems, and consciously adapt the psychotherapeutic technique to the deficit in the particular patient.

The task of psychotherapy with the patient with brain damage is to assess his or her capability for each step in the cognitive sequence of defense against threat, to help break down difficult steps into subroutines, and to assist in bridging gaps with the psychiatrist's own analytic functions. Hamburg (1985) outlined a sequence of cognitive defenses, which includes 11 elements: 1) regulate the timing and dosage of the threat; 2) deal with stresses one at a time; 3) seek information from multiple sources; 4) formulate expectations; 5) delineate manageable goals; 6) rehearse coping strategies and practice in safe situations; 7) test coping strategies in situations of moderate risk; 8) appraise feedback from those situations; 9) try more than one approach, keeping several options open; 10) commit to one approach; and 11) develop buffers against disappointment and develop contingency plans.

Consider how the person stressed with brain damage is deprived of these optimal mental and psychosocial mechanisms of mastery. The stress arises from within and cannot be eliminated by avoidance or flight. The organic disease cannot be viewed at a distance from the self because it is in the very organ's self-perception. On the other hand, the cognitively distorted perceptions of a paralyzed limb involve highly metaphorical removals from the self and illustrate the difficulty one has in grasping an illness of one's own brain. The virtual impossibility of clearly grasping the disease of the perceiving organ itself renders the regulation of the timing, dosage, and sequence of multiple threats as formidable problems for psychotherapy. Formulation of expectations and delineation of goals are frequently impossible when the requisite cognitive skills are absent. "Safe" and "moderate risk" situations are lacking for the patient haunted by a global sense of impairment that intrudes into every pleasurable aspect of life. Finally, the choice of multiple options, the use of feedback from situations, and the possibility of contingency plans are all techniques that may be quite unreachable for the patient with brain damage.

Sexual Disturbances After Brain Injury

Sexual disturbances may follow brain injury, especially damage to the limbic system. According to Weinstein (1974), "Changes in sexual behavior observed in brain-damaged patients are often abnormal by reason of the [inappropriate] circumstances in which they occur, rather than their intrinsic nature" (p. 16) or by their being different from the person's habitual conduct. It is often helpful to make it clear to the family that the patient with a brain injury has not become oversexed and that the patient is just enacting a normal sexuality in the wrong context because of a more general disorder of judgment.

Sexual behavior in individuals with brain damage is usually marked by a loss of specificity as to objects or forms of excitation, rather than a new focus. Although specific behavior such as fetishism has been linked to temporal lobe seizure activity (as well as hyper- and hyposexuality), intermediary personality factors and learning are more probably the cause than postulated so-called sexual centers, as has recently been suggested for heterosexual pursuit.

Verbal seductiveness frequently occurs in a situation of stress, such as when a patient is asked about his or her illness or is being tested, and thus may have a defensive, avoidant quality. Another stress-related phenomenon is ludic play, which appears as punning or joking about illness, caricaturing disabilities, or imitating or mimicking the examiner's behavior. Often patients classify their disabilities in sexual terms, or sex enters into the content of their confabulations and delusions in the acute state, which Weinstein (1974) declared are useful signs that sexual behavior will be acted out later in a real-life situation. Some patients seek relatedness through physical contact that may "put off" visitors or staff, all the more so when the dementia is secondary to a contagious disease.

A study of the psychosexual consequences of brain injury by Kreutzer and Zasler (1989) showed most patients reported a lessening of sexual drive, erectile function, and frequency of intercourse; reduced self-esteem and self-perceived sex appeal; and no relationship between the level of affect and sexual behavior. Despite the changes, the quality of the patients' marital relationships appeared preserved.

STROKE

According to a study of stroke survivors by Kotila et al. (1984), clear improvement could be expected from the acute stage to 3 months, continuing to a lesser degree to 12 months. At 12 months, 78% of these patients were living at home and 58% were independent in activities of daily living. Of those patients who were gainfully employed before having a stroke, 55% had returned to work after 12 months. The authors emphasized that emotional reactions as well as neurological deficits influence outcome and should be considered in assessing prognosis. A stroke is unwelcome at any age, but Goodstein (1983) noted that for the older patient, a stroke activates preexisting fears of losing control or sanity, dying, and becoming disfigured or impaired physically or sexually. The elderly are also more insecure about sudden recurrences, long stays away from home, and running out of retirement funds.

If the capability for empathic, loving relatedness is lost, the patient may not be able to invest an inner representation of the spouse with emotion. The tragic result late in the course of the disease may be a lack of appreciation of the spouse's loving care. A patient in an advanced stage of the disease may not even miss the caregiving spouse on his or her death if the patient's practical needs are satisfied. This can alienate or demoralize the most important caregiver. Often the psychiatrist must sensitively weigh the couple's unequal relationship, including the need of the spouse who is not the patient to recognize the discouraging lack of emotional mutuality.

Postdischarge Planning

A number of studies have underscored the importance of social support in the patient's adjustment to physical deficits from a stroke. Evans and Northwood (1983) related the wide variation in individual differences in adjustment to expressed interpersonal needs for social support. Labi et al. (1980) studied long-term stroke survivors and found a significant proportion manifested social disability, despite complete physical restoration. The parameters of social function in the study were socialization inside and outside the home, hobbies, and interests; much of the subjects' disability could not be accounted for by age, physical impairment, or specific neurological deficits. The distribution of documented functional disabilities suggested that, in addition to organic deficits, psychosocial factors were major determinants.

The psychiatrist should be aware, as Wilson and Smith (1983) determined, that poststroke patients will often attempt to drive. However, these patients may have special difficulty handling all aspects of driving. Many of these problems are predictable from the clinical examination, and the patient should be warned. In addition to these deficits, problems with diminished vision, personality change, the prominence of denial and projection as mental defenses, and alcoholism are likely to increase the risks of driving for these patients.

Defenses and Object Relations in Hemiplegia

Critchley's discussion (1979) of patients' reactions to hemiplegia contains observations of a variety of defensive maneuvers that epitomize the possibilities of "neurologizing" the dynamic defenses of psychiatry. In the loss of the sensation and control of parts of the body, the most remarkable changes occur in relatedness to those parts that Critchley calls "personification of the paralyzed limbs." This develops after an initial period of anosognosia and may be an overcompensation. The patient becomes a detached onlooker and the limb a foreign body outside the self. A patient may refer to the paralyzed limb as if it were an object such as a pet or a plaything, or a person of another gender. Splitting and lateralization into good and bad sides of the body, which ordinarily require a psychotic personality to be manifested in the absence of neurological disease, become accessible, readily used defenses against the changed representation of the impaired body part, in brain and mind. Beneath the level of denotative meaning and concrete representation that neurology comprehends, metaphors appear that speak to psychiatrists in fuller connotations about the state of the personality in relation to the diseased limb.

Approach to Patients Who Are Unstable on Their Feet

The fearful, usually elderly patient who feels unstable on his or her feet is a common neuropsychiatric problem. An educational therapeutic approach is often helpful and may serve as a model of that approach within the context of an ongoing therapeutic relationship. The patient is taught that there are at least six components of balance, any and all of which, once improved, will contribute to them all. This immediately begins to dispel the sense of helplessness and maps a multipronged offensive effort that the patient can marshal.

The neuromental dimension is often the most important. The patient may express the feeling of a lack of support in symbolic somatic language of unsteadiness and a fear of falling. Frequently the patient has become isolated through the deaths of relatives and friends, and therapy must deal with a resistance to affiliate that usually expresses the sentiment that the loved ones cannot be replaced. This sentiment must be given its due, as it is a form of loving memorial. But progress is rapid once the patient sees associating with others as compatible with loving memories. Even the acquisition of a pet that stays in the home can improve the sense of security. Physical immobility diminishes the patient's sense of participation in life. While not working on the gait in the ways described above, patients are encouraged to correspond with distant friends, authors whose books and articles they have enjoyed, and new contacts through clubs and interests that encourage correspondence.

SPINAL CORD INJURY

A quarter of a million Americans live permanently paralyzed from spinal cord injuries, with 10,000 new cases each year (most often young persons), with devastating career impact and emotional cost for the patients and their families (National Advisory Neurological Disorders and Stroke Council 1990). These patients, insofar as they are brain intact, may exhibit emotional reactions that are similar to those of mourning in the death of a loved one or other situations of severe loss (Bracken and Shepard 1980). Consequently, premorbid personality and the influence of significant others play a central role in coping with injury.

Manifest depression is not an inevitable psychological sequel to spinal cord injury. Howell et al. (1981) found diagnosable depression in only 5 of 22 patients with spinal cord injuries of less than 6 months' duration. Bodenhamer et al. (1983) found that patients with spinal cord injuries reported less depression and more anxiety and optimism than their caregivers predicted. Bodenhamer et al. (1983) also pointed out that traditional stage theories of what is said to be a mourning-like adjustment must be individualized.

The best predictor of future self-care by these patients was past self-care behavior, augmented by knowledge of personality tendencies. Green et al. (1984), studying persons who had had spinal cord injuries at least 4 years previously, administered the Tennessee Self-Concept Scale (Fitts 1965) and found, in comparison with scale norms, that the respondents had significantly *higher* personal self, moral-ethical self, and social self scores, although they had significantly lower physical self scores. The higher-than-normal self-concept scores were related to perceived independence, provision of one's own transportation, assistance needed, and living arrangements. These findings suggest the possibility of *enhanced* self-concepts through mastery of handicaps and that the psychiatrist often need not settle for limitations in the patient's mental health.

In a longitudinal study, Rosenstiel and Roth (1981) found that their best adjusted patients with spinal cord injuries predominantly employed the defenses of rationalization and denial, in keeping with the notion that the psychiatrist ought to respect the so-called more primitive defenses, if they work. Other traits that favored adjustment were avoidance of catastrophizing and of worrying what their life would be like, thinking about goals to be achieved after leaving the rehabilitation center, and employment of internal forms of mental rehearsal in anticipation of going home. DeJong et al. (1984) found that the best predictors of independent living outcome were marital status, education, transportation barriers, economic disincentives, and severity of disability. Table 27–5 summarizes management issues for patients who have spinal cord injuries.

Sexual Therapy for Patients With Spinal Cord Injury

Sexual therapy for the patient with a spinal cord injury, like sexual counseling for other patients, requires that the psychiatrist be comfortable and specially trained in such work. Schuler (1982) culled the techniques from five programs. The myth that patients with spinal cord injuries are asexual should be dispelled, and these patients should be helped to derive satisfaction from their sexual relations. The psychiatrist should emphasize resolving the high rate of marital discord. This includes not provoking guilt in the spouses with homilies about mutual responsibility, but instead giving close attention to the spouse's role in the vital area of sexuality. Ovulation still occurs in women, and testicular atrophy is avoided in many men who receive excellent care. Pregnancy is possible with artificial insemination. Attitudes toward sexuality may be changed with the exploration of neglected erogenous zones in each partner, and sexuality should be redefined as any activity that is mutually stimulating.

A person with spinal cord injuries can be taught to prepare a new partner by explaining the physical condition and improving communication. New techniques that use mechanical devices for stimulation and the expanded use of fantasy may be introduced. The psychiatrist should be sensitive to a patient's embarrassment and should be willing to spend sufficient time to discuss the topics. A psychosexual history may be used to obtain information that initially may be controversial (e.g., prosthetic devices, oral sex, and masturbation). Disabled male patients and their spouses must be helped to overcome any rigid sex-role stereotypes of male domination and female passivity.

The Family Model in Spinal Cord Injury

Whereas family attitudes about the injured person's entitlements are pervasive, all members of the family are affected differently according to their roles. Children must be specially prepared for their first confrontation with their parent's disability

---

Table 27–5. Managing patients with spinal injury

1. Recognize injured patients are not generally greater risk-takers.
2. Expect mourning reactions to loss of use of body.
3. Evaluate premorbid personality to understand coping techniques.
4. Consider anxiety and optimism as well as depression.
5. Individualize traditional stage theories of mourning.
6. Avoid giving priority to medication over psychotherapy.
7. Gauge self-care ability based on past self-care.
8. Expect enhanced self-concepts with experience of mastery.
9. Avoid learned helplessness with early rehabilitation.
10. Treat interfering affective reactions before discharge.
11. Respect "primitive" rationalization and denial if they work.
12. Help avoid catastrophizing and worrying.
13. Encourage mental rehearsal for goals after discharge.
14. Consider spouse and socioeconomic and educational level in plans.

(Romano 1976), especially in dealing with fantasies of divine punishment. Children and other family members who construe human relationships in overly corporeal terms may also fear that with paralysis, the disabled parent has lost all effectiveness as an authority to admire or control them. Questions about the meaning of suffering almost always arise in persons with strong religious beliefs; often persons whose religiousness is less than mature have fantasies that they or their entire families are being punished for their intrinsic badness. Steinglass et al. (1982) considered the suddenness of the impact of spinal cord injury on families and how an overemphasis on short-term stability of family life may lead patients to sacrifice family needs for growth and development. Family involvement with the rehabilitation process decreases feelings of anxiety, helplessness, and isolation.

EPILEPSY

Twenty million Americans will have at least one seizure during their lives, and 2 million will have spontaneously recurrent seizures. Although seizures can generally be controlled and patients remain relatively well-adjusted, in one study of patients with epilepsy, Roberts and Guberman (1989) found 33% had been treated for mental disorder.

In formulating psychotherapy, the neuropsychiatrist may consider the functional context (Sands 1982) in which epilepsy occurs. Differing age-related needs and tasks may be delayed or arrested at each stage of life by seizures, which usually have a regressive, exhibitionistic, and shame-producing impact. In the preschooler, it is important to consider the impact on the affective climate of the family and whether the family reaction manifests enlightenment or neurotic enmeshment. In the school-age child, the psychiatrist should consider the effects of peer acceptance or scapegoating on medication compliance; in the adolescent, issues related to epilepsy and driving, dating, sexuality, employability, and substance abuse should be explored. It is also important to determine if there is any linkage of seizure occurrence to menstruation and, if so, what the teenage girl's ideas about this relationship may be. The visibility of medication side effects may be mortifying for an adolescent. For a young adult, the psychiatrist should help the patient consider the degree of autonomy as opposed to inhibition of independence. Travel becomes relevant for such a patient, as well as issues regarding the pursuit of a career and the acceptance of seizures by employers, prospective mates, or the patient's own family. In the older adult, the psychiatrist needs to help the patient accept any necessary limitations on living alone or to face issues such as forced retirement or placement in a nursing home.

Management of Interictal Behavior and Personality Changes

From Blumer (1982), we may adapt hints for the management of the behavior and personality changes that he associated with the interictal states of temporal lobe epilepsy (complex partial seizure state) and that may occur in other seizure states:

1. Viscosity, or stickiness, to a subject in conversation (or to the interviewer) by a laborious, detailed, and emphatic conversation and delay at the door on the way out, may be worked with, if the psychiatrist is neither rejecting nor overly passive.

Self-critical patients with left temporal foci accept this better than patients with right temporal foci, who tend to deny.

2. Deepened emotionality is associated with conflict around a hyperreligious over-preoccupation with righteousness and a Dostoevskian concern with crime and punishment. In these patients, cheerful hypermoralism alternates with briefer episodes of explosive verbalized anger and threatened violence, followed by remorse or denial. A patient may benefit from the psychiatrist's explaining how others learn to avoid the patient because of this deepened emotionality. These patients may also be coached to drop the proselytizing mode and remove themselves physically from entanglements.

3. Hyposexuality is seldom complained of, but further isolates patients with temporal lobe epilepsy, especially males. Although the hyposexuality may be drug responsive, the psychiatrist should address the isolation and the needs of the spouse and encourage closeness.

4. Mood swings, especially those that build up over several days to a seizure, may be difficult for relatives, who try to avoid outbursts.

5. Schizophrenia-like psychosis may occur after many years in the presence of a personality more like that of the patient with temporal lobe epilepsy than that of the schizoid patient. The psychiatrist should adapt the treatment approach to specific features, as with patients who are schizophrenic. Psychosis may diminish when anticonvulsants are discontinued for a few days.

6. Memory disorders, related in severity to seizure severity and bitemporality, occur retrograde and anterograde during postictal confusion. Having the patient write memos at the first sign of an aura may help. Psychomotor automatisms also are a postictal phenomenon to be identified and explained.

ALZHEIMER'S DISEASE

The neuropsychiatrist should approach the impact of Alzheimer's disease on the patient and his or her family in a way that is comprehensive yet sensitive to the stage of the disease. The following suggestions are adapted and amplified from Aronson (1984), Jenicke (1985), and Rabins et al. (1982):

Because attention and memory are impaired in patients with Alzheimer's disease, a dyadic psychotherapeutic learning process is usually impossible. But in speaking with the patient and the family together, the psychiatrist should convey by affects directed toward the patient that the patient is valued by the psychiatrist. This provides for attitudinal modeling by the family and helps prevent retaliatory behavior by the patient against the family. Genuine feelings of appreciation of the Alzheimer's patient may be difficult for physicians and other professionals to have because we are selected and trained to overvalue intellect and memory in ourselves.

The single overriding principle for treatment of the family unit of the Alzheimer's patient is the maintenance of family homeostasis and equilibrium despite the great changes in roles that result. Both patient and family benefit most if the family life can preserve its function as a holding environment for all its members and a social entity in which the members can feel loved and loving.

Sleep is the first consideration in home care. The family cannot care for the patient and will resent the patient more if family members are suffering from sleep deficits caused by the patient's reversed sleep cycle. A strict diurnal schedule is prescribed as with any insomnia, with sufficient daily activity and exercise so that the characteristically physically vigorous patient does not have an unusual amount of leftover energy during the night.

Quality-of-life considerations for the family should be immediately addressed by the psychiatrist. Discussions should counter the family's irrational feelings of guilt, family shame, punitive self-denial, and taking responsibility for the disease, all of which may lead to resentment and the potential for abuse of the patient. The physician must *prescribe* family fun with and without the patient.

Financial planning based on clinical reality should be addressed as soon as possible after diagnosis. Early consultation with a social worker to access available care resources and legal advice about the shifting of financial responsibility can help avoid bankrupting the family. The psychiatrist neither shuns relevant financial concerns nor takes sides in financial disputes. Aspects of the patient's clinical condition may enter into court proceedings, and the psychiatrist should keep clinical notes grounded in specific observations, quotes, and evaluations.

Care of the patient, a new dependent, requires help from the whole family, but children and other immature members may find it especially taxing and may be less than helpful because of their own unanswered needs for support and inability to tolerate a situation that does not conform with ideal expectations. The psychiatrist should assist the family in avoiding situations stressful to the patient's diminished processing ability. Just as a person with cardiac failure should not be physically overtaxed, a person with brain failure should not be pressed to evaluate multiple inputs or negotiate complex interpersonal situations, compensate for changes in plans or schedules that were attuned to bodily cycles, or weather a physical illness without special help.

The family can prevent the patient from making errors and straying by eliminating dangerous choices. Weapons, dangerous tools, or substances that could erroneously be ingested by the patient must be locked away and outside door locks installed that cannot be opened at night. Keys to the car can be made unavailable, knobs can be removed from stoves, and matches hidden. The patient should not be left alone with minors who would be vulnerable to molestation. Secondary systems of memory enhancement may be employed, such as posted signs, arrows, daily schedules, and identifying labels on objects or clothes. Simple syntax should be used in all conversations so that the patient's memory and attention are not taxed.

Frank fear in the patient should be investigated as a possible index of victimization by the family. The psychiatrist should employ knowledge of the 15 predictable functional assessment stages in the progression both of normal aging and of Alzheimer's disease as described by Reisberg (1985) to weigh the presence of other, treatable factors. For example, incontinence should only occur late in Alzheimer's disease; if the patient experiences this sooner, there may be a treatable infection. Loss of the ability to dress properly never precedes loss of the ability to choose clothing properly, and could mean the patient is misbehaving. However, skills that the patient had yesterday may be gone today, and the family should be helped to accept the deterioration. As the sad saying goes, first it's forgetting names; then forgetting to zip up; then forgetting to zip down.

It is an emotional reality that families may premourn the loss of the personality of Alzheimer's patients before the death of these patients and may thereby devalue what is left of the person. Often the patient is protected by the disease from awareness of this emotional abandonment, but at times when sensibility lingers the caring doctor remains the last real representative of "other people." Table 27–6 summarizes management issues for Alzheimer's patients.

PARKINSON'S DISEASE

In describing the "shaking palsy" as a purely motor rather than mental degeneration, Parkinson (1817) referred to depression and terminal delirium. Reflecting the more recent recognition of concomitant mental involvement, Mayeux and Stern (1983) described some of the specific mental processes that are impaired. Building on such observations, the psychiatrist may make a more educated psychotherapeutic approach to the patient with this syndrome.

Table 27–6.   Management issues for patients with Alzheimer's disease

 1. Convey valuation of patient for attitudinal modeling.
 2. Maintain equilibrium of family when roles must shift.
 3. Prescribe sleep and exercise schedule so patient sleeps at night.
 4. Discuss family guilt and shame about affected member.
 5. Prescribe family fun with and without patient.
 6. Refer to social worker to access care resources.
 7. Suggest legal help with financial responsibility.
 8. Avoid taking sides in family financial disputes.
 9. Encourage log of incapacities in advanced patient.
10. Note effect of newly dependent patient on dependent family members.
11. Attend to age-specific needs of children, teenagers.
12. Encourage substitute role models for children.
13. Discuss wounded pride about loss of ideal family image.
14. Assist family in avoiding situations that tax brain failure.
15. Coach family in avoiding changes in plans and schedules.
16. Give added help at times of stress like physical illness.
17. Capitalize on poor memory to distract patient from stress.
18. Lock up weapons, poisons, money, and car keys.
19. Remove matches, lighters, and knobs from stove.
20. Do not leave patient alone with minors vulnerable to molesting.
21. Set timers for comforting radio and TV programs in patient's room.
22. Post signs, labels, and arrows as memory reinforcers.
23. Avoid household clutter and distracting background sounds.
24. Speak in short clauses and simple syntax to patient.
25. Investigate frank fear in patient for possible abuse.
26. Check emerging problems against known stages to see if avoidable.
27. Help patient find appropriate substitute activities with friends.
28. Attend closely to mental health needs of spouse.
29. Note overconcern about care, concealing feeling of family that patient would be "better off dead."
30. Recognize family may premourn physical death of patient.

Because the degree of intellectual impairment tends to increase as the severity of motoric symptoms increases (Mayeux and Stern 1983), the psychiatrist should also assume that the patient will have greater impairment in the ability to make therapeutic contact if motor ability is more impaired. Furthermore, the psychiatrist should not conclude that all psychopathology is reactive to impairment, or that the constriction of the patient's life is due solely to motoric limitations. Beatty et al. (1989) found the Mini-Mental State Exam (MMSE; Folstein et al. 1975) useful in assessing the cognitive impairments of Parkinson's disease, and they also found that tests of frontal lobe function such as the Wisconsin Card Sorting Test (Heaton 1985) did not indicate that the cognitive impairments these patients experienced arose principally from typical frontal lobe dysfunction. Instead, such tests suggested that cerebral dysfunction extended beyond subcortical-frontal circuits.

Mayeux and Stern (1983) found that bradykinesia and rigidity, but not tremor, gait disturbance, or posture, predicted overall intellectual performance for a patient taking the MMSE. The neuropsychiatrist should not hesitate to examine the patient neurologically to gauge potential areas of mental difficulty. Although this would appear to be a roundabout approach compared with doing a mental status, it is often less threatening and efficiently yields a preliminary clinical impression. The types of motor impairments tell us much about the patient's quality of thought, insight, and ability to relate to the therapist. Mayeux and Stern (1983) and Hallet (1979) have noted that the activities that are impaired require directed attention to the task, sequencing of cognitive processes, and often additional motor interaction. In more psychiatric terms, these activities involve an inherent motoric or spatial mental action.

Other disturbances characteristic of patients with Parkinson's disease are impaired perceptual motor or visuospatial functions, especially the inability to perform sequential or predictive voluntary movements (Stern et al. 1984). This results in impaired internal spatial representation (from which may arise the initiation of independent thought and mental action) and articulatory difficulty without impaired language reception or production. In fact, Parkinson's disease is distinct from other neuropsychiatric disorders because of the paucity of language impairment, a significant boon to the psychiatrist trying to do psychotherapeutic work.

Memory in these patients is often slowed without being impaired. Trouble with word finding, which worsens with increased motoric symptoms in some parkinsonian patients, was considered a form of the "tip of the tongue" phenomenon similar to anomia in aphasic patients with frontal lesions. Mayeux (1984) summarized a review of the literature on Parkinson's disease and Huntington's disease by stating that "nearly every patient with a movement disorder has some type of behavioral dysfunction, whether it is personality change or intellectual impairment" (p. 537). The close linkage of motor and mental action may be turned to advantage by using a number of behavioral techniques, as described below.

Patients should be encouraged to keep fit by regular moderate exercise, especially if their occupations are sedentary. Fitness does not stop the progression of Parkinson's disease but helps patients cope with symptoms. Free moving calisthenics and sports such as swimming are best, but safety, especially with patients who freeze motorically, must be considered.

It is important to employ sensory, rhythmic, and other cues and reminders to keep the bradykinetic patient moving. A patient can put taplike nails in the shoes to provide an auditory cue to keep the rhythm of walking constant and prevent festination. A small piece of raw carrot in the mouth may remind the patient to swallow and prevent drooling. Many techniques helpful to movement and mental state seem mechanical: wearing slippery rather than rubber soles to permit shuffling without falling, dispensing with canes and walkers when there is retropulsion, raising the back legs of chairs and toilet seats 2 inches to facilitate rising, and removing doorsills to prevent a patient from freezing in a doorway. An L-shaped extension at the tip of a cane can be stepped over so that the patient can keep moving. A simple device to quantify tremor (Forrest 1990) reassures patients of preserved control of intentional movements.

Parkinson's disease is a disorder of knife-edge tolerances and balances. The response to levodopa (L-dopa) is so dramatic that the patient and family are exquisitely conscious of the central role of drug effects. Patient and family, building on this medication response, may try to convey the idea that the psychiatrist is dealing with a cumbersome apparatus—a thing rather than a person. The psychiatrist should avoid becoming so totally immersed in the intricacies of compelling medicomotor phenomena such as on-off reactions and sudden transient freezing that the emotional issues are neglected.

A previous strategy of being reluctant to make the diagnosis or treat it in the earliest stages may be changing as deprenyl and antioxidant therapy may now be used to slow the course and keep the patient employed (National Advisory Neurological Disorders and Stroke Council 1990). The early parkinsonian patient should be watched closely for symptoms of depression. The psychiatrist should seriously consider the increased suicide risk, especially in males who overvalue physical mobility and power and are extremely anxious about their continued performance in competitive and exacting sports such as tennis and golf. Activities less aggravating for the mild parkinsonian patient may be chosen. More confusion than meets the eye (because of the preservation of language) contributes to the consternation that these patients feel over adaptation to the new challenge of disability. Further, the early pharmacotherapy of the disorder often employs anticholinergic agents with their additional potential for confusion.

Often, antiparkinsonian drugs lose their efficacy with time. This can result in severe disillusionment to parkinsonian patients and their families, or increasing the doses can aggravate side effects. Emotional sequelae of L-dopa treatment may include domineering behavior, increased libido, manic hyperactivity or depression, confused irrational behavior, and activation of latent psychosis or of vivid nightmares that may disturb sleep and visual hallucinations. Psychiatrists may be called on to help with these effects. Attention to the requirements for a patient's orientation (e.g., night-lights and familiar schedules), decreasing the stimulus level to diminish irritability, encouraging the beleaguered spouse to set limits, informing the spouse that the libidinal changes seldom persist, and most of all, assuring compliance with the times of dosing may all be helpful.

Starkstein et al. (1990) studied patients with Parkinson's disease and found that 40% had major or minor depression and that depression was associated with left-hemisphere involvement in patients with unilateral symptoms. Thus depression in the early stages of Parkinson's disease may be generally related to left-hemisphere dysfunction. Another peak of depression late in the course of the disease correlated with impairment of activities of daily living and of cognitive function.

The psychiatrist should explore the patient's image of the disease process. Parkinson's disease is common enough to be a vivid caricature on the minds of patients, who fear they will become an exaggeration of the motor tendencies of the aged that are assumed by stage actors and comics who portray shuffling old duffers. Fear of humiliation because of such an image may be allayed by emphasizing the medical manageability of the condition, its usual slow progression, and intense research efforts including transplantation that are based on knowledge of the pathophysiology of the disease. Later symptoms of emotional flattening, apathy, and impoverishment of the ability to relate to loved ones can be especially painful for the spouse.

Dopamine and Personality in Parkinson's Disease

Personality is not only a learned and habitual phenomenon simply to be unlearned in the psychotherapeutic analysis of character defenses. Evidence is growing that neurotransmitters have specific influences on personality. Dopamine has been associated with novelty seeking (analogous to exploratory behavior in animals), serotonin with harm avoidance, and norepinephrine with reward dependence. Menza et al. (1990), viewing Parkinson's disease with its low dopamine levels as a natural experiment, have shown by rating scales completed by patients and their families that there is significantly less novelty-seeking behavior in Parkinson's patients both currently and premorbidly as compared with control subjects from rheumatology and orthopedics, and no differences in the serotonin- and norepinephrine-mediated behaviors. The psychotherapeutic approach to the "reflective, rigid, stoic, slow-tempered, frugal, and orderly behaviors," as Menza et al. (1990, p. 286) characterized them, can include admiration of these traits as virtues. Table 27–7 summarizes management issues for patients with Parkinson's disease.

HUNTINGTON'S DISEASE

In a large kindred of Huntington's disease families from Venezuela, in whom the G8 DNA marker was localized to chromosome 4, all descendants were said to "inherit" the disease and only those who were affected by it were said to "have" it (Gusella et al. 1983). Wexler (1985) pointed out that although this distorts genetic truth, it expresses the experience of being at risk as a distinct state of mind. Because this state is stressful and conflict-ridden, the psychiatrist may be consulted on various issues.

Ambiguity about whether one will be affected, as with any later-onset autosomal dominant disease, may dominate the mental life of people at risk. Administration of the genetic test for persons at risk requires much sensitivity to the emotional dimensions of determining whether an individual possesses the gene, and the test should always be administered as part of a personal physician-patient relationship. Only a tiny percentage of those at risk have taken the test, for a variety of reasons including cost and fears of discrimination, especially by insurers (Mechcatie 1990).

The overlap of initial symptoms of Huntington's disease and everyday experience, such as incidences of clumsiness, irritability, nocturnal myoclonus, emotional instability, or infrequent lapses of memory or judgment, can lead to hypochondriacal worries. The psychiatrist may help the patient by taking over the responsibility of the symptom search, distinguishing between those symptoms that overlap with normality and the disease, or by teaching the patient to delegate this function to the neurologist.

Management of Affected Patients

Knowing one has Huntington's disease and knowing which parent is affected often leads to an unreasonable conscious or unconscious blaming of the gene-donating parent. This can disrupt vital processes of internalization of character from that present during development. Psychotherapy can help patients deal with their longings for a healthy parental model and control primitive, envious rage against unaffected siblings. Positive aspects of the affected parent as a model should be sought. Psychotherapy can help with fantasies that the disease is a punishment, that anyone is to blame, and that alternative behaviors could have prevented it, while recognizing such thoughts are defenses against helplessness and lack of control. There are also instances when knowledge of the risk of the disorder has been denied by persons at risk, and even their professional caregivers, with the result of needless transmission of the gene to another generation (Table 27–8).

The disease itself adds the further incapacitation of a movement disorder to a progressive unremitting dementia affecting higher intellectual skills and judgment. Frequently, speech is impaired. Patients with Huntington's disease remain oriented to their surroundings, are able to recognize family and caregivers, and are able to convey their likes and dislikes somewhat better than patients with Alzheimer's disease and other dementias. In keeping with this, they have more depression and less psychosis.

Table 27–7.   Management issues for patients with Parkinson's disease

1. Estimate problems of therapeutic contact by motor impairment.
2. Estimate cognitive impairment by bradykinesia and rigidity.
3. Employ neurological exam readily as less threatening than cognitive exam.
4. Capitalize on language preservation without underestimating impairment of spatial planning.
5. Coordinate psychotherapy with occupational and physical therapy sessions.
6. Encourage exercise and fitness to help cope with symptoms.
7. Employ sensory, mechanical, and cognitive aids to movement.
8. Anticipate symbiotic relationship with pharmacotherapy process.
9. Avoid neglecting emotional issues amidst dosing schedule.
10. Observe early in course for depression and suicide risk.
11. Choose activities and sports appropriate to abilities.
12. Distinguish early neuropsychiatric depression from later reaction to impairment.
13. Explore patient's embarrassment about image of appearance.
14. Emphasize manageability and slow progression of illness.
15. Anticipate disillusionment as drugs lose efficacy in time.
16. Anticipate side effects of levodopa treatment.
17. Aid orientation with night-lights and schedules.
18. Decrease stimulus level to decrease irritability.
19. Anticipate spouse's pain confronted by affective flattening.
20. Praise reflective, stoic, frugal, and orderly premorbid personality.

Table 27–8. Management issues for Huntington's disease: affected patients

1. Interpret blaming of gene-donating parent.
2. Help patient internalize healthy heritage from affected patient.
3. Ventilate wishes for healthy parental model.
4. Work with envy and rage against unaffected siblings.
5. Discuss fantasies that disease is a punishment.
6. Recognize ideas of blame and prevention are strategies for control.
7. Do not participate in denial of transmissibility.
8. Recognize movement disorder adds disability to dementia.
9. Note preservation of recognition may lead to depression.
10. See family has aid of physiatrists and nutritionists.
11. Improvise mechanical assistances to movement function.
12. Discuss family ambivalence about preserving life in downhill course.
13. Help family take pride in giving nutrition and learning Heimlich maneuver for choking.
14. Encourage caregivers to pace themselves and take recreation.

Choreic movements eventually may increase a patient's caloric needs to 6,000 calories/day while the coordination required to eat and swallow the food is impaired.

Family and staff ambivalence may arise around the sad irony of the daily struggle to keep the patient adequately nourished, in view of the disease's progressive downhill course and the likelihood that the patient will one day die of choking. But there is comfort for the family and staff in treating the patient properly, managing nutrition in an efficient way, and knowing the Heimlich maneuver. Care of patients with Huntington's disease is a great burden, and those who do it need to monitor and pace themselves to avoid undue discouragement while deriving the satisfaction of having been compassionate and useful.

MULTIPLE SCLEROSIS

Whitlock (1984) reviewed the variety of affective conditions in multiple sclerosis (MS) and concluded that it is difficult to separate the reactive from the organic (frontal and limbic) sources. The influential view of Cottrell and Wilson (1926) that 63% of the patients were unusually euphoric has been supplanted by numerous studies, beginning with that of Braceland and Giffin (1950), which showed more depression among these patients.

Minden and Schiffer (1990), in reviewing affect disorders in MS, stated that the euphoria is usually described as a mental serenity, a cheerful feeling of physical well-being found more frequently later in the course, an affect disassociated from the cognitive awareness of the disability. This is not a fluctuating, reversible affect but a persistent change of personality. Although a positive affect is unlikely to stir a clamor for psychotherapy, it is advisable to have a close look to address the patient's possible pain beneath the euphoria in view of the frequent depressive symptoms that do respond to psychotherapy. Minden and Schiffer (1990) have noted a higher rate of bipolar disorder in MS patients. Emotional instability of a labile nature responds so well to antidepressants that psychotherapy alone should not be considered.

Ron and Logsdail (1989) found no evidence that psychiatric symptoms in isolation were the first manifestation of MS, and that whereas elation correlated with widespread magnetic resonance imaging (MRI) abnormalities, flattening of affect, delusions, and thought disorder correlated with temporoparietal pathology on MRI. Grant et al. (1989) found that 77% of new MS patients, as compared to only 35% of control subjects, experienced marked life stress in the year before onset of symptoms, perhaps explaining the timing of symptom exacerbation for some patients by a psychosomatic process of further destabilizing an already unstable neuroimmunological system.

Psychiatrists should help the patient focus on the lack of certainty in prognosis in a positive sense, rather than on the myriad of possible symptoms. It is important to point out that the absence of sure knowledge reflects the general uncertainty of life, including variability of the disease over time. The psychiatrist should emphasize the presence of medical support and treatment rather than the lack of cure and be aware that the mysterious nature of the disease encourages magical theories of self-blame and of taking the illness as an ominous metaphor (Simons 1984).

The psychiatrist should not reinforce the sick role for these patients; rather, it is necessary to reiterate the concept that, although suffering from a disease, the MS patient is not ill in the traditional sense. Thus encouraging the realistic, but temporary and selective, omission of activities that are onerous for the patient becomes important. But family fun needs to be preserved as well. Psychiatrists should recognize differences in patients' expectations about self-reliance and involvement in their own care, versus passivity toward medical authority, in this illness, which has a great capacity to stimulate dependence upon doctors.

If direct questioning reveals that the MS patient has sexual difficulties, the psychiatrist should distinguish between degrees of organic and psychogenic sexual dysfunction in males by nocturnal penile tumescence monitoring. Many people have erectile difficulties and inorgasmia unrelated to MS. A spouse's resistance to the labeling of a partner as "disabled" may indicate a lesser likelihood of marital breakdown than immediate acceptance.

In assessing the potential of MS for creating disappointment with the self, the psychiatrist needs to recognize that MS is a disease of young adults that occurs in the prime of their lives, when they may have the highest performance expectations of themselves. Because extensive frontal lobe involvement of MS greatly impairs analytic ability, planning and organizing, flexibility, and emotional lability and limits the value of psychotherapy, it is important not to reach beyond reasonable therapeutic goals or to attempt sweeping revision of defenses when neuropsychiatric assessment suggests such involvement of the frontal lobe. Psychiatrists should help these patients to manage fatigue and other limitations by assisting them in selecting and planning participation in activities, rather than seeing the patients withdraw or regress as a result of frustration at attempting too much. It is imperative to focus on what the patient is able to do, not what he or she is unable to do. This means that the psychiatrist should advise the patient to avoid undue stress, which temporarily worsens symptoms, and reassure the patient that these flare-ups do not permanently advance the disease. Table 27–9 summarizes management issues for MS patients.

BRAIN TUMOR

The brain tumors most likely to produce behavioral difficulties in patients for which a psychiatrist might be consulted are those of the temporal lobe, and the tumors do so by becoming an irritative focus for temporal lobe epilepsy. Blumer and Benson (1975) noted the difficulties for psychotherapy that are caused by the viscous type of verbal expression in patients with temporal lobe epilepsy, including a deepening of emotional response that is not reversed by anticonvulsant therapy, as are the changes in sexuality and episodic aggressivity. These authors argue in favor of nondrug psychiatric management of temporal lobe emotional features.

Blumer and Benson (1975) stated that the "pseudodepressed" change in personality caused by lesions of the convexity of the frontal lobes warrants early and ongoing rehabilitative efforts and mobilization; that is, patients should not be allowed to sit around. Patients with the "pseudopsychopathic" alteration of personality, more attributed to lesions of the orbital surface, have misbehavior that tries the patience of family members, who may benefit by psychiatric support. In patients with recurrent or intractable central nervous system (CNS) tumors, more diffuse signs of increased intracranial pressure sometimes supplant the specific personality changes already mentioned.

Jaffe (personal communication, August 1990) found that psychiatric consultation in several hundred neurosurgical brain tumor and arteriovenous malformation cases led to an appreciation of how much warm understanding and explanation by a consis-

---

Table 27–9.   Management issues for patients with multiple sclerosis

---

1. Expect more depression than euphoria, especially early.
2. Look past euphoria for coexistent depressive symptoms.
3. Consider possible bipolar disease or steroid effects during psychotherapy.
4. Avoid relying on psychotherapy alone for emotional instability.
5. Avoid unnecessarily medicating euphoria.
6. Note likely presence of life stress before episode.
7. Suggest psychotherapy, especially after diagnosis.
8. Disclose diagnosis to significant others, not to all.
9. Assist those who are dating with disclosure after rapport with partner.
10. Help patient see uncertainty of prognosis in a positive sense of possibility.
11. Plan for the possibility of disability, as in choosing a new home, but hope for the best.
12. Anticipate magical theories of self-blame in view of mysterious nature of the disease's etiology and fluctuations.
13. Avoid reinforcing sick or disabled role.
14. Select activities to substitute for those posing difficulties.
15. Accept differences in patients' relying on self versus doctors.
16. Inquire directly about sexual difficulties.
17. Approach sexual area cautiously and involve spouse eventually.
18. Consider urological treatment options for male patients.
19. Adapt therapeutic goals and discourse in impaired planning ability.
20. Help to manage fatigue by selection and planning.
21. Focus on capacities, not disabilities.
22. Advise avoidance of stresses that worsen symptoms.
23. Reassure that flare-ups do not permanently advance the disease.
24. Keep newly diagnosed patients from support groups for wheelchair bound, blind, or incontinent cases.

Source.   Items 7–9 and 11 were adapted from Scheinberg 1983.

tent figure can minimize the distress before and after surgery. Certain communications are frequently useful. For example, the CNS anatomic basis of puzzling peripheral symptoms can be explained, because patients are not so familiar with brain symptoms as they are with cardiac symptoms. In cases that face a terminal course, reassurance may be given to these patients about competency, with assistance in arranging for their wishes to be respected. The patient who has fears of a painful and frightening death can be told death will likely come after lapsing into a coma and (with the exception of certain headache patients) will bring little or controllable pain. Table 27–10 summarizes management issues for patients with brain tumors.

CONCLUSIONS

Neuropsychiatry has been thought to involve poor prognoses; but when the statistics are in the patient's favor, they may aid the psychiatrist's supportive role. For example, in Thorngren et al.'s study (1990) of stroke patients discharged from the hospital to independent living, 1 year later 90% were still in their own homes, 99% could walk independently, 92%–95% could climb a staircase, and 90% could manage their daily hygiene. Six percent had died, and 25% had had a rehospitalization.

When the statistics are not so favorable, the psychiatrist's objective and relativistic viewpoint may be tested. Frequently, psychiatrists and other physicians have such high demands for their own performance that they must guard against identifying too easily with suicidal impulses in patients who might later be grateful for aggressive intervention against depression and suicide. Lessons that can be learned from this include the need for a relativistic viewpoint that can adopt the patients' differing standards for acceptable living. It is also imperative to recognize that emotional exhaustion and burnout may sometimes affect young professionals with high standards more than most people, who have more relaxed standards of performance and may be better able to contemplate enduring life with prolonged morbidity and a chronic downhill course. In general, patients with neurological deficits affecting their performance may be better able to accept them than some of their physicians, and it is up to us to help them make the most of living.

Table 27–10.   Management issues for patients with brain tumors

1. Correlate observations of specific impairments with tumor location, as in the case of temporal lobe involvement.
2. Expect diffuse difficulties and trouble with novel situations.
3. Mobilize patients with frontal "pseudodepressed" changes.
4. Watch for communication of fears, sometimes nonverbally.
5. Provide warmth, understanding, and explanation as a consistent figure before and after surgery.
6. Explain puzzling anatomic symptoms, such as contralateral effects.
7. Discuss permissibility of exertion and sex in arteriovenous malformations.
8. Distinguish between growth and malignancy of tumor.
9. Explain that malignancy may differ in degree and is not black and white.
10. Invite reporting of psychotic symptoms on high-dose steroids.
11. Reassure about competency and arrange for wishes to be respected in terminal patients.
12. Reassure that death will come after a coma and there will be little or controllable pain.

REFERENCES

Aronson MK: Alzheimer's and other dementias (Carrier Letter #102). Belle Meade, NJ, Carrier Foundation, November 1984

Beatty WW, Staton RD, Weir WS, et al: Cognitive disturbances in Parkinson's disease. J Geriatr Psychiatry Neurol 2:22–33, 1989

Benson DF: Disorders of verbal expression, in Psychiatric Aspects of Neurological Disease. Edited by Benson DF, Blumer D. New York, Grune & Stratton, 1975, pp 121–135

Berry V: Partners/Families and Professionals Together: A Model of Posttraumatic Rehabilitation. Austin, TX, Ranch Treatment Center, 1984

Blumer D: Specific psychiatric complications in certain forms of epilepsy and their treatment, in Epilepsy: A Handbook for the Mental Health Professional. Edited by Sands H. New York, Brunner/Mazel, 1982, pp 97–111

Blumer D, Benson DF: Personality changes with frontal and temporal lobe lesions, in Psychiatric Aspects of Neurologic Disease, Vol 1. Edited by Benson DF, Blumer D. New York, Grune & Stratton, 1975, pp 151–170

Bodenhamer E, Achterberg-Lawlis J, Kevorkian G, et al: Staff and patient perceptions of the psychosocial concerns of spinal cord injured persons. Am J Phys Med 62(4):182–193, 1983

Braceland FJ, Giffin ME: The mental changes associated with MS (an interim report; ARNMD 28:450–455). Baltimore, MD, Williams & Wilkins, 1950

Bracken MB, Shepard MJ: Coping and adaptation following acute spinal cord injury: a theoretical analysis. Paraplegia 18(2):74–85, 1980

Childs AH: Brain injury: "now what shall we do?": problems in treating brain injuries. Psychiatric Times, April 1985, pp 15–17

Cottrell SS, Wilson SAK: The affective symptomatology of disseminated sclerosis. Journal of Neurology and Psychopathology 7:1, 1926

Critchley M: The Divine Banquet of the Brain and Other Essays. New York, Raven, 1979

DeJong G, Branch LG, Corcoran PJ: Independent living outcomes in spinal cord injury: multivariate analyses. Arch Phys Med Rehabil 65(2):66–73, 1984

Evans RL, Northwood LK: Social support needs in adjustment to stroke. Arch Phys Med Rehabil 64(2):61–64, 1983

Fitts WH: Manual for Tennessee Self-Concept Scale. Nashville, TN, Counselor Recordings and Tests, 1965

Folstein MF, Folstein SE, McHugh PR: "Mini-Mental State": a practical method of grading the cognitive state of patients for the clinician. J Psychiatr Res 12:189–198, 1975

Forrest DV: Selected American Expressions for the Foreign-Born Psychiatrist and Other Professionals. New York, Educational Research, 1982

Forrest DV: Therapeutic adaptations to the cognitive features of schizophrenia, and Therapeutic adaptations to the affective features of schizophrenia, in Treating Schizophrenic Patients. Edited by Stone MH, Albert HD, Forrest DV, et al. New York, McGraw-Hill, 1983

Forrest DV: The tremometer: a convenient device to measure postural tremor from lithium and other causes. Journal of Neuropsychiatry and Clinical Neurosciences 2:391–394, 1990

Goodstein RK: Overview: cerebrovascular accident and the hospitalized elderly: a multidimensional clinical problem. Am J Psychiatry 140:141–147, 1983

Grant I, Brown GW, Harris T, et al: Severely threatening events and marked life difficulties preceding onset or exacerbation of multiple sclerosis. J Neurol Neurosurg Psychiatry 52:8–13, 1989

Green BC, Pratt CC, Grigsby TE: Self-concept among persons with long-term spinal cord injury. Arch Phys Med Rehabil 65(12):751–754, 1984

Gusella JF, Wexler NS, Coneally PM, et al: A polymorphic DNA marker genetically linked to Huntington's disease. Nature 306:234–238, 1983

Hallet M: Physiology and pathophysiology of voluntary movement. Current Neurology 2:351–376, 1979

Hamburg D: Brain, behavior and health (VanGieson Award Address). Presented at the New York State Psychiatric Institute, New York, November 1985

Heaton R: Wisconsin Card Sorting Test. Odessa, TX, Psychological Assessment Resources, 1985

Howell T, Fullerton DT, Harvey RF, et al: Depression in spinal cord injured patients. Paraplegia 19(5):284–288, 1981

Jenicke MA: Alzheimer's Disease: Diagnosis, Treatment and Management. Philadelphia, PA, Clinical Perspectives on Aging, Wyeth Labs Div American Home Products Corp, 1985

Kotila M, Waltimo O, Niemi ML, et al: The profile of recovery from stroke and factors influencing outcome. Stroke 15:1039–1044, 1984

Kreutzer JS, Zasler ND: Psychosexual consequences of traumatic brain injury: methodology and preliminary findings. Brain Inj 3:177–186, 1989

Labi MJ, Phillips TF, Greshman GE: Psychosocial disability in physically restored long-term stroke survivors. Arch Phys Med Rehabil 61:561–565, 1980

Luria AR: The Working Brain: An Introduction to Neuropsychology. New York, Basic Books, 1973

Mayeux R: Behavior manifestations of movement disorders: Parkinson's and Huntington's disease. Neurol Clin 2:527–540, 1984

Mayeux R, Stern Y: Intellectual dysfunction and dementia in Parkinson disease, in The Dementias. Edited by Mayeux R, Rosen WG. New York, Raven, 1983

Mechcatie E: Guidelines for Huntington's genetic testing, follow up. Clinical Psychiatry News 18(2):2, 22, 1990

Menza MA, Forman NE, Goldstein HS, et al: Parkinson's disease, personality and dopamine. Journal of Neuropsychiatry 2:282–287, 1990

Minden SL, Schiffer RB: Affective disorders in multiple sclerosis: review and recommendations for clinical research. Arch Neurol 47:98–104, 1990

National Advisory Neurological Disorders and Stroke Council: Implementation Plan: Decade of the Brain. Washington, DC, National Institute of Neurological Disorders and Stroke, 1990

Oddy M, Humphrey M, Uttley D: Subjective impairment and social recovery after closed head injury. J Neurol Neurosurg Psychiatry 41:611–616, 1978

Parkinson J: An Essay on the Shaking Palsy. London, Sherwood, Neely and Jones, 1817

Rabins PV, Mace NL, Lucas MJ: The impact of dementia on the family. JAMA 248:333–335, 1982

Reisberg B: Alzheimer's disease update. Psychiatric Annals 15:319–322, 1985

Roberts JK, Guberman A: Religion and epilepsy. Psychiatr J Univ Ottawa 14:282–286, 1989

Romano MD: Preparing children for parental disability. Soc Work Health Care 1:309–315, 1976

Ron MA, Logsdail SJ: Psychiatric morbidity in multiple sclerosis: a clinical and MRI study. Psychol Med 19:887–895, 1989

Rosenstiel AK, Roth S: Relationship between cognitive activity and adjustment in four spinal cord-injured individuals: a longitudinal investigation. Journal of Human Stress 7:35–43, 1981

Sands H: Psychodynamic management of epilepsy, in Epilepsy: A Handbook for the Mental Health Professional. Edited by Sands H. New York, Brunner/Mazel, 1982, pp 135–157

Sarno MT: The nature of verbal impairment after closed head injury. J Nerv Ment Dis 168:685–692, 1980

Scheinberg LC: Multiple Sclerosis: A Guide for Patients and Their Families. New York, Raven, 1983

Schiffer RB: Psychiatric aspects of clinical neurology. Am J Psychiatry 140:205–211, 1983

Schuler M: Sexual counseling for the spinal cord injured: a review of 5 programs. J Sex Marital Ther 8:241–252, 1982

Simons AF: Problems of providing support for people with MS and their families, in Multiple Sclerosis: Psychological and Social Aspects. Edited by Simons AF. London, Heinemann Medical Books, 1984, pp 1–20

Starkstein SE, Preziosi TJ, Bolduc PL, et al: Depression in Parkinson's disease. J Nerv Ment Dis 178:27–31, 1990

Steinglass P, Temple S, Lisman SA, et al: Coping with spinal cord injury: the family perspective. Gen Hosp Psychiatry 4:259–264, 1982

Stern Y, Mayeux R, Rosen J: Contribution of perceptual motor dysfunction to construction and tracing disturbances in Parkinson's disease. J Neurol Neurosurg Psychiatry 47:987–989, 1984

Thorngren M, Westling B, Norrving B: Outcome after stroke in patients discharged to independent living. Stroke 21:236–240, 1990

Weinstein EA: Sexual disturbances after brain injury. Medical Aspects of Human Sexuality 8(10):10–31, 1974

Wexler NS: Genetic jeopardy and the new clairvoyance, in Progress in Medical Genetics, Vol 6. New York, Praeger, 1985

Whitlock A: Emotional disorder in multiple sclerosis, in Multiple Sclerosis: Psychological and Social Aspects. Edited by Simons AF. London, Heinemann Medical Books, 1984, pp 72–81

Wilson T, Smith T: Driving after stroke. International Rehabilitation Medicine 5(4):170–177, 1983

Woods BT, Short MP: Neurological dimensions of psychiatry. Biol Psychiatry 20:192–198, 1985

Chapter 28

Cognitive Rehabilitation and Behavior Therapy of Neuropsychiatric Disorders

Mark R. Lovell, Ph.D.
Christopher Starratt, Ph.D.

As psychiatry's role in the assessment and treatment of individuals with neurological impairment has expanded dramatically over the last decade, so has the need for a broad-based understanding of methods of promoting recovery from brain injury and disease. The role of the psychiatrist in the diagnosis and treatment of the sequelae of central nervous system (CNS) dysfunction has become a crucial one and promises to become even more central with the continued development of sophisticated neuropharmacological treatments for both cognitive and psychosocial components of brain impairment (Gualtieri 1988). In addition to these exciting new developments, an understanding of non-pharmacological, behavioral methods of assessment and treatment can greatly enhance the patient's recovery from cognitive deficits as well as provide a useful adjunct treatment for behavioral deficits and excesses that are commonly associated with CNS dysfunction.

COGNITIVE REHABILITATION OF NEUROPSYCHIATRIC DISORDERS

The terms *cognitive rehabilitation* and *cognitive retraining* have been variously used to describe treatments designed to maximize recovery of the individual's abilities in the areas of intellectual functioning, visual processing, language, and, particularly, memory.

Techniques to improve cognitive functioning after a neurological event represent an extremely heterogeneous group of procedures that vary widely in their focus depending on the nature of the patient's cognitive difficulties, the specific skills and training of the staff members, and the medium through which the information is presented (i.e., computer versus individual therapy versus group therapy). Because patients with different neurological or neuropsychiatric syndromes often have different cognitive deficits, the focus of the treatment is likely to vary a great deal.

Despite the recent surge in interest in psychiatric problems in patients with neurological impairment, there has been little systematic research concerning the effectiveness of cognitive and behavioral treatment strategies in this group. Most of our information comes from experience with patients in pure rehabilitation settings. The following is a brief review of cognitive rehabilitation strategies to treat specific cognitive deficits that may be associated with neuropsychiatric disorders.

Attentional Processes

Disorders of attention are common sequelae of a number of neurological disorders and are particularly common after traumatic brain injury. Recognition and treatment of attentional disorders are extremely important because an inability to focus and sustain attention may directly limit the patient's ability to actively participate in the rehabilitation program and may, therefore, affect progress in other areas of cognitive functioning.

Rehabilitation programs designed to improve attentional processes usually attempt to address all of these processes. One such program is the Orientation Remedial (OR) module (Ben-Yishay and Diller 1981). The OR program consists of five separate tasks that are presented by microcomputer and vary in degree of difficulty. These tasks involve 1) training the patient to attend and react to environmental "signals," 2) training the patient to time his or her responses in relation to changing environmental cues, 3) training the patient to be actively vigilant, 4) training in time estimation, and 5) training the patient to synchronize responding with complex rhythms.

Memory

Within the field of cognitive rehabilitation, much emphasis has been placed on the development of treatment approaches to improve memory. Rehabilitation strategies for improving memory can be divided into three primary categories depending on whether the technique involves 1) the use of mnemonic strategies, 2) the use of repetitive practice and drills, or 3) approaches that rely on external devices or procedures to improve memory.

Mnemonic strategies.   Mnemonic strategies are specifically designed to promote the encoding and remembering of a specific type of information depending on the patient's particular memory impairment. A number of different types of mnemonic strategies may be of use in neuropsychiatric settings. *Visual imagery,* one of the most commonly used strategies (Glisky and Schacter 1986), involves the use of visual images to assist in the learning and retention of verbal information.

A related method of learning and remembering new information is *peg mnemonics,* which requires the patient to learn a list of peg words and to associate these words with a given visual image. Sequential information can then be remembered in order by association with the visual image (Gouvier et al. 1986). However, this approach may not be highly effective because of an inability of patients with brain injury to generate visual images (Crovitz et al. 1979) and because of difficulty maintaining this information over time.

Another widely used visual imagery procedure is *face-name association.* This procedure has been used with brain injury patients to promote the remembering of peoples' names based on visual cues and involves association of components of the name with a distinctive visual image. For example, the name *Angela Harper* might be encoded by the patient visualizing an angel playing a harp. Overall, visual imagery strategies may be useful for specific patients (i.e., patients with impairment in verbal memory who need nonverbal cues to assist in recall) and in patients whose impairments are mild enough to allow them to recall the series of steps necessary to spontaneously use these strategies once they return to their natural environments.

Verbally based mnemonic strategies has also become quite popular, particularly with patients who have difficulty employing visual imagery. One such procedure, *semantic elaboration,* involves constructing a story out of new to-be-remembered information. This type of procedure may be particularly useful in cases where the patient may be unable to use imagery strategies because of a reduced ability to generate internal visual images.

Rhyming strategies involve remembering verbal information by incorporating the information into a rhyme. This procedure was originally demonstrated by Gardner (1977) with a globally amnestic patient. For patients who have difficulty learning and remembering written information, Glasgow et al. (1977) used a structured procedure for approaching the information called *PQRST*. This strategy involves application of five steps: 1) *P*review the information, 2) form *Q*uestions about the information, 3) *R*ead the information, 4) *S*tate the questions, and 5) *T*est for retention by answering the questions after the material has been read.

Repetitive practice.   Repetitive practice strategies rely heavily on the use of drills and appear to be based on a "mental muscle" conceptualization of memory (Harris and Sunderlund 1981), which infers that memory can be improved merely by repeated exposure to the information that is to be learned. Although it is generally accepted that patients with brain injury can learn specific pieces of information through repeated exposure, studies designed to demonstrate generalization of this training to new settings or tasks has not been encouraging. Glitsky and Schacter (1986) suggested that attempts to remedy memory disorders focus on the acquisition of "domain-specific knowledge" that is likely to be specifically relevant to the patient's ability to function in everyday life.

External memory aids.   External aids to memory generally fall into two categories: memory-storage devices and memory-cuing strategies (Harris 1984). Probably the most basic memory-storage devices take the form of written lists and memory books. Lists and memory books are widely used with brain injury patients and often include the patient recording information vital to his or her daily function and then consulting this information at a given time. These strategies are not designed to provide a general improvement in the patient's ability to learn and retain new information.

With recent advances in the field of microelectronics, hand-held electronic storage devices have become increasingly popular. However, their oftentimes complicated operations requirements may obviate their use in all but the mildest cases of brain injury or disease. Since the device must be consulted at the appropriate time to be useful, cuing strategies which involve prompts designed to remind the patient to engage in a specific behavioral sequence at a given time. One particularly useful cuing device that is currently in use is the alarm wristwatch. This device can be set to sound an alarm at a given time.

Visual-Perceptual Disorders

Deficits in visual perception most commonly occur in patients who have suffered right-hemisphere cerebral vascular accidents (Gouvier et al. 1986). Given the importance of visual perceptual processing to many occupational tasks and to the safe operation of an automobile (Sivak et al. 1985), the rehabilitation of deficits in this area could have important implications for the recovery of the neuropsychiatric patient.

One deficit that is particularly common in stroke patients is the hemispatial neglect syndrome, characterized by an inability to recognize stimuli in the contralateral visual field. One strategy that has been used extensively to treat hemispatial neglect is visual scanning training (Diller and Weinberg 1977; Gianutsos et al. 1983). This approach uses a light board with 20 colored lights and a target that can be moved around the board at different speeds. The patient can be systematically trained to attend to the neglected visual field.

Intellectual and Executive Functions

Patients who have sustained a brain injury often suffer a breakdown in their ability to reason, form concepts, solve problems, execute and terminate behavioral sequences, and engage in other complex cognitive activities (Goldstein and Levin 1987). Deficits in these areas are among the most debilitating to the neuropsychiatric patient because they often underlie changes in the patient's basic abilities to function interpersonally, socially, and vocationally.

Intellectual and executive functioning cannot be conceptualized as unitary constructs, but rather involve a number of processes that include motivation, abstract thinking, and concept formation, as well as the ability to plan, reason, and execute and terminate behaviors. Therefore, breakdowns in intellectual and executive functioning can occur for a number of different reasons depending on the underlying core deficit(s) and can vary based on the area of the brain that is injured.

An apparent breakdown in the patient's ability to function intellectually can also occur secondary to deficits in other related areas of neuropsychological functioning such as attention, memory, and language. The type of rehabilitation strategy chosen depends on the underlying core deficit that needs to be addressed. For example, rehabilitation efforts with a frontal lobe patient might emphasize impulse control and execution of the appropriate behavioral sequence to solve the problem.

Because of the multitude of factors that can result in intellectual and executive functioning difficulties in patients with brain injury, programs designed to rehabilitate these deficits have necessarily involved attempts to address them in a hierarchical manner, as originally proposed by Luria (1963). One such program (Ben-Yishay and Diller 1983) defines five basic deficit areas (arousal and attention, memory, impairment in underlying skill structure, language and thought, and feeling tone) and two domains of higher-level problem solving. This model proposes that deficits in the higher-level skills are often produced by core deficits and that the patient's behavior is likely to depend on an interaction between the two domains (Goldstein and Levin 1987).

Speech and Language

Disorders of speech and language are common sequelae of neurological damage, particularly when the dominant (usually left) hemisphere is injured. As the ability to communicate is often central to the patient's personal, social, and vocational readjustment after brain injury or disease, rehabilitation efforts in this area are extremely important. In most rehabilitation settings, speech and language therapies have traditionally been the province of speech pathologists. Therapy has often involved a wide variety of treatments depending on the training, interest, and theoretical orientation of the therapist.

USE OF COMPUTERS IN COGNITIVE REHABILITATION

The use of the microcomputer in cognitive rehabilitation has increased dramatically over the last decade, just as its use has increased in many other facets of everyday life. The microcomputer has a great deal of potential for use in rehabilitation settings and may offer several advantages over more conventional, therapist-based treatments (Grimm and Bleiberg 1986). Microcomputers may have the advantage of being potentially self-instructional and self-paced, of requiring less direct staff time, and of accurately providing direct feedback to the patient regarding his or her performance. Microcomputers also facilitate research by accurately and consistently recording the large amounts of potentially useful data that are generated during the rehabilitation process.

Several cautions must be mentioned concerning the use of microcomputers in the rehabilitation process. First, the microcomputer is merely a tool (albeit a highly sophisticated one) whose usefulness is limited by the availability of software that meets the needs of the individual patient and the skill of the therapist in implementing the program or programs. Second, microcomputers are not capable of simulating human social interaction and should not be used in lieu of human therapeutic contact.

BEHAVIORAL DYSFUNCTION AFTER BRAIN INJURY

Our understanding of the full range of behavioral dysfunction in individuals with brain injury or disease remains far from complete. To date, relatively few follow-up studies have systematically investigated the efficacy of neuropsychiatric treatment programs. In addition, much of what we know comes from studies conducted in rehabilitation settings rather than in hospitals specifically designed to treat patients with neuropsychiatric disorders. Despite the relatively sparse literature on treatment outcome in this area, the studies that have been reported have been useful in guiding the development of practical strategies for dealing with the behavioral-psychiatric consequences of brain injury. In particular, behaviorally based treatments have been heavily used.

Behavioral dysfunction after brain injury can have a marked impact on the recovery process itself, as well as on the more general aspects of psychosocial adjustment. It is indeed a tragedy that the patients most needing cognitive rehabilitation services are often kept out of many treatment facilities because of their disruptive behavior. In fact, research studies (Levin et al. 1982; Weddell et al. 1980) have shown that behavioral dysfunction is often associated with reduced ability to comply with rehabilitation programs, return to work, engage in recreational and leisure activities, and sustain positive interpersonal relationships.

Behavioral dysfunction is not limited to individuals with traumatic brain injury. Patients with lesions in specific brain regions secondary to various pathological conditions can exhibit characteristic patterns of dysfunctional behavior as well. For example, frontal lobe dysfunction secondary to stroke, tumor, or other disease processes is often associated with a cluster of symptoms including social disinhibition, reduced attention and distractibility, impaired judgment, affective lability, and more pervasive mood disorder (Bond 1984; Stuss and Benson 1984). In contrast, Prigatano (1987) noted that individuals who have temporal lobe dysfunction can display heightened interpersonal sensitivity, which can evolve into frank paranoid ideation.

Adjustment (and failure to adjust) after brain injury appears to be related to a multitude of neurological and nonneurological factors, each requiring consideration when deciding on an appropriate course of intervention for any observed behavioral dysfunction. Other factors that can contribute to the presence and type of behavioral dysfunction include time since injury, premorbid psychiatric and psychosocial adjustment, financial resources, social supports, and personal awareness of (and reaction to) acquired deficits (Eames 1988; Meier et al. 1987).

Given the large number of factors that are known to influence recovery from brain injury, a multidimensional approach to the behavioral treatment of patients with brain injury is likely to result in an optimal recovery. This approach should take into consideration the patient's premorbid level of functioning (both in terms of psychological adjustment and neuropsychological functioning), as well as his or her current psychological and neuropsychological resources.

BEHAVIORAL THERAPY WITH BRAIN-IMPAIRED PATIENTS

The domain of behavioral therapies has undergone considerable expansion over the past 20 years. Current behavioral assessment and treatment methods extended far beyond the early roots of classical and operant conditioning and have been adapted for use with numerous special populations, most recently including persons with brain injury (Haynes 1984; Hersen and Bellack 1985).

Despite a broadening scope that has included the treatment of neurologically impaired patients, behavioral approaches remain committed to the original principles derived from experimental and social psychology. They also emphasize the empirical and objective implementation and evaluation of treatment (Bellack and Hersen 1985).

The general assumptions that form the basis of behavioral approaches include the following (Haynes 1984):

1. Disordered behavior can be expressed through overt actions, thoughts, verbalizations, and physiological reactions.
2. These reactions are not necessarily going to vary in the same way for different individuals or for different behavioral disorders.
3. Changing one specific behavior may result in changes in other, related behaviors.
4. Environmental conditions play an important role in the initiation, maintenance, and alteration of behavior.

These assumptions lead to approaches that emphasize the objective evaluation of "observable" aspects of the individual and his or her interaction with the environment. The range of observable events is bounded only by the clinician's ability to establish a reliable, valid quantification of the target behavior or environmental condition.

Intervention focuses on the active interaction between the individual and environment. The goal of treatment is to alter those aspects of the environment that have become associated with the initiation or maintenance of maladaptive behaviors or to alter the patient's response to those aspects of the environment in some way.

The application of a behavioral intervention with a neuropsychiatric patient requires careful consideration of both the neuropsychological and environmental aspects of the presenting problem. At present, the accumulated body of evidence remains limited regarding the specific types of behavioral interventions that are most effective in treating the various dysfunctional behaviors observed in individuals with different kinds of brain injuries. Despite this, there is optimism, based on the current literature, that behavior therapy can be effectively used with brain injury patients (Horton and Miller 1985).

As outlined below, behavioral approaches can be broadly classified into at least three general models (Calhoun and Turner 1981): 1) a traditional behavioral approach, 2) a social learning approach, and 3) a cognitive-behavioral approach.

Traditional Behavioral Approach

This approach emphasizes the effects of environmental events that occur after (consequences), as well as before (antecedents), a particular behavior of interest.

Interventions aimed at the consequences of behavior.   Any *consequence* that increases the probability of a specific behavior occurring again under similar circumstances is termed a *reinforcer.* Consequences can have the effect of either increasing or decreasing the likelihood of a particular behavior occurring again.

When a behavior is followed by an environmental consequence that increases the likelihood that the behavior will occur again, this event is called a *positive reinforcer.* When a behavior is followed by the *removal* of a negative or aversive environmental condition it is called a *negative reinforcer.* When a behavior is followed by an aversive environmental event, that condition is termed a *punisher.* The effect of punishers is to reduce the probability that the behavior will occur under similar conditions. There has often been confusion concerning the difference between negative reinforcers and punishers. It is useful to remember that reinforcers (positive or negative) always increase the likelihood of the behavior occurring again, whereas punishers decrease the likelihood of a behavior occurring again. When the reliable relationship between a specific behavior and an environmental consequence is removed, the behavioral effect is to reduce the target behavior to a near zero level of occurrence. This process is called *extinction.*

Interventions aimed at the antecedents of behavior.   Behavior is controlled or affected not only by the consequences that follow a behavior but also by events that precede the behavior. These events are called *antecedents.* For example, an aggressive patient may only have outbursts in the presence of the nursing staff but never in the presence of the physician. In this case, failure to search for potential antecedents that may be eliciting (e.g., female gender or physical size) may leave half of the behavioral assessment undone and may result in difficulty decreasing the aggressive behavior.

Social Learning Approach

With this approach, cognitive processes that mediate between environmental conditions and behavioral response are included in explanations of the learning process. Social learning approaches take advantage of learning through "modeling" by systematically arranging opportunities for patients to observe socially adaptive examples of social interaction. Practice of the components of social skills in role-playing situations where the patient can receive corrective feedback is also stressed. Intervention that focuses on "social skills training" is one example of a treatment that is often useful with brain injury patients who have lost the ability to effectively monitor their behavior and respond appropriately in a given situation. Socially skilled behavior is generally divided into three components: social perception, social problem solving, and social expression. Training can occur at any one of these levels (Bandura 1977).

Cognitive-Behavioral Approach

The term *cognitive-behavioral approach* represents a heterogeneous group of procedures that emphasize the individual's cognitive mediation (self-messages) in explaining behavioral responses within environmental contexts. The thoughts, beliefs, and predictions about one's own actions and potential environmental consequences are emphasized. Treatment focuses on changing maladaptive beliefs and increasing the amount of self-control an individual has within the current social environment by changing maladaptive thoughts or beliefs. This approach is particularly useful when used with patients who have relatively intact language and self-evaluative abilities.

CONCLUSIONS

Neuropsychological and behavioral dysfunction associated with brain injury is varied and complex. Effective intervention requires an integrated interdisciplinary approach that focuses on the individual patient and his or her specific needs. Behaviorally based formulations can provide a valuable framework from which to understand the interaction between an individual with compromised physical, neuropsychological, and emotional functioning, and the psychosocial environment in which he or she is trying to adjust. Much work remains to define the most effective cognitive and behaviorally based treatments for various neuropsychiatric disorders. The evidence to date suggests that this area is indeed an area worthy of continued pursuit.

REFERENCES

Bandura A: Social Learning Theory. Englewood Cliffs, NJ, Prentice-Hall, 1977
Bellack AS, Hersen M: General considerations, in Handbook of Clinical Behavior Therapy With Adults. Edited by Hersen M, Bellack AS. New York, Plenum, 1985, pp 3–19
Ben-Yishay Y, Diller L: Rehabilitation of cognitive and perceptual deficits in people with traumatic brain damage. Int J Rehabil Res 4:208–210, 1981

Ben-Yishay Y, Diller L: Cognitive deficits, in Rehabilitation of the head-injured adult. Edited by Griffith, EA, Bond, M, Miller, J. Philadelphia, Davis, 1983

Bond M: The psychiatry of closed head injury, in Closed Head Injury: Psychosocial, Social and Family Consequences. Oxford, England, Oxford University Press, 1984

Calhoun KS, Turner SM: Historical perspectives and current issues in behavior therapy, in Handbook of Clinical Behavior Therapy. Edited by Turner SM, Calhoun KS, Adams HE. New York, Wiley, 1981, pp 1–11

Crovitz H, Harvey M, Horn R: Problems in the acquisition of imagery mnemonics: three brain damaged cases. Cortex 15:225–234, 1979

Diller L, Weinberg J: Hemi-inattention in rehabilitation: the evolution of a rational remediation program. Adv Neurol 18:63–82, 1977

Eames P: Behavior disorders after severe head injury: their nature, causes and strategies for management. Journal of Head Trauma Rehabilitation 3:1–6, 1988

Gardner H: The Shattered Mind: The Person After Brain Damage. London, Routledge & Kegan Paul, 1977

Gianutsos R, Glosser D, Elbaum J, et al: Visual imperception in brain injured adults: multifacted measures. Arch Phys Med Rehabil 64:456–461, 1983

Glasgow RE, Zeiss RA, Barrera M, et al: Case studies on remediating memory deficits in brain damaged individuals. J Clin Psychol 33:1049–1054, 1977

Glisky EL, Schacter DL: Remediation of organic memory disorders: current status and future prospects. Journal of Head Trauma Rehabilitation 4:54–63, 1986

Goldstein FC, Levin HS: Disorders of reasoning and problem solving ability, in Neuropsychological Rehabilitation. Edited by Meier MJ, Benton AL, Diller L. New York, Guilford, 1987, pp 327–354

Gouvier WD, Webster JS, Blanton PD: Cognitive retraining with brain damaged patients, in The Neuropsychology Handbook: Behavioral and Clinical Perspectives. Edited by Wedding D, Horton AM, Webster J. New York, Springer, 1986, pp 278–324

Grimm BH, Bleiberg J: Psychological rehabilitation in traumatic brain injury, in Handbook of Clinical Neuropsychology, Vol 2. Edited by Filskov SB, Boll TJ. New York, Wiley, 1986, pp 495–560

Gualtieri CT: Pharmacotherapy and the neurobehavioral sequelae of traumatic brain iniury. Brain Inj 2:101–109, 1988

Harris JE: Methods of improving memory, in Clinical Management of Memory Problems. Edited by Wilson BA, Moffat N. Rockville, MD, Aspen, 1984, pp 46–62

Harris JE, Sunderland A: A brief survey of the management of memory disorders in rehabilitation units in Britain. International Rehabilitation Medicine 3:206–209, 1981

Haynes SN: Behavioral assessment of adults, in Handbook of Psychological Assessment. Edited by Goldstein G, Hersen M. New York, Pergamon, 1984, pp 369–401

Hersen M, Bellack AS: Handbook of Clinical Behavior Therapy With Adults. New York, Plenum, 1985

Horton AM, Miller WA: Neuropsychology and behavior therapy, in Progress in Behavior Modification. Edited by Hersen M, Eisler R, Miller PM. New York, Academic Press, 1985, pp 1–55

Levin HS, Benton AL, Grossman RG: Neurobehavioral Consequences of Closed Head Injury. New York, Oxford University Press, 1982

Luria AR: Restoration of Function After Brain Injury. New York, Macmillian, 1963

Meier MJ, Strauman S, Thompson WG: Individual differences in neuropsychological recovery: an overview, in Neuropsychological Rehabilitation. Edited by Meier MJ, Benton AL, Diller L. New York, Guilford, 1987, pp 71–110

Prigatano GP: Personality and psychosocial consequences after brain injury, in Neuropsychological Rehabilitation. Edited by Meier MJ, Benton AL, Diller L. New York, Guilford, 1987, pp 355–378

Sivak M, Hill C, Henson D, et al: Improved driving performance following perceptual training of persons with brain damage. Arch Phys Med Rehabil 65:163–167, 1985

Stuss DT, Benson DF: Neuropsychological studies of the frontal lobes. Psychol Bull 95:3–28, 1984

Weddell R, Oddy M, Jenkins D: Social adjustment after rehabilitation: a two year follow up of patients with severe head injury. Psychol Med 10:257–263, 1980

Family Caregivers of Persons With Neuropsychiatric Illness: A Stress and Coping Perspective

Frederick E. Miller, M.D., Ph.D.
William Borden, Ph.D.

Family caregivers of persons with neuropsychiatric illness have emerged as an important group in social-psychological research efforts over the last decade, and investigators have documented a range of problems in living associated with the strain of the caregiving experience in such disparate conditions as Alzheimer's disease, stroke, traumatic brain injury, mental retardation, and acquired immunodeficiency syndrome (AIDS).

From the perspective of stress and coping theory, neuropsychiatric disorders may be viewed as adverse life events that tax adaptive resources and threaten the well-being of the family caregivers, placing them at risk for stress-related dysfunction and psychopathology. Rabins et al. (1982) showed that some family members develop discrete signs of physical or mental distress (notably depression, anxiety, demoralization, depletion, and psychosomatic symptoms) after onset and progression of illness and disability. Other investigations (e.g., Cohler et al. 1989), however, have suggested that many family members appear to manage the demands of the illness experience without overt signs of dysfunction. A third area of work (Borden 1991a, 1991b) indicated that some family members report personal growth and enduring positive changes as a consequence of the illness experience. Increasingly, researchers and clinicians have recognized the significance of individual differences among family caregivers in determining levels of functioning and well-being and, in turn, have realized the need to develop multivariate models of caregiver adaptation.

In this chapter we 1) provide an overview of work to date in the study of neuropsychiatric illness and family caregivers; 2) describe a model of stress, coping, and adaptation that provides an organizing frame of reference for identification of core tasks in psychiatric intervention; and 3) consider the implications of research to date for psychosocial intervention with family caregivers.

STRESS RESEARCH

Over the years a growing number of reports, informed by findings in the stress and illness literature, have suggested that family members of persons with chronic neuropsychiatric illness commonly experience symptoms of depression, anxiety, and depletion, as well as feelings of helplessness and hopelessness (Rabins et al. 1982). In addition, various physical conditions, such as hypertension, peptic ulcer, migraine, and colitis, as well as exacerbation of chronic illness, such as diabetes mellitus, coronary artery disease, and rheumatoid arthritis, have been associated with the stress of caring for a chronically ill member (Borden 1991a). The central question integrating such studies is what characteristics best predict development of physical or mental symptoms in family members. Basic lines of research have examined variables in five areas: 1) severity of illness, as determined by extent of physical and mental impairment; 2) social support; 3) family characteristics; 4) gender and social roles; and 5) developmental stages of the illness experience.

Severity of Illness

The earliest line of research, based largely on conceptual models of life events study, set out to explore the relationship between characteristics of chronic illness and burden in family caregivers. Studies relied largely on objective measures of patient functional status and focused generally on two aspects of neuropsychiatric illness: behavioral symptoms and physical impairment. A series of British studies compared the effects of dementing conditions and functional psychiatric disorders on family members. Hoenig and Hamilton (1966) reported significant degrees of burden in 80% of the families of elderly patients with functional psychiatric or cognitive impairment. They noted that dementing conditions caused more problems than any other disorders. Severity of symptomatology, inferred by global measures of behavioral disturbance and functional status, was associated with greater degrees of burden in dementing illness.

In a study of family members that provided home care for patients with functional psychiatric disorders and dementing illnesses, Grad and Sainsbury (1968) identified a series of patient behaviors that appeared to predict degree of burden. Aggressive behaviors, delusions, hallucinations, confusion, and inability to provide self-care were correlated with family stress. Family members specified frequent somatic complaints, threats of self-harm or harm of others, and excessive demands for attention as the most provocative behaviors. Severity of dementia was identified as a potential determinant of family burden.

Greene et al. (1982) found that the highest levels of caregiver distress were significantly associated with apathetic or withdrawn patient behavior. Caregivers of dementia patients with depression reported experiencing the most negative feelings about the patients. Wilder et al. (1983) reported that noxious behaviors associated with dementia, such as expressions of anger and aggression as well as excessive demands for attention, appeared to correlate with family stress. Further, the study indicated that such behaviors often precipitated institutionalization of the patient. Patient demands for attention and emotional management were associated with caregiver strain, anxiety, and depression in studies by Gelleard and Boyd-Watts (1982), and Poulshock and Deimling (1984).

Social Support

Research examining the family efforts to mediate stressors associated with chronic illness is based on the assumption that social support buffers potentially harmful effects of stressor events and strengthens coping capacity and adaptive ability (M. Johnson 1985; Sarason 1985). Although evidence for the mediating effect of social support is equivocal (Cohen and Syme 1985; Henderson 1981), reviews have suggested that support variables exert a direct effect on a number of mental health measures (Lin et al. 1985).

In a global study of psychosocial stressors and dementia, Zarit et al. (1980) found that the only variable significantly related to perceived caregiver burden was the number of visits from children, grandchildren, or siblings. Similarly, C. L. Johnson (1983) found that caregiving spouses who reported frequent contact with their adult children experienced less depression than those with irregular or minimal interaction, presumably because of varying degrees of social support.

Zarit et al. (1985) suggested that lack of social support is more predictive of family stress than specific symptoms or impairment associated with the dementing process. They reported that family members tended to become isolated over the course of the illness, initiating social contact less frequently and receiving fewer visits from persons outside the household. Their clinical studies supported earlier findings that family members who continued to receive emotional support experienced less strain than those who reported diminished social contact.

Findings in this area have provided a rationale for the development of family support groups, self-help groups, and formal support services such as day care and respite programs (Groves et al. 1984). Some studies have indicated that formal support services help to relieve stress in family members (Frankfather 1977; Kahn and Tobin 1981), whereas other reports did not show significant relationships between burden and support services (Noelker and Poulshock 1982). Groves (1988) suggested that support from family and friends exerts a greater influence on caregiver distress than support from formal service programs.

Family Characteristics

A third focus of investigation examines the influence of family characteristics on stress and adaptation in members. Instrumental and affective problem-solving processes, communication processes, affective responsiveness, and behavior control are important issues in this area of study (Borden 1988). Although most reports have been based on single case studies or preliminary empirical research, reviews of the literature have suggested that the increased dependency of the person with neuropsychiatric impairment leads to shifts in the power or authority structure of the family, thereby necessitating major role changes (Lansky 1984; Niederehe and Fruge 1985).

Tasks and responsibilities must be reassigned as the illness progresses, and the process of reorganizing power within the family system may precipitate tension, conflict, and disequilibrium. For example, differences may emerge between the primary caregiver and other family members about the most effective way to care for the patient or about the veracity of the caregiver's perception of patient deficits and needs (Koopman-Boyden and Wells 1979; Rabins et al. 1982).

Neuropsychiatric illness in a parent or sibling may inhibit other members' efforts to separate from the family, particularly in enmeshed systems, and members may find it difficult to maintain a sense of separateness in their caregiving activities. Families showing evidence of rigid role assignments, maladaptive communication patterns, chronic marital conflict, and reliance on defenses such as repression and denial appear to be especially vulnerable to breakdown and dysfunction (Lansky 1984; Niederehe and Fruge 1985). The structure and function of the family, accordingly, are hypothesized to serve as important mediating variables in the process of adaptation (Bruhn 1977).

Some accounts have suggested that the preexisting quality of family relationships, especially the marital relationship, is a major determinant of the spouse's ability to tolerate the stress of caregiving (Borden 1988; Niederehe and Fruge 1985). The hypothesis is that greater degrees of satisfaction in the relationship buffer illness-related stressors. This line of thinking is supported by findings that showed a significant relationship between quality of affective relations and caregiver strain (Cantor 1983; Robinson 1983; Zarit et al. 1985).

Finally, some authors have hypothesized that the strain of the illness intensifies preexisting intrapsychic conflict in family members, thereby leading to development of stress-related dysfunction. Groves et al. (1984) observed that unconscious conflict related to loss, such as the death of a parent, may be unmasked by losses inherent in the disease process or in senescence. They suggested that family members with unresolved issues are at greatest risk of developing stress-related difficulties.

Gender and Social Roles

The differential effects of gender on coping and adaptation in family caregivers have received little attention to date. However, there is some evidence that women tend to report higher levels of psychological distress than do men (Borden 1991a; Borden and Berlin 1990; Cantor 1983; C. L. Johnson 1983; Noelker and Poulshock 1982). Fitting et al. (1986) reported that husband and wife caregivers experienced similar degrees of burden but found that wives exhibited more symptoms of depression and demoralization. Interestingly, 25% of husbands reported an improved relationship with their spouse since assuming the caregiver role, whereas about a third of the wives reported a deterioration in the marital relationship. The authors cast potential explanations for such a finding in terms of developmental role changes associated with gender (Neugarten and Gutmann 1968), husbands' repayment of support and nurturance received through the marriage, and guilt associated with the recognition of sacrifices wives had made.

In a longitudinal study of subjective burden in husbands and wives caring for spouses with chronic dementing disorders, Zarit et al. (1985) found that women initially reported more distress than men, although no differences were found at the end of a 2-year follow-up period. They hypothesized that wives may have emphasized distress at the outset but assumed a stoic attitude over time or adopted more effective coping strategies.

The influence of social norms on caregiving is implicit in discussions of role conflict. Brody (1985) described the norm that offspring should provide their aging parents with care of comparable quality and quantity to what they received from their parents during childhood. Adherence to such a norm, she suggested, leads to disappointment and guilt because the expectation is an unattainable ideal. George (1986) proposed two contradictory norms as potential sources of stress in caring for a demented parent: reciprocity, which holds that family members should experience equitable levels of gain and loss; and solidarity, which holds that members should be given as much help as they need on an unconditional basis. In a study of family caregivers George (1986) found that such norms appeared to contribute to feelings of distress and diminished self-esteem in adult children, although spouses appeared to experience relatively little normative conflict in assuming the role of primary caregiver.

Developmental Stages of the Illness Experience

Clinicians have described phases of family adjustment and adaptation, seeking to understand stress responses in the context of developmental issues associated with various disorders. The work of Teusink and Mahler (1984) is representative. They developed a stage model of family adjustment in dementing illness consisting of five phases: 1) initial denial of difficulty associated with dementing condition; 2) overinvolvement with the patient in an effort to compensate for symptoms of the illness; 3) anger, when compensatory efforts fail; 4) guilt, in response to feelings of anger; and 5) acceptance of the illness. Such stages parallel phases of adaptation in the demented patient as described by Cohen et al. (1984).

Several investigators have considered specific aspects of the adjustment process. In studies of traumatic brain injury and degenerative neurological disorders, Romano (1974) and Falek (1979) noted that families often denied the nature or extent of cognitive impairment at the outset, moving toward acceptance of the condition in stages resembling those hypothesized for the acceptance of terminal illness. Borden (1988) considered the implications of the diagnostic process and noted that family members may alter or cease normal patterns of interaction with the patient once they learn that a condition is irreversible. At the same time, diagnosis of the condition may help to account for seemingly inexplicable behaviors and thereby reduce anxiety in members, particularly in early stages of the illness.

In the context of such models, stress-related symptoms in family members are seen as normative reactions in efforts to adjust to progressive losses associated with the illness. Developmental processes, rather than specific stressor variables, are viewed as primary determinants of stress and adaptation. Although stage models have been criticized on the grounds that they oversimplify adaptive processes, prospective study is needed to document shifts in caregiver perceptions, needs, resources, and coping strategies over the course of the illness experience.

STRESS AND COPING

Two constructs, coping and psychological well-being, emerge as central concepts in the development of further study and clinical intervention.

Coping

In critical reviews of the literature, Moos and Billings (1982) and Lazarus and Folkman (1984) distinguished two approaches in work on the concept of coping. The earliest line of thinking, based on animal models of stress, focused on the notion of arousal and defined coping as acts that control aversive situations and reduce drive or activation. Avoidance and escape behaviors were emphasized.

Critics noted that such approaches failed to address cognitive and affective processes that figure in human coping efforts.

The second line of development, drawing on concepts of ego psychology, was concerned with thoughts, feelings, and actions that persons used to mediate difficulties in relationships and situations. Hierarchies of coping strategies, ranging from immature to mature mechanisms, were conceptualized by numerous theoreticians and clinicians over the last quarter century (Vaillant 1977). Such models emphasized traits or styles that presumably predisposed persons to cope in particular ways over the life course. Empirical work has suggested, however, that ego psychological formulations underestimated the complexity and the variability of coping processes. Further difficulties emerged from the equation of coping with positive adaptational outcomes; less successful efforts to manage stressors were seen as defensive or primitive in character.

Coping should not be equated with mastery over the environment, according to social-psychological views, because many sources of stress cannot be mastered. Commentators have suggested that denial, minimization, or acceptance of stressful situations may be adaptive in some instances. The implication of such arguments is that no strategy can be considered inherently better or worse than any other. Judgments concerning the adaptiveness of a strategy must be made in the context of the person-situation configuration.

In an effort to extend traditional formulations of coping processes, Lazarus and Folkman (1984) conceptualized coping as ongoing cognitive and behavioral efforts to manage specific internal and external demands that are perceived as taxing or exceeding the adaptive resources of the person. As Lazarus's and Folkman's use of the word *effort* suggests (1984), coping may include anything the person thinks or does in an attempt to deal with a stressful experience, independent of outcome. Use of the word *manage* is intended to avoid the equation of coping with mastery. Managing may mean minimization, avoidance, tolerance, or acceptance of stressful conditions as well as attempts to master the environment.

Problem-focused coping efforts attempt to eliminate sources of stress or deal with the tangible consequences of a problem. Strategies in this category include seeking information, advice, or concrete sources of assistance and initiation of problem-solving actions, such as development of plans or skills in efforts to resolve difficulties. Emotion-focused coping efforts, on the other hand, involve attempts to neutralize emotion aroused by the problem and thereby maintain affective equilibrium. Strategies in this category include direct attempts to control emotion, such as detachment, wishful thinking, emphasizing positive aspects of a situation, acceptance, and efforts to discharge emotions, such as letting off steam, crying, or exercise (Lazarus and Folkman 1984; Moos and Billings 1982).

Although there has been little consideration of coping processes in study of neuropsychiatric illness and family caregivers, several investigators have examined features of coping experience in global study of organic brain syndrome and psychosocial stressors. C. L. Johnson (1983) found that family caregivers frequently attempted to deal with the strain of dementing illness either by psychological distancing from the patient or by extreme involvement with the patient, often marked by withdrawal from other relationships. Clinicians have pointed out that excessive involvement with the patient may preclude engagement of informal and formal sources of social support that potentially help to reduce the burden.

Levine et al. (1983) reported that family members best able to cope with caregiving demands attempted to develop specific strategies for solving illness-related problems, such as wandering and activities of daily living. Use of prayer was also associated with positive outcomes in their study. Similarly, reliance on problem-solving strategies and emotion-focused strategies that emphasize positive elements of the caregiving situation emerged as salient predictors of psychological well-being in a study by Borden (1991a). Capacity to see beyond the illness, or futurity, was associated with reduced role strain in dementia caregivers.

Psychological Well-Being

Researchers have increasingly assumed that stress and coping are important determinants of health status, and that greater degrees of stress, unmediated by effective coping strategies, are manifested in physical or mental signs of illness. In limiting evaluation of adaptational outcomes to assessment of distinct pathological signs, however, investigators have failed to consider psychological and social indicators of functional status beyond the boundary of discrete symptom configurations or illness states.

Psychological well-being has been defined as a cognitive appraisal of functional status and outcome along multiple dimensions, including emotional states, morale, life satisfaction, and perceptions of relationships. Psychological well-being would appear to be an important indicator of adaptational outcome in research on neuropsychiatric illness and caregiver functioning. Researchers have inferred "health" or "well-being" in the absence of distinct symptom configurations or illness states. However, such assessments have failed to distinguish absence of illness from perceptions of relative health status (e.g., from feeling "so-so" to feeling "good enough" to feeling "wonderful"). Spouses may experience diminished states of well-being without developing signs of mental or physical illness, as suggested in numerous clinical accounts (Borden 1992), just as they may show symptoms of diagnosable conditions without experiencing distressing degrees of strain.

TRANSACTIONAL MODEL OF STRESS AND COPING

Much of the work on impairment associated with neuropsychiatric illness and caregiver functioning has been based on relatively simple antecedent-consequent or stimulus-response models. That is, researchers have attempted to identify global antecedent variables (e.g., neuropsychiatric symptoms) as causes of unitary outcomes (e.g., ill-effects), without examining specific aspects of such characteristics or mediating processes. Such designs fail to reflect the interactive configuration of person and environment and overlook specific processes such as perception and coping that would appear to be central mediators of stress and adaptation.

The Lazarus-Folkman model (Lazarus and Folkman 1984), developed in an effort to extend traditional antecedent-consequent frameworks, shifts the focus from stress and pathology to coping and adaptation. Stress is understood as a particular relationship between the person and the environment that is appraised by the individual as taxing or exceeding adaptive resources and endangering well-being. In this model, coping, as noted earlier, is defined as ongoing cognitive and behavioral efforts to mediate internal and external demands that are appraised as taxing or exceeding the

adaptive resources of the person. Given the emphasis on perceptual and coping processes, the model is especially useful in conceptualizing areas of research and intervention with family caregivers in neuropsychiatric illness.

Figure 29–1, based on the Lazarus-Folkman model, conceptualizes the interactive pattern of patient, caregiver, family, and environmental characteristics in terms of
antecedent factors and mediating processes. As the schema shows, caregiver outcome
is mediated by 1) caregiver perception and appraisal of physical, psychological, and
social characteristics, specified as antecedent conditions, and 2) caregiver coping
strategies. Physical, mental, and social outcomes in caregiver functioning, in turn, are
believed to influence caregiver perception of conditions and coping strategies over
time. Units of intervention may involve the caregiver, the caregiver-patient dyad, the
family, or the social-environmental field.

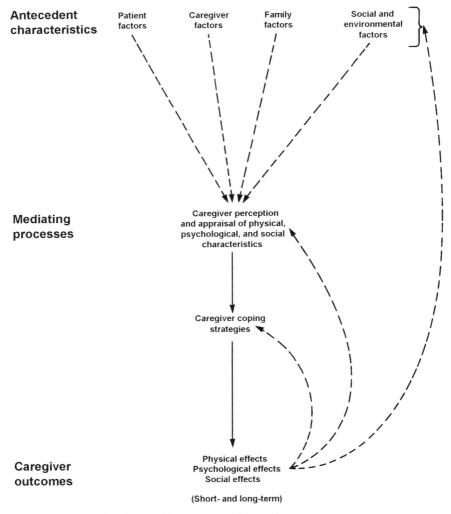

Figure 29–1. Multivariate model of caregiver functioning.

CLINICAL INTERVENTION

Caregiving is a heterogeneous process, and there is considerable variation in the ways family members deal with the demands of the role over the course of the illness experience. Although varying degrees of strain appear to be inevitable, research and clinical practice suggest that development of coping skills and mobilization of social support work to buffer the negative impact of caregiving demands.

Assessment

Caregivers vary widely in their abilities to deal with the demands of the illness experience, and individual differences in appraisal of illness characteristics, social relationships, and coping strategies are important factors in determining levels of well-being (Borden 1991a). Accordingly, assessment strategies must focus not only on objective phenomena, but also on subjective perceptions and meanings of illness characteristics, appraisals of family and peer relationships, and use of coping strategies. Assessment should specify the conditions under which the caregiver experiences strain and determine whether the difficulty is located primarily in the appraisal process, or the coping process.

Intervention

In the context of psychotherapeutic treatment, three tasks emerge from review of work to date. First, intervention should specifically seek to reduce distress in appraisal of illness characteristics. Second, intervention should facilitate development of coping skills that help caregivers solve specific problems and alter stressful circumstances in the context of the illness experience. Third, intervention efforts should promote use of social networks in efforts to mobilize sources of emotional and instrumental support.

Educational, psychotherapeutic, and supportive modes of intervention are key to the development of comprehensive service programs. Education of family members about the nature and course of neuropsychiatric conditions would appear to provide the basis for management of illness-related problems. Instructing caregivers in specific problem-solving techniques, such as behavioral and cognitive procedures, may help them reduce behavioral problems associated with neuropsychiatric conditions such as dementia, stroke, and traumatic brain injury. Further, education in stress management and other self-care procedures may provide varying degrees of relief from caregiving burdens.

Clinicians have developed a series of intervention approaches in their efforts to help family caregivers of persons with neuropsychiatric illness, ranging from provision of respite care, education, and social support to skills training and formal psychotherapy. Presently, however, there is no consistent evidence to suggest the superiority of any one approach (Montgomery and Borgatta 1985). Although we emphasize the value of interventions from the perspective of caregiver burden, it is important to note that any reduction in caregiver distress may also be expected to have a positive effect on patient psychiatric symptoms as well.

Self-help organizations such as the Alzheimer's Disease and Related Disorders Association (ADRDA) and the National Alliance for the Mentally Ill (NAMI) have emerged as major forces, paving the way for legislation and public funding favorable to care for neuropsychiatrically ill patients and, in many cases, offering support groups facilitated by members. Although no studies have demonstrated the social and psychological effects of these grass-roots organizations, the relationship between social isolation and caregiver distress has been documented in a number of studies, and it is reasonable to assume that participation in such groups fosters development of supportive relationships.

Research suggests that most family caregivers do not request formal assistance for themselves, and often appear reluctant to make use of family support services (Montgomery and Borgatta 1985). Anderson et al. (1986) described the empathic stance that should guide clinicians in engaging family caregivers in the treatment process. Clinicians must demonstrate an understanding of the hardships caregivers face and be willing to bear the brunt of the family's frustrations in initial contacts.

Most support programs involve some form of education. Systematic programs include didactic presentations on the diagnosis, course, and treatment of conditions and specific coping and management strategies. Studies have documented the effectiveness of such programs in reducing the frequency of psychiatric hospitalizations and in increasing the community tenure of patients who will eventually be hospitalized (Eisdorfer and Cohen 1981). Some studies have suggested that family educational programs facilitate engagement of persons in rehabilitation programs and, in doing so, promote recovery after stroke and traumatic brain injury. Educational programs also appear to be effective in reducing family strain and increasing coping skills in caregivers (Chiverton and Caine 1989).

Respite services seek to lessen the burden of daily care by temporarily relieving family members from caregiving responsibilities. Although there may be a high degree of satisfaction with such programs from the perspective of the family, formal studies of the impact of family respite on patient community tenure and caregiver burden are equivocal (Montgomery and Borgatta 1985).

A number of intervention programs have employed family caregivers in cognitive and physical rehabilitation of their ill relative. Giving family caregivers explicit rehabilitative tasks to perform may help prevent them from placing unrealistic demands on the patient and thereby reduce frustration and aggressive behavior. Quayhagen and Quayhagen (1989) documented the effectiveness of a program in which family caregivers received training in communication, memory, and problem-solving skills. Subjects showed diminished burden and higher levels of psychological well-being. Other studies have demonstrated ways in which family members may usefully maintain behaviorally based treatment programs initiated during hospitalization and promote adjustment and adaptation (Pinkston and Linsk 1984).

CONCLUSIONS

Commentators have acknowledged the potential conflict between "research" and "service" objectives in discussion of chronic illness and caregiver burden (Borden 1988), and writers have questioned the costs and benefits of extended empirical study in the face of what would appear to be self-evident problems and solutions. Little progress will be made, however, until we achieve a better understanding of caregiving experience as seen in specific types of illness. Researchers must continue to move beyond global descriptions of persons, problems, and outcomes and consider the effects of biological, psychological, and social characteristics on caregiver functioning in the context of multidimensional models of stress and coping.

REFERENCES

Anderson C, Reiss D, Hogarty G: Schizophrenia and the Family. New York, Guilford, 1986

Borden W: Stress, appraisal, and coping in spouses of demented elderly: Predictors of psychological well-being. Doctoral dissertation, University of Chicago Press, Chicago, IL, 1988

Borden W: Stress, coping, and adaptation in spouses of older adults with chronic dementia: predictors of psychological well being. Social Work Research and Abstracts 27:14–22, 1991a

Borden W: Beneficial outcomes in adjustment to HIV seropositivity. Social Service Review September 3:601–603, 1991b

Borden W: Psychosocial intervention following adverse life events: a narrative perspective. Social Work 37(2):135–144, 1992

Borden W, Berlin S: Gender, coping, and psychological well-being in spouses of older adults with chronic dementia. Am J Orthopsychiatry 60:605–610, 1990

Brody EM: Parent care as a normative family stress. Gerontologist 25:19–29, 1985

Bruhn JG: Effects of chronic illness on the family. J Fam Pract 4:1057–1060, 1977

Cantor M: Strain among caregivers: a study of the experience in the United States. Gerontologist 23:597–604, 1983

Chiverton P, Caine ED: Education to assist spouses in coping with Alzheimer's Disease. J Am Geriatr Soc 37:593–598, 1989

Cohen D, Kennedy G, Eisdorfer C: Phases of change in the patient with Alzheimer's dementia: a conceptual dimension for defining health care management. J Am Geriatr Soc 32:11–15, 1984

Cohen S, Syme SL: Social Support and Health. Orlando, FL, Academic Press, 1985

Cohler B, Borden W, Groves L, et al: Caring for family members with Alzheimer's Disease, in Alzheimer's Disease Treatment and Family Stress. Edited by Lebowitz B, Light E. Washington, DC, U.S. Government Printing Office, 1989

Eisdorfer C, Cohen D: Management of the patient and family coping with dementing illness. J Fam Pract 12:831–837, 1981

Falek A: Observations on patient and family coping with Huntington's Disease. Omega 10:35–42, 1979

Fitting M, Rabins P, Lucas M, et al: Caregivers for demented patients: a comparison of husbands and wives. Gerontologist 26:248–252, 1986

Frankfather D: The Aged in the Community: Managing Senility and Deviance. New York, Praeger, 1977

Gelleard CJ, Boyd-Watts WD: Problems in caring for the elderly mentally infirm at home. Archives of Gerontology and Geriatrics 1:151–158, 1982

George LK: Caregiver burden: conflict between norms of reciprocity and solidarity, in Elder Abuse: Conflict in the Family. Edited by Pillemer K, Wolf R. Dover, MA, Auburn House, 1986

Grad J, Sainsbury P: The effects that patients have on their families in a community care and a control psychiatric service: a two-year follow-up. Br J Psychiatry 114:265–278, 1968

Greene JG, Smith R, Gardiner M, et al: Measuring behavioural disturbance of elderly demented patients in the community and its effects on relatives: a factor analytic study. Age Ageing 11:121–126, 1982

Groves L: Psychological distress of caregivers in Alzheimer's Disease. Unpublished doctoral dissertation, Northwestern University, Chicago, IL, 1988

Groves L, Lazarus LW, Newton N, et al: Brief psychotherapy with families of patients with Alzheimer's disease, in Clinical Approaches to Psychotherapy with the Elderly. Edited by Lazarus LW. Washington, DC, American Psychiatric Press, 1984, pp 37–53

Henderson S: Social relationships, adversity, and neurosis. Br J Psychiatry 138:391–398, 1981

Hoenig J, Hamilton MW: Elderly psychiatric patients and the burden on the household. Psychiatria Neurologia [Basel] 154:281–293, 1966

Johnson CL: Dyadic family relations and social support. Gerontologist 23:377–383, 1983

Johnson M: Interweaving of informal and formal care: a challenge to some of the myths. Paper presented at the International Congress of Gerontology, New York, July 12, 1985

Kahn RL, Tobin S: Community treatment for aged persons with altered brain function, in Clinical Aspects of Alzheimer's Disease and Senile Dementia. Edited by Miller N, Cohen G. New York, Raven, 1981

Koopman-Boyden P, Wells L: The problems arising from supporting the elderly at home. N Z Med J 89:265–269, 1979

Lansky J: Family psychotherapy of the patient with chronic organic brain syndrome. Psychiatric Annals 14:2–17, 1984

Lazarus R, Folkman S: Stress, Appraisal, and Coping. New York, Springer, 1984

Levine N, Dastorr D, Gendron C: Coping with dementia: a pilot study. J Am Geriatr Soc 31:12–18, 1983

Lin N, Woelfel MW, Light SC: The buffering effect of social support subsequent to an important life event. J Health Soc Behav 26:247–263, 1985

Montgomery RJ, Borgatta EF: Family support project: final report, Administration on Aging. Seattle, WA, University of Washington Press, 1985

Moos R, Billings AG: Conceptualizing and measuring coping resources and processes, in Handbook of Stress. Edited by Goldberger L, Breznitz S. New York, Macmillan, 1982, pp 212–230

Neugarten B, Gutmann D: Age-sex roles and personality in middle age: a thematic apperception study, in Middle Age and Ageing. Edited by Neugarten B. Chicago, IL, University of Chicago Press, 1968, pp 54–73

Niederehe G, Fruge E: Dementia and family dynamics. J Geriatr Psychiatry 17:21–56, 1985

Noelker LS, Poulshock SW: The Effects on Families of Caring for Impaired Elderly in Residence (Final Report, Administration on Aging Grant 90-AR-2112). Cleveland, OH, Benjamin Rose Institute, 1982

Pinkston E, Linsk N: Behavioral family intervention with the impaired elderly. Gerontologist 24:576–583, 1984

Poulshock SW, Deimling GT: Families caring for elders in residence: issues in measurement of burden. J Gerontol 39:230–239, 1984

Quayhagen MP, Quayhagen M: Differential effects of family-based strategies in Alzheimer's Disease. Journal of the Geriatric Society of America 29:150–155, 1989

Rabins P, Mace NL, Lucas MJ: The impact of dementia on the family. JAMA 248:333–335, 1982

Robinson BC: Validation of a caregiver strain index. J Gerontol 38:344–348, 1983

Romano M: Family response to traumatic head injury. Scand J Rehabil Med 6:1–4, 1974

Sarason IG: Social support: conceptual and methodological issues. Paper presented at the 93rd conference of the American Psychological Association, Los Angeles, CA, August 1985

Teusink JP, Mahler S: Helping families cope with Alzheimer's Disease. Hosp Community Psychiatry 35:152–156, 1984

Vaillant G: Adaptation to Life. Boston, MA, Little, Brown, 1977

Wilder D, Teresi J, Bennett R: Family burden and dementia, in The Dementias. Edited by Mayeur P, Rosen H. New York, Raven, 1983, pp 87–101

Zarit SH, Reever KE, Bach-Peterson J: Relatives of the impaired elderly: Correlates of feelings of burden. Gerontologist 20:649–655, 1980

Zarit SH, Orr NK, Zarit JM: Families Under Stress: The Hidden Victims of Alzheimer's Disease. New York, New York University Press, 1985

Chapter 30

Ethical and Legal Issues in Neuropsychiatry

Robert I. Simon, M.D.

The term *neuropsychiatrist* refers to a psychiatrist who diagnoses patients with organic and other mental disorders and treats them with somatic therapies. The body of law applied to the practice of psychiatry does not differ for the treatment of functional or organic mental disorders. The diagnosis, treatment, and management of patients with organic mental disorders, however, presents not only unique clinical and ethical concerns, but legal considerations as well. For example, an assessment of competency may be required to determine a neuropsychiatric patient's capacity to make health care decisions or ability to manage his or her personal affairs.

Individuals who have been criminally charged must be legally competent to stand trial. Defendants with neuropsychiatric impairments may not meet that standard. Therefore, these defendants are likely candidates for pretrial evaluations of their mental status and cognitive capability for understanding the charges against them and their ability to assist in their legal defense. Moreover, depending on the nature and duration of a neuropsychiatric disorder, a criminal defendant may seek acquittal or have the charges reduced based on the argument that the defendant was legally insane at the time the offense occurred. This chapter presents a brief review of some of the salient clinical, ethical, and legal issues that link neuropsychiatry to criminal law and civil personal injury litigation.

ETHICAL CONSIDERATIONS

Since the late 1950s and early 1960s, the medical profession has moved away from an authoritarian, physician-oriented stance toward a more collaborative relationship with patients concerning their health care decisions. This is especially reflected in contemporary ethical principles (1). Thus on ethical grounds, psychiatry endorses granting competent patients the legal right to autonomy in determining their medical care. Quite apart from any legal compulsion, most psychiatrists disclose truthful and pertinent medical information to their patients as a way of enhancing the therapeutic alliance (2,3).

The ethical principles of beneficence, nonmaleficence, and the respect for the dignity and autonomy of the patient provide the moral-ethical foundation for the doctor-patient relationship. Accordingly, patients with dementia or other brain disorders that significantly interfere with the capacity to make decisions require more active intervention by the psychiatrist. For example, the psychiatrist has a legal and ethical duty to obtain consent from substitute decision makers when a patient is incapable of making an informed decision. The rights of all patients are the same—only how these rights are exercised is different (4).

The ethics of social justice call for the fair allocation of medical resources in accord with medical need (5). Although seemingly a new development, the ethical concerns about equitable health care distribution are found in the *Hippocratic Oath* and in the tradition of medicine and psychiatry (6). Thus neuropsychiatric patients are ethically entitled to have access to the same medical resources available to other patients. For example, it would be unethical to discriminate against patients with AIDS-related dementia by not providing adequate treatment and management resources.

Ethical issues arise daily for psychiatrists who become involved in the critical care of neuropsychiatric patients. Medical decision making, informed consent, resuscitation, "brain death," organ transplantation, the withholding and withdrawing of life support, and the allocation of medical resources all give rise to complex ethical and legal problems (7). Moreover, that which is considered ethical in clinical practice today may become a legal requirement tomorrow.

LEGAL ISSUES

Nearly every area of human endeavor is affected by the law and, as a fundamental condition, requires one to be mentally competent. Essentially, *competent* is defined as "having sufficient capacity, ability [or] possessing the requisite physical, mental, natural, or legal qualifications" (8). This definition is deliberately vague and ambiguous because the term *competent* is a broad concept encompassing many different legal issues and contexts. As a result, its definition, requirements, and application can vary widely depending on the circumstances in which it is being measured (e.g., health care decisions, executing a will, or confessing to a crime).

In general, competency refers to some *minimal* mental, cognitive, or behavioral ability, trait, or capability required to perform a particular legally recognized act or to assume some legal role. The term *capacity*, which is often interchanged with the word *competency*, refers to an individual's actual ability to understand or to form an intention with regard to some act. In patients with traumatic brain injuries, fluctuation in mental capacity is common, particularly in the days or even months following injury. Generally, patients with brain disorders of diverse etiologies often manifest considerable variability in mental functioning from day to day.

As a distinction, the term *incompetent* is applied to an individual who fails one of the tests of capacity and is therefore considered by law not mentally capable of performing a particular act or assuming a particular role. The adjudication of incompetence is subject or issue specific. In other words, the fact that a neuropsychiatric patient is adjudicated incompetent to execute a will does not automatically render that patient incompetent to do other things, such as consent to treatment, testify as a witness, marry, drive, or make a legally binding contract.

Generally, the law will recognize only those decisions or choices that have been made by a competent individual. The law seeks to protect incompetent individuals from the harmful effects of their acts. Persons over the age of majority, which is now 18, are presumed to be competent (9). This presumption is rebuttable, however, by evidence of an individual's incapacity (10). For the neuropsychiatric patient, evidence of impaired perception, short- and long-term memory, judgment, language comprehension, verbal fluency, and reality orientation are the most likely areas of cerebral functioning to be implicated when questions regarding capacity and competency are raised.

However, lack of capacity or competency *cannot* be presumed from either treatment for mental disorders (11) or from institutionalization of such persons (12). Mental disability or disorder does *not* necessarily render a person incompetent or incompetent in all areas of functioning. Nor do idiosyncratic or foolish decisions, by themselves, denote mental incompetence. Instead, a determination must be made whether there are specific functional incapacities that render a person incapable of making a particular kind of decision or performing a particular type of task.

Respect for individual autonomy demands that individuals be allowed to make decisions of which they are capable, even if seriously mentally ill, developmentally arrested, or organically impaired. As a rule, a patient with a neuropsychiatric disorder that produces mental incapacity must be declared incompetent judicially before that patient's exercise of his or her legal rights can be abridged. The person's current or past history of physical and mental illness is but one factor to be weighed in determining whether a particular test of competency is met.

Informed Consent

Because neuropsychiatric patients frequently suffer from impaired mental capacity, the difficulty associated with obtaining a valid informed consent to proposed diagnostic procedures and treatments can be both challenging and frustrating. The capacity to consent, particularly following head injury, may be present one moment and gone the next. Lucid intervals may permit the obtaining of competent consent for health care decisions. The legal requirement to obtain competent, informed consent is not negated simply because it "appears" that the patient is in need of medical intervention or would likely benefit from it. Instead, clinicians must assure themselves that the patient or an appropriate substitute decision maker has given a competent consent before proceeding with treatment.

Under the doctrine of informed consent, health care providers have a legal duty to abide by the treatment decisions made by competent patients unless a compelling state interest exists. The term *informed consent* is a legal principle in medical jurisprudence that holds that a physician must disclose to a patient sufficient information to enable the patient to make an "informed" decision about a proposed treatment or procedure (13). In order for a patient's consent to be considered informed, it must adequately address three essential elements: competency, information, and voluntariness (Table 30–1).

The law recognizes several specific exceptions to the requirement of informed consent (14). The most notable is the "emergency exception," which states that consent is implied in circumstances in which the patient is unable to give consent (e.g., unconsciousness) and is suffering from an acute, life-threatening crisis that requires immediate medical attention.

Only a competent person is legally recognized as being able to give informed consent. This is particularly important for health care providers working with patients who sometimes are of questionable competence because of mental illness, narcotic abuse, or alcoholism. When clinicians treat patients with neuropsychiatric deficits, the responsibility to obtain a valid informed consent can be clinically daunting due to the vacillating and unpredictable mental status associated with many central nervous system diseases (15) and lesions (16).

The psychiatrist planning to treat a patient suspected of having neuropsychiatric deficits should conduct a thorough and systematic assessment of cognitive functioning. The sole objective of such an evaluation should be the determination of the neuropsychiatric patient's ability to meet the minimum requirements for consent. At the very least, a mental status assessment of the patient's language, memory, judgment, insight, affect, orientation, and attention span should be performed (17). Certain neuropsychiatric patients may be cognitively intact but manifest such severe affective lability that they are rendered mentally incompetent.

Except in an emergency, the patient lacking health care decision-making capacity will need an authorized or appointed guardian to make health care decisions on his or her behalf (18). Table 30–2 lists a number of consent options that may be available for such patients, depending on the jurisdiction.

Table 30–1.   Informed consent: reasonable information to be disclosed

Although there exists no consistently accepted set of information to be disclosed for any given medical or psychiatric situation, as a rule of thumb, five areas of information are generally provided:

1. Diagnosis—description of the condition or problem
2. Treatment—nature and purpose of proposed treatment
3. Consequences—risks and benefits of the proposed treatment
4. Alternatives—viable alternatives to the proposed treatment including risks and benefits
5. Prognosis—projected outcome with and without treatment

Source.   Reprinted from Simon RI: *Clinical Psychiatry and the Law,* 2nd Edition. Washington, DC, American Psychiatric Press, 1992, p. 128. Used with permission.

Table 30–2.   Common consent options for patients lacking the mental capacity for health care decisions

1. Proxy consent of next of kin
2. Right-to-die statutory surrogate laws (spouse or court appointed guardian when treatment wishes of patient unstated)
3. Advance directives (living will or durable power of attorney)
4. Adjudication of incompetence; appointment of guardian
5. Institutional administrators or committees
6. Treatment review panels
7. Substituted consent of the court

Source.   Reprinted from Simon RI: *Clinical Psychiatry and the Law,* 2nd Edition. Washington, DC, American Psychiatric Press, 1992, p. 109. Used with permission.

Incompetent Patients

Right to die. Legal decisions addressing the issue of a patient's "right to die" fall into one of two categories: 1) those dealing with individuals incompetent at the time that removal of life-support systems is sought and 2) those dealing with competent patients.

In what was hoped to be the final word on the very difficult and personal question of autonomy for *incompetent patients*, the United States Supreme Court ruled in *Cruzan v. Director, Missouri Department of Health* (19) that the state of Missouri may refuse to remove a food and water tube surgically implanted in the stomach of Nancy Cruzan without clear and convincing evidence of her wishes. She had been in a persistent vegetative state for 7 years. In other words, without clear and convincing evidence of a patient's decision to have life-sustaining measures withheld in a particular circumstance, the state has the right to maintain that individual's life, even at the exclusion of the wishes of the family.

The importance of the *Cruzan* decision for clinicians treating severely or terminally impaired neuropsychiatric patients is that they must seek clear and competent instructions regarding foreseeable treatment decisions. For example, psychiatrists treating patients with progressive degenerative diseases should attempt to obtain the patient's wishes regarding the use of life-sustaining measures while that patient can still competently articulate those wishes. This information is best provided in the form of a living will or durable power of attorney agreement. Any written manifestation, however, that clearly and convincingly documents the patient's wishes would serve the same purpose. Although physicians fear civil or criminal liability for stopping life-sustaining treatment, liability may now arise from overtreating critically or terminally ill patients (20).

A small but growing body of cases has emerged involving *competent patients*— usually suffering from excruciating pain and terminal diseases—that seek the termination of further medical treatment. The single most significant influence in the development of this body of law is the doctrine of informed consent. Beginning with the fundamental tenet that "no right is held more sacred . . . than the right of every individual to the possession and control of his own person" (21; p. 250), courts have fashioned the present day "informed consent" doctrine and applied it to "right-to-die" cases.

Notwithstanding these principles, the right to decline life-sustaining medical intervention, even for a competent person, is not absolute. As noted in *In re Conroy* (22), four countervailing state interests generally exist that may limit the exercise of that right: preservation of life, prevention of suicide, safeguarding the integrity of the medical profession, and the protection of innocent third parties. In each of these situations, and depending on the surrounding circumstances, the trend has been to support a competent patient's right to have artificial life-support systems discontinued (23).

As a result of the *Cruzan* decision, courts will focus primarily on the reliability of the evidence proffered in establishing the patient's competence, specifically the clarity and certainty with which a decision to withhold medical treatment is made. Assuming that a terminally ill patient has chosen to forgo any further medical intervention *and* the patient is competent at the time this decision is made, courts will be reluctant to overrule or subvert the patient's right to privacy and autonomy.

Do-not-resuscitate (DNR) orders.   Cardiopulmonary resuscitation (CPR) is a medical lifesaving technology. To be effective it must be applied immediately, leaving no time to think about the consequences of reviving a patient. Ordinarily, patients requiring CPR have not thought about or expressed a preference for or against its use.

With chronic degenerative brain disease, terminal brain tumors, or end-stage traumatic head injury, the psychiatrist and the substitute medical decision maker have time to consider whether CPR should be offered based on the patient's earlier expressed wishes. The ethical principle of patient autonomy justifies the position that the patient or substitute decision maker should make the final decision regarding the use of CPR. However, some patients and families who are not offered a CPR option may feel helpless and abandoned. Psychiatrists must remain mindful of this reaction to properly assist the patient and family. Malpractice liability for not offering or providing futile care is unlikely, whereas the clinician is exposed to greater liability if such care is provided (24). Hospital CPR policies make DNR decisions discretionary (7). Psychiatrists should be familiar with the specific hospital policy, however, whenever a DNR order is written.

Advance directives.   The use of advance directives such as a living will, a health care proxy, or a durable medical power of attorney is highly recommended to avoid ethical and legal complications associated with requests to withhold life-sustaining treatment measures (25,26). The Patient Self-Determination Act that took effect December 1, 1991, requires hospitals, nursing homes, hospices, managed care organizations, and home health care agencies to advise patients or family members of their right to accept or refuse medical care and to execute an advance directive (27). These advance directives provide a method for individuals, while competent, to choose proxy health care decision makers in the event of future incompetency. A living will can be contained as a subsection of a durable power of attorney agreement. In the ordinary power of attorney created for the management of business and financial matters, the power of attorney generally becomes null and void if the person creating it becomes incompetent.

In a durable power of attorney, general or specific directions about how future decisions should be made in the event one becomes unable to make these decisions are set forth. The determination of a patient's competence, however, is not specified in most durable power of attorney statutes. Because this is a medical or psychiatric question, the examination by two physicians concerning the patient's ability to understand the nature and consequences of the proposed treatment or procedure, ability to make a choice, and ability to communicate that choice are usually minimally sufficient. This information, like all significant medical observations, should be clearly documented in the patient's file.

The application of advance directives to neuropsychiatric patients presents some difficulties. The classic example arises when the manic-depressive patient who is currently asymptomatic draws up a durable power of attorney or health care proxy directing that, "If I become manic again, administer lithium even if I strenuously object or resist." However, when mania recurs, the bipolar patient may strenuously object to lithium treatment. Because durable power of attorney agreements or health care proxies can be easily revoked, the treating psychiatrist or institution has no choice but to honor the patient's refusal, even if there is reasonable evidence that the patient is incompetent. If the patient is grossly disordered and is an immediate danger to self and others, the physician or hospital is on firmer ground medically and legally to temporarily override the patient's treatment refusal. Otherwise, it is better to seek a court order for treatment than risk legal entanglement with the patient over an advance directive. Typically, unless there are compelling medical reasons to do otherwise, courts will honor the patient's original treatment directions given while competent.

Guardianship. Guardianship is a method of substitute decision making for individuals who have been judicially determined as unable to act for themselves (28). Historically, the state or sovereign possessed the power and authority to safeguard the estate of incompetent persons (29).

Guardianship arrangements are increasingly used with patients suffering from dementia, particularly AIDS-related dementia and Alzheimer's disease (30). Under the Anglo-American system of law, an individual is presumed to be competent unless adjudicated incompetent. Thus incompetence is a legal determination made by a court of law based on evidence provided by health care providers and others that the individual's functional mental capacity is significantly impaired. The Uniform Guardianship and Protective Proceeding Act (UGPPA) or the Uniform Probate Code (UPC) is used as a basis for laws governing competency in many states (31). The threshold requirement of incompetency, as defined by the UGPPA, means impaired by reason of mental illness, mental deficiency, physical illness or disability, advanced age, chronic use of drugs, chronic intoxication, or other cause (except minority) to the extent of lacking sufficient understanding or capacity to make or communicate reasonable decisions. (32)

A significant number of patients suffering from neuropsychiatric disorders meet the above definition. A guardian is needed only when there is some question whether the individual is de facto (or actually) incompetent. The standard of proof required for a judicial determination of incompetency is clear and convincing evidence. Although the law does not assign percentages to proof, clear and convincing evidence is in the range of 75% certainty (33).

Substituted judgment. Psychiatrists often find that the time required to obtain an adjudication of incompetence is unduly burdensome to providing quality treatment on a timely basis. Moreover, families are often reluctant to face the formal court proceedings necessary to declare their family member incompetent, particularly when sensitive family matters are disclosed. A common solution to both of these problems is to seek the legally authorized proxy consent of a spouse or relative serving as guardian, when the refusing patient is believed to be incompetent. Proxy consent, however, is not available in every state.

Perr (34) noted the advantages associated with having family members serve as decision makers. First, use of responsible family members as surrogate decision maker maintains the integrity of the family unit and relies on the sources that are most likely to know the patient's wishes. Second, it is more efficient and less costly. However, there are some disadvantages. Ambivalent feelings, conflicts within the family and with the patient, and conflicting economic interest may make certain family members suspect as guardians (35). Also, relatives may not be available or want to get involved.

A number of states permit proxy decision making by statute, mainly through their informed consent statute (25). Some state statutes specify that another person may authorize consent on behalf of the incompetent patient; others mention specific relatives. Unless proxy consent by a relative is provided by statute or by case law authority in the state where the psychiatrist practices, it is not recommended that the good faith consents of next of kin be relied on in treating a patient believed to be incompetent (36). The legally appropriate procedure to follow is to seek judicial recognition of the family member as the substitute or proxy decision maker.

Some patients treated in an emergency may be expected to recover competency within a few days. As soon as the patient is able to competently consent to further treatment, such consent should be obtained directly from the patient. For the patient who continues to lack mental capacity for health care decisions, an increasing number of states provide administrative procedures authorized by statute that permit involuntary treatment of the incompetent and refusing mentally ill patient who does not meet current standards for involuntary civil commitment (37,38). In most jurisdictions, a durable power of attorney agreement permits the next of kin to consent through durable power of attorney statutes (25). In some instances, however, this procedure may not meet judicial challenge.

Criminal proceedings.   Neuropsychiatrists are frequently requested to evaluate the mental competency of criminal defendants. Individuals charged with committing crimes frequently display significant psychiatric and neurological impairment. A history of severe head injury may be present. The possibility of a neuropsychiatric disorder must be thoroughly investigated in criminal defendants. For example, Lewis et al. (39) studied 15 death row inmates who were chosen for examination because of imminent execution rather than evidence of neuropathology. In each case, evidence of severe head injury and neurological impairment was found.

Criminal intent (mens rea).   Under the common law, the constituent elements of a crime are 1) the mental state or level of intent to commit the act (known as the *mens rea*, or guilty mind), 2) the act itself or conduct associated with committing the crime (known as *actus reus*, or guilty act), and 3) a concurrence in time between the guilty act and the guilty mental state (40). To convict a person of a particular crime, the state must prove beyond a reasonable doubt that the defendant committed the criminal act with the requisite intent. All three elements are necessary to satisfy the threshold requirements for the imposition of criminal sanctions. In addition to *mens rea*, a person's mental status and reality testing can play a deciding role in whether the defendant will be ordered to stand trial to face the criminal charges (41) or be acquitted of the alleged crime (42), or whether the person accused is sent to prison, is hospitalized (43), or, in some extreme cases, sentenced to death (44). Before any defendant can be criminally prosecuted, the court must be satisfied that the accused is competent to stand trial (i.e., understand the charges brought against him or her and be capable rationally of assisting counsel with the defense).

Competency to stand trial.   The legal standard for assessing pretrial competency was established by the United States Supreme Court in *Dusky v. United States* (41). Throughout involvement with the trial process, the defendant must have "sufficient present ability to consult with his lawyer with a reasonable degree of rational understanding (and have) a rational as well as factual understanding of the proceedings against him. Conviction of an accused person while he is legally incompetent deprives him of his liberty without due process of law" (41).

Any disorder, whether psychiatric or neuropsychiatric, that significantly impairs a defendant's cognitive and communicative abilities is likely to have impact on a defendant's competency. Nevertheless, it is the actual functional capability to meet the minimal standard of trial competency and not the severity of the deficits that will determine whether an individual is cognitively capable to be tried.

Numerous commentators have sought to identify clinical guides that could be used in assessing the general standards established in *Dusky*. One such attempt is the Competency to Stand Trial Instrument (CSTI), the purpose of which is to standardize, objectify, and qualify relevant criteria for the determination of an individual's competency to stand trial (45).

Psychiatrists and psychologists who testify as expert witnesses regarding the effect of neuropsychiatric problems on a defendant's competency to stand trial will be most effective if their findings are framed according to the degree to which the defendant is cognitively capable of meeting the standards enunciated in *Dusky*. Use of instruments such as the CSTI to pragmatically illustrate actual functional conformity to competency standards is especially helpful.

Insanity defense. In American jurisprudence, one of the most controversial issues is the insanity defense. Defendants with mental or neuropsychiatric disabilities who are found competent to stand trial may seek acquittal on the basis that they were not criminally responsible for their actions due to insanity at the time the offense was committed.

The vast majority of criminals choose to commit crimes for a number of reasons, but the law presumes all of them to do so rationally and of their own free will. As a result, the law concludes that they are deserving of some form of punishment. Some offenders, however, are so mentally disturbed in their thinking and behavior that they are thought to be incapable of acting rationally. Under these circumstances, civilized societies have deemed it unjust to punish a "crazy" or insane person (46). This is in part due to fundamental principles of fairness and morality. Additionally, the punishment of a person who cannot rationally appreciate the consequences of his or her actions thwarts the two major tenets of punishment: retribution and deterrence.

The threshold issue in making an insanity determination is not the existence of a mental disease or defect, per se, but the lack of substantial mental capacity because of it. Therefore, lack of capacity due to causes other than mental illness may be sufficient. For instance, mental retardation may represent an adequate basis for the insanity defense under certain circumstances. There are less commonly considered disorders that may be related to central nervous dysfunction that could potentially render a defendant legally incapable of conforming his or her behavior to the dictates of the law. These disorders include metabolic conditions (e.g., functional hypoglycemia) (47), premenstrual syndrome (PMS) (48), and episodic dyscontrol syndrome (49,50).

Diminished capacity. Diminished capacity permits the accused to introduce medical and psychological evidence that relates directly to the *mens rea* for the crime charged, without having to assert a defense of insanity (51). For example, for the crime of assault with the intent to kill, psychiatric testimony would be permitted to address whether the offender acted with the purpose of committing homicide at the time of the assault. When a defendant's *mens rea* for the crime charged is nullified by clinical evidence, the defendant is acquitted only of that charge. Patients suffering from neuropsychiatric disorders who commit criminal acts may be eligible for a diminished capacity defense.

Ordinarily, *intoxication* is not a defense to a criminal charge. Because intoxication, unlike mental illness, mental retardation, and most neuropsychiatric conditions, is usually the product of a person's own actions, the law is naturally cautious about viewing it as a complete defense or a mitigating factor. Most states view voluntary alcoholism as relevant to the issue of whether the defendant possessed the *mens rea* necessary to commit a specific intent crime or whether there was premeditation in a crime of murder. Generally, however, the mere fact that the defendant was voluntarily intoxicated will not justify a finding of automatism or insanity. A distinct difference does arise when, because of chronic, heavy use of alcohol, the defendant is suffering from an alcohol-induced organic mental disorder, such as alcohol hallucinosis, withdrawal delirium, amnestic disorder, or dementia associated with alcoholism. If competent neuropsychiatric evidence is presented that an alcohol-related neuropsychiatric disorder caused significant cognitive or volitional impairment, a defense of insanity or diminished capacity could be upheld.

NEUROPSYCHIATRIC MALPRACTICE

Neuropsychiatric malpractice is medical malpractice. Malpractice is the provision of substandard professional care that causes a compensable injury to a person with whom a professional relationship existed. Although this concept may seem relatively clear and simple, it has its share of conditions and caveats. For example, the essential issue is not the existence of substandard care, per se, but whether there is actual compensable liability. For a physician to be found liable to a patient for malpractice, several fundamental concepts must be established.

Medical malpractice is a tort or civil wrong (i.e., a noncriminal or noncontract-related wrong) committed as a result of negligence by physicians or other health care professionals that causes injury to a patient in their care. *Negligence*, the fundamental concept underlying a malpractice lawsuit, is simply described as doing something that a person with a duty of care (to the patient) should not have done or failing to do something that a person with a duty of care should have done. The fact that a psychiatrist commits an act of negligence does not automatically make him or her liable to the patient bringing the lawsuit. Liability for malpractice is based on the plaintiff's (e.g., patient's) establishing by a preponderance of the evidence that 1) there was a duty of care owed by the defendant (duty), 2) that duty of care was breached (deviation), 3) the plaintiff suffered actual damages (damages), and 4) the deviation was the direct cause of the damages (direct causation). These elements are sometimes referred to as the four Ds of malpractice.

Each of these elements must be met or there can be no finding of liability, regardless of any finding of negligence. In other words, a physician can actually have been negligent but still not be found liable. For example, if the plaintiff suffered no real injuries because of the negligence or if there was an injury but it was not directly due to the doctor's negligence, then a claim of malpractice will be defeated.

Critical to the establishment of a claim of professional negligence is the requirement that the defendant's conduct was substandard or was a deviation in the standard of care owed to the plaintiff. The law presumes and holds all physicians (psychiatrists) to a standard of ordinary care, which is measured by its reasonableness according to the clinical circumstances in which it is provided.

Somatic Therapies

Generally speaking, psychiatric intervention with neuropsychiatric patients, especially those exhibiting serious affective, delusional, or aggressive disorders, is essentially composed of drug therapy and electroconvulsive therapy (ECT). It is generally acknowledged within the psychiatric profession that there is no absolute standard protocol for the administration of psychotropic medication or ECT. The existence of certain guidelines, procedures, and authoritative resources regularly accepted or used by a significant percentage of psychiatrists, however, should alert clinicians to consider them as a reference and counsel. For example, APA published comprehensive findings in the form of task force reports on ECT (52) and tardive dyskinesia (53).

These or any other publications, do not, per se, establish the standard of care by which a court might evaluate a psychiatrist's treatment. They do represent, however, a credible source of information with which a reasonable psychiatrist should at least be familiar and have considered (54). It is the failure to consider these and other sources (e.g., current reviews of the clinical literature) that the courts will most likely look to in establishing contemporary psychiatric practices and determining the standard of care.

Normally, the "reasonable care" standard that is applied to psychiatric treatment is construed in a fairly broad manner because psychiatry is currently considered inexact. Some psychiatric treatments such as ECT, however, appear to be more rigidly regulated than others (55). The "standard" for judging the use and administration of medication, on the other hand, appears to be consistent with the more flexible and general "reasonable care" requirement. The *Physicians' Desk Reference (PDR)* is often used to establish or dispute a psychiatrist's pharmacotherapy procedures. However, although numerous courts have cited *PDR* as a credible source of medication-related information in the medical profession (56), it does not by itself establish *the* standard of care. Instead, the *PDR* may be used as one piece of evidence to establish the standard of care in a particular situation (57). The *PDR* or any other reference, however, cannot serve as a substitute for a clinician's judgment.

The standard of care associated with the use of a somatic therapy to treat a neuropsychiatric patient should, at a minimum, include some variation of the following considerations and measures:

1. Pretreatment
   - Complete clinical history (e.g., medical and psychological) (58)
   - Complete physical examination, if needed
   - Administration of necessary laboratory tests and review of past test results (59)

- Disclosure of sufficient information to obtain informed consent, including information regarding the consequences of *not* receiving treatment
- Thorough documentation of all decisions, informed consent information, patient responses, and any other relevant treatment data

2. Posttreatment
   - Careful monitoring of the patient's response to treatment, including frequent patient interviews and appropriate laboratory testing (60)
   - Prompt adjustments in treatment, as needed
   - Obtaining a renewed informed consent when appreciably altering treatment or initiating new treatment

Fortunately, courts recognize the importance of professional judgment and will give psychiatrists and other medical specialists some latitude in explaining any special diagnostic or treatment considerations that guided their decision making. For example, the research data regarding pharmacologic treatment of aggression in neurologically impaired patients indicate that there is a variety of potentially useful drug therapies—some that are considered experimental or on the cutting edge (61). However, no drug is presently approved by the FDA for the treatment of aggression (62).

Theories of Liability in Neuropsychiatry

The term *psychiatric malpractice* is a misnomer because the same basic legal principles will be applied to any lawsuit alleging malpractice by a patient, regardless of medical subspecialty. Adjectives such as *psychiatric* or *neuropsychiatric* reflect the general recognition that the theories of liability to be discussed represent the most common areas of malpractice associated with that subspecialty. The following is a limited review of the most common litigation areas in treating neuropsychiatric patients.

Medication.   The potential for negligence by a psychiatrist would appear greatest in clinical situations involving the use of psychotropic medications. Although no reliable compilation of malpractice claims data has been published, anecdotal information suggests that medication-related lawsuits constitute a significant share of the litigation filed against psychiatrists. For example, insurance data collected by the Medical Protective Company revealed that medication-related injuries constituted 20% of the total claims against psychiatrists between 1980 and 1985 (63). Similar figures are reported by APA's insurance committee and other commentators studying the incidence of psychiatric malpractice claims (64).

A review of the relevant case law indicates that a variety of mistakes, omissions, and poor pharmacological treatment practices that commonly result in malpractice actions brought against a psychiatrist or other physician:

1. *Failure to properly evaluate.* Sound clinical practice requires that the patient be properly examined before any form of somatic treatment is initiated.
2. *Failure to monitor or supervise.* Probably the most common act of negligence associated with pharmacotherapy is the failure to supervise the patient's progress on the medication, including monitoring the patient for adverse side effects.

3. *Negligent prescription practices.* These include exceeding recommended dosages and then failing to adjust the medication level to therapeutic levels, negligent mixing of drugs (or polypharmacy), prescribing medication for unapproved uses, prescribing "unapproved" medications, and failing to disclose medication effects.
4. *Other.* These practices include failure to treat side effects once they have been recognized or should have been recognized, failure to monitor a patient's compliance with prescription limits, failure to prescribe medication or appropriate levels of medication according to the treatment needs of the patient, failure to refer a patient for consultation or treatment by a specialist, and negligent withdrawal from medication.

Tardive dyskinesia. Shortly after the introduction of neuroleptic medications as therapeutic agents, however, researchers and clinicians observed unusual muscle movements (later referred to as tardive dyskinesia [TD]) in certain patients treated with these drugs. It is estimated that at least 10%–20% (96) and perhaps as many as 50% of all patients (65) exposed to neuroleptic drugs for more than 1 year exhibit some degree of probable TD. These projections are even higher for elderly patients (66). Despite the possibility of numerous TD-related suits, however, relatively few psychiatrists have been sued under this cause of action.

Cases involving allegations of negligence after a patient developed TD are based on the same legal elements as any other malpractice action. Moreover, the bases for negligence mirror those that have been previously identified with general medication cases including (but not limited to) failure to properly evaluate a patient, failure to obtain informed consent, and negligent diagnosis of a patient's condition. For example, in *Hyde v. University of Michigan Board of Regents* (67), a woman was awarded $1,000,000 from a medical center that misdiagnosed her condition—TD—as Huntington's chorea. This verdict was later reversed on the basis of a subsequent case that expanded the state's sovereign immunity coverage (68).

The defenses and preventive measures applicable to TD-related malpractice claims are consistent with those used in any case alleging negligent drug treatment. Generally speaking, the application of sound clinical practice that is appropriately communicated to the patient and documented in the treatment chart will serve as an effective foil to any allegation of negligence should TD develop (69).

ECT. Although a significant proportion of psychiatrists believe ECT is a viable treatment for certain mental disorders (70), it has been estimated that no more than 3%–5% of all psychiatric inpatients in the United States receive this form of treatment (71). Although these figures suggest that the potential number of legal actions alleging negligence associated with ECT is likely to be low, lawsuits involving ECT are occasionally brought.

These cases can be categorized into three groups: pretreatment, treatment, and posttreatment. Generally five procedures—recommended by the APA Task Force on ECT (52)—should be observed: 1) a psychiatric history and examination to evaluate the indications for ECT, 2) a medical examination to determine risk factors, 3) an anesthesia evaluation, 4) informed consent (written), and 5) an evaluation by a physician privileged to administer ECT.

Failure to adequately conduct one of these *pretreatment* procedures could endanger the welfare of the patient and ultimately result in a lawsuit for negligence. It is well established that a psychiatrist will not be held liable for a mere mistake in judgment, nor will a psychiatrist be held to a standard of 100% accuracy or perfect performance (72). Therefore, a bad result does not automatically establish a claim for malpractice (73). Instead, a patient must prove, by a preponderance of the evidence, that the physician deviated from the standard of care and that deviation proximately caused the patient some injury or damage. The procedure for evaluating the care and treatment afforded a patient when ECT is used is no different.

Cases involving ECT-related injuries in which the negligence has centered around the actual *treatment* process include 1) failure to use a muscle relaxant to reduce the chance of a bone fracture, 2) negligent administration of the procedure, and 3) failure to conduct an evaluation of an injured patient, including the failure to obtain X rays, before continuing treatment.

It is not uncommon for patients being treated with ECT to experience certain side effects such as temporary confusion, disorientation, and memory loss following its administration (70). Due to this temporary debilitating effect, sound clinical practice requires that the psychiatrists provide reasonable *posttreatment* care and safeguards. Courts have held that the failure to properly attend to a patient for a period of time following the administration of ECT can result in malpractice liability. Posttreatment circumstances in which legal liability may occur include 1) failure to evaluate complaints of pain or discomfort following treatment, 2) failure to evaluate a patient's condition before resuming ECT treatments, 3) failure to properly monitor a patient to prevent falls, and 4) failure to properly supervise a patient who had been injured as a result of ECT.

The violent patient.   Aggressive and violent behaviors are common among patients exhibiting neuropsychiatric disorders and often precipitate admissions to psychiatric hospitals. In one survey it was found that 10% of patients at a state psychiatric facility had had assaultive behavior in the 2 weeks before admission (74). Also, it is not uncommon for neuropsychiatric patients to exhibit aggression after hospitalization (75).

For psychiatrists who treat violent or potentially violent patients, probably the greatest risk of a lawsuit involves *failure to control aggressive outpatients* and *the discharge of violent inpatients*. Psychiatrists can be sued for failing to protect society from the violent acts of their patients if it was reasonable for the psychiatrist to have known about the patient's dangerous proclivities and if he or she was in a position to do something that may have safeguarded the public. Since the landmark case *Tarasoff v. Regents of the University of California* (76), in which the California Supreme Court held that mental health professionals had a duty to protect third parties from imminent threats of serious harm made by their patients, courts and state legislatures have increasingly held psychiatrists to a fictional standard of having to predict the future behavior (dangerousness) of potentially violent patients whom they are treating.

Psychiatrists who treat violent, aggressive, or potentially dangerous outpatients must be cognizant of their responsibility not only to the patient but also to any person or persons that might be a foreseeable victim of the patient's aggression. Accordingly, psychiatrists must adequately assess the patient's risk of violence to self or others as part of the general psychiatric examination. Furthermore, the mental capacity of patients at risk for violence must also be evaluated. This is particularly critical for neuropsychiatric patients manifesting cognitive deficits and diminished impulse control. Serious depression may be a consequence of compromised brain functioning that may go undetected. Patients with brain disorders may lack the capacity to properly inform the psychiatrist of violent intentions. Generally, the psychiatrist must exercise close supervision of patients lacking full mental capacity, both cognitively and affectively.

If a patient threatens harm to a third party, a majority of states require that the psychiatrist perform some act that might prevent the harm from occurring. In states with duty-to-warn statutes, the responses available to psychiatrists and psychotherapists are defined by law. In states offering no such guidance, health care providers are required to use clinical judgment appropriate to the situation that will accomplish the objective of safeguarding the object of the patient's threat. Typically, a variety of options are clinically and legally available including voluntary hospitalization, involuntary hospitalization (if civil commitment requirements are met), warning the intended victim of the threat, notifying the police, adjusting medication, and seeing the patient more frequently (77). Seclusion and restraint as clinical management modalities have both indications and contraindications (Tables 30–3 and 30–4). The legal regulation of seclusion and restraint has become increasingly stringent over the past decade.

Lawsuits stemming from the release of a foreseeably dangerous patient who subsequently injures or kills himself or someone else are a source of considerable litigation. Psychiatrists should not discharge patients and then forget about them. The patient's willingness to cooperate with the psychiatrist, however, is critical to maintaining follow-up treatment. The psychiatrist's obligation focuses on structuring the

---

Table 30–3.   Indications for seclusion and restraint

1. Prevent clear, imminent harm to the patient or others
2. Prevent significant disruption to treatment program or physical surroundings
3. Assist in treatment as part of ongoing behavior therapy
4. Decrease sensory overstimulation[a]
5. At patient's voluntary reasonable request

---

[a]Seclusion only.
Source.   Reprinted from Simon RI: *Concise Guide to Clinical Psychiatry and the Law.* American Psychiatric Press, Washington, DC, 1988, p. 185. Used with permission.

Table 30–4.   Contraindications to seclusion and restraint

1. Extremely unstable medical and psychiatric conditions[a]
2. Delirious or demented patients unable to tolerate decreased stimulation[a]
3. Overtly suicidal patients[a]
4. Patients with severe drug reactions, overdoses, or requiring close monitoring of drug dosages[a]
5. For punishment or convenience of staff

---

[a]Unless close supervision and direct observation provided.
Source.   Reprinted from Simon RI: *Concise Guide to Clinical Psychiatry and the Law.* American Psychiatric Press, Washington, DC, 1988, p. 187. Used with permission.

follow-up visits in a fashion that encourages compliance. A study of Veteran's Administration (VA) outpatient referrals showed that of 24% of inpatients referred to the VA mental health clinic, approximately 50% failed to keep their first appointments (78). Limitations do exist, however, on the extent of the psychiatrist's ability to ensure follow-up care. This must be acknowledged by both the psychiatric and legal communities (79).

While professional standards do exist for the assessment of the risk factors for violence (80), no standard of care exists for the prediction of violent behavior. The clinician should assess the risk of violence frequently, updating the risk assessment at significant clinical junctures (e.g., room and ward changes, passes, and discharge). A risk-benefit assessment should be conducted and recorded before issuing a pass or discharge.

Involuntary hospitalization.   A person may be involuntarily hospitalized only if certain statutorily mandated criteria are met. Three main substantive criteria serve as the foundation to all statutory commitment requirements: the individual must be 1) mentally ill, 2) dangerous to self or others, and/or 3) unable to provide for his or her basic needs. Generally, each state spells out which criteria are required and what each means.

In addition to individuals with mental illness, certain states have enacted legislation that permits the involuntary hospitalization of three other distinct groups: developmentally disabled (mentally retarded) persons, persons addicted to substances (alcohol and drugs), and mentally disabled minors. Special commitment provisions may exist governing requirements for the admission and discharge of mentally disabled minors as well as numerous due process rights afforded these individuals. Clinicians must remember that they do not commit the patient. This is done solely under the jurisdiction of the court. The psychiatrist merely initiates a medical certification that brings the patient before the court, usually after a brief period of evaluation.

The most common type of lawsuit involving involuntary hospitalization relates to a physician's or psychiatrist's failure to adhere to the statutory requirements in good faith, which results in a wrongful commitment. Oftentimes, these lawsuits are brought under the theory of false imprisonment. Other areas of liability that may arise from wrongful commitment include assault and battery, malicious prosecution, abuse of authority, and intentional infliction of emotional distress.

In many states, psychiatrists are granted immunity from liability as long as they use reasonable professional judgment and act in good faith when petitioning for commitment (31). However, evidence of willful, blatant, or gross failure to adhere to statutorily defined commitment procedures will not likely immunize a psychiatrist from a lawsuit.

Personal Injury Litigation

Traumatic head injury is an enormous medical, social, and economic problem. It is estimated that the annual incidence of serious head injury is over 500,000 new cases (81). The National Head Injury Foundation estimated that at least 50,000 of these patients suffer chronic disability each year (82). Patients with compromised brain function may manifest difficulties in judgment, mood regulation, memory, orientation, insight, impulse control, and the maintenance of a clear sensorium. In addition, they are likely to suffer from a plethora of psychiatric symptoms. The plaintiff's (person bringing suit) organic and psychiatric injuries are likely to produce large economic losses due to unemployment, which may be permanent. In combination with current and future medical expenses, it is easy to see that compensable damages from head trauma can be substantial.

To establish in court the nature and extent of any psychiatric and neurological problems and to determine their relationship to the event causing the head trauma, expert testimony is needed. Litigation in head injury cases generally requires the evaluation and testimony of a psychiatrist, as well as neurologist, neuropsychologist, and other mental health professionals. These professionals can become involved in litigation as witnesses in two ways: as *treating physicians* or as *forensic experts*.

Psychiatrists who venture into the legal arena must be aware of the fundamentally different roles between a treating psychiatrist and the forensic psychiatric expert. Unlike the orthopedist who possesses objective, concrete information, such as the X ray of a broken limb to demonstrate orthopedic damages in court, the treating psychiatrist must rely heavily on the subjective reporting of the patient. In a clinical context, psychiatrists are interested primarily in the patient's perception of difficulties, not necessarily objective reality. As a consequence, many psychiatrists do not speak to third parties to gain information about a patient or corroborate their statements. The law, however, is only interested in what can reasonably be established as fact. Uncorroborated, subjective patient data are frequently attacked in court as being speculative, self-serving, and unreliable. The treating psychiatrist usually is not well equipped to counter these charges.

Credibility issues also abound. The treating psychiatrist is, and must be, a total ally of the patient. This bias toward the patient is a proper treatment stance that fosters the therapeutic alliance. Furthermore, to effectively treat psychiatric patients, the patient must be "liked" by the psychiatrist. No patient can be effectively treated for long who is fundamentally disliked by the therapist. Moreover, the therapist looks for psychiatric disorders. This again is an appropriate bias for the treating psychiatrist.

In court, credibility is a critical virtue to possess when testifying. Opposing counsel will take every opportunity to portray the treating psychiatrist as a subjective mouthpiece for the plaintiff, which may or may not be true. Also, court testimony by the treating psychiatrist may compel the disclosure of information that may not be legally privileged but is nonetheless seen as private and confidential by the patient. This disclosure by the trusted therapist is bound to cause psychological damage to the therapeutic relationship (83). In addition, psychiatrists must be careful to inform patients about the consequences of releasing treatment information, particularly in legal matters.

Finally, when the treating psychiatrist testifies concerning the need for further treatment, a conflict of interest is readily apparent. In making such treatment prognostications, the therapist stands to benefit economically from further treatment. Although this may not be the psychiatrist's intention, opposing counsel is sure to point out that the psychiatrist has a financial interest in the case.

Although opposing counsel may attempt to depict the forensic expert as a "hired gun," he or she is usually free of these encumbrances. No doctor-patient relationship is created during forensic evaluation with its treatment biases toward the patient. The expert can review various records and speak to numerous people who know the litigant. Furthermore, the forensic expert is not as easily distracted from considering exaggeration or malingering because of a clear appreciation of the litigation context and the absence of treatment bias. Finally, the forensic psychiatrist is not placed in a conflict-of-interest position of recommending treatment from which the treating psychiatrist would necessarily benefit.

The treating psychiatrist should attempt to remain solely in a treatment role. If it becomes necessary to testify on behalf of the patient, the psychiatrist should testify as a fact witness rather than as an expert witness. As a fact witness, the psychiatrist will be asked to describe the number and length of visits and the diagnosis and treatment. No opinion evidence will be requested concerning causation of the injury or extent of damages. In some jurisdictions, however, the court may convert a fact witness into an expert at the time of trial.

CONCLUSIONS

The neuropsychiatrist today must be informed concerning the legal regulation of psychiatric practice. Without a working knowledge of the law, the neuropsychiatrist's ability to provide good clinical care will be significantly impaired by fear and uncertainty. Neuropsychiatrists who are forensically knowledgeable are in a much better position to practice relatively unencumbered within the requirements of the law while also minimizing the potential adverse clinical impacts of burgeoning legal regulation.

NOTES

1. American Psychiatric Association: Opinions of the Ethics Committee on the Principles of Medical Ethics with Annotations Especially Applicable to Psychiatry. Washington, DC, American Psychiatric Press, 1989
2. Simon RI: Clinical Psychiatry and the Law. Washington, DC, American Psychiatric Press, 1987, p 113
3. Simon RI: Beyond the doctrine of informed consent: a clinician's perspective. The Journal for the Expert Witness, The Trial Attorney, The Trial Judge 4 (Fall):23–25, 1989
4. Parry JW, Beck JC: Revisiting the civil commitment/ involuntary treatment stalemate using limited guardianship, substituted judgment and different due process considerations: a work in progress. Medical and Physical Disability Law Reporter 14:102–114, 1990
5. Ruchs VR: The "rationing" of medical care. N Engl J Med 311:1572–1573, 1984
6. Dyer AR: Ethics and Psychiatry: Toward Professional Definition. Washington, DC, American Psychiatric Press, 1988, p 34
7. Luce JM: Ethical principles in critical care. JAMA 263:696–700, 1990
8. Black HC: Black's Law Dictionary, 6th Edition. St Paul, MN, West Publishing, 1990, p 284
9. Meek v City of Loveland, 85 Colo 346, 276 P 30 (1929)
10. Scaria v St Paul Fire & Marine Ins Co, 68 Wis2d 1, 227 NW2d 647 (1975)
11. Wilson v Lehman, 379 SW2d 478, 479 (Ky 1964)
12. Rennie v Klein, 462 FSupp 1131 (DNJ 1978), modified, 653 F2d 836 (3d Cir 1981), vacated, 458 US 1119 (1982), on remand, 720 F2d 266 (3d Cir 1983)
13. Black HC: Black's Law Dictionary, 6th Edition. St Paul, NM, West Publishing, 1990, p 779

14. Rozovsky FA: Consent to Treatment: A Practical Guide. Boston, MA, Little, Brown, 1984, pp 87–122

15. Snider WD, Simpson DM, Nielsen S, et al: Neurological complications of acquired immune deficiency syndrome: analysis of 50 patients. Ann Neurol 14:403–418, 1983

16. Carlson RJ: Frontal lobe lesions masquerading as psychiatric disturbances. Canadian Psychiatric Association Journal 22:315–318, 1977

17. Folstein MF, Folstein SW, McHugh PR: "Mini-Mental State": a practical method of grading the cognitive state of patients for the clinician. J Psychiatr Res 12:189–198, 1975

18. Aponte v United States, 582 FSupp 555, 566-69 (D PR 1984)

19. Cruzan v Director, Missouri Depart of Health, 110 S Ct 2841 (1990)

20. Weir RF, Gostin L: Decisions to abate life-sustaining treatment for nonautonomous patients: ethical standards and legal liability for physicians after Cruzan. JAMA 264:1846–1853, 1990

21. Union Pacific Ry Co v Botsford, 141 US 250, 251 (1891); Schloendorff v Society of New York Hosp, 211 NY 125, 105 NE 92 (1914)

22. In re Conroy, 98 NJ 321, 486 A2d 1209, 1222-23 (1985)

23. Tune v Walter Reed Army Medical Hosp, 602 FSupp 1452 (DDC 1985); Bartling v Superior Court, 163 Cal App 3d 186, 209 Cal Rptr 220 (1984); Bouvia v Superior Court, 179 Cal App 3d 1127, 225 Cal Rptr 297 (1986); in re Farrell, 108 NJ 335, 529 A2d 404 (1987); in re Peter, 108 NJ 365, 529 A2d 419 (1987); in re Jobes, 108 NJ 365, 529 A2d 434 (1987)

24. Marsh FH, Staver A: Physician authority for unilateral DNR orders. J Leg Med 12:115–165, 1991

25. Solnick PB: Proxy consent for incompetent nonterminally ill adult patients. J Leg Med 6:1–49, 1985

26. Simon RI: Clinical Psychiatry and the Law. Washington, DC, American Psychiatric Press, 1987, pp 500–504

27. LaPuma J, Orentlicher D, Moss RJ: Advance directives on admission: clinical implications and analysis of the Patient Self-Determination Act of 1990. JAMA 266:402–405, 1991

28. Brakel SJ, Parry J, Weiner BA: The Mentally Disabled and the Law, 3rd Edition. Chicago, IL, American Bar Foundation, 1985, p 370

29. Regan M: Protective services for the elderly: commitment, guardianship, and alternatives. William and Mary Law Review 13:569–573, 1972

30. Overman W, Stoudemire A: Guidelines for legal and financial counseling of Alzheimer's Disease patients and their families. Am J Psychiatry 145:1495–1500, 1988

31. Mishkin B: Determining the capacity for making health care decisions. Adv Psychosom Med 19:151–166, 1989

32. Uniform Guardianship and Protective Proceeding Act (UGPPA). Section 1-101(7); see also Uniform Probate Code (UPC) Section 5-101

33. Simon RI: Clinical Psychiatry and the Law. Washington, DC, American Psychiatric Press, 1987, p 451; citing, Addington v Texas, 441 US 418 (1979)

34. Perr IN: The clinical considerations of medication refusal. Legal Aspects of Psychiatric Practice 1:5–8, 1984

35. Gutheil TG, Appelbaum PS: Substituted judgment and the physician's ethical dilemma: with special reference to the problem of the psychiatric patient. J Clin Psychiatry 41:303–305, 1980

36. Klein J, Onek J, Macbeth J: Seminar on Law in the Practice of Psychiatry. Washington, DC, Onek, Klein & Farr, 1983, p 28

37. Zito JM, Lentz SL, Routt WW, et al: The treatment review panel: a solution to treatment refusal? Bull Am Acad Psychiatry Law 12:349–358, 1984

38. Hassenfeld IN, Grumet B: A study of the right to refuse treatment. Bull Am Acad Psychiatry Law 12:65–74, 1984

39. Lewis DO, Pincus JH, Feldman M, et al: Psychiatric, neurological, and psychoeducational characteristics of 15 death row inmates in the United States. Am J Psychiatry 143:838–845, 1986

40. Bethea v United States, 365 A2d 64, (DC 1976) cert denied, 433 US 911 (1977)

41. Dusky v United States, 362 US 402 (1960)

42. M'Naughten's Case, 10 Cl F 200, 8 Eng Rep 718 (HL 1943); United States v Brawner, 471 F2d 969 (DC Cir 1972)

43. Note, Mental Aberration and Post Conviction Sanctions, 15 Suffolk University Law Review: 1219 (1981); State v Hehman, 110 Ariz 459, 520 P2d 507 (1974); Commonwealth v Robinson, 494 Pa 372, 431 A2d 901 (1981)

44. Ford v Wainwright, 477 US 399 (1986); Note, The eighth amendment and the execution of the presently incompetent. Stanford Law Review 32:765, 1980

45. McGarry AL: Competency to Stand Trial and Mental Illness (a monograph sponsored by the Center for Studies of Crime and Delinquency, National Institute of Mental Health, DHEW Publ No (HSM) 73–910). Washington, DC, U.S. Government Printing Office, 1973 p 73

46. Blackstone W: Commentaries, Vol 4. pp 24–25 (1769); Coke E: Third Institute, 6th Edition. 1680

47. Moyer KE: The Psychobiology of Aggression. New York, Harper & Row, 1976

48. Dalton K: Once A Month: Premenstrual Syndrome. Pomona, CA, Hunter House, 1979

49. Monroe RR: Brain Dysfunction in Aggressive Criminals, Lexington, MA, Lexington Books, 1978

50. Elliot FA: Neurological findings in adult minimal brain dysfunction and the dyscontrol syndrome. J Nerv Ment Dis 170:680–687, 1982

51. Melton GB, Petrila J, Poythress NG, et al: Psychological Evaluation for the Courts. New York, Guilford, 1987, p 128

52. American Psychiatric Association: The Practice of Electroconvulsive Therapy: Recommendations for Treatment, Training and Privileging: A Task Force Report of the American Psychiatric Association. Washington, DC, American Psychiatric Association, 1990

53. American Psychiatric Association: Tardive dyskinesia: a task force report of the American Psychiatric Association. Washington DC, 1992.

54. Stone v Proctor, 259 NC 633, 131 SE2d 297 (1963)

55. Joint Commission on Accreditation of Healthcare Organizations: Consolidated Standards Manual for Child, Adolescent, and Adult Psychiatric, Alcoholism and Drug Abuse Facilities and Facilities Serving the Mentally Retarded/Developmentally Disabled (1989). Chicago, IL, Joint Commission on Accreditation of Healthcare Organizations, 1988

56. Witherell v Weimer, 148 Ill App 3d 32, 499 NE2d 46 (1986) Revised on other grounds, 118 Ill2d 515 NE2d 68 (1987); Gowan v United States, 601 FSupp 1297 (D Or 1985)

57. Doerr v Hurley Medical Center, No 82-674-39 NM (Mich Aug (1984); Callan v Norland, 114 Ill App 3d 196, 448 NE2d 651 (1983)

58. Taylor MA, Sierles FS, Abrams R: The neuropsychiatric evaluation, in Textbook of Neuropsychiatry. Edited by Hales RE, Yudofsky SC. Washington, DC, American Psychiatric Press, 1987, pp 3–16

59. Rosse RB, Owen CM, Morihisa JM: Brain Imaging and Laboratory Testing in Neuropsychiatry, in Textbook of Neuropsychiatry. Edited by Hales RE, Yudofsky SC. Washington, DC, American Psychiatric Press, 1987, pp 17–39

60. Rosse RB, Owen CM, Morihisa JM: Brain Imaging and Laboratory Testing in Neuropsychiatry, in Textbook of Neuropsychiatry. Edited by Hales RE, Yudofsky SC. Washington, DC, American Psychiatric Press, 1987, pp 17–39

61. American Psychiatric Association: Clinical perspectives. Managing Aggression in Elderly Patients 3:9–10, July 1990

62. Yudofsky SC, Silver JM, Schneider SE: Pharmacologic treatment of aggression. Psychiatric Annals 17:397–407, 1987

63. Psychiatry claims closed. Medical Protective Co Protector 3(3):2, 1986

64. Hogan DB: The Regulation of Psychotherapists, Vol III. Cambridge, MA, Ballinger, 1979, p 382

65. Gardos G, Cole JO: Overview: public health issues in tardive dyskinesia. Am J Psychiatry 137:776–781, 1980

66. Klawans HL, Barr A: Prevalence of spontaneous lingual-facial–buccal dyskinesia in the elderly. Neurology 32:558–559, 1982; Kane JM, Weinhold P, Kinon B, et al: Prevalence of abnormal involuntary movements ("spontaneous dyskinesia") in the normal elderly. Psychopharmacology 77:105–108, 1982

67. Hyde v University of Michigan Bd of Regents, 426 Mich 223, 393 NW2d 847 (1986)

68. Hyde v University of Michigan Bd of Regents, 426 Mich 223, 393 NW2d 847 (1986)

69. Radank v Heyl, No F4-2316 Wisc Comp Bd (1986); Frasier v Department of Health and Human Resources, 500 So2d 858 (La Ct App 1986); Rivera v NYC Health and Hospitals, No 27536/82 New York Sup Ct (NY 1988)

70. O'Connell RA: A review of the use of electroconvulsive therapy. Hosp Community Psychiatry 33:469–473, 1982

71. Weiner RD: The psychiatric use of electrically induced seizures. Am J Psychiatry 136:1507–1517, 1979

72. Smith JT: Medical Malpractice: Psychiatric Care. Colo Springs, CO, Shepards-McGraw Hill, 1986, p 68; Holton v Pfingst, 534 SW2d 786, 789 (Ky 1976)

73. Howe v Citizens Memorial Hosp, 426 SW2d 882 (Tex Civ App 1968), revised 436 SW2d 115 (Tex 1968)

74. Tardiff K, Sweillam A: Assault, suicide and mental illness. Arch Gen Psychiatry 73:164–169, 1980

75. Tardiff K, Sweillam A: Assaultive behavior among chronic inpatients. Am J Psychiatry 139:212–215, 1982; Reid HW, Bollinger MF, Edwards G: Assaults in hospitals. Bull Am Acad Psychiatry Law 13:13–14, 1985

76. Tarasoff v Regents of the University of California, 17 Cal 3d 425, 131 Cal Rptr 14, 551 P2d 334 (1976)

77. Simon RI: Concise Guide to Clinical Psychiatry and the Law. Washington, DC, American Psychiatric Press, 1988, pp 99–121

78. Zeldow PB, Taub HA: Evaluating psychiatric discharge and aftercare in a VA medical center. Hosp Community Psychiatry 32:57–58, 1981

79. Simon RI: Clinical Psychiatry and the Law. Washington, DC, American Psychiatric Press, 1987, pp 119–120

80. Simon RI: Concise Guide to Clinical Psychiatry and the Law. Washington, DC, American Psychiatric Press, 1988, pp 117

81. Frankowski RF, Anngers JF, Whitman S: Epidemiological and descriptive studies, part I: the descriptive epidemiology of head trauma in the United States, in Central Nervous System Trauma Status Report—1985. Edited by Becker DP, Poulishock JT. Washington, DC, National Institute of Neurological and Communicative Disorders and Stroke, 1985, pp 23–43

82. Clifton GL: Head injury incidence and organization of pre-hospital care, in Head Injury: Principles of Modern Management. Edited by Appel SH. Princeton, NJ, Geigy Pharmaceuticals, 1982, pp 3–5

83. Strasburger LH: "Crudely, without any finesse:" the defendant hears his psychiatric evaluation. Bull Am Acad Psychiatry Law 15:229–233, 1987

Index

Page numbers printed in **boldface** type refer to tables or figures.